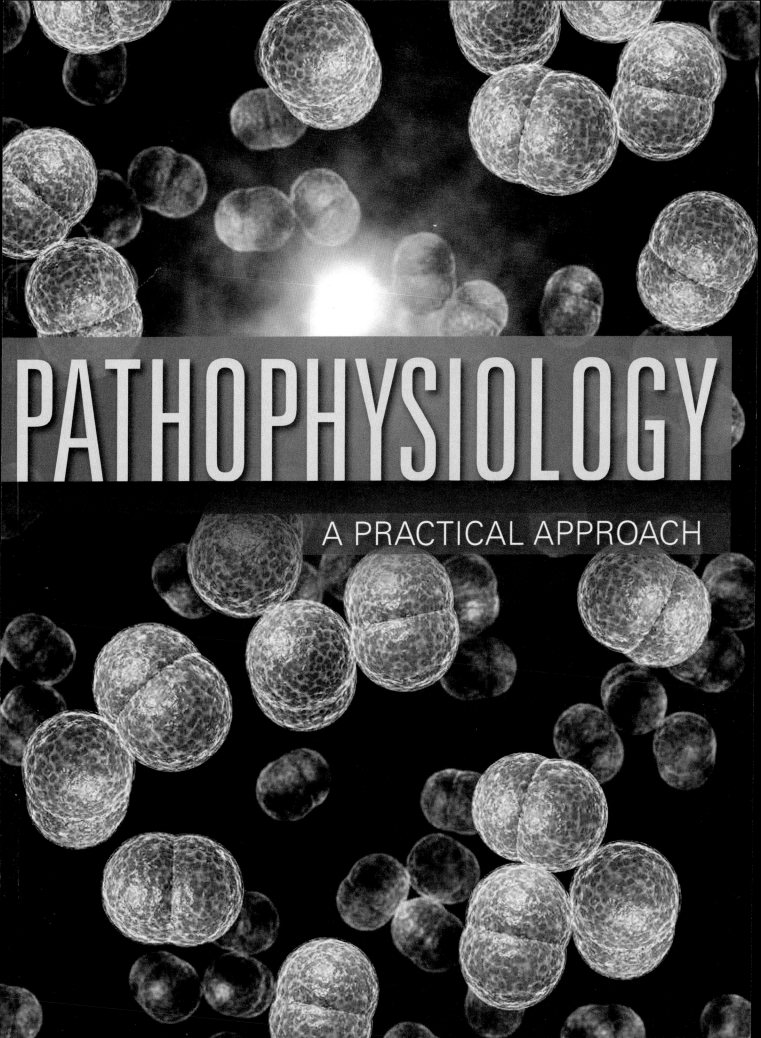

PATHOPHYSIOLOGY

A PRACTICAL APPROACH

The Pedagogy

Pathophysiology: A Practical Approach, Third Edition focuses on driving comprehension through a variety of strategies that meet the learning needs of students while generating enthusiasm about the topic. This interactive approach addresses different learning styles, making this the ideal text to ensure mastery of key concepts. The pedagogical aids that appear in most chapters include the following:

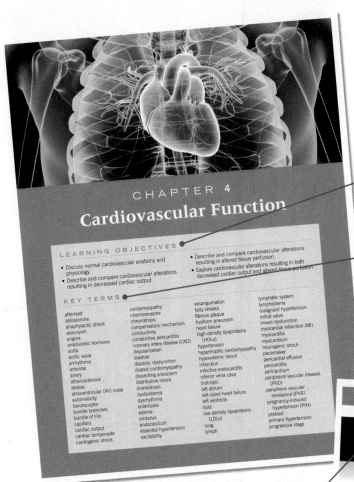

CHAPTER 4
Cardiovascular Function

LEARNING OBJECTIVES

- Discuss normal cardiovascular anatomy and physiology.
- Describe and compare cardiovascular alterations resulting in decreased cardiac output.
- Describe and compare cardiovascular alterations resulting in altered tissue perfusion.
- Explore cardiovascular alterations resulting in both decreased cardiac output and altered tissue perfusion.

KEY TERMS

afterload
aldosterone
anaphylactic shock
aneurysm
angina
antidiuretic hormone
aorta
aortic valve
arrhythmia
arteriole
artery
atherosclerosis
atresia
atrioventricular (AV) node
automaticity
baroreceptor
bundle branches
bundle of His
capillary
cardiac output
cardiac tamponade
cardiogenic shock

cardiomyopathy
chemoreceptor
chronotropic
compensatory mechanism
conductivity
constrictive pericarditis
coronary artery disease (CAD)
depolarization
diastole
diastolic dysfunction
dilated cardiomyopathy
dissecting aneurysm
distributive shock
dromotropic
dyslipidemia
dysrhythmia
eclampsia
edema
embolus
endocardium
essential hypertension
excitability

exsanguination
fatty streaks
fibrous plaque
fusiform aneurysm
heart failure
high-density lipoproteins (HDLs)
hypertension
hypertrophic cardiomyopathy
hypovolemic shock
infarction
infective endocarditis
inferior vena cava
inotropic
left atrium
left-sided heart failure
left ventricle
lipid
low-density lipoproteins (LDLs)
lung
lymph

lymphatic system
lymphedema
malignant hypertension
mitral valve
mixed dysfunction
myocardial infarction (MI)
myocarditis
myocardium
neurogenic shock
pacemaker
pericardial effusion
pericarditis
pericardium
peripheral vascular disease (PVD)
peripheral vascular resistance (PVR)
pregnancy-induced hypertension (PIH)
preload
primary hypertension
progressive stage

> **Learning Objectives** These objectives provide instructors and students with a snapshot of key information they will encounter in each chapter. They can serve as a checklist to help guide and focus study.

> **Key Terms** Found in a list at the beginning of each chapter and in bold throughout, these terms will create an expanded vocabulary in pathophysiology.

> **Concept-Based Learning** Each chapter is organized by overarching concepts, providing a framework for study and deepening understanding of content.

UNDERSTANDING CONDITIONS THAT AFFECT THE CARDIOVASCULAR SYSTEM

When considering alterations in the cardiovascular system, organizing them based on their basic underlying pathophysiology can increase understanding. These concepts are based on the two major cardiac-related nursing diagnoses—decreased cardiac output and altered tissue perfusion. Understanding what each of those diagnoses means facilitates understanding of the conditions that lead to their development.

Decreased cardiac output refers to states in which the amount of blood being pumped by the heart is less than normal. Decreased cardiac output can be associated with changes in preload, afterload, contractility, or dysrhythmias. Typical manifestations reflect the inability to meet the body's needs and may include fatigue, oliguria, cyanosis, fluid accumulation, and decreased peripheral pulses.

Altered tissue perfusion refers to a state in which there is a decrease in nutrition and oxygenation at the cellular level due to a deficit in capillary blood flow supply. Altered tissue perfusion can be associated with an interruption of blood flow, decreased cellular exchange, or fluid shifts. Typical manifestations reflect cellular ischemia and may include pain, skin changes, and signs of organ necrosis.

ALTERATIONS RESULTING IN DECREASED CARDIAC OUTPUT

Pericarditis

Pericarditis refers to an inflammation of the pericardium—the sac that surrounds, protects, and supports the heart. This inflammation is most commonly triggered by viral infections (usually after a respiratory infection), but it may also result from other infections, thoracic trauma (e.g., surgery, radiation, accidents), myocardial infarction, malignancy, tuberculosis, uremia, and autoimmune conditions (e.g., systemic lupus erythematosus, rheumatoid arthritis, scleroderma). In this inflammatory process (see the *Immunity* chapter), fluid shifts from the capillaries to the space between the pericardial sac and the heart. This fluid may be serous (resulting from heart failure), purulent (resulting from infections), serosanguineous (resulting from neoplasms or uremia), or hemorrhagic (resulting from aneurysms or trauma). As the pericardial tissue becomes inflamed, the swollen pericardial tissue rubs against the swollen cardiac tissue, creating friction.

Fluid can accumulate in the pericardial cavity, creating a pericardial effusion. This condition can eventually progress to life-threatening cardiac tamponade (FIGURE 4-13). In cardiac tamponade, the fluid accumulates in the pericardial cavity to the point that it compresses the heart. This compression prevents the heart from stretching and filling during diastole, resulting in decreased cardiac output. Arterial pressures then fall (because of the decreased cardiac output), venous pressures rise (because of the accumulation of blood within the systemic circulation), and the pulse pressure narrows (because of the arterial and venous pressure changes). Additionally, the heart sounds are muffled upon auscultation because the excess fluid drowns out the sound. Heart failure, cardiogenic shock, and death can result from cardiac tamponade.

Chronic inflammation can lead to constrictive pericarditis. In constrictive pericarditis, the pericardium becomes thick and fibrous from the chronic inflammation and adheres to the heart. Essentially, the pericardium resembles a restrictive rubber band that has lost its elasticity. The loss of elasticity restricts cardiac filling.

Learning Points Quick facts called out to highlight important topics within each chapter.

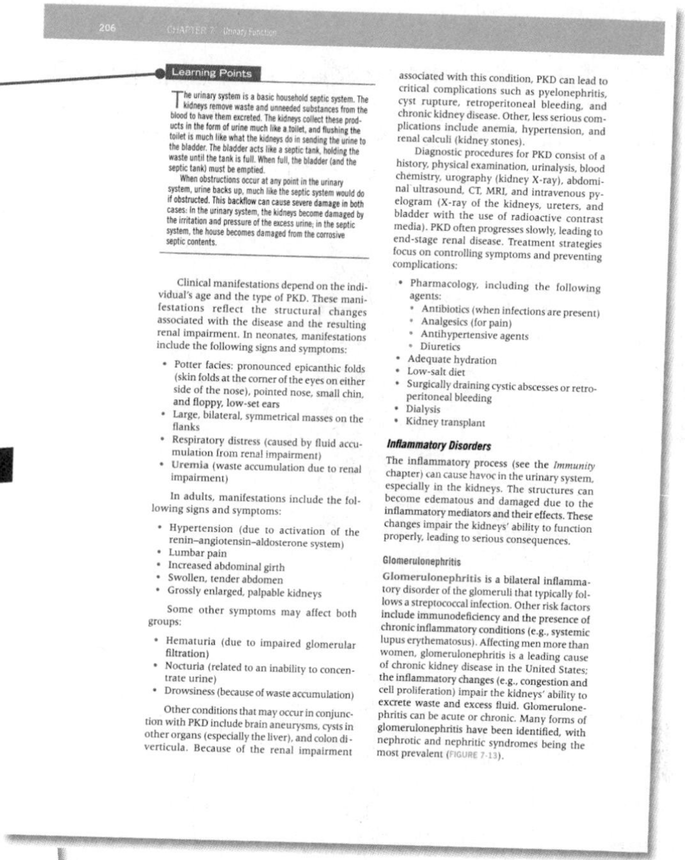

Learning Points

The urinary system is a basic household septic system. The kidneys remove waste and unneeded substances from the blood to have them excreted. The kidneys collect these products in the form of urine much like a toilet, and flushing the toilet is much like what the kidneys do in sending the urine to the bladder. The bladder acts like a septic tank, holding the waste until the tank is full. When full, the bladder (and the septic tank) must be emptied.

When obstructions occur at any point in the urinary system, urine backs up, much like the septic system would do if obstructed. This backflow can cause severe damage in both cases: In the urinary system, the kidneys become damaged by the irritation and pressure of the excess urine; in the septic system, the house becomes damaged from the corrosive septic contents.

Clinical manifestations depend on the individual's age and the type of PKD. These manifestations reflect the structural changes associated with the disease and the resulting renal impairment. In neonates, manifestations include the following signs and symptoms:

- Potter facies: pronounced epicanthic folds (skin folds at the corner of the eyes on either side of the nose), pointed nose, small chin, and floppy, low-set ears
- Large, bilateral, symmetrical masses on the flanks
- Respiratory distress (caused by fluid accumulation from renal impairment)
- **Uremia** (waste accumulation due to renal impairment)

In adults, manifestations include the following signs and symptoms:

- Hypertension (due to activation of the renin–angiotensin–aldosterone system)
- Lumbar pain
- Increased abdominal girth
- Swollen, tender abdomen
- Grossly enlarged, palpable kidneys

Some other symptoms may affect both groups:

- Hematuria (due to impaired glomerular filtration)
- Nocturia (related to an inability to concentrate urine)
- Drowsiness (because of waste accumulation)

Other conditions that may occur in conjunction with PKD include brain aneurysms, cysts in other organs (especially the liver), and colon diverticula. Because of the renal impairment associated with this condition, PKD can lead to critical complications such as pyelonephritis, cyst rupture, retroperitoneal bleeding, and chronic kidney disease. Other, less serious complications include anemia, hypertension, and renal calculi (kidney stones).

Diagnostic procedures for PKD consist of a history, physical examination, urinalysis, blood chemistry, urography (kidney X-ray), abdominal ultrasound, CT, MRI, and intravenous pyelogram (X-ray of the kidneys, ureters, and bladder with the use of radioactive contrast media). PKD often progresses slowly, leading to end-stage renal disease. Treatment strategies focus on controlling symptoms and preventing complications:

- Pharmacology, including the following agents:
  - Antibiotics (when infections are present)
  - Analgesics (for pain)
  - Antihypertensive agents
  - Diuretics
- Adequate hydration
- Low-salt diet
- Surgically draining cystic abscesses or retroperitoneal bleeding
- Dialysis
- Kidney transplant

Inflammatory Disorders

The inflammatory process (see the *Immunity* chapter) can cause havoc in the urinary system, especially in the kidneys. The structures can become edematous and damaged due to the inflammatory mediators and their effects. These changes impair the kidneys' ability to function properly, leading to serious consequences.

Glomerulonephritis

Glomerulonephritis is a bilateral inflammatory disorder of the glomeruli that typically follows a streptococcal infection. Other risk factors include immunodeficiency and the presence of chronic inflammatory conditions (e.g., systemic lupus erythematosus). Affecting men more than women, glomerulonephritis is a leading cause of chronic kidney disease in the United States; the inflammatory changes (e.g., congestion and cell proliferation) impair the kidneys' ability to excrete waste and excess fluid. Glomerulonephritis can be acute or chronic. Many forms of glomerulonephritis have been identified, with nephrotic and nephritic syndromes being the most prevalent (FIGURE 7-13).

Myth Busters Common myths and misconceptions highlighted and debunked.

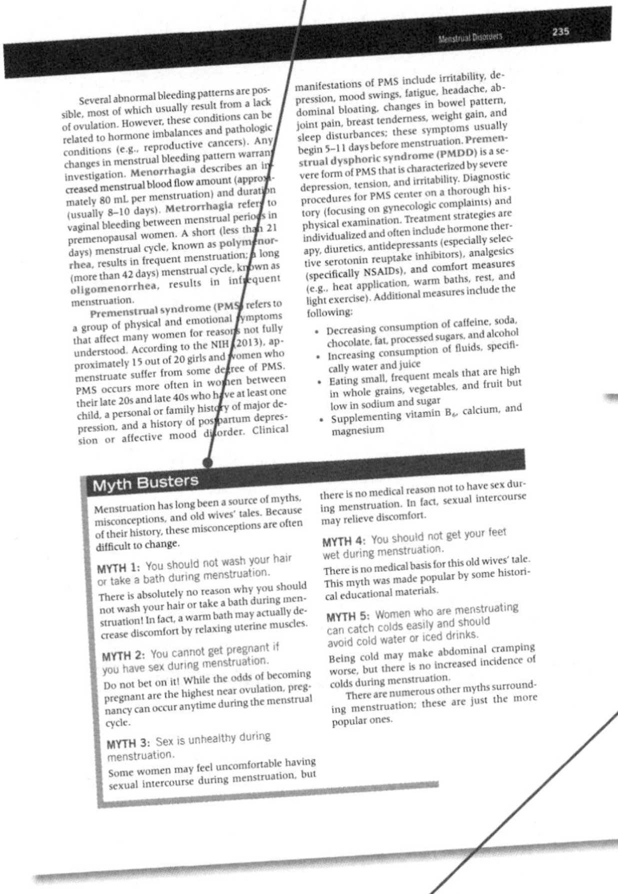

Several abnormal bleeding patterns are possible, most of which usually result from a lack of ovulation. However, these conditions can be related to hormone imbalances and pathologic conditions (e.g., reproductive cancers). Any changes in menstrual bleeding pattern warrant investigation. **Menorrhagia** describes an increased menstrual blood flow amount (approximately 80 mL per menstruation) and duration (usually 8–10 days). **Metrorrhagia** refers to vaginal bleeding between menstrual periods in premenopausal women. A short (less than 21 days) menstrual cycle, known as **polymenorrhea**, results in frequent menstruation; a long (more than 42 days) menstrual cycle, known as **oligomenorrhea**, results in infrequent menstruation.

Premenstrual syndrome (PMS) refers to a group of physical and emotional symptoms that affect many women for reasons not fully understood. According to the NIH (2013), approximately 15 out of 20 girls and women who menstruate suffer from some degree of PMS. PMS occurs more often in women between their late 20s and late 40s who have at least one child, a personal or family history of major depression, and a history of postpartum depression or affective mood disorder. Clinical manifestations of PMS include irritability, depression, mood swings, fatigue, headache, abdominal bloating, changes in bowel pattern, joint pain, breast tenderness, weight gain, and sleep disturbances; these symptoms usually begin 5–11 days before menstruation. **Premenstrual dysphoric syndrome (PMDD)** is a severe form of PMS that is characterized by severe depression, tension, and irritability. Diagnostic procedures for PMS center on a thorough history (focusing on gynecologic complaints) and physical examination. Treatment strategies are individualized and often include hormone therapy, diuretics, antidepressants (especially selective serotonin reuptake inhibitors), analgesics (specifically NSAIDs), and comfort measures (e.g., heat application, warm baths, rest, and light exercise). Additional measures include the following:

- Decreasing consumption of caffeine, soda, chocolate, fat, processed sugars, and alcohol
- Increasing consumption of fluids, specifically water and juice
- Eating small, frequent meals that are high in whole grains, vegetables, and fruit but low in sodium and sugar
- Supplementing vitamin B_6, calcium, and magnesium

Myth Busters

Menstruation has long been a source of myths, misconceptions, and old wives' tales. Because of their history, these misconceptions are often difficult to change.

MYTH 1: You should not wash your hair or take a bath during menstruation.

There is absolutely no reason why you should not wash your hair or take a bath during menstruation! In fact, a warm bath may actually decrease discomfort by relaxing uterine muscles.

MYTH 2: You cannot get pregnant if you have sex during menstruation.

Do not bet on it! While the odds of becoming pregnant are the highest near ovulation, pregnancy can occur anytime during the menstrual cycle.

MYTH 3: Sex is unhealthy during menstruation.

Some women may feel uncomfortable having sexual intercourse during menstruation, but there is no medical reason not to have sex during menstruation. In fact, sexual intercourse may relieve discomfort.

MYTH 4: You should not get your feet wet during menstruation.

There is no medical basis for this old wives' tale. This myth was made popular by some historical educational materials.

MYTH 5: Women who are menstruating can catch colds easily and should avoid cold water or iced drinks.

Being cold may make abdominal cramping worse, but there is no increased incidence of colds during menstruation.

There are numerous other myths surrounding menstruation; these are just the more popular ones.

Application to Practice Found in select chapters, these vignettes provide critical-thinking challenges for students.

Chapter Summary Summaries are included at the end of each chapter to provide a concise review of material covered in each chapter.

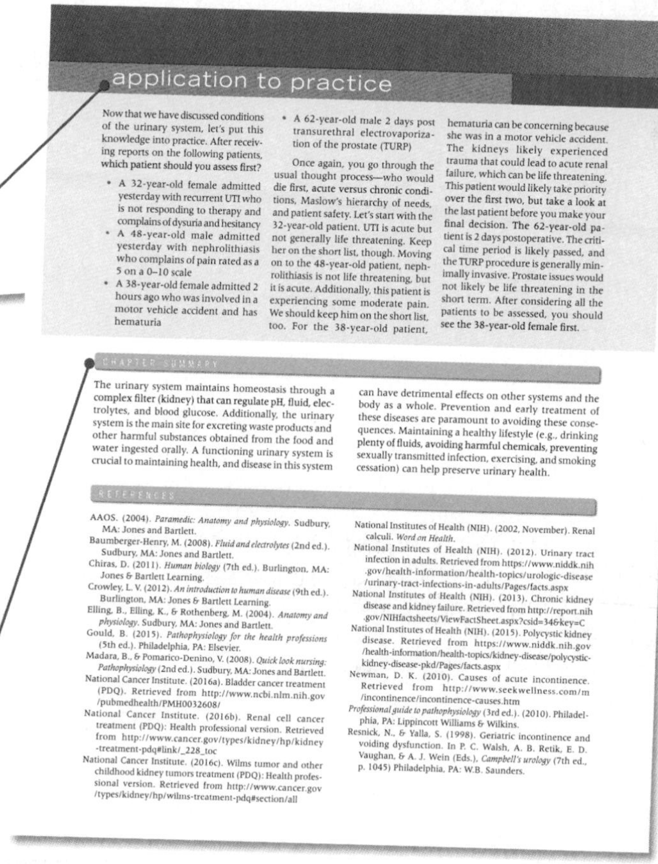

application to practice

Now that we have discussed conditions of the urinary system, let's put this knowledge into practice. After receiving reports on the following patients, which patient should you assess first?

- A 32-year-old female admitted yesterday with recurrent UTI who is not responding to therapy and complains of dysuria and hesitancy
- A 48-year-old male admitted yesterday with nephrolithiasis who complains of pain rated as a 5 on a 0–10 scale
- A 38-year-old female admitted 2 hours ago who was involved in a motor vehicle accident and has hematuria
- A 62-year-old male 2 days post transurethral electrovaporization of the prostate (TURP)

Once again, you go through the usual thought process—who would die first, acute versus chronic conditions, Maslow's hierarchy of needs, and patient safety. Let's start with the 32-year-old patient. UTI is acute but not generally life threatening. Keep her on the short list, though. Moving on to the 48-year-old patient, nephrolithiasis is not life threatening, but it is acute. Additionally, this patient is experiencing some moderate pain. We should keep him on the short list, too. For the 38-year-old patient, hematuria can be concerning because she was in a motor vehicle accident. The kidneys likely experienced trauma that could lead to acute renal failure, which can be life threatening. This patient would likely take priority over the first two, but take a look at the last patient before you make your final decision. The 62-year-old patient is 2 days postoperative. The critical time period is likely passed, and the TURP procedure is generally minimally invasive. Prostate issues would not likely be life threatening in the short term. After considering all the patients to be assessed, you should see the 38-year-old female first.

CHAPTER SUMMARY

The urinary system maintains homeostasis through a complex filter (kidney) that can regulate pH, fluid, electrolytes, and blood glucose. Additionally, the urinary system is the main site for excreting waste products and other harmful substances obtained from the food and water ingested orally. A functioning urinary system is crucial to maintaining health, and disease in this system can have detrimental effects on other systems and the body as a whole. Prevention and early treatment of these diseases are paramount to avoiding these consequences. Maintaining a healthy lifestyle (e.g., drinking plenty of fluids, avoiding harmful chemicals, preventing sexually transmitted infection, exercising, and smoking cessation) can help preserve urinary health.

REFERENCES

AAOS. (2004). *Paramedic: Anatomy and physiology*. Sudbury, MA: Jones and Bartlett.
Baumberger-Henry, M. (2008). *Fluid and electrolytes* (2nd ed.). Sudbury, MA: Jones and Bartlett.
Chiras, D. (2011). *Human biology* (7th ed.). Burlington, MA: Jones & Bartlett Learning.
Crowley, L. V. (2012). *An introduction to human disease* (9th ed.). Burlington, MA: Jones & Bartlett Learning.
Elling, B., Elling, K., & Rothenberg, M. (2004). *Anatomy and physiology*. Sudbury, MA: Jones and Bartlett.
Gould, B. (2015). *Pathophysiology for the health professions* (5th ed.). Philadelphia, PA: Elsevier.
Madara, B., & Pomarico-Denino, V. (2008). *Quick look nursing: Pathophysiology* (2nd ed.). Sudbury, MA: Jones and Bartlett.
National Cancer Institute. (2016a). Bladder cancer treatment (PDQ). Retrieved from http://www.ncbi.nlm.nih.gov/pubmedhealth/PMH0032608/
National Cancer Institute. (2016b). Renal cell cancer treatment (PDQ): Health professional version. Retrieved from http://www.cancer.gov/types/kidney/hp/kidney-treatment-pdq#link/_228_toc
National Cancer Institute. (2016c). Wilms tumor and other childhood kidney tumors treatment (PDQ): Health professional version. Retrieved from http://www.cancer.gov/types/kidney/hp/wilms-treatment-pdq#section/all
National Institutes of Health (NIH). (2002, November). Renal calculi. *Word on Health*.
National Institutes of Health (NIH). (2012). Urinary tract infection in adults. Retrieved from https://www.niddk.nih.gov/health-information/health-topics/urologic-disease/urinary-tract-infections-in-adults/Pages/facts.aspx
National Institutes of Health (NIH). (2013). Chronic kidney disease and kidney failure. Retrieved from http://report.nih.gov/NIHfactsheets/ViewFactSheet.aspx?csid=34&key=C
National Institutes of Health (NIH). (2015). Polycystic kidney disease. Retrieved from https://www.niddk.nih.gov/health-information/health-topics/kidney-disease/polycystic-kidney-disease-pkd/Pages/facts.aspx
Newman, D. K. (2010). Causes of acute incontinence. Retrieved from http://www.seekwellness.com/m/incontinence/incontinence-causes.htm
Professional guide to pathophysiology (3rd ed.). (2010). Philadelphia, PA: Lippincott Williams & Wilkins.
Resnick, N., & Yalla, S. (1998). Geriatric incontinence and voiding dysfunction. In P. C. Walsh, A. B. Retik, E. D. Vaughan, & A. J. Wein (Eds.), *Campbell's urology* (7th ed., p. 1045) Philadelphia, PA: W.B. Saunders.

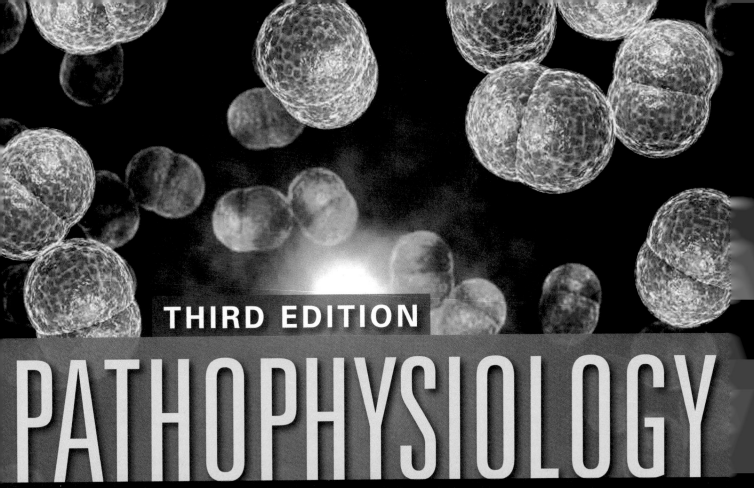

THIRD EDITION

PATHOPHYSIOLOGY

A PRACTICAL APPROACH

Lachel Story, PhD, RN

Assistant Dean for Research and Evaluation
PhD Program Director
Associate Professor
College of Nursing
The University of Southern Mississippi
Hattiesburg, Mississippi

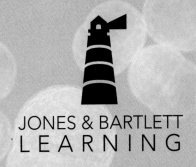

JONES & BARTLETT
LEARNING

World Headquarters
Jones & Bartlett Learning
5 Wall Street
Burlington, MA 01803
978-443-5000
info@jblearning.com
www.jblearning.com

Jones & Bartlett Learning books and products are available through most bookstores and online booksellers. To contact Jones & Bartlett Learning directly, call 800-832-0034, fax 978-443-8000, or visit our website, www.jblearning.com.

The content, statements, views, and opinions herein are the sole expression of the respective authors and not that of Jones & Bartlett Learning, LLC. Reference herein to any specific commercial product, process, or service by trade name, trademark, manufacturer, or otherwise does not constitute or imply its endorsement or recommendation by Jones & Bartlett Learning, LLC and such reference shall not be used for advertising or product endorsement purposes. All trademarks displayed are the trademarks of the parties noted herein. *Pathophysiology: A Practical Approach, Third Edition* is an independent publication and has not been authorized, sponsored, or otherwise approved by the owners of the trademarks or service marks referenced in this product.

There may be images in this book that feature models; these models do not necessarily endorse, represent, or participate in the activities represented in the images. Any screenshots in this product are for educational and instructive purposes only. Any individuals and scenarios featured in the case studies throughout this product may be real or fictitious, but are used for instructional purposes only.

The author, editor, and publisher have made every effort to provide accurate information. However, they are not responsible for errors, omissions, or for any outcomes related to the use of the contents of this book and take no responsibility for the use of the products and procedures described. Treatments and side effects described in this book may not be applicable to all people; likewise, some people may require a dose or experience a side effect that is not described herein. Drugs and medical devices are discussed that may have limited availability controlled by the Food and Drug Administration (FDA) for use only in a research study or clinical trial. Research, clinical practice, and government regulations often change the accepted standard in this field. When consideration is being given to use of any drug in the clinical setting, the health care provider or reader is responsible for determining FDA status of the drug, reading the package insert, and reviewing prescribing information for the most up-to-date recommendations on dose, precautions, and contraindications, and determining the appropriate usage for the product. This is especially important in the case of drugs that are new or seldom used.

12113–1

Production Credits
VP, Executive Publisher: David D. Cella
Executive Editor: Amanda Martin
Editorial Assistant: Christina Freitas
Senior Production Editor: Amanda Clerkin
Senior Marketing Manager: Jennifer Scherzay
Product Fulfillment Manager: Wendy Kilborn
Composition: codeMantra
Cover Design: Scott Moden
Rights & Media Specialist: Wes DeShano
Media Development Editor: Troy Liston
Cover Image (Title Page): © Ezume Images/Shutterstock
Printing and Binding: LSC Communications
Cover Printing: LSC Communications

Library of Congress Cataloging-in-Publication Data
Names: Story, Lachel, author.
Title: Pathophysiology : a practical approach / Lachel Story.
Description: Third edition. | Burlington, Massachusetts : Jones & Bartlett
    Learning, [2018] | Includes bibliographical references and index.
Identifiers: LCCN 2016047299 | ISBN 9781284120196
Subjects: | MESH: Pathology | Physiology | Nurses' Instruction
Classification: LCC RB113 | NLM QZ 140 | DDC 616.07–dc23
LC record available at https://lccn.loc.gov/2016047299

6048

Printed in the United States of America
21 20 19 18 17   10 9 8 7 6 5 4 3 2

Contents

Preface

While teaching pathophysiology for more than 13 years and nursing for more than 21 years, I noticed a lack of pathophysiology books that students could relate to, and high student frustration in learning the convoluted material. Pathophysiology—while being the foundation of much of nursing education, from medical–surgical to pharmacology—is often an insurmountable barrier for students. They are faced with a copious amount of complicated information to weed through. While some students become bogged down in an information marsh, others seek more information than is provided in a skeleton book that has been cut to the bone. Nursing faculty join the students on this frustrating, Goldilocks journey by trying to make the available resources fit. Unfortunately, nursing students and faculty often have pathophysiology books available that provide either far too much information or far too little.

This text provides the right fit: it is a practical guide to pathophysiology that presents information in a student-friendly, understandable way. Here, extraneous information is omitted, leaving only necessary information. The information in this text is also presented in a more accessible manner by considering readability, providing colorful graphics, and giving the content context and meaning.

This ground-breaking text will provide a springboard for faculty and students to come together as co-learners to explore this fascinating content. When such co-learning is stimulated, pathophysiology is no longer just mindlessly deposited into the students in a stifling manner; rather, learning for the students and the faculty becomes an empowerment pedagogy. This approach has been supported by experts at the Institute of Medicine (2011), the Robert Wood Johnson Foundation (Committee on the Robert Wood Johnson Foundation Initiative on the Future of Nursing at the Institute of Medicine, 2010), and nursing leaders (Benner, Sutphen, Leonard, & Day, 2010), among others, who have sought to change how nurses are educated to meet the changing landscape of health care and needs of new generations.

The third edition of this text organizes content in a conceptual manner to provide students with an understandable and practical resource for learning pathophysiology. New and updated material has been added to every chapter. An increased focus on pediatric content and considerations has been threaded throughout. New and updated case studies add to students' understanding and ability to apply their learning on a practical level. Instructor resources have been expanded to include active learning activities that support the "flipped" classroom approach. Faculty will appreciate having a resource that speaks to and engages students. Health professionals will also be able to refer the text to refresh their memory on concepts in a pragmatic way.

References

Benner, P., Sutphen, M., Leonard, V., & Day, L. (2010). *Educating nurses: A call for radical transformation.* San Francisco, CA: Jossey-Bass.

Committee on the Robert Wood Johnson Foundation Initiative on the Future of Nursing at the Institute of Medicine. (2010). A summary of the February 2010 forum on the future of nursing: Education [Chapter 2: What to teach]. Retrieved from http://www.nap.edu/catalog/12894.html

Institute of Medicine. (2011). *The future of nursing education: Leading change, advancing health.* Washington, DC: National Academies Press.

Acknowledgments

First, I would like to thank my husband, Tom, and children, Clayton and Mason, for their never-ending love and encouragement. I would also like to express my deepest gratitude to my mom, Carolyn, and dad, Tommy, because I would not be who I am today without them. I would also like to acknowledge all my students past, present, and future for constantly teaching me more than I could ever teach them and for all their feedback—I heard it and I hope this is more what you had in mind. Finally, I would like to convey my appreciation to my colleagues for their gracious mentoring and support.

Reviewers

Judy Anderson, PhD, RN, CNE
Associate Professor
School of Nursing
Viterbo University
La Crosse, Wisconsin

Margaret Hamilton Birney, PhD, RN
Associate Professor
School of Nursing
University of Delaware
Newark, Delaware

Patsy E. Crihfield, DNP, APRN, FNP-BC
Associate Professor of Nursing and Director of Nurse
  Practitioner Program
School of Nursing
Union University
Germantown, Tennessee

Jennifer Donwerth, MSN, RN, ANP-BC, GNP-BC
Instructor
Department of Nursing
Tarleton State University
Stephenville, Texas

Julie Eggert, PhD
Associate Professor and Healthcare Genetics Doctoral
  Program Coordinator
School of Nursing
Clemson University
Clemson, South Carolina

Masoud Ghaffari, MSN/RN, MEd, MT (ASCP), CMA
Associate Professor
College of Nursing
East Tennessee State University
Johnson City, Tennessee

Kathleen A. Goei, PhD, RN, MSN
Assistant Professor
School of Nursing and Health Professions
University of the Incarnate Word
San Antonio, Texas

Christine Henshaw, EdD, RN, CNE
Associate Dean, Undergraduate Program
School of Health Sciences
Seattle Pacific University
Seattle, Washington

Patricia R. Keene, DNP, ACNP, CS, BC
Associate Professor of Nursing
School of Nursing
Union University
Germantown, Tennessee

Linda Keilman, DNP(c), MSN, GNP-BC
Assistant Professor
College of Nursing
Michigan State University
East Lansing, Michigan

Barbara McClaskey, PhD, MN, ARNP-CNS
Associate Professor
Department of Nursing
Pittsburg State University
Pittsburg, Kansas

Joan Niederriter, PhD, RN
Assistant Professor
Department of Nursing
Cleveland State University
Cleveland, Ohio

Tanya L. Rogers, APRN, BC, MSN, EdD
Associate Professor of Nursing
School of Nursing and Allied Health Administration
Fairmont State University
Fairmont, West Virginia

Jennifer K. Sofie, MSN, ANP, FNP
Adjunct Assistant Professor
College of Nursing
Montana State University
Bozeman, Montana

Joan Stokowski, MSN
Assistant Professor
Department of Health Careers
Illinois Central College
Peoria, Illinois

Brenda D. Tilton, RN, MSN, FNP-BC
Assistant Professor of Nursing
School of Nursing
Southern State Community College
Hillsboro, Ohio

Vickie Walker, DNP, RN
Assistant Professor of Nursing
School of Nursing
Gardner-Webb University
Boiling Springs, North Carolina

Introduction to Pathophysiology

LEARNING OBJECTIVES

- Define pathophysiology and identify its importance for clinical practice.
- Identify key health and disease concepts.

KEY TERMS

acute	epidemic	inflammatory	pathophysiology
chronic	epidemiology	insidious	positive feedback systems
compensatory mechanism	etiology	manifestation	predisposing factor
complication	exacerbation	metabolic	prevention
congenital	genetic	morbidity	prognosis
convalescence	health	mortality	remission
degenerative	hereditary	negative feedback system	signs
developmental	homeostasis	neoplastic	symptoms
diagnosis	iatrogenic	pandemic	syndrome
disease	idiopathic	pathogenesis	treatment

Pathophysiology Concepts

What is meant by **pathophysiology**? And why is it so important to understand, especially for nurses? Essentially, pathophysiology is the study of what happens when normal anatomy and physiology go wrong. Veering off this normal path can cause diseases or abnormal states. Pathophysiology is the foundation upon which all of nursing is built. It is the "why" that unlocks all the mysteries of the human body and its response to medical and nursing therapies. Understanding pathophysiology provides insight into why patients look the way they do when they have a certain disease, why the medicines we give them work, why the side effects of treatments occur, and why complications sometimes transpire. Pathophysiology provides the rationale for evidence-based medicine.

Why are so many students mystified by pathophysiology? Unfortunately, students often get lost in the minute details and the complicated nuances of pathophysiology. Pathophysiology, when brought back to the basics and framed in a practical context, can bring meaning and understanding to the world of health and disease in which people live.

Health and Disease

To understand disease, first the definition of health must be clarified. **Health** may be considered the absence of disease, but this concept can also be expanded to include wellness of mind, body, and spirit. The normal state may vary due to genetic, age, and gender differences, and it becomes relative to the individual's baseline. Negative events in any one of these three areas can cause issues in the others—these areas coexist. Humans are complicated and do not exist in a vacuum. Just as the mind, body, and spirit are interrelated, so humans are interrelated with their environment, including their physical ecology as well as social factors. These external factors play a significant role in an individual's health, whether negatively or positively.

On the flip side of health is disease. **Disease** is a state in which a bodily function is no longer occurring normally. The severity of diseases ranges from merely causing temporary stress to causing life-changing complications. Health and disease may be considered as two ends of a continuum. At one end are severe, life-threatening disease states that cause significant physical and emotional issues; at the other end is optimal health that supports mind, body, and spirit well-being.

Diseases can be classified in several ways. First, a disease may be **hereditary**, meaning it is transmitted before birth. Disease may also be present at birth, or **congenital**. **Genetic** diseases are caused by abnormalities in the individual's genetic makeup (e.g., chromosomal numbers or mutations) (see the *Cellular Function* chapter). **Developmental** diseases occur as a result of an issue that arises during embryonic or fetal development. Other diseases may develop over the life span. **Inflammatory** diseases are those that trigger the inflammatory response (see the *Immunity* chapter). **Degenerative** diseases include conditions that cause parts of the body to deteriorate (e.g., arthritis). Conditions that affect metabolism are referred to as **metabolic** diseases (e.g., diabetes mellitus). **Neoplastic** diseases are caused by abnormal or uncontrolled cellular growth, which can lead to benign and malignant tumors (see the *Cellular Function* chapter).

Exploring concepts of homeostasis is a good place to start in understanding the origins of disease.

Homeostasis

Many words can be used to describe **homeostasis**, such as *equilibrium, balance, consistency,* and *stability.* Some examples of this relative consistency can be seen in vital signs such as blood pressure, pulse, and temperature. Every part of the human body—from the smallest cells to the largest organs—needs balance to maintain its usual functions. In some cases, such as with pH, even minimal changes can cause significant and life-threatening problems. The human body is constantly engaging in multiple strategies to maintain this balance and addressing external stressors such as injury or organism invasion that might tip the balance in one direction or another.

Homeostasis is a self-regulating, give-and-take system that responds to minor changes in the body through compensation mechanisms. Compensation mechanisms attempt to counteract those changes and return the body to its normal state (**FIGURE I-1**). Several brain structures are instrumental in maintaining this balance, including the medulla oblongata, hypothalamus, reticular formation, and pituitary gland. The medulla oblongata is located in the brain stem and controls vital functions such as blood pressure, temperature, and pulse. The reticular

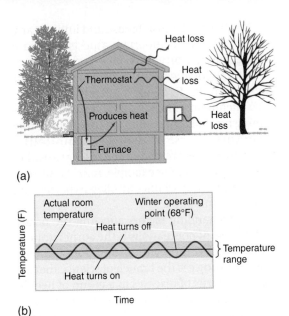

FIGURE I-1 Homeostasis is like a house. (a) Heat is maintained in a house by a furnace, which compensates for heat loss. (b) A hypothetical temperature graph.

formation is a network of nerve cells in the brain stem and the spinal cord that also controls vital functions; it relays information to the hypothalamus. The hypothalamus, in turn, controls homeostasis by communicating information to the pituitary gland. The pituitary gland, also known as the master gland, regulates other glands that contribute to growth, maturation, and reproduction.

Two types of feedback systems exist to maintain homeostasis: negative and positive. A **negative feedback system**—the most common type—works to maintain a deficit in the system. Such negative feedback mechanisms work to resist any change from normal. Examples include temperature and glucose regulation. **Positive feedback systems**, though few in number, move the body away from homeostasis. With this type of feedback, an amplified response occurs in the same direction as the original stressor. Examples of positive feedback systems include childbirth, sneezing, and blood clots.

Disease Development

Etiology is the study of disease causation. Etiologic factors may include infectious agents, chemicals, and environmental influences, to name a few. Etiologic factors may also be unknown, or **idiopathic**. Additionally, diseases can be caused by an unintended, or **iatrogenic**, effect of a medical treatment. **Predisposing factors** are tendencies that put an individual at

risk for developing certain diseases. Examples of predisposing factors are similar to etiologic factors and may include dietary imbalances and carcinogen exposure. Identifying the etiology and predisposing factors for a disease can be instrumental in preventing the disease by distinguishing at-risk populations who can be targeted with prevention measures. Today, the healthcare system is focusing more on disease prevention because investing resources before a disease develops can decrease the long-term financial burden associated with its treatment.

How a disease develops is referred to as **pathogenesis**. Some diseases are self-limiting, whereas others are chronic and never resolve. Some diseases cause reversible changes, while others cause irreparable damage. The body attempts to limit the damage from diseases by activating compensatory mechanisms. **Compensatory mechanisms** are physiological strategies the body employs in the midst of homeostatic imbalance to maintain normalcy. When those mechanisms can no longer maintain relative consistency, disease occurs.

The onset of the disease may be sudden or acute. Acute onset of a disease may include pronounced indicators such as pain or vomiting, whereas a gradual, or **insidious**, onset may be associated with only vague signals. Hypertension, for example, can occur in this subtle manner.

Disease duration is another important concept to consider. A disease may be short term, or **acute**, occurring and resolving quickly. Gastroenteritis and tonsillitis are examples of acute diseases. When an acute disease does not resolve after a short period, it may move into a chronic state. A **chronic** disease often has less notable signs and occurs over a longer period. Chronic diseases may not ever resolve but may sometimes become manageable. Diabetes mellitus and depression are examples of chronic diseases. Additionally, people with chronic diseases can experience an acute event of that disease, complicating care. An example of this phenomenon can be seen when a patient with asthma (a chronic disease) has an acute asthma attack.

Recognition of a disease when it is encountered is important in diagnosis, or identification, of disease. **Manifestations** are the clinical effects or evidence of a disease. They may include both **signs**—what can be seen or measured—and **symptoms**—what the patient describes but is not visible to the healthcare practitioner. Manifestations may include issues identified during a physical assessment (e.g., heart murmur), diagnostic results (e.g., laboratory levels), patient complaints (e.g., pain), and family reports (e.g., unusual behavior). A **syndrome** comprises a group of signs and symptoms that occur together. Some chronic diseases may include episodes of remission and exacerbation. **Remission** occurs when the manifestations subside, and **exacerbation** occurs when the manifestations increase again. Systemic lupus erythematosus and heart failure are examples of diseases that demonstrate remissions and exacerbations. Manifestations may vary depending on the point at which they occur in the pathogenesis. For instance, an early sign of shock may be tachycardia, whereas bradycardia occurs late in the disease process. Manifestations are often a critical component of disease **diagnosis**, or identification. Additionally, a detailed patient history may be used to facilitate accurate diagnosis.

Treatment refers to strategies used to manage or cure a disease. Treatment may be specific to the cause of the disease or used to alleviate the disease's clinical manifestations. For example, an antibiotic may be used to target the specific organism causing a patient's pneumonia or an antiemetic may be administered to relieve vomiting associated with acute pancreatitis. Treatment regimens often require the services of an interdisciplinary team (e.g., nurses, nurse practitioners, dietitians, respiratory therapists, physical therapists, occupational therapists, physiotherapists, physicians, and pharmacists). Such a team is often necessary when a swift, aggressive approach is required or when long-term management is needed.

Some of the same treatment strategies are used for disease prevention. **Prevention** includes strategies to avoid the development of disease in individuals or groups. Such strategies may include screening, vaccinations, lifestyle changes, or prophylactic interventions (e.g., medication to reduce high cholesterol levels to prevent strokes, mastectomy in a person at high risk of breast cancer).

Recovering from a disease and limiting any residual effects are important aspects of disease management. **Convalescence** is the stage of recovery following a disease, which may last for days or months. **Prognosis** refers to an individual's likelihood of making a full recovery or regaining normal functioning. The death rate from a particular disease is referred to as **mortality**. **Complications** are new problems that arise because of a disease. For example, renal failure can be a complication of uncontrolled hypertension or diabetes mellitus.

Understanding factors affecting the health and disease of populations is the cornerstone to understanding prevention and containment. **Epidemiology** is the branch of science that analyzes patterns of diseases in a group of people. Such tracking of disease patterns includes occurrence, incidence, prevalence, transmission, and distribution of a disease. **Morbidity** refers to disease rates within a group. **Epidemics** occur when there are increasing numbers of people with a certain disease within a specific group. When the epidemic expands to a larger population, it becomes a **pandemic**.

Summary

Pathophysiology is the basis for understanding the intricate world of the human body, its response to disease, and the rationale for treatment. Understanding pathophysiology can assist the nurse to better anticipate situations, correct issues, and provide appropriate care. The concepts of health and disease, although complex, need not cause stress to nursing students or patients. Instead, these concepts can open a world of wonder of which to be in awe.

References

Crowley, L. (2017). *An introduction to human disease: Pathology and pathophysiology correlations* (10th ed.). Burlington, MA: Jones & Bartlett Learning.

Mosby's dictionary of medicinal, nursing, and health professionals (9th ed.). (2012). St. Louis, MO: Mosby.

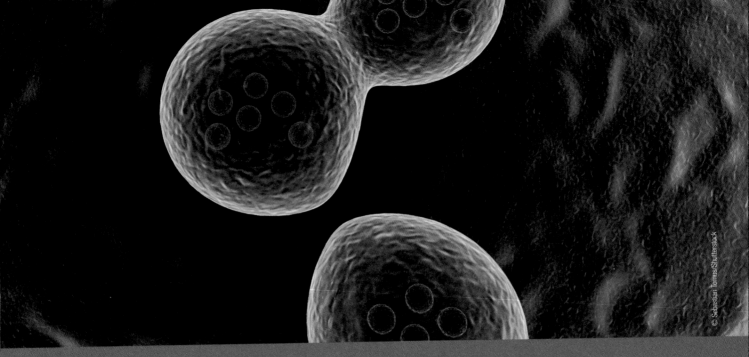

CHAPTER 1
Cellular Function

LEARNING OBJECTIVES

- Describe basic cellular structures and function.
- Describe common cellular adaptations and possible reasons for the occurrence of each.
- List common causes of cell damage. Discuss cancerous cellular damage.
- Describe common genetic and congenital alterations.

KEY TERMS

active transport
adaptation
alleles
anaphase
anaplasia
apoptosis
atrophy
autosomal dominant
autosomal recessive
autosome
benign
cancer
carcinogenesis
caseous necrosis
cell membrane
chromosome
coagulative necrosis
congenital
crenation
curative
cytoplasm
deoxyribonucleic acid (DNA)

differentiation
diffusion
dominant
dry gangrene
dysplasia
electrolyte
endocytosis
enzyme
exocytosis
facilitated diffusion
fat necrosis
free radicals
gangrene
gas gangrene
genes
genetics
glucose
grading
heterozygous
homozygous
hyperplasia
hypertrophy

initiation
ischemia
karyotype
lipid bilayer
liquefaction necrosis
lysis
malignant
meiosis
metaphase
metaplasia
metastasize
mitosis
multifactorial disorders
necrosis
neoplasm
nucleotide
nucleus
oncogene
organelle
osmosis
osmotic pressure
palliative

phagocytosis
phenotype
pinocytosis
plasma membrane
programmed cell death
prognosis
progression
proliferation
promotion
prophase
prophylactic
protoplasm
recessive
remission
selectively permeable
sex-linked
telophase
teratogens
TNM staging
tumor
wet gangrene

Pathophysiology inquiry begins with exploring the basic building blocks of living organisms. Cells give organisms their immense diversity. Organisms can be made up of a single cell, such as with bacteria or viruses, or billions of cells, such as with humans. In humans, these building blocks work together to form tissues, organs, and organ systems. These basic units of life are also the basic units of disease. As understanding increases about specific diseases, these diseases can be reduced to their cellular level. Diseases are likely to occur due to some loss of homeostatic control, and the impact is evident from the cellular level up to the system level. Understanding the various cellular dysfunctions associated with diseases has led to improved prevention and treatment of those diseases. Therefore, understanding basic cellular function and dysfunction is essential to understanding pathophysiology.

Basic Cell Function

Cells are complex miniorganisms resulting from millions of years of evolution. Cells can arise only from a preexisting cell. Although they vary greatly in size and shape (FIGURE 1-1), cells have the remarkable ability to exchange materials with their immediate surroundings, obtain energy from organic nutrients, synthesize complex molecules, and replicate themselves.

The basic components of cells include the cytoplasm, nucleus, and cell membrane. The **cytoplasm**, or **protoplasm**, is a colorless, viscous liquid containing water, nutrients, ions, dissolved gases, and waste products; this liquid is where the cellular work takes place. The cytoplasm supports all of the internal cellular structures called **organelles** (FIGURE 1-2). Organelles ("little organs") perform the work that maintains the cell's life (**TABLE 1-1**). The cytoplasm also surrounds the nucleus. The **nucleus**, which is the control center of the cell, contains all the genetic information (DNA) and is surrounded by a double membrane (FIGURE 1-3). The nucleus regulates cell growth, metabolism, and reproduction. The **cell membrane**, also called the **plasma membrane**, is the semipermeable boundary containing the cell and its components (FIGURE 1-4). A **lipid bilayer**, or fatty double covering, makes up the membrane. The interior surface of the bilayer is uncharged and primarily made up of lipids. The exterior surface of the bilayer is charged and is less fatty than the interior surface. This fatty cover protects the cell from the aqueous environment in which it exists, while allowing it to be permeable to some molecules but not others.

Exchanging Material

Cellular permeability is the ability of the cell to allow passage of some substances through the membrane, while not permitting others to enter or exit. To accomplish this process, cells have gates that may be opened or closed by proteins, chemical signals, or electrical charges. Being **selectively permeable** allows the cell to maintain a state of internal balance, or homeostasis. Some substances have free passage in and out of the cells, including enzymes, glucose, and electrolytes. **Enzymes** are proteins that facilitate chemical reactions in cells, while **glucose** is a sugar molecule that provides energy. **Electrolytes** are chemicals that are charged conductors when dissolved in water. Passage across the cell membrane is accomplished through several mechanisms, including diffusion, osmosis, facilitated diffusion, active transport, endocytosis, and exocytosis.

Diffusion is the movement of solutes—that is, particles dissolved in a solvent—from an area of higher concentration to an area of lower concentration (FIGURE 1-5). The degree of diffusion depends on the permeability of the membrane and the concentration gradient, which is the difference in concentrations of substances on either side of the membrane. Smaller particles diffuse more easily than larger ones, and less viscous solutions diffuse more rapidly than thicker solutions. Many substances, such as oxygen, enter the cell through diffusion.

Learning Points

To illustrate diffusion, consider an elevator filled beyond capacity with people. When the door opens, the people near the door naturally fall out—moving from an area of high concentration to an area with less concentration with no effort, or energy. In the body, gases are exchanged in the lungs by diffusion. Unoxygenated blood enters the pulmonary capillaries (low concentration of oxygen; high concentration of carbon dioxide), where it picks up oxygen from the inhaled air of the alveoli (high concentration of oxygen; low concentration of carbon dioxide), while dropping off carbon dioxide to the alveoli to be exhaled.

Learning Points

To understand osmosis, envision a plastic bag filled with sugar water and with holes punched in it that allow only water to pass through them. If this bag is submerged in distilled water (contains no impurities), the bag will begin to swell because the water is attracted to the sugar. The water shifts to the areas with higher concentrations of sugar in an attempt to dilute the sugar concentrations (FIGURE 1-6). In our bodies, osmosis allows the cells to remain hydrated.

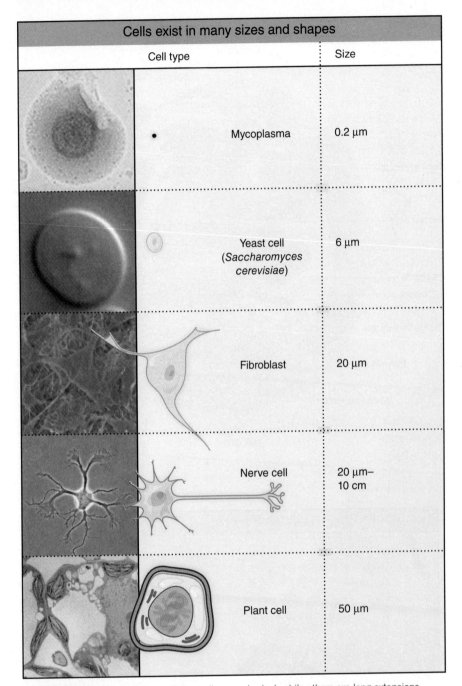

FIGURE 1-1 Cells vary greatly in size and shape. Some cells are spherical, while others are long extensions.

Courtesy of Tim Pietzcker, Universitat Ulm University

Courtesy of Fred Winston, Harvard Medical School

Courtesy of Junzo Desaki, Ehime University School of Medicine

Courtesy of Gerald J. Obermair and Bernhard E. Flucher, Innsbruck Medical Unversity

Courtesy of Ming H. Chen, University of Alberta

Osmosis is the movement of water or another solvent across the cellular membrane from an area of low solute concentration to an area of high solute concentration. The membrane is permeable to the solvent (liquid) but not to the solute (dissolved particles). The movement of the solvent usually continues until concentrations of the solute equalize on both sides of the membrane. **Osmotic pressure** refers to the tendency of water to move by osmosis. If too much water enters the cell membrane, the cell will swell and burst (**lysis**). If too much water moves out of the cell, the cell will shrink (**crenation**). Osmosis helps regulate fluid balance in the body; an example can be found in the functioning of the kidneys.

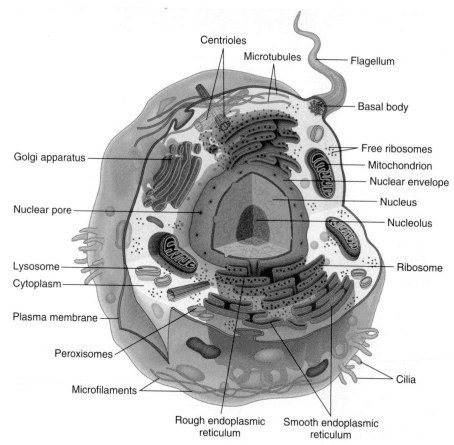

FIGURE 1-2 The cytoplasm contains several organelles.

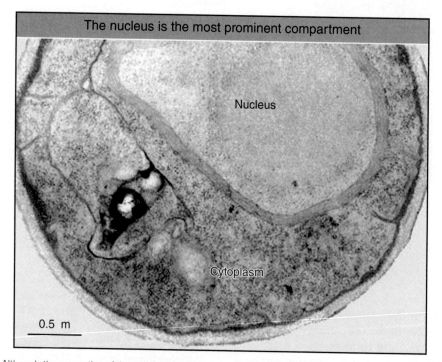

FIGURE 1-3 Although the proportion of the cell that is taken up by the nucleus varies according to cell type, the nucleus is usually the largest and most prominent cellular compartment.

TABLE 1-1	Overview of Cell Organelles

Organelle	Structure	Function
Nucleus	Round or oval body; surrounded by nuclear envelope.	Contains the genetic information necessary for control of cell structure and function; DNA contains hereditary information.
Nucleolus	Round or oval body in the nucleus consisting of DNA and RNA.	Produces ribosomal RNA.
Endoplasmic reticulum (ER)	Network of membranous tubules in the cytoplasm of the cell. Smooth endoplasmic reticulum (SER) contains no ribosomes. Rough endoplasmic reticulum (RER) is studded with ribosomes.	SER is involved in the production of phospholipids and has many different functions depending on the cells; RER is the site of the synthesis of lysosomal enzymes and proteins for extracellular use.
Ribosomes	Small particles found in the cytoplasm; made of RNA and protein.	Aid in protein production on the RER and polysomes.
Golgi complex	Series of flattened sacs usually located near the nucleus.	Sorts, chemically modifies, and packages proteins produced on the RER.
Secretory vesicles	Membrane-bound vesicles containing proteins produced by the RER and repackaged by the Golgi complex; contain protein hormones or enzymes.	Store protein hormones or enzymes in the cytoplasm awaiting a signal for release.
Food vacuole	Membrane-bound vesicle containing material engulfed by the cell.	Stores ingested material and combines with lysosomes.
Lysosome	Round, membrane-bound structure containing digestive enzymes.	Combines with food vacuoles and digests materials engulfed by cells.
Peroximomes	Small structures containing enzymes.	Break down various potentially toxic intracellular molecules.
Mitochondria	Round, oval, or elongated structures with a double membrane. The inner membrane is shaped into folds.	Complete the breakdown of glucose, producing nicotine adenine dinucleotide (NADH) and adenosine triphosphate (ATP).
Cytoskeleton	Network of microtubules and microfilaments in the cell.	Gives the cell internal support, helps transport molecules and some organelles inside the cell, and binds to enzymes of metabolic pathways.
Cilia	Small projections of the cell membrane containing microtubules; found on a limited number of cells.	Propel materials along the surface of certain cells.
Flagella	Large projections of the cell membrane containing microtubules; in humans, found only on sperm cells.	Provide motive force for sperm cells.
Centrioles	Small cylindrical bodies composed of microtubules arranged in nine sets of triplets; found in animal cells, not plants.	Help organize spindle apparatus necessary for cell division.

Facilitated diffusion is the movement of substances from an area of higher concentration to an area of lower concentration with the assistance of a carrier molecule (**FIGURE 1-7**). Energy is not required for this process, and the number of molecules that can be transported in this way is directly equivalent to the concentration of the carrier molecule. Insulin transports glucose into the cells using this method. **Active transport** is the movement of a substance from an area of lower concentration to an area of higher concentration, against a concentration gradient (Figure 1-7). This movement requires a carrier molecule and energy because of the effort necessary to go against the gradient. This energy is usually in the form of adenosine triphosphate (ATP).

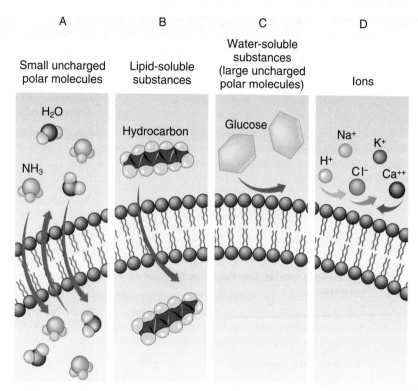

A	B	C	D
Small uncharged polar molecules	Lipid-soluble substances	Water-soluble substances (large uncharged polar molecules)	Ions

FIGURE 1-4 A selectively permeable membrane maintains homeostasis by allowing some molecules to pass through, while others may not.

Endocytosis is the process of bringing a substance into the cell (**FIGURE 1-8**). The cell membrane surrounds the particles, engulfing them. **Phagocytosis**, or cell eating, occurs when this process involves solid particles. **Pinocytosis**, or cell drinking, takes place when this process involves a liquid. Components of the immune system use endocytosis, particularly phagocytosis, to consume and destroy bacteria and other foreign material. **Exocytosis** is the release of materials from the cell, usually with the assistance of a vesicle (a membrane-bound sac) (Figure 1-8). Often glands secrete hormones using exocytosis.

Learning Points

To understand active transport, consider the overfilled elevator again. If the door opens and someone from outside the elevator attempts to get in, it will require a great deal of effort (energy) to enter the full elevator. The sodium–potassium pump is an example of active transport in the body. Energy is required to move sodium out of the cell where the concentrations are high and move potassium into the cell where the concentrations are high.

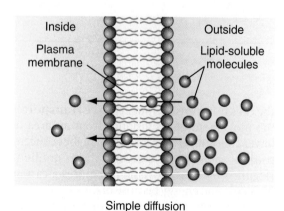

Simple diffusion

FIGURE 1-5 Lipid-soluble substances pass through the membrane directly via simple diffusion.

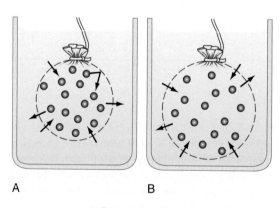

● Sucrose molecules

FIGURE 1-6 (a) When a bag of sugar water is immersed in a solution of pure water, (b) water will diffuse into the bag toward the lower concentrations of water, causing the bag to swell.

Energy Production

Energy can be a mystery to many of us. To understand energy, first we must understand that it comes in many forms. Cells can obtain energy from two main sources—the breakdown of glucose (a type of carbohydrate) and the breakdown of triglycerides (a type of fat). Food enters the gastrointestinal tract, where it is broken down into sugars, amino acids, and fatty acids. These substances then are either converted to larger molecules (e.g., glucose to glycogen, amino acids to proteins, and fatty acids to triglycerides and fats), stored until needed, or metabolized to make ATP. When used to make ATP, all three sources of energy must first be converted to acetyl coenzyme A (acetyl CoA). Acetyl CoA enters the Krebs cycle, a high-electron-producing process, of the mitochondria. During the Krebs cycle, these molecules go through a complex series of reactions that result in the production of large amounts of ATP.

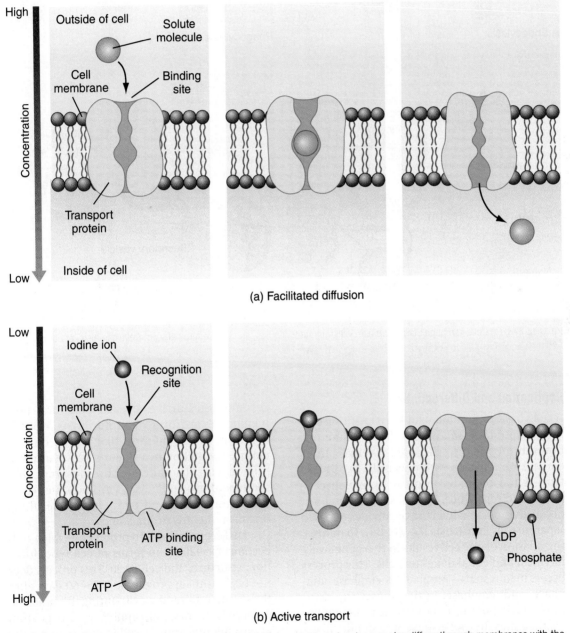

(a) Facilitated diffusion

(b) Active transport

FIGURE 1-7 Facilitated diffusion and active transport. (a) Water-soluble molecules can also diffuse through membranes with the assistance of proteins in facilitated diffusion. (b) Other proteins use energy from ATP to move against concentration gradients in a process called active transport.

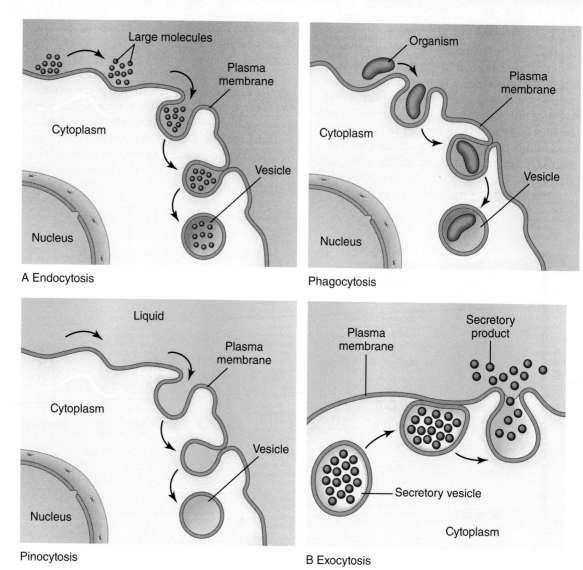

FIGURE 1-8 (a) Cells can engulf large particles, cell fragments, liquids, and even entire cells. (b) Cells can also get rid of large particles.

Replication and Differentiation

A cell's basic requirement for life is ensuring that it can reproduce. Many cells divide numerous times throughout the life span, whereas others die and are replaced with new cells. **Proliferation** is the regulated process by which cells divide and reproduce. The most common form of cell division, in which the cell divides into two separate cells, is **mitosis** (FIGURE 1-9). In mitosis, the division of one cell results in two genetically identical and equal daughter cells. This process occurs in four steps—prophase, metaphase, anaphase, and telophase. In **prophase**, the chromosomes condense and the nuclear membrane disintegrates. In **metaphase**, the spindle fibers attach to centromeres and the chromosomes align. The chromosomes separate and move to opposite poles in **anaphase**. Finally, the

chromosomes arrive at each pole, and new membranes are formed in **telophase**. **Meiosis** is a form of cell division that occurs only in mature sperm and ova (Figure 1-9). Normally, human cells contain 46 chromosomes, but sperm and ova contain 23 chromosomes each. When the sperm and ova join, the resulting organism has 46 chromosomes.

Differentiation is a process by which cells become specialized in terms of cell type, function, structure, and cell cycle. This process does not begin until approximately 15–60 days after the sperm fertilizes the ova. During this time, the embryo is the most susceptible to damage from environmental influences. Differentiation is the process by which the primitive stem cells of the embryo develop into the highly specialized cells of the human (e.g., cardiac cells and nerve cells).

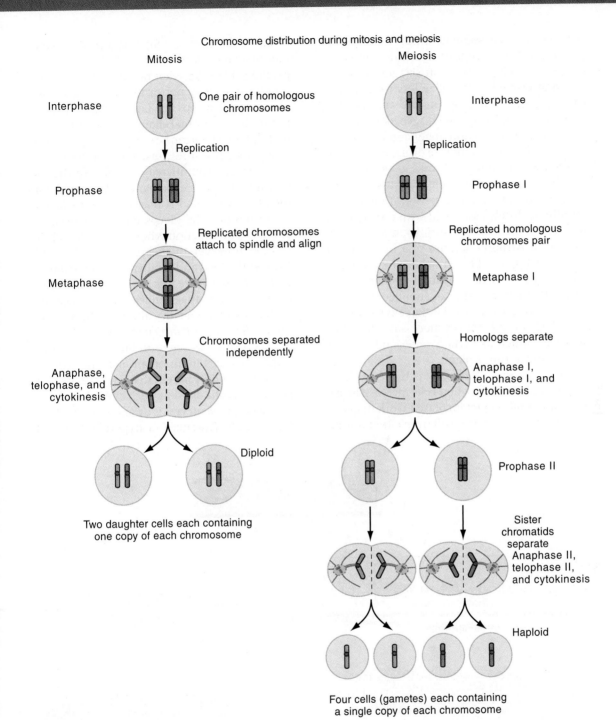

FIGURE 1-9 Mitosis and meiosis.

Cellular Adaptation and Damage

Cellular Adaptation

Cells are constantly exposed to a variety of environmental factors that can cause damage. Cells attempt to prevent their own death from environmental changes through **adaptation**. They may modify their size, numbers, or types in an attempt to manage these changes and maintain homeostasis. Adaptation may involve one or a combination of these modifications. These modifications may be normal or abnormal depending on whether they were mediated through standard pathways. They may also be permanent or reversible. Nevertheless, once the stimulus is removed, adaptation ceases. Specific types of adaptive changes include atrophy, hypertrophy, hyperplasia, metaplasia, and dysplasia (**FIGURE 1-10**).

Atrophy occurs because of decreased work demands on the cell. The body attempts to work as efficiently as possible to conserve energy and resources. When cellular work demands decrease, the cells decrease in size and number. These atrophied cells utilize less oxygen, and their organelles decrease in size and number. Causes of atrophy include disuse, denervation, endocrine hypofunction, inadequate nutrition, and ischemia. An example of disuse atrophy can be seen when a muscle shrinks in an extremity that has been in an immobilizing cast due to a fracture for an extended period. Denervation atrophy is closely associated with disuse; it can be seen when a muscle shrinks in a paralyzed extremity. Atrophy because of a loss of endocrine function can be seen when the reproductive organs of postmenopausal women shrink. When these organs are not supplied with adequate nutrition and blood flow, cells shrink due to a lack of substances necessary for their survival—much like when water and fertilizer are withheld from a plant.

The opposite of atrophy is **hypertrophy**. Hypertrophy occurs when cells increase in size in an attempt to meet increased work demand. This size increase may result from either normal or abnormal changes. Such changes are commonly seen in cardiac and skeletal muscle. For example, consider what happens when a body builder diligently performs biceps curls with weights—the biceps gets larger. This type of hypertrophy is a normal change. An abnormal hypertrophic change can be seen with hypertension (high blood pressure). Just as the biceps muscle grows larger from increased work, so the cardiac muscle will thicken and enlarge when an increased workload is placed on it because of hypertension. The biceps muscle increases in strength and function when its workload is increased; however, the heart loses the flexibility to fill with blood and pump the blood when the cardiac muscle increases in size. This abnormal hypertrophic change can lead to complications such as cardiomyopathy and heart failure (see the *Cardiovascular Function* chapter).

Hyperplasia refers to an increase in the number of cells in an organ or tissue. This increase occurs only in cells that have the ability to perform mitotic division, such as epithelial cells. The hyperplasia process is usually a result of normal stimuli. Examples of hyperplasia include

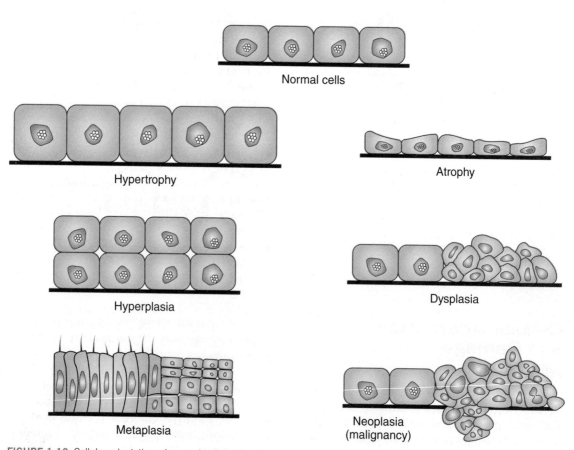

Normal cells

Hypertrophy

Atrophy

Hyperplasia

Dysplasia

Metaplasia

Neoplasia (malignancy)

FIGURE 1-10 Cellular adaptation: abnormal cellular growth patterns.

menstruation, liver regeneration, wound healing, and skin warts. Hyperplasia is different from hypertrophy, but these processes often occur together because they have similar triggers.

The process in which one adult cell is replaced by another cell type is called **metaplasia**. This change is usually initiated by chronic irritation and inflammation, such that a more virulent cell line emerges. The cell types do not cross over the overarching cell type. For instance, epithelial cells may be converted into another type of epithelial cell, but they will not be replaced with nerve cells. Examples of metaplastic changes are the ciliary changes that occur in the respiratory tract because of chronic smoking or vitamin A deficiency. Metaplasia does not necessarily lead to cancerous changes; however, if the stimulus is not removed, cancerous changes will likely occur.

The final cellular adaption is **dysplasia**. In dysplasia, cells mutate into cells of a different size, shape, and appearance. Although dysplasia is abnormal, it is potentially reversible by removing the trigger. Dysplastic changes are often implicated as precancerous cells. The reproductive and respiratory tracts are common sites for this type of adaptation because of their increased exposure to carcinogens (e.g., human papillomavirus and cigarette smoke).

Cellular Death and Injury

Cellular injury can occur in many ways and is usually reversible up to a point. Whether the injury is reversible or irreversible usually depends on the severity of the injury and intrinsic factors (e.g., blood supply and nutritional status). Cell injury can occur because of (1) physical agents (e.g., mechanical forces and extreme temperature), (2) chemical injury (e.g., pollution, lead, and drugs), (3) radiation, (4) biologic agents (e.g., viruses, bacteria, and parasites), and (5) nutritional imbalances.

Death is a normal part of the human existence, and it is no different at the cellular level. When cellular injury becomes irreversible, it usually results in cell death. The process of eliminating unwanted cells, called **programmed cell death**, usually occurs through the **apoptosis** mechanism (FIGURE 1-11). Programmed cell death occurs at a specific point in development; apoptosis specifically occurs because of morphologic (structure or form) changes. This mechanism of cell death is not limited to developmental causes, but rather may also result from environmental triggers. Apoptosis is important in tissue development, immune defense, and cancer prevention. However, this mechanism can result in inappropriate destruction of cells if it is unregulated. Such inappropriate activation of apoptosis can occur in degenerative neurologic diseases such as Alzheimer's disease (see the *Neural Function* chapter).

Not all cell death is apoptotic, however. Cell death can also occur because of ischemia or necrosis (Figure 1-11). **Ischemia** refers to inadequate blood flow to tissue or an organ. This lack of blood flow essentially strangles the tissue or organ by limiting the supply of necessary nutrients and oxygen. Ischemia can leave cells damaged to the extent that they cannot survive, a condition called **necrosis**. The difference between apoptosis and necrosis lies mostly in the cell's morphologic changes. In apoptosis, the cells condense or shrink; in necrosis, the cells swell and burst.

Necrosis can take one of several pathways. **Liquefaction necrosis** (FIGURE 1-12) occurs when caustic enzymes dissolve and liquefy necrotic cells. The most common site of this type of necrosis is the brain, which contains a plentiful supply of these enzymes. **Caseous necrosis** (FIGURE 1-13) occurs when the necrotic cells disintegrate but the cellular debris remains in the area for months or years. This type of necrosis has a cottage cheese–like appearance, and it is most commonly noted with pulmonary tuberculosis. **Fat necrosis** (FIGURE 1-14) occurs when lipase enzymes break down intracellular triglycerides into free fatty acids. These fatty acids then combine with magnesium, sodium, and calcium, forming soaps. These soaps give fat necrosis an opaque, chalky appearance. **Coagulative necrosis** (FIGURE 1-15) usually results from an interruption in blood flow. In such a case, the pH drops (acidosis), denaturing the cell's enzymes. This type of necrosis most often occurs in the kidneys, heart, and adrenal glands.

Gangrene is a form of coagulative necrosis that represents a combination of impaired blood flow and a bacterial invasion. Gangrene usually occurs in the legs because of arteriosclerosis (hardening of the arteries) or in the gastrointestinal tract. Gangrene can take any of three forms—dry, wet, and gas. **Dry gangrene** (FIGURE 1-16) occurs when bacterial presence is minimal, and the skin has a dry, dark brown, or black appearance. **Wet gangrene** (FIGURE 1-17) occurs with liquefaction necrosis. In this condition, extensive damage from bacteria and white blood cells produces a liquid

Apoptosis versus necrosis

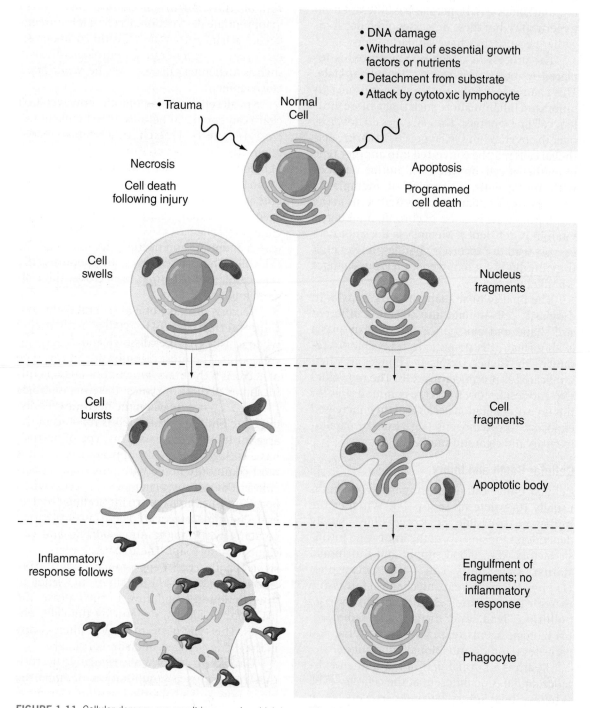

FIGURE 1-11 Cellular damage can result in necrosis, which has a different appearance than apoptosis, as organelles swell and the plasma membrane ruptures.

wound. Wet gangrene can occur in extremities and internal organs. **Gas gangrene** (**FIGURE 1-18**) develops because of the presence of *Clostridium*, an anaerobic bacterium. This type of gangrene is the most serious and has the greatest potential to be fatal. The bacterium releases toxins that destroy surrounding cells, so the infection spreads rapidly. The gas released from this

process bubbles from the tissue, often underneath the skin.

Another important mechanism of cellular injury is free radicals. **Free radicals** are injurious, unstable agents that can cause cell death. A single unbalanced atom initiates this pathway, which can rapidly produce a wide range of damage. Such an atom has an unpaired electron,

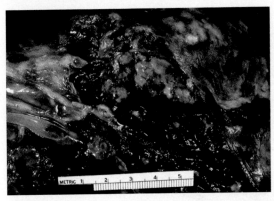

FIGURE 1-12 Liquefaction necrosis.
© University of Alabama at Birmingham Department of Pathology PEIR Digital Library (http://peir.net)

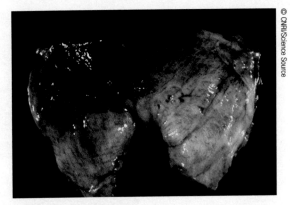
© CNRI/Science Source

FIGURE 1-15 Coagulative necrosis.

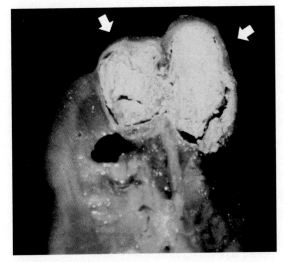

FIGURE 1-13 Caseous necrosis.
Reproduced from Gibson, M. S., Pucket, M. L., & Shelly, M. E. (2004). Renal tuberculosis. *Radiographics, 24*(1), 251–256.

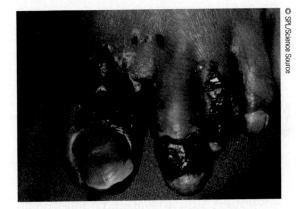
© SPL/Science Source

FIGURE 1-16 Dry gangrene.

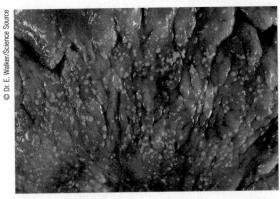
© Dr. E. Walker/Science Source

FIGURE 1-14 Fat necrosis.

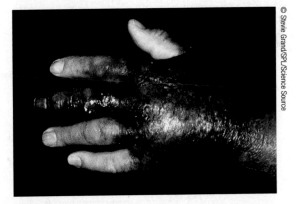
© Stevie Grand/SPL/Science Source

FIGURE 1-17 Wet gangrene.

making it unstable. In an attempt to stabilize itself, the atom borrows an electron from a surrounding atom, usually rendering it unstable. This newly unstable atom will then borrow an electron from its neighbor, creating a domino effect that continues until the atom giving the electron is stable without it. The extent of damage that this process causes depends on how long this chain of events continues. The immune system is equipped with agents to protect or limit the damage (see the *Immunity* chapter) that might occur because of this process, and certain dietary components can aid in this fight (e.g., vitamins C and E and beta-carotene). Free radicals have been linked to cancer, aging, and a variety of other conditions.

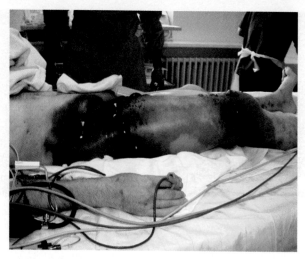

FIGURE 1-18 Gas gangrene.

Reproduced from Schröpfer, E., Rauthe, S., & Meyer, T. (2008). Diagnosis and misdiagnosis of necrotizing soft tissue infections: Three case reports. *Cases Journal*, 1, 252.

Neoplasm

When the process of cellular proliferation or differentiation goes wrong, neoplasms can develop. A **neoplasm**, or **tumor**, is a cellular growth that is no longer responding to normal regulator processes, usually because of a mutation. The disease state associated with this uncontrolled growth is termed **cancer**. Cancer's key features include rapid, uncontrolled proliferation and a loss of differentiation. Thus cancer cells differ from normal cells in size, shape, number, differentiation, purpose, and function.

Carcinogenesis, the process by which cancer develops, occurs in three phases: initiation, promotion, and progression (**FIGURE 1-19**). **Initiation** involves the exposure of the cell to a substance or event (e.g., chemicals, viruses, or

radiation) that causes DNA damage or mutation. Usually the body has enzymes that detect these events and repair the damage. If the event is overlooked, however, the mutation can become permanent and is passed on to future cellular generations. **Promotion** involves the mutated cells' exposure to factors (e.g., hormones, nitrates, or nicotine) that promote growth. This phase may occur just after initiation or years later, and it can be reversible if the promoting factors are removed. In **progression**, the tumor invades, metastasizes (spreads), and becomes drug resistant. This final phase is permanent or irreversible.

A healthy body is equipped with the necessary defenses to shield it against cancer (see the *Immunity* chapter). When those defenses fail, however, cancer prevails. Evidence suggests that these defenses may fail because of a

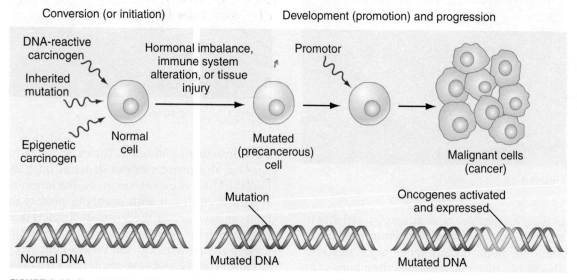

FIGURE 1-19 Carcinogenesis: the stages leading to cancer.

TABLE 1-2	Characteristics of Benign and Malignant Tumors	
	Benign Tumors	**Malignant Tumors**
Cells	Similar to normal cells Differentiated Mitosis fairly normal	Varied in size and shape Many undifferentiated Mitosis increased and atypical
Growth	Relatively slow Expanding mass Frequently encapsulated	Rapid growth Cells not adhesive, infiltrate tissue No capsule
Spread	Remains localized	Invades nearby tissue or metastasizes to distant sites through blood and lymph vessels
Systemic effects	Rare	Common
Life threatening	Only in certain locations (e.g., brain)	Yes, by tissue destruction and spread

combination of complex interactions between carcinogen exposure and genetic mutations. Numerous genes have been identified as causing cancers. **Oncogenes** activate cell division and influence embryonic development. Some of these cancer-producing genes may remain harmless until altered by a genetic or acquired mutation. Common causes of acquired mutations include viruses, radiation, environmental and dietary carcinogens, and hormones. Other factors that can increase a person's likelihood of developing cancer include age, nutritional status, hormonal balance, and stress response. As we age, statistically there is a higher likelihood of a DNA transcription error occurring; we are also more likely to have more carcinogen exposure. Examples of how changes in nutritional status increase the likelihood of cancer can be seen in free radical damage. Some cancers almost feed off of hormones, meaning they grow faster in the presence of particular hormones. Finally, the immune system is impaired during stress states, which can affect its ability to find and respond to carcinogenesis.

The loss of differentiation that occurs with cancer is referred to as **anaplasia**. Anaplasia occurs in varying degrees. The less the cell resembles the original cell, the more anaplastic the cell. Anaplastic cells may begin functioning as completely different cells, often producing hormones or hormone-like substances.

Benign and Malignant Tumors

The two major types of neoplasms are benign and malignant (**TABLE 1-2**; FIGURE 1-20). **Benign** tumors usually consist of differentiated (less anaplastic) cells that are reproducing more rapidly than normal cells. Because of their differentiation, benign tumors are more like normal cells and cause fewer problems. Benign cells

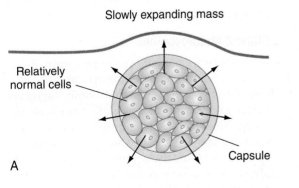
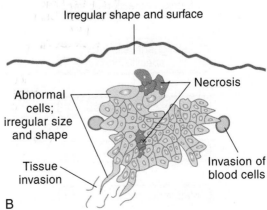

FIGURE 1-20 Characteristics of (a) benign and (b) malignant tumors.

are usually encapsulated and are unable to **metastasize**. The tumor, however, can compress surrounding tissue as it grows. Benign tumors usually cause problems due to that compression. Regardless of its size, if the tumor arises in a sensitive area such as the brain or spinal cord, it can cause devastating problems.

Malignant tumors usually are undifferentiated (more anaplastic), nonfunctioning cells that are reproducing rapidly. Malignant tumors often penetrate surrounding tissue and spread to secondary sites. The tumor's ability to metastasize (**FIGURE 1-21**; **FIGURE 1-22**) depends on its ability to access and survive in the circulatory or the lymphatic system. Most commonly, the

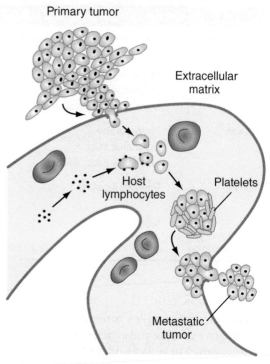

FIGURE 1-22 Pathogenesis of metastasis.

tumor metastasizes to tissue or organs near the primary site, but some tumor cells may travel to distant sites (**TABLE 1-3**).

Regardless of the type of tumor, several factors are essential for the tumor's progression and survival. The tumor must have an adequate blood supply, and sometimes it will divert the blood supply from surrounding tissue to meet those needs. The tumor will grow only as large as what the blood supply will support. Location is critical because it determines the cytology of the tumor as well as the tumor's ability to survive and metastasize. Host factors including age, gender, health status, and immune function will also affect the tumor. Alterations in some of these host factors can create a prime environment for the tumor to grow and prosper.

Clinical Manifestations

In most cases, a patient's prognosis improves the earlier the cancer is detected and treated. Healthcare providers, patients, and family members detect many cases of cancer first through the recognition of manifestations. Heeding these warning signs is vital to initiating treatment early. Unfortunately, people often ignore or do not recognize the warning signs for a variety of reasons (e.g., denial and symptom ambiguity).

As the cancer progresses, the patient may present with manifestations of advancing disease,

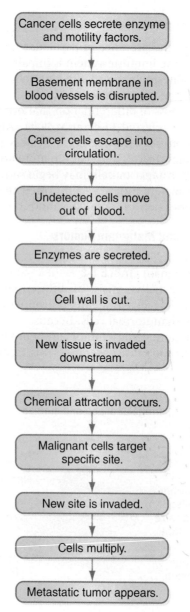

FIGURE 1-21 How cancer metastasizes.

TABLE 1-3   **Common Sites of Metastasis**

Cancer Type	Main Sites of Metastasis*
Bladder	Bone, liver, lung
Breast	Bone, brain, liver, lung
Colorectal	Liver, lung, peritoneum
Kidney	Adrenal gland, bone, brain, liver, lung
Lung	Adrenal gland, bone, brain, liver, other lung
Melanoma	Bone, brain, liver, lung, skin/muscle
Ovary	Liver, lung, peritoneum
Pancreas	Liver, lung, peritoneum
Prostate	Adrenal gland, bone, liver, lung
Stomach	Liver, lung, peritoneum
Thyroid	Bone, liver, lung
Uterus	Bone, liver, lung, peritoneum, vagina

*In alphabetical order.

Reproduced from National Cancer Institute. (2016). Metastatic cancer. Retrieved from http://www.cancer.gov/about-cancer/what-is-cancer/metastatic-fact-sheet

including anemia, cachexia, fatigue, infection, leukopenia, thrombocytopenia, and pain. Anemia—that is, decreased red blood cells—can be a result of the bloodborne cancers (e.g., leukemias), chronic bleeding, malnutrition, chemotherapy, or radiation. Cachexia, a generalized wasting syndrome in which the person appears emaciated, often occurs due to malnutrition. Fatigue, or feeling of weakness, is a result of the parasitic nature of a tumor, anemia, malnutrition, stress, anxiety, and chemotherapy. Factors that can increase the risk for infection include bone marrow depression, chemotherapy, and stress. Leukopenia (low leukocyte levels) and

Myth Busters

Myth 1: Standing in front of a microwave oven while it is cooking food can increase your risk for cancer.

This is a common myth that may hold a grain of truth. An increased cancer risk has been linked to increased levels of ionizing radiation (e.g., X-rays) because such radiation detaches electrons from atoms. Microwaves use non-ionizing microwave radiation to heat food. Early microwave ovens emitted higher levels of this radiation, which may have increased users' cancer risk to a slight extent. Research has never been able to determine whether cancer risk increases with exposure to non-ionizing radiation. Currently, Food and Drug Administration guidelines limit the amount of the non-ionizing radiation microwave ovens can emit, further decreasing the cancer risk associated with these devices.

Myth 2: Using cell phones can increase your risk of cancer.

This is another common myth. Cell phones use the same non-ionizing microwave radiation as microwave ovens to emit a signal. Even though these devices may be in close proximity to your head while in use, evidence does not support that they promote an increased risk of brain cancer. Using a cell phone for an extended period at one time will heat your ear for the same reason that the microwave heats your food, but no clear evidence suggests that this extended use increases cancer risk.

thrombocytopenia (low platelet levels) are common side effects of chemotherapy and radiation due to bone marrow depression. Pain is often associated with cancer due to tissue pressure, obstructions, tissue invasion, visceral stretching, tissue destruction, and inflammation.

Diagnosis

Diagnosis of cancer is complex and is specific to the type of cancer suspected. This chapter provides a basic overview of cancer diagnostic procedures; more specifics are presented in other chapters as specific cancers are discussed. A set of diagnostic procedures usually follows a thorough history and physical examination. These diagnostic procedures may vary depending on the type of cancer suspected. The intention of these diagnostic tests is to identify cancer cells, establish the cytology, and determine the primary site and any secondary sites; however, all these goals are not always accomplished. The healthcare provider will gather as much

information as possible to paint the clearest and most complete picture possible of the patient so as to develop an appropriate treatment plan.

Some screening tests are used for early detection of cancer cells as well as staging the cancer (**TABLE 1-4**). These screening tests include X-rays, radioactive isotope scanning, computed tomography scans, endoscopies, ultrasonography, magnetic resonance imaging, positron emission tomography scanning, biopsies, and blood tests. Some of the blood tests may include tumor markers—substances secreted by the cancer cells—for specific cancers (**TABLE 1-5**). These tumor markers not only aid in cancer detection, but also assist in tracking disease progression and treatment response.

Malignant cancer cells are classified based on the degree of differentiation (grading) and extent of disease (staging). The **grading** system determines the degree of differentiation on a scale of 1 to 4, in order of clinical severity. For instance, grade 1 cancers are well differentiated,

TABLE 1-4	Cancer Screening Guidelines
Screening Area	**Recommendations**
Breast	
Mammogram	Every year age 40 and older
Clinical breast examination	Every year age 40 and older; every 3 years for ages 20 to 39
Breast self-examination	Suggested monthly for age 20 and older
Cervix	
Papanicolaou (Pap) test	Every 3 years between the ages of 21 and 29
	Every 5 years between the ages of 30 and 65
	Not necessary after age 65 unless serious cervical precancer or cancer present in the last 20 years
Human papillomavirus (HPV)	Every 5 years between the ages of 30 and 65
Endometrium	
Endometrial biopsy	Yearly beginning at age 35 for those women at risk for colon cancer
Prostate	
Prostate-specific antigen (PSA)	Frequency depends on risk factors; may begin as early as age 40
Digital rectal examination	Frequency depends on risk factors; may begin as early as age 40
Colon and Rectum	
Fecal occult blood test	Yearly age 50 and older
Fecal immunochemical test	Yearly age 50 and older
Stool DNA test	Every 3 years for age 50 and older
Flexible sigmoidoscopy	Every 5 years age 50 and older
Barium enema	Every 5 years age 50 and older
Colonoscopy	Every 10 years age 50 and older
Virtual colonography	Every 5 years age 50 and older

Data from American Cancer Society. (2016). American Cancer Society guidelines for the early detection of cancer. Retrieved from http://www.cancer.org/; National Cancer Institute. www.cancer.gov.

TABLE 1-5 | **Common Tumor Cell Markers**

Marker	Malignant Condition	Nonmalignant Condition
Alpha-fetoprotein	Liver cancer Ovarian germ cell cancer Testicular germ cell cancer	Ataxia telangiectasia Cirrhosis Hepatitis Pregnancy
Anaplastic lymphoma kinase (ALK)	Lung cancer Large-cell lymphoma	Unknown
BCR-ABL	Chronic myeloid leukemia Acute lymphocytic leukemia	Unknown
Beta$_2$ microglobulin (B2M)	Multiple myeloma Chronic lymphocytic leukemia Some lymphomas	Kidney disease
Carcinoembryonic antigen	Bladder cancer Breast cancer Cervical cancer Colorectal cancer Kidney cancer Liver cancer Lung cancer Lymphoma Melanoma Ovarian cancer Pancreatic cancer Stomach cancer Thyroid cancer	Inflammatory bowel disease Liver disease Pancreatitis Chronic obstructive pulmonary disease Rheumatoid arthritis Tobacco use
CA 15-3	Breast cancer Lung cancer Ovarian cancer Prostate cancer	Benign breast disease Endometriosis Hepatitis Lactation Benign ovarian disease Pelvic inflammatory disease Pregnancy
CA 19-9	Bile duct cancer Colorectal cancer Pancreatic cancer Stomach cancer	Thyroid disease Rheumatoid arthritis Cholecystitis Inflammatory bowel disease Cirrhosis Pancreatitis
CA 27-29	Breast cancer Colon cancer Kidney cancer Liver cancer Lung cancer Ovarian cancer Pancreatic cancer Stomach cancer Uterine cancer	Benign breast disease Endometriosis Kidney disease Liver disease Ovarian cysts Pregnancy (first trimester)

(continues)

TABLE 1-5 Common Tumor Cell Markers (*continued*)

Marker	Malignant Condition	Nonmalignant Condition
CA 125	Colorectal cancer Gastric cancer Ovarian cancer Pancreatic cancer	Endometriosis Liver disease Menstruation Pancreatitis Pelvic inflammatory disease Peritonitis Pregnancy
Human chorionic gonadotropin	Choriocarcinoma Embryonic cell carcinoma Liver cancer Lung cancer Pancreatic cancer Stomach cancer Testicular cancer	Marijuana use Pregnancy
Lactate dehydrogenase	Almost all cancers Ewing's sarcoma Leukemia Non-Hodgkin's lymphoma Testicular cancer	Anemia Heart failure Hypothyroidism Liver disease Lung disease
Neuron-specific enolase	Kidney cancer Melanoma Neuroblastoma Pancreatic cancer Small-cell lung cancer Testicular cancer Thyroid cancer Wilms' tumor	Unknown
Prostatic acid phosphatase	Prostate cancer	Benign prostate conditions
Prostate-specific antigen	Prostate cancer Multiple myeloma Lung cancer	Benign prostatic hyperplasia Prostatitis

meaning they are less likely to cause serious problems because they are more like the original tissue. By comparison, grade 4 cancers are undifferentiated, meaning they are highly likely to cause serious problems because they do not share any characteristics of the original tissue. The **TNM staging** system evaluates the tumor size, nodal involvement, and metastatic progress (FIGURE 1-23).

Cancer treatment usually consists of a combination of chemotherapy, radiation, surgery, targeted therapy, hormone therapy, immunotherapy, hyperthermia, stem cell transplants, photodynamic therapy, and laser treatment. Additionally, other strategies may include watchful waiting and alternative therapies (e.g., herbs,

diet, and acupuncture). The goal of treatment may be either **curative** (eradicate the disease), **palliative** (treat symptoms to increase comfort), or **prophylactic** (prevent the disease).

When surgery is undertaken, attempts are made to remove the tumor and surrounding tissue. Chemotherapy involves the administration of a wide range of medications that destroy replicating tumor cells. Radiation includes the use of ionizing radiation to cause cancer cellular mutation and interrupt the tumor's blood supply. Radiation may be administered by external sources or via internally implanted sources. Targeted therapy is a newer treatment that uses drugs to identify and attack cancer cells; this drug therapy differs from the traditional

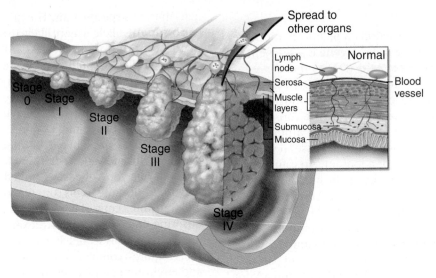

FIGURE 1-23 TNM staging system. The example shown is staging of colorectal cancer.

chemotherapy. Hormone therapy involves administering specific hormones that inhibit the growth of certain cancers. Immunotherapy involves administering specific immune agents (e.g., interferons and interleukins) to alter the host's biological response to the cancer. Hyperthermia precisely delivers heat to a small area of cells or part of the body to destroy tumor cells. This technique can also increase the effectiveness of radiation, immunotherapy, and chemotherapy. Stem cell transplants may include peripheral blood, bone marrow, or umbilical cord blood. These transplants are used to restore stem cells in bone marrow destroyed by disease or treatment. In photodynamic therapy, specific drugs are combined with light to kill cancer cells; these drugs work only when they are activated by certain types of light. Lasers may be used to shrink or destroy a tumor through application of heat, perform precise cuts in surgery, or activate a chemical.

Prognosis

A cure for cancer is usually defined as a 5-year survival without recurrence after diagnosis and treatment. **Prognosis** refers to the patient's likelihood for surviving the cancer. Prognosis is heavily dependent on the cancer's ability to metastasize. The more the cancer spreads to other sites by way of the circulation or lymph system, the worse the patient's prognosis. Early diagnosis and treatment usually improve the prognosis by treating the cancer before metastasis has occurred.

Remission refers to a period when the cancer has responded to treatment and is under control. Remission may occur with some cancers, and generally the patient does not exhibit any manifestations of cancer during that time.

Many cancers are preventable, so health-promoting education (e.g., smoking cessation, proper nutrition, and weight management) is vital to decrease the incidence and prevalence of all cancers. Although the likelihood of these cancers can be diminished with these strategies, it is noteworthy that cancer can develop in people with no risk factors. This unpredictable development contributes to the mystery and challenges surrounding cancer.

Genetic and Congenital Alterations

Genetic and congenital defects are important to understand because of the encompassing nature of these disorders. These diseases affect all levels of health care and people in all age groups, by involving almost any tissue type and organs. **Genetics** is the study of heredity—the passing of physical, biochemical, and physiologic traits from biological parents to their children. Disorders and mutations can result in serious disability or death and can be transmitted through genetic material. Genetic disorders may or may not be present at birth. **Congenital** defects, often referred to as birth defects, usually develop during the prenatal phase of life and are apparent at birth or shortly thereafter.

Genetics

The cellular instructions and information are carried with our **genes**. A gene is a segment of **deoxyribonucleic acid (DNA)** that serves as a template of protein synthesis. DNA is a long double-stranded chain of nucleotides called **chromosomes**. Each **nucleotide** consists of a five-carbon sugar (deoxyribose), a phosphate group, and one of four nitrogen bases (cytosine, thymine, guanine, or adenine). An estimated 3 billion nucleotides make up the human genome, and each gene can contain hundreds to thousands of these nucleotides. Of the 46 chromosomes, the 22 sets of paired chromosomes are called **autosomes**, and the remaining 2 chromosomes are the sex chromosomes (a pair of X chromosomes for females and an X and a Y for males). The representation of a person's unique set of chromosomes is referred to as the **karyotype**, and the physical expression of those genes is referred to as the **phenotype** (e.g., blue eyes). Not all genes in the code are expressed.

Patterns of Inheritance

During reproduction, each parent contributes one set of chromosomes to the fertilized egg. Some characteristics, or traits, are determined by one gene that may have many variants (**alleles**) (**TABLE 1-6**). A person who has identical alleles of each chromosome is **homozygous** for that gene; if the alleles are different, then the person is said to be **heterozygous** for that gene. For unknown reasons, one allele on a chromosome may be more influential than the other in determining a specific trait. The more powerful, or **dominant**, allele is more likely to be expressed in the offspring than the less influential, or **recessive**, allele. Offspring will express the dominant allele in both homozygous and heterozygous allele pairs. In contrast, offspring will express the recessive allele only in homozygous pairs.

The sex chromosomes (X and Y) can pass on genes when they are linked, or attached, to one of the sex chromosomes. For example, a male will transmit one copy of each X-linked gene to his daughter but none to his son, whereas a female will transmit a copy of her X-linked gene to each offspring, male or female. An example of an X-linked disorder is Klinefelter's syndrome. Some traits require a combination of two or more genes and environmental factors, or multifactorial inheritance. Examples of this type of inheritance include height, diabetes mellitus, and obesity.

Autosomal Dominant Disorders

Autosomal dominant disorders are single-gene mutations that are passed from an affected parent to an offspring regardless of sex. These disorders occur with both homozygous and heterozygous allele pairs. In most cases, offspring with the homozygous pair will have a more severe expression of the disorder, as compared to offspring with the heterozygous pair, because the homozygous pair provides a "double dose" of the gene. Autosomal dominant disorders typically involve abnormalities with structural proteins. Examples of autosomal dominant disorders include Marfan syndrome and neurofibromatosis.

TABLE 1-6	Genetic Disorders and Inheritance	
Single-Gene Disorders	**Multifactorial Disorders**	**Chromosomal Disorders**
Autosomal Dominant	Anencephaly	Cri du chat syndrome
Adult polycystic kidney disease	Cleft lip and palate	Down syndrome
Familial hypercholesterolemia	Clubfoot	Monosomy X (Turner's syndrome)
Huntington's disease	Congenital heart disease	Polysomy X (Klinefelter's syndrome)
Marfan's syndrome	Myelomeningocele	Trisomy 18 (Edwards' syndrome)
	Schizophrenia	
Autosomal Recessive		
Albinism		
Color blindness		
Cystic fibrosis		
Phenylketonuria		
Sickle cell anemia		
Tay-Sachs disease		
X-Linked Recessive		
Duchenne muscular dystrophy		
Hemophilia A		

History

Mrs. Turner is a 47-year-old Caucasian female who has been admitted to the general surgical floor with a lump in her right breast. She generally has enjoyed good health up to this admission. Mrs. Turner neither smokes nor drinks, and she follows a daily exercise regimen. Approximately 2 months ago, Mrs. Turner's husband noticed a small lump in her right breast. She gave this finding little attention, assuming that the lump was like the many others she tended to experience around her menses. The lump failed to resolve after her menses, and Mrs. Turner became concerned when it seemed to grow bigger.

Mrs. Turner is the mother of two children, 8 and 6 years old. Mrs. Turner took birth control pills for 5 years after the birth of her second child. Last year she chose to discontinue birth control pill use and turned to an alternative method of birth control.

Mrs. Turner is an only child, born to her parents late in their life. Her father is alive and well, but her mother died of breast cancer 5 years ago. A family history revealed a strong history of both heart disease and cancer on both sides of Mrs. Turner's family.

Current Status

On exam, a 2- to 3-cm mass was palpated in the upper quadrant of Mrs. Turner's right breast. This mass felt firm, was fixed to the chest wall, and was tender to the touch. The remaining breast skin was normal in appearance with no discoloration or retraction of the skin. One node, approximately the size of a pea, was palpated under the right axilla. Palpation of the left breast revealed two 1- to 2-cm soft, movable masses. Mrs. Turner said that she noticed these lumps in her left breast 2 weeks ago but stated the lumps in her left

breast became palpable and bothersome about 12 days from the start of menses. A reproductive history disclosed the onset of menses occurred at the age of 10. There is no history of dysmenorrhea associated with her periods, although Mrs. Turner states her breasts become tender and lumpy 1 to 2 weeks before her menses. She has had no pregnancies that were delivered by cesarean section. Her one and only Papanicolaou (Pap) smear was done 2 years ago and produced a normal result. The remaining exam findings were unremarkable. Mammography confirmed the presence of a 3-cm mass in the upper quadrant of the right breast and three 1.5-cm masses in the left breast. The result of a bone scan and other diagnostic procedures were negative.

1. Mrs. Turner is considered to be at increased risk for developing breast cancer. Which of the following factors is most positively related to this high-risk profile?

   A. History of breast cancer in family members
   B. History of cystic breast disease
   C. Early onset of menarche
   D. Trauma related to birth of her children

2. Which of the following best explains the existence of an enlarged right axillary lymph node in Mrs. Turner?

   A. The lymph node is the result of an inflammatory reaction that normally occurs with the onset of her current menses.
   B. The existence of the node is the result of an increased strain on the lymphatic system as a result of cellular degeneration.
   C. The lymph node exists to provide nutrients to the rapidly growing cancer cells.

   D. The lymph node is the result of cancer cells spreading to different tissues within the body.

Mrs. Turner was taken to surgery 3 days later, and a modified radical mastectomy was performed. A histological exam was used to classify the tumor using the TNM staging system. An estrogen receptor assay performed on the removed tissue confirmed Mrs. Turner's tumor was estrogen dependent. She returned to her room with a drain in place. Her dressing was dry and intact. She was able to turn, cough, and breathe deeply on her own. Her temperature remained within normal limits after surgery. Progesterone therapy was initiated daily. Ambulation was started on the second postoperative day.

3. Mrs. Turner's tumor was staged at stage III using the TNM staging system. Pathological exam of the surgically removed tissue sample placed Mrs. Turner's tumor in category type II. Characterizing and classifying tumors is important for which of the following reasons?

   A. Treatment is based on the knowledge of tumor size, extent, and tissue type.
   B. Tumor staging is useful for studying a number of researchable factors, from survival to treatment response.
   C. A consistent classification system provides a way to catalogue individuals with breast tumors for statistical analysis.
   D. All of the above.

4. Which activities by Mrs. Turner increase her likelihood for a good prognosis?

5. What was the rationale for hormone therapy with Mrs. Turner?

Marfan Syndrome

Marfan syndrome is a degenerative generalized disorder of the connective tissue with an incidence of 1 in 5,000 persons (FIGURE 1-24). The condition results from a single-gene mutation (*FBN1*) on chromosome 15. This gene provides instructions for making a protein called fibrillin-1. Fibrillin-1 binds to other fibrillin-1 proteins and other molecules to form threadlike filaments called microfibrils. Microfibrils provide strength and flexibility to connective tissue as well as store and release growth factors to control growth and tissue repair. The mutation causes excess growth factors to be released, and elasticity in many tissues is decreased; together, these two processes lead to overgrowth and instability of tissues. These defects produce a variety of ocular, skeletal, and cardiovascular disorders. Clinical manifestations of Marfan syndrome vary widely in their severity, timing of onset, and rate of progression. These manifestations include the following:

- Aortic defects (e.g., coarctation, aneurysm, dissection) (most life threatening)
- Myopia (nearsightedness) and lens displacement (ocular hallmark)
- Increased height
- Long extremities
- Arachnodactyly (long, spiderlike fingers)
- Sternum defects (e.g., funnel chest or pigeon breast)
- Chest asymmetry
- Spine deformities (e.g., scoliosis or kyphosis)
- Flat feet
- Hypotonia and increased joint flexibility
- Highly arched palate, crowded teeth, small lower jaw
- Thin, narrow face
- Valvular defects (e.g., redundancy of leaflets, stretching of the chordae tendineae, mitral valve regurgitation, and aortic regurgitation)

Multiple complications can occur with Marfan syndrome, including the following:

- Aortic rupture and internal bleeding
- Weak joints and ligaments that are prone to injury
- Cataracts
- Glaucoma
- Retinal detachment
- Severe mitral regurgitation
- Spontaneous pneumothorax
- Inguinal hernia

A thorough history and physical examination are vital in diagnosing Marfan syndrome. In most cases, the family history is positive for the disease or the symptoms, but as many as 25% of patients have no family history of this condition. A physical examination would reveal the presence of the hallmark lens displacement and other symptoms of the disease. Diagnostic procedures include a skin biopsy that would be positive for fibrillin, X-rays that would confirm the skeletal abnormalities, an echocardiogram that would reveal the cardiac abnormalities, and a DNA analysis for the gene. Typical treatment focuses on relieving symptoms and may include the following measures:

- Surgical repair of aneurysms and valvular defects
- Surgical correction of ocular deformities
- Steroid and sex hormone therapy to aid in closure of long bones, thereby limiting height
- Beta-adrenergic blockers (which decrease blood pressure and heart rate) to limit complications from cardiac deformities
- Bracing and physical therapy for mild scoliosis, and surgical correction for severe cases

Other strategies include avoiding contact sports, supportive care for the patient and family, and frequent checkups.

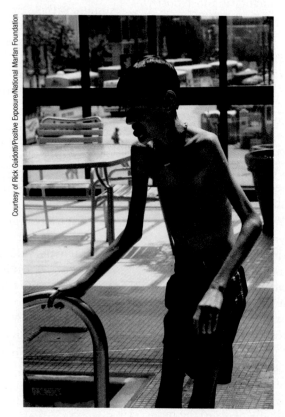

Courtesy of Rick Guidotti/Positive Exposure/National Marfan Foundation

FIGURE 1-24 Marfan syndrome.

Neurofibromatosis

Neurofibromatosis is a condition involving neurogenic (nervous system) tumors that arise from Schwann cells and other similar cells. Schwann cells keep peripheral nerve fibers alive. Although most cases of neurofibromatosis are inherited, 30% to 50% occur spontaneously. There are two main types.

Type 1 neurofibromatosis (FIGURE 1-25) results from mutations in the *NF1* gene on chromosome 17. This gene provides instructions for making a protein called neurofibromin that acts to suppress tumor development. The defect caused by the mutations results in cutaneous lesions that may include raised lumps, café au lait spots (brown pigmented birthmarks), and freckling. Type 1 neurofibromatosis occurs in 1 in 3,000 to 4,000 people.

Type 2 neurofibromatosis results from mutations in the *NF2* gene on chromosome 22. This gene provides the instructions for making a protein called merlin that acts to suppress tumor development. The defect caused by the mutations results in bilateral acoustic (eighth cranial nerve) tumors that cause hearing loss. Type 2 neurofibromatosis occurs in 1 in 33,000 people.

People with neurofibromatosis can be affected in many ways. For example, this genetic disorder is associated with an increased incidence of learning disabilities and seizure disorders. Vision (e.g., optic gliomas and cataracts), skeletal (e.g., scoliosis), and cardiac (e.g., hypertension) issues may also be present, particularly with type 1. Some individuals with type 1 neurofibromatosis may develop cancerous tumors, and neurofibromatosis increases risk of developing other cancers (e.g., brain and leukemia). The appearance of the lesions may vary between individuals, but the lesions can be disfiguring in some cases. There is no cure for neurofibromatosis, but surgeries may be necessary to remove the lesions for palliative or safety reasons.

Autosomal Recessive Disorders

Autosomal recessive disorders are single-gene mutations passed from an affected parent to an offspring regardless of sex, but they occur only in homozygous allele pairs. Those persons with heterozygous pairs are carriers only and exhibit no symptoms. The age of onset for these disorders is usually early in life, and they occur most commonly as deficiencies in enzymes and inborn errors in metabolism. Examples of autosomal recessive disorders include phenylketonuria (PKU) and Tay-Sachs disease.

Phenylketonuria

PKU is a deficiency of phenylalanine hydroxylase, the enzyme necessary for the conversion of phenylalanine to tyrosine, due to a mutation in the *PAH* gene on chromosome 12. Phenylalanine is a building block of proteins that is obtained in the diet (all proteins and aspartame), and it plays a role in melanin production. A deficiency of phenylalanine hydroxylase leads to toxic levels of phenylalanine in the blood, causing central nervous system damage. The occurrence of PKU varies worldwide, but it is found in 1 in 10,000 to 15,000 newborns.

If untreated, PKU leads to severe intellectual disability. Symptoms develop slowly and can go undetected. Because untreated cases almost always lead to intellectual disability, all newborns in the United States are screened for PKU shortly after birth by testing for high serum phenylalanine levels. If untreated, children can develop the following clinical manifestations:

- Failure to meet milestones
- Microcephaly
- Progressive neurologic decline
- Seizures

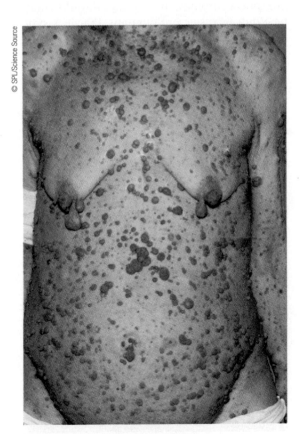

© SPL/Science Source

FIGURE 1-25 Neurofibromatosis type 1.

- Hyperactivity
- Electrocardiograph (EKG) abnormalities
- Learning disability
- Mousy-smelling urine, skin, hair, and sweat
- Lighter skin and hair than unaffected family members
- Eczema
- Behavioral problems (e.g., hyperactivity disorders)
- Psychiatric disorders

In addition to diagnosis after birth, prenatal screening through chorionic villus sampling and amniocentesis can be done for at-risk women. Treatment for PKU involves consumption of a diet low in phenylalanine. Newborns may be breastfed, but the quantity of breastmilk taken in has to be monitored. Special infant formulas are available for supplementation. Dietary restrictions include avoiding proteins and aspartame as well as minimizing starches. Oral medications are available to lower phenylalanine (e.g., sapropterin [Kuvan]). Additionally, gene and enzyme therapy have demonstrated promise in treating PKU.

Tay-Sachs Disease

Tay-Sachs disease is a progressive disorder that results from a mutation in the *HEXA* gene on chromosome 15. This gene provides the instructions for making part of a lysosomal enzyme called hexosaminidase A. Hexosaminidase A is necessary to metabolize certain lipids called gangliosides. These lipids accumulate in the lysosomes of nerve cells and gradually destroy and demyelinate nerve cells. This destruction of nerve cells leads to a progressive mental and motor deterioration, often causing death by 5 years of age.

Tay-Sachs disease is very rare in the general population and almost exclusively affects individuals of Jewish descent, of whom about 1 in every 27 is a carrier. The mutation is also more common in certain French Canadian communities in Quebec, the Old Older Amish community in Pennsylvania, and the Cajun population in Louisiana.

Tay-Sachs disease is divided into three forms based on symptom onset—infantile (most common), juvenile, and adult (extremely rare). Clinical manifestations of Tay-Sachs usually appear between 3 to 10 months and include the following:

- Exaggerated Moro reflex (startle reflex) at birth
- Apathy to loud sounds by age 3–6 months
- Inability to sit up, lift head, or grasp objects

- Difficulty turning over
- Progressive vision loss
- Deafness and blindness
- Seizure activity
- Paralysis
- Spasticity
- Pneumonia

This genetic disorder is diagnosed by a thorough history and physical examination as well as deficient serum and amniotic hexosaminidase A levels. Because of the devastating nature of Tay-Sachs disease, genetic counseling is important for persons of Jewish ancestry and individuals with a positive family history. No cure for the disease exists; most treatments are supportive. Those supportive approaches include parenteral nutrition (tube feedings), pulmonary hygiene (e.g., suctioning and postural drainage), skin care, laxatives, and psychological counseling.

Sex-Linked Disorders

Genes located on the sex chromosomes cause a variety of genetic disorders. Most **sex-linked** disorders are X-linked. Females are frequently carriers of the trait because they have two X chromosomes, whereas men with the defective X gene will be affected because they have only one X chromosome. X-linked disorders may be either recessive or dominant. Fragile X syndrome is an example of an X-linked disorder.

Fragile X Syndrome

Fragile X syndrome (**FIGURE 1-26**) is an X-linked dominant disorder associated with a single trinucleotide gene sequence (*FMR1*) on the X chromosome. Normally, this sequence is repeated about 5 to 40 times, but in people with fragile X syndrome, it is repeated more than 200 times,

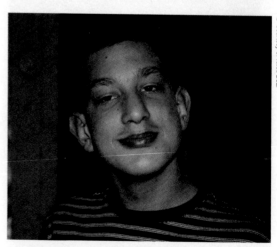

© Courtesy of Nikki Deal

FIGURE 1-26 Fragile X syndrome.

turning off the *FMR1* gene. The *FMR1* gene provides the instructions for making a protein called FMRP that regulates production of other proteins and plays a role in synapses development. Synapses are critical in relaying nerve impulses. The more repeats of this gene sequence, the more severe the condition.

Fragile X syndrome is more common and usually more severe in males (it occurs in 1 in 4,000 males and 1 in 8,000 females). Clinical manifestations of fragile X syndrome include the following:

- Intellectual, behavioral, and learning disabilities
- Prominent jaw and forehead
- Long, narrow face with long or large ears
- Connective tissue abnormalities
- Large testes
- Hyperactivity and inattentiveness
- Seizures
- Speech and language delays
- Tendency to avoid eye contact
- Autism spectrum disorders

Diagnosis of fragile X syndrome involves the identification of clinical manifestations and a positive genetic test. No cure for this condition exists, so treatment focuses on controlling individual symptoms. Genetic counseling is appropriate for persons with a positive family history. Behavioral and psychological support may be indicated for both parents and the affected child. Other supportive interventions include physical, speech, and occupational therapy.

Multifactorial Disorders

Most **multifactorial disorders** are the result of an interaction between genes and environmental factors. These disorders do not follow a clear-cut pattern of inheritance. Multifactorial disorders may be present at birth, as with cleft lip or palate, or they may be expressed later in life, as with hypertension. Environmental factors that play roles in these disorders may include any of a number of **teratogens** (birth defect–causing agents) such as infections, chemicals, or radiation.

Cleft Lip and Cleft Palate

Cleft lip and palate are birth defects that occur when soft tissue of the lip or mouth do not form properly. Cleft lip and palate may occur either together or separately. These conditions usually develop in the second month of pregnancy, when the facial structures are forming. Every year in the United States, approximately 2,650 babies are born with cleft palate and approximately 4,440 babies are born with a cleft lip with or without a cleft palate. Maternal smoking, preexisting diabetes, and seizure medication use (especially the first trimester) are significant risk factors. Additionally, these defects are more prevalent in Native Americans and Asian Americans, with African Americans having the lowest prevalence.

The deformities with cleft lip and palate may be unilateral or bilateral. The severity of the deformity ranges from a mild notch to involvement of the lip, palate, and tongue (**FIGURE 1-27**). Feeding and nutritional issues may occur because of these structural problems, which affect the ability to nurse/eat.

Clinical manifestations are obvious at birth and can be detected with a prenatal ultrasound. A series of surgeries are performed to close the gap in the lip and palate. Speech therapy and feeding devices can minimize speech delays and nutritional deficits. Parental support is important to ensure the child's proper care and minimize caregiver stress.

Chromosomal Disorders

Chromosomal disorders are a major category of genetic disorders that result most often from alteration in chromosomal duplication or number. Oftentimes these disorders occur in utero because of some environmental influences (e.g., maternal age, drugs, and infections). The most vulnerable time for the fetus is at 15–60 days' gestation. This period immediately follows fertilization and implantation, when much of the cellular differentiation is occurring. More than

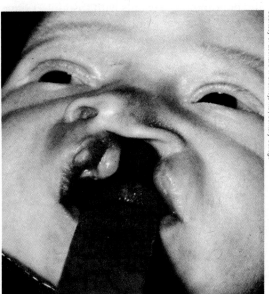

Courtesy of Leonard V. Crowley, MD, Century College

FIGURE 1-27 Cleft lip and palate.

60 disorders fall in this category, many of which result in first-trimester abortions. The more common examples of these disorders include trisomy 21, monosomy X, and polysomy X.

Trisomy 21

Trisomy 21, or Down syndrome, is a spontaneous chromosomal mutation that results in three copies of chromosome 21 (**FIGURE 1-28**). These extra copies are thought to disrupt the course of normal development. The risk of this mutation increases with greater parental age and environmental teratogen exposure. Trisomy 21 occurs in about 1 in 800 births. Clinical manifestations can vary widely and are apparent at birth and often in utero. These manifestations typically include the following characteristics:

- Hypotonia
- Distinctive facial features (e.g., low nasal bridge, epicanthic folds, protruding tongue, low-set ears, and small, open mouth)
- Congenital heart defects
- Single crease on the palm (simian crease)
- White spots on the iris
- Varying intellectual disability that typically worsens with age
- Developmental delay
- Behavioral issues (e.g., inattention, obsessive/compulsive behavior, stubbornness, and tantrums)
- Strabismus and cataracts
- Poorly developed genitalia and delayed puberty

Early death can occur due to cardiac and pulmonary complications (e.g., hypertension and pneumonia). Persons with trisomy 21 have increased susceptibility to leukemia and infections. These individuals are also at increased risk for developing gastrointestinal (e.g., intestinal obstruction, gastroesophageal reflux disease, and celiac disease) and thyroid (e.g., hypothyroidism) issues. Approximately half of all persons with trisomy 21 will develop Alzheimer's disease, usually starting around age 50. Clinical manifestations can be detected using four-dimensional ultrasounds. Other prenatal testing includes amniocentesis and serum hormone levels. No cure for trisomy 21 exists. Treatment strategies focus on symptom and complication management.

Monosomy X

Monosomy X, or Turner's syndrome, is the result of a deletion of part or all of an X chromosome (**FIGURE 1-29**). This abnormality usually occurs spontaneously during the formation of reproductive cells (eggs and sperm) in the parents. It is not completely understood which genes on the X chromosome are associated with the features of Turner's syndrome. This condition occurs in about 1 of every 2,500 live births, but

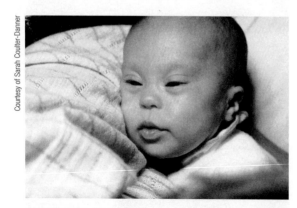

Courtesy of Sarah Coulter-Danner

FIGURE 1-28 Down syndrome.

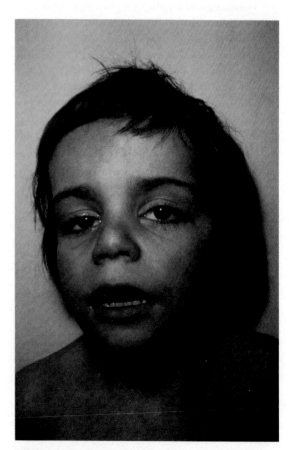

FIGURE 1-29 Turner's syndrome.
© Medical Images RM/Giancarlo Zuccotto

is much more common among pregnancies that do not survive to term.

Turner's syndrome affects only females. Affected females develop gonadal streaks instead of ovaries; therefore, they will not menstruate. Other clinical manifestations may vary but often include the following:

- Short stature
- Lymphedema (swelling) of the hands and feet
- Broad chest with widely spaced nipples
- Low-set ears
- Small lower jaw
- Drooping eyelids
- Increased weight
- Small fingernails
- Webbing of the neck
- Coarctation of the aorta
- Horseshoe kidney
- Ear infections
- Reduced bone mass

Complications of monosomy X include vision (e.g., cataracts), skeletal (e.g., osteoporosis, pathological fractures, and scoliosis), hearing, metabolic (e.g., diabetes and thyroid), cardiac (e.g., hypertension and valvular defects), and renal (e.g., kidney failure) issues. Diagnosis is usually accomplished through a history, physical examination, serum hormone levels, and genetic testing (either before or after birth).

Turner's syndrome is treated by administering female sex hormones to promote development of secondary sex characteristics and skeletal growth. Growth hormones may also be administered to improve skeletal growth. Identification of this condition is often delayed until late childhood or early adolescence if the clinical presentation is more subtle, but chromosomal analysis can confirm the diagnosis. Early treatment allows for early hormone replacement to minimize problems and detect complications.

Polysomy X

Polysomy X, or Klinefelter's syndrome, is a relatively common abnormality that results from an extra X chromosome, which creates an XXY sex chromosome. Because of the presence of a Y chromosome, persons with this syndrome are male (FIGURE 1-30). Klinefelter's syndrome affects 1 in 500 to 1,000 newborn males. The syndrome usually becomes apparent at puberty when testicles fail to mature, rendering affected boys infertile. The extra copies of the X chromosome interfere with male sexual

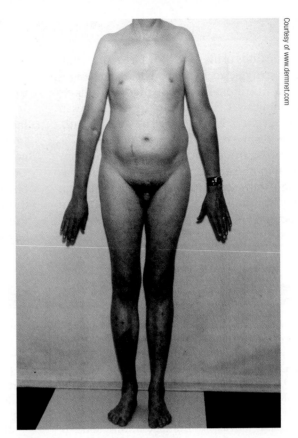

Courtesy of www.dermnet.com

FIGURE 1-30 Klinefelter's syndrome.

development. Clinical manifestations of Klinefelter's syndrome include the following:

- Small penis, prostate gland, and testicles
- Sparse facial and body hair
- Sexual dysfunction (e.g., impotence, decreased libido)
- Gynecomastia (female-like breasts)
- Long legs with a short, obese trunk
- Tall stature
- Behavioral problems
- Learning disabilities
- Delayed speech and language development
- Increased incidence of pulmonary disease and varicose veins

Other problems that can develop include osteoporosis and breast cancer.

Diagnostic procedures consist of a history, physical examination, hormone levels, and chromosomal testing. Treatment includes male hormone replacement to promote secondary sex characteristics. A mastectomy may be performed in cases of gynecomastia and breast cancer. Psychological counseling and support may be beneficial to the patient and the parents.

CHAPTER SUMMARY

Cells are the basic units of life, and they face many challenges in their struggle to survive. These challenges include hypoxia, nutritional changes, infection, inflammation, and chemicals. Cells adapt to the challenges in an attempt to prevent or limit damage as well as death. This adaptation may be reversible or permanent.

Neoplasms arise from abnormal cellular proliferation or differentiation. They can be either benign or malignant. Benign neoplasms are more differentiated; therefore, they are more like the parent cells. Benign tumors are less likely to cause problems in the host or metastasize except in terms of location. Malignant tumors are less differentiated; therefore, they are more like the parent cells. Malignant tumors are more likely to cause problems in the host and metastasize.

Genetic and congenital disorders can develop from factors that disrupt normal fetal development or interact with defective genes. These factors, or teratogens, can include radiation, infections, or chemicals. Genetic and congenital disorders may be present at birth or may not appear until later in life. Exploring these basic cellular and genetic concepts and issues lays the foundation for understanding where disease begins.

REFERENCES

AAOS. (2004). *Paramedic: Anatomy and physiology.* Sudbury, MA: Jones and Bartlett.

Berry, T., & Workman, L. (2011). *Genetics and genomics in nursing and health care.* Philadelphia, PA: F. A. Davis.

Chiras, D. (2011). *Human biology* (7th ed.). Burlington, MA: Jones & Bartlett Learning.

Crowley, L. (2013). *An introduction to human disease: Pathology and pathophysiology correlations.* Burlington, MA: Jones & Bartlett Learning.

Elling, B., Elling, K., & Rothenberg, M. (2004). *Anatomy and physiology.* Sudbury, MA: Jones and Bartlett.

Lewin, B., Cassimeris, L., Lingappa, V., & Plopper, G. (Eds.). (2007). *Cells.* Sudbury, MA: Jones and Bartlett.

Mosby's dictionary of medicine, nursing, and health professionals (9th ed.). (2012). St. Louis, MO: Mosby.

Porth, C. (2010). *Essentials of pathophysiology* (3rd ed.). Philadelphia, PA: Lippincott Williams & Wilkins.

Professional guide to pathophysiology (3rd ed.). (2010). Philadelphia, PA: Lippincott Williams & Wilkins.

Schropfer, E., Rauthe, S., & Meyer, T. (2008). Diagnosis and misdiagnosis of necrotizing soft tissue infections: Three case reports. *Cases Journal, 1,* 252.

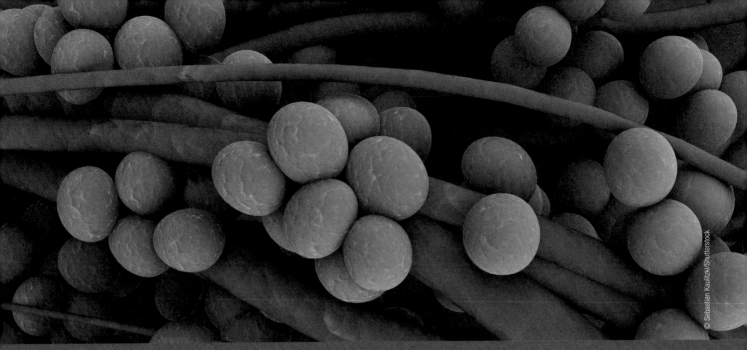

CHAPTER 2
Immunity

LEARNING OBJECTIVES

- Describe the effect of stress on the body.
- Explain the role of the body's normal defenses in preventing disease.
- Differentiate between innate and adaptive immunity.
- Discuss some examples of altered immune responses.
- Identify factors that enhance and impair the body's defenses.

KEY TERMS

acquired immunity
active acquired immunity
acute tissue rejection
adaptive or acquired defenses
alarm
allogeneic
antibody-producing cell
antigen
autoimmune
autologous
B cell

chronic tissue rejection
cytotoxic cell
effector cell
exhaustion
general adaptation syndrome
graft-versus-host rejection
helper cell
host-versus-graft rejection
hyperacute tissue rejection
hypersensitivity
immunodeficiency

inflammatory response
innate immunity
interferon
killer cell
local adaptation syndrome
memory cell
opportunistic infections
passive acquired immunity
primary deficit
pyrogen
regulator cell
resistance

secondary or acquired immunodeficiency
suppressor cell
syngenic
systemic lupus erythematosus (SLE)
T cell
type I hypersensitivity
type II hypersensitivity
type III hypersensitivity
type IV hypersensitivity
xenogenic

variety of entities that have the potential to cause harm constantly bombard the human body. These entities include things such as stressors and organisms. The body's ability to resist damage and deal with these events will determine the effects of such events. Humans can arm themselves with an arsenal of health behaviors that can help defend against these adversaries, yet humans often increase their vulnerability to harm through other behaviors. All patients we encounter as healthcare providers are affected by this constant state of warfare. These patients have either fallen victim to such an attack or they are attempting to defend against it. Healthcare providers can identify those persons at risk or under attack and help them take up arms to defeat these persistent adversaries.

Stress

Stress is a universal experience of human existence that can negatively affect the body's fragile homeostasis state (see the *Introduction to Pathophysiology* section at the beginning of the text). Stress can contribute directly to the development or exacerbation of disease, as well as contribute to negative behaviors such as smoking and drug abuse as individuals attempt to cope with this state. Stress can arise from many events, even those that may be perceived as positive (e.g., weddings and vacations). Understanding the nature of stress and the effects that it can have on the body is vital for healthcare providers in their interactions with patients.

The Stress Response

Hans Selye first described the bodily changes associated with stress in the 1930s. He noted that the body responds to any stimuli, or stressor, with a series of nonspecific events (**FIGURE 2-1**). Selye described this protective stress response as the **general adaptation syndrome**, which is a cluster of systemic manifestations that represent an attempt to cope with a stressor. Several factors can affect adaptation, including natural reserves, time, genetics, age, gender, health status, nutrition, sleep–wake cycles, hardiness, and psychosocial factors.

The general adaptation syndrome includes three stages: alarm, resistance, and exhaustion (**FIGURE 2-2**). The **alarm** stage includes the generalized stimulation of the sympathetic nervous system resulting in the release of catecholamines and cortisol, also known as the fight-or-flight response. In the **resistance** stage, the body

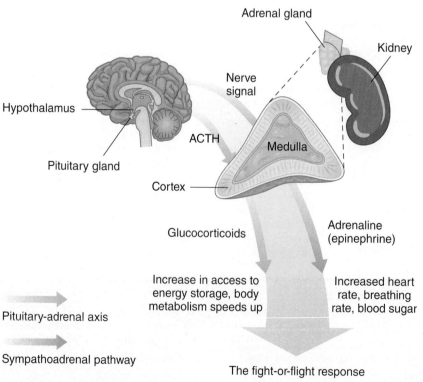

FIGURE 2-1 Physiological response to stress.

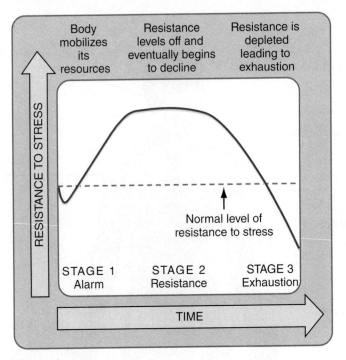

FIGURE 2-2 General adaptation syndrome.

chooses the most effective and advantageous defense. Cortisol levels and the sympathetic nervous system return to normal, causing the fight-or-flight symptoms to disappear. The body either adapts or alters its workings in an attempt to limit problems or become desensitized to the stressor. Stress management techniques (e.g., meditation and relaxation) can assist in the desensitization process. If the stressor is prolonged or overwhelms the body, the **exhaustion** phase is initiated. During this phase, the body becomes depleted and damage may appear, as homeostasis can no longer be maintained through compensatory mechanisms. As the body's defenses are utilized, disease or death results. Diseases and ailments that have been attributed to stress include anxiety, depression, headaches, insomnia, infections, and cardiovascular disease (**FIGURE 2-3**).

The **local adaptation syndrome** is the localized version of the general adaptation syndrome. In this syndrome, the body attempts to limit the damage associated with the stressor by confining the stressor to one location. An example of this response can be seen in the local inflammatory reaction that results from tissue trauma. The inflammatory response is discussed in an upcoming section.

Although the stress response is predictable to some extent, individual variability exists due to conditioning factors. These conditioning factors may include genetics, age, gender, life experiences, dietary status, and social support. The positive presence of these factors can limit or eliminate the likelihood of damage, disease, or death. The implementation of one or more coping strategies can also minimize and eliminate negative stress effects. These strategies include lifestyle modifications such as physical activity, adequate sleep, and optimal dietary status. Other strategies include relaxation, distraction, and biofeedback.

Unfortunately, maladaptive coping strategies may sometimes be used instead of such positive strategies. These maladaptive strategies cause more problems than benefits and include activities such as smoking, substance abuse, and overeating. Healthcare professionals can assist patients to replace those negative strategies with more positive ones.

Immunity

The body is under constant assault by life-threatening microbes. Although the vast majority of microbes are harmless, occasionally they are not. The immune system is responsible for protecting the body against an array of microorganisms (e.g., bacteria, viruses, fungi, protozoans, and prions) as well as removing damaged cells and destroying cancer cells. The immune system provides this protection

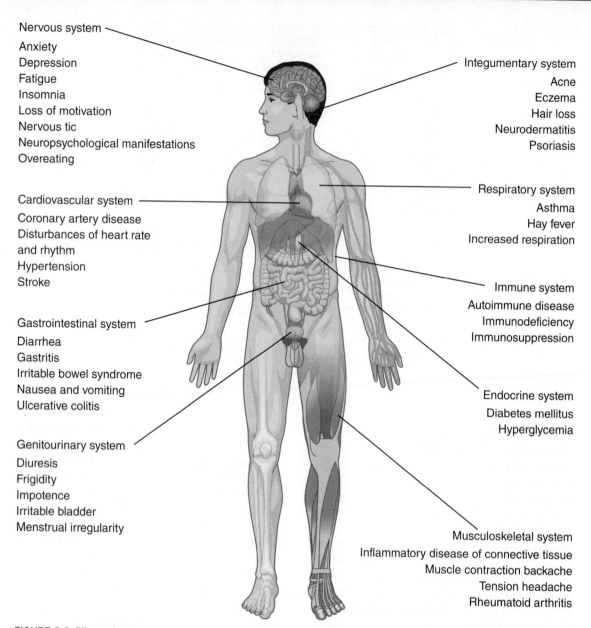

Nervous system
Anxiety
Depression
Fatigue
Insomnia
Loss of motivation
Nervous tic
Neuropsychological manifestations
Overeating

Cardiovascular system
Coronary artery disease
Disturbances of heart rate
and rhythm
Hypertension
Stroke

Gastrointestinal system
Diarrhea
Gastritis
Irritable bowel syndrome
Nausea and vomiting
Ulcerative colitis

Genitourinary system
Diuresis
Frigidity
Impotence
Irritable bladder
Menstrual irregularity

Integumentary system
Acne
Eczema
Hair loss
Neurodermatitis
Psoriasis

Respiratory system
Asthma
Hay fever
Increased respiration

Immune system
Autoimmune disease
Immunodeficiency
Immunosuppression

Endocrine system
Diabetes mellitus
Hyperglycemia

Musculoskeletal system
Inflammatory disease of connective tissue
Muscle contraction backache
Tension headache
Rheumatoid arthritis

FIGURE 2-3 Effects of stress.

through two major actions—defending and attacking. A functioning immune system is essential for survival. Optimal immunity requires intact nonspecific defenses (e.g., skin, mucous membranes, phagocytes, complement systems), a functional lymphatic system, an efficient innate immune response, an operational inflammatory response, and an appropriate and adaptive acquired immunity. Fundamental to a properly functioning immune system is the ability to recognize and respond to a foreign agent, or **antigen**. Some immune cells circulate constantly, always on alert for an invasion, whereas others remain passively in tissue and organs, waiting to be

activated (**TABLE 2-1**). Additionally, some of the body's structures serve as barriers to antigens, preventing invasion.

Innate and Adaptive Defenses

The immune system takes multiple approaches to protect the body from antigens, including the use of innate and adaptive defenses. **Innate immunity** provides immediate protection and is nonspecific, meaning it provides protection against all invaders. Adaptive or acquired immunity can take 7 to 10 days to provide protection, but it is specific to the antigen.

TABLE 2-1	Major Components of the Immune System
Antigen	A foreign agent that triggers the production of antibodies by the immune system.
Antibody	A protein used by the immune system to identify and neutralize foreign agents, such as viruses and bacteria.
Autoantibody	An antibody made by the immune system that attacks an individual's own proteins.
Thymus	A gland located in the anterior superior mediastinum; develops T lymphocytes and thymosins.
Lymphatic tissue	Connective tissue containing many lymphocytes; transports immune cells, antigen-presenting cells, fatty acids, and fats; filters body fluids.
Bone marrow	Soft, fatty tissue found inside of bones; contains stem cells and leukocytes.
Cells	
Neutrophils	Infection-fighting agents; usually the first to arrive on the scene of an infection; attracted by various chemicals released by infected tissue; escape from the capillary wall, migrate to the site of infection, and phagocytize microorganisms.
Basophils	White blood cells that bind immunoglobulin E (IgE) and release histamine in anaphylaxis.
Eosinophils	White blood cells involved in allergic reactions.
Monocytes	White blood cells that replenish macrophages and dendritic cells in normal states and respond to inflammation by migrating to infected tissue to become macrophages and dendritic cells; their conversion elicits an immune response.
Macrophages	White blood cells within tissues, produced by differentiation of monocytes; phagocytize and stimulate lymphocytes and other immune cells to respond to pathogens.
Mast cells	Connective tissue cells that contain histamine, heparin, hyaluronic acid, slow-reacting substance of anaphylaxis (SRS-A), and serotonin.
B cells (B lymphocytes)	Cells that mature in the bone marrow, where they differentiate into memory cells or immunoglobulin-secreting (antibody) cells; eliminate bacteria, neutralize bacterial toxins, prevent viral reinfection, and produce immediate inflammatory response.
Plasma cells	White blood cells that develop from B cells and produce large volumes of specific antibodies.
T cells (T lymphocytes)	Produced in the bone marrow and mature in the thymus—hence "T" cell; include two major types that work to destroy antigens—regulator cells and effector cells.
Killer T cells	T cells that destroy cells infected with viruses by releasing lymphokines that degrade cell walls; also called cytotoxic cells and effector cells.
Memory B cells	B cells that stimulate a quick response with subsequent exposures to an antigen; recall the antigen as foreign, leading to rapid antibody production.
Helper B cells	Regulator cells that activate, or call up, B cells to produce antibodies.
NK lymphocytes	Natural killer cells that destroy cancer cells, foreign cells, and virus-infected cells.
Chemical Mediators	
Complement	A group of inactive proteins in the circulation that, when activated, stimulate the release of other chemical mediators, promoting inflammation, chemotaxis, and phagocytosis.
Histamine	Released by mast cells and basophils, especially during allergic reactions, triggering the inflammatory response; increases the permeability of the capillaries to white blood cells and other proteins, thereby allowing them to engage foreign invaders in the infected tissues.
Kinins (e.g., bradykinin)	Induce vasodilation and contraction of smooth muscle.
Prostaglandins	A group of lipid compounds that have a variety of effects, including constriction or dilation of vascular smooth muscle cells, control of cell growth, and sensitization of spinal neurons to pain.
Leukotrienes	Fatty molecules of the immune system that contribute to contraction of bronchiolar smooth muscle.
Cytokines (messengers)	Small cell-signaling protein molecules that are extensively involved in intracellular communication; include interleukins, interferons, and lymphokines.
Tumor necrosis factor (TNF)	A group of cytokines that can cause cell death (apoptosis).
Chemotactic factors	Attract phagocytes to the area of inflammation.

Innate Defenses

Barriers

The first innate or nonspecific approach relies on physical and chemical barriers that indiscriminately protect against all invaders. The most prominent barriers used in this approach are the skin and mucous membranes. The skin is a thick, impermeable layer of epidermal cells overlying a rich vascular layer known as the dermis. As newly produced skin cells push the dead ones outward, the dead cells produce a waterproof layer because of the keratin contained in those dead cells. Although the skin does protect the human body from microbe invasions, some passageways allow direct access to the body's interior (respiratory, digestive, and genitourinary tracts). These passageways are lined with a protective mucous membrane that is not as thick as skin but does provide a moderate layer of protection.

The physical barriers also include chemical barriers to prevent invasion. The skin, for example, produces a slightly acidic substance that inhibits bacterial growth. Hydrochloric acid in the stomach destroys many ingested bacteria. Tears and saliva contain lysozyme, an enzyme that dissolves bacterial cell walls.

The physical and chemical barriers are not completely impenetrable. Tiny breaks in the skin or in the lining of the respiratory, digestive, or genitourinary tracts may permit an antigen invasion. Additional bloodborne innate defenses are in place to respond to those antigens, including the inflammatory response, pyrogens, interferons, and complement proteins.

Inflammatory Response

Damage or trauma to body tissue triggers a series of reactions referred to as the **inflammatory response**. The inflammatory reaction is characterized by erythema (redness), edema (swelling), heat, and pain at the site of injury (**FIGURE 2-4**). This response is triggered by a set of mediators, or mast cells, including histamine

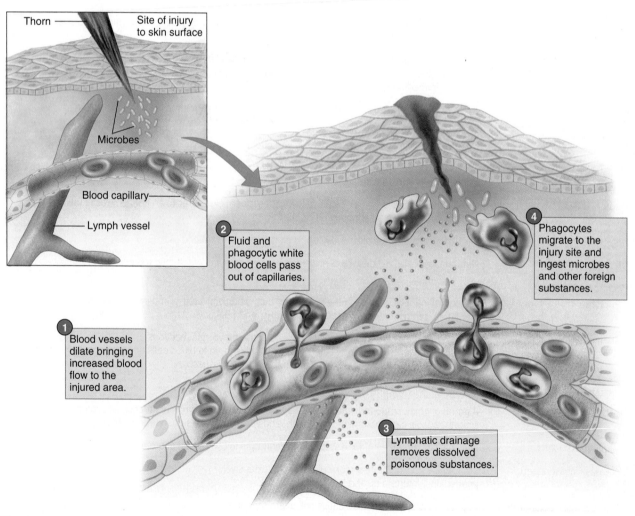

FIGURE 2-4 Inflammatory response.

(stimulates vasodilation) and prostaglandins (stimulates pain receptors in the area). Immediately after the injury, arterioles in the area briefly go into spasm and constrict to limit bleeding and the extent of injury. This vasoconstriction is immediately followed by vasodilation, which increases blood flow to the injured area in an attempt to dilute toxins and provide the area with essential immune cells (e.g., neutrophils and monocytes), nutrients, and oxygen. The vasodilation increases capillary permeability; as permeability increases, leukocytes line the vessel wall in preparation for migration into the surrounding tissue. While the leukocytes are lining the vessel walls, endothelial cells in the vessel walls react to biochemical mediators that cause these vessels to retract. This retraction gives the leukocytes enough room to migrate into the interstitial space and begin the cleanup process of phagocytosis, or the engulfing and digestion of foreign substances and cellular debris. In conjunction with phagocytosis, fibrinogen is transformed into fibrin. This fibrin is used to wall off the injured area so that foreign substances are contained. A meshwork of new cells forms to provide support for the healing process. Blood clotting begins if blood vessels have been damaged.

Pyrogens

Pyrogens are molecules released by macrophages that have been exposed by bacteria. Pyrogens travel to the hypothalamus, the portion of the brain primarily responsible for controlling body temperature. There, they turn the heat up on the bacteria, producing fever and creating an unpleasant environment for bacterial growth. Mild fevers cause the spleen and liver to remove iron from the blood, which is required by many bacteria to reproduce. Fever also increases metabolism, which facilitates healing and accelerates phagocytosis. However, severe fever (more than 105°F) can be life threatening because it begins to denature vital proteins, especially enzymes needed for biochemical reactions.

Interferons

Interferons are small proteins released from cells infected by viruses (**FIGURE 2-5**). These molecules diffuse away from the site of invasion through the interstitial tissue and bind to receptors on the plasma membranes of uninfected cells. The binding of interferons to uninfected cells triggers the synthesis of enzymes that inhibit viral replication. Consequently, when viruses enter the previously uninfected cells,

they cannot replicate and spread. Interferons do not protect cells already infected by a virus but rather stop the spread of the virus to new cells. In essence, interferon production is the dying cells' attempt to protect other cells.

Complement Proteins

The complement system is a process that involves blood plasma proteins (approximately 20) and enhances the action of antibodies. Complement proteins circulate in the blood in an inactive state. When foreign substances invade the body, these proteins become activated. Only a few activities in this complex process are described here.

Five complement system proteins join together to form a large molecule, or membrane-attack complex. The membrane-attack complex becomes embedded in the plasma membrane of bacteria, creating an opening into which water flows. The influx of water causes the bacterial cells to swell, burst, and die. Other complement proteins stimulate vasodilation in an infected area as a part of the inflammatory response. Some complement proteins increase the permeability of vessels, allowing white blood cells and plasma to pass quickly through them to the infected area. Other complement proteins serve as chemical attractants, drawing macrophages, monocytes, and neutrophils to the infected area, where they phagocytize foreign cells. Still other complement proteins bind to microbes, forming a rough coat on the invader that promotes phagocytosis.

Adaptive Defenses

Adaptive or acquired defenses are the body's own individual immune system. These defenses recognize and attack antigens that make it through the innate defenses. These approaches include two major approaches—cellular and humoral immunity. Key players in these approaches are T cells and B cells (**FIGURE 2-6**). **T cells** and **B cells** mingle with antigens as they circulate throughout the body's fluids and peripheral lymphoid tissue (e.g., tonsils, lymph nodes, spleen, and intestinal lymphoid tissue). This interaction serves either to destroy the antigen (T-cell function or cellular immunity) or to produce antibodies against the antigen (B-cell function or humoral immunity).

Cellular Immunity

Cellular immunity is a defense approach that is mediated by T cells, which recognize the presence of the antigen, bind to the antigen, and trigger a response by other immune cells.

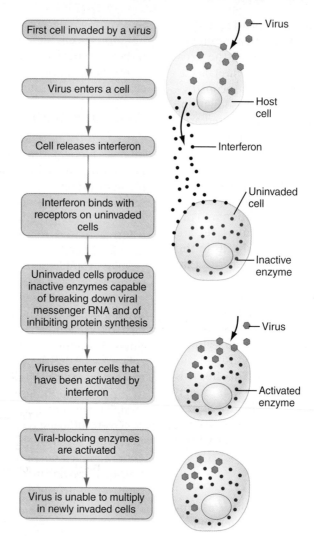

First cell invaded by a virus

↓

Virus enters a cell

↓

Cell releases interferon

↓

Interferon binds with receptors on uninvaded cells

↓

Uninvaded cells produce inactive enzymes capable of breaking down viral messenger RNA and of inhibiting protein synthesis

↓

Viruses enter cells that have been activated by interferon

↓

Viral-blocking enzymes are activated

↓

Virus is unable to multiply in newly invaded cells

FIGURE 2-5 How interferon works.

T cells get their name from the place where they mature, the thymus. T cells are produced in the bone marrow, but then enter the bloodstream and travel to the thymus for maturation.

Two major types of T cells work to destroy antigens: (1) **regulator cells**, including helper T cells and suppressor T cells, and (2) **effector cells**, or killer cells. **Helper cells** activate, or call up, B cells to produce antibodies. **Suppressor cells** turn that antibody production off. **Killer cells**, or **cytotoxic cells**, destroy cells infected with viruses by releasing lymphokines that degrade cell walls. T cells work to protect the body against viruses and cancer cells, and they are responsible for hypersensitivity and transplant rejection.

Humoral Immunity

B cells mature in the bone marrow, where they differentiate into either memory cells or immunoglobulin (Ig)-secreting (antibody) cells (**TABLE 2-2**). These cells eliminate bacteria, neutralize bacterial toxins, prevent viral reinfection, and produce immediate inflammatory response. Each B cell has receptor sites for a specific antigen; when it encounters this antigen, the B cell becomes activated and multiplies into either **antibody-producing cells** or **memory cells**. The antibody-producing cells produce millions of antibody molecules during their 24-hour life span. B cells can begin this antigen production within 72 hours after initial antigen exposure. Subsequent exposures to the antigen then trigger a quick response because memory cells recall the antigen as foreign, and antibody production occurs rapidly. This reaction is referred to as **acquired immunity** (**TABLE 2-3**).

Active acquired immunity refers to immunity gained by actively engaging with the antigen—that is, through invasion or

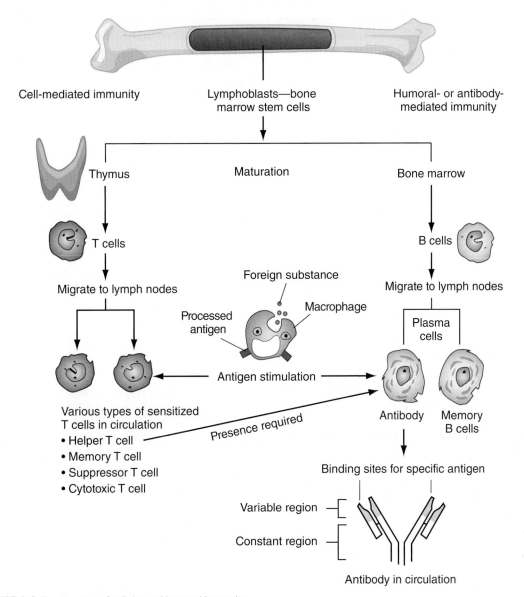

FIGURE 2-6 Development of cellular and humoral immunity.

Modified from Gould, B. (2014). *Pathophysiology for the health professions* (5th ed.). Philadelphia, PA: Elsevier. Copyright Elsevier 2015.

TABLE 2-2	Immunoglobulins and Their Functions
IgG	Main defense against bacteria; can cross the placenta to protect the fetus against infections (passive immunity).
IgM	Fights blood infections and triggers additional production of IgG; present in lymphocyte cells; first antibody made by a developing fetus.
IgA	Found in membranes of respiratory and gastrointestinal tract, tears, saliva, mucus, and colostrum; important in local immunity.
IgE	Protects the body through its presence in mucous membranes and skin; triggers allergic reactions.
IgD	Present in blood serum (in small amounts) and B-cell surfaces; receptor for antigens; helps anchor cell membranes.

Modified from Gould, B. (2014). *Pathophysiology for the health professions* (5th ed.). Philadelphia, PA: Elsevier. Copyright Elsevier 2015.

TABLE 2-3	Types of Acquired Immunity		
Type	**Mechanism**	**Memory**	**Example**
Natural active	Pathogens enter the body and cause illness; antibodies form.	Yes	Person has rubella once
Artificial active	Vaccine (live or attenuated organisms) is injected into the body. No illness results, but antibodies form.	Yes	Person receives measles vaccine
Natural passive	Antibodies are passed directly from mother to child to provide temporary protection.	No	Passage through placenta during pregnancy; consumption of breastmilk
Artificial passive	Antibodies are injected into the body (antiserum) to provide temporary protection or to minimize the severity of an infection.	No	Gamma globulin injection to treat immunological disease, such as idiopathic thrombocytopenia purpura (ITP)

Modified from Gould, B. (2014). *Pathophysiology for the health professions* (5th ed.). Philadelphia, PA: Elsevier. Copyright Elsevier 2015.

vaccination. In active immunity, the person makes his or her own antibodies, and protection is usually long term. Examples of active immunity include both the case in which a person has a condition such as varicella infection (chickenpox) and does not have it again and the case in which a person receives the varicella vaccine and never has the condition.

Passive acquired immunity refers to immunity gained by receiving antibodies made outside the body by another person, animal, or recombinant DNA. In passive immunity, the person is not actively producing antibodies, and protection is short lived. Examples of passive immunity include mother-to-fetus transfer through placenta and breastfeeding transference of antibodies.

Altered Immune Response

Malfunction at any point in any of the numerous and highly complex immune responses can create a pathologic state. Malfunctions may include exaggeration (hypersensitivity), misdirection (autoimmune), or diminution (immunodeficiency).

Hypersensitivity

Hypersensitivity is an inflated or inappropriate response to an antigen. The result is inflammation and destruction of healthy tissue. Hypersensitivity reactions may be immediate, occurring within minutes to hours of reexposure to the antigen, or delayed, occurring several hours after reexposure. There are four types of hypersensitivity reactions: type I (IgE mediated), type II (tissue specific), type III (immune complex mediated), and type IV (cell mediated) (**TABLE 2-4**).

With **type I hypersensitivity**, allergens activate T cells (usually helper cells), which bind to mast cells. These T cells stimulate B cells to produce IgE antibodies specific to the antigen. The difference between a normal immune response and a type I hypersensitivity response is that the antibody produced is IgE instead of IgA, IgG, or IgM. The IgE coats the mast cell and basophils, making them sensitive to the allergen. At the next exposure to the same antigen, the antigen binds with the surface IgE, releasing mediators (e.g., histamines, cytokines, and prostaglandins) and triggering the complement system. The effects of type I reactions include immediate inflammation and pruritus. Repeated exposure to relatively large doses of the allergens is usually necessary to cause this response. Examples of type I reactions include hay fever, food allergies, and anaphylaxis. Treatment of type I reactions may include epinephrine, antihistamines, corticosteroids, and desensitizing injections, all of which will suppress the inflammatory activity.

Type II hypersensitivity generally involves the destruction of a target cell by an antibody-directed, cell-surface antigen. IgG or IgM binds with an antigen on the individual's own cell, activating the complement system. The antigens may be intrinsic (self) or extrinsic (absorbed through exposure). Recognition of these cells by macrophages triggers antibody production. The effects of type II

TABLE 2-4 **Overview of the Hypersensitivity Reactions**

Hypersensitivity Type	Origin of Hypersensitivity	Antibody Involved	Cells Involved	Mediators Involved	Evidence of Hypersensitivity	Examples
Type I IgE-mediated	B lymphocytes	IgE	Mast cells Basophils	Histamine Serotonin Leukotrienes Prostaglandins	30 minutes or less	Hay fever Systemic anaphylaxis Asthma
Type II Cytotoxic	B lymphocytes	IgG, IgM	RBC, WBC	Complement	5–8 hours	Transfusion reactions Hemolytic disease of newborns
Type III Immune complex	B lymphocytes	IgG	Host tissue cells	Complement	2–8 hours	Serum sickness Arthus phenomenon SLE Rheumatic fever Rheumatoid arthritis
Type IV Cellular	T lymphocytes	None	Host tissue cells	Cytokines	1–3 days	Contact dermatitis Infection allergy

reactions include cell lysis and phagocytosis. Examples of type II reactions include blood transfusion reactions and erythroblastosis fetalis. Treatment focuses on prevention and includes ensuring blood compatibility prior to transfusions and administering medication to suppress immune activity (e.g., corticosteroids and cyclosporine) and prevent maternal antibody development (e.g., Rho[D] immune globulin [RhoGAM]).

In **type III hypersensitivity**, circulating antigen–antibody complexes that have not been adequately cleared by the innate bloodborne immune cells accumulate and become deposited in tissues. Tissues often affected in this way include the kidneys, joints, skin, and blood vessels. The accumulation of the complexes triggers the complement system, causing local inflammation and increased vascular permeability; in turn, more complexes accumulate. Examples of type III reactions include autoimmune disorders (e.g., systemic lupus erythematosus and glomerulonephritis). Treatment for type III reactions is disease specific.

Type IV hypersensitivity involves a delayed processing of the antigen by macrophages. Once processed, the antigen is presented to the T cells (usually helper or cytotoxic cells), resulting in the release of cytokines that cause inflammation and antigen destruction. These reactions can cause severe tissue injury and fibrosis. Examples of type IV reactions include tuberculin skin testing, transplant reactions, and contact dermatitis. Treatment for type IV reactions is disease specific.

Transplant Reactions

The immune system's protective nature presents challenges for patients who require tissue and organ transplants and blood transfusions. Transplant success is closely tied to ensuring the best possible tissue match. Four types of tissue transplants are possible: allogeneic, syngenic, autologous, and xenogenic. **Allogeneic** transplants are those in which the tissue used is from the same species and is of similar tissue type, but is not identical. Most transplants use allogeneic tissue. **Syngenic** transplants use tissue from the identical twin of the host. With **autologous** transplants, the host and the donor are the same person. An example of this type of transplant is someone storing up his or her own blood prior to a scheduled surgery. **Xenogenic** transplants use tissue from another species. An example of this type of transplant is the use of pig heart valves to replace diseased valves in a human. Donors may be live or a cadaver, but no matter which source is used, making a close tissue match is fundamental to preventing rejection.

Rejection reactions are classified based on their timing. **Hyperacute tissue rejections** occur immediately to 3 days after the transplant. Such reactions occur due to a complement response in which the recipient has antibodies against the donor tissue. This complement response triggers a systemic inflammatory reaction. The response is so quick that often the tissue has not had a chance to establish vascularization; as a result, the tissue becomes permanently necrotic.

Acute tissue rejections are the most common and treatable type of rejection. These reactions usually occur between 4 days and 3 months following the transplant. Acute reactions are cell mediated and result in transplant cell destruction (lyses) or necrosis. The patient exhibits manifestations of the inflammatory process including fever, redness, swelling, and tenderness at the graft site. Additionally, the patient may experience impaired functioning of the transplanted organ.

Chronic tissue rejection occurs from about 4 months to years after the transplant. This reaction is most likely due to an antibody-mediated immune response. Antibodies and complement molecules become deposited in the transplanted tissue vessel walls, resulting in decreased blood flow and ischemia.

Most rejection reactions are classified as **host-versus-graft rejection**; in other words, the host is fighting the graft. The graft fights the host in another type of reaction, known as **graft-versus-host rejection**. This potentially life-threatening type of reaction occurs *only* with bone marrow transplants. The immunocompetent graft cells recognize the host cells as foreign and organize a cell-mediated attack. The host is usually immunocompromised and unable to fight the graft cells' actions.

Identifying the rejection reaction quickly is crucial to reversing it. Assessment including manifestations of a healthy and unhealthy transplant organ is paramount. For example, when the transplanted organ is a kidney, decreased urine output may indicate a failing transplant. Diagnostic procedures include laboratory tests to identify immune and inflammatory activity (e.g., white blood count and erythrocyte sedimentary rate) and specific tests to determine functioning of the transplanted organ (e.g., renal panel and urinalysis).

Treatment for transplant rejection usually begins with prevention. Prevention starts with ensuring a tissue match and initiating immunosuppressive therapy (e.g., corticosteroids and cyclosporine). The transplant patient will likely require immunosuppressive therapy for life. Once a rejection is suspected, immunosuppression therapy is intensified to reverse it.

Autoimmune Disorders

In **autoimmune** reactions, the body's normal defenses become self-destructive—that is, they perceive the self as foreign. What causes this misdirected response is unclear. Some theories include etiologies that are viral, genetic, medicinal, hormonal, and environmental in nature. Autoimmune disorders affect women more often than men. They can affect any tissue or organ in the body, and some are systemic. These disorders are characterized by frequent, progressive periods of exacerbations (worsening of symptoms) and remissions (easing of symptoms). Physical and emotional stressors frequently trigger exacerbations. Examples of autoimmune disorders include systemic lupus erythematosus, rheumatoid arthritis, and Guillain-Barré syndrome.

Because of the somewhat mysterious nature of autoimmune disorders, diagnostic procedures often begin by eliminating all other causes. Sometimes laboratory tests are used that are specific to the suspected autoimmune disorder (e.g., rheumatoid factor for rheumatoid arthritis). Treatment for autoimmune disorders is disease specific but often includes coping and stress management strategies to prevent exacerbations.

Systemic Lupus Erythematosus

Systemic lupus erythematosus (SLE) is a chronic, inflammatory, autoimmune disorder that can affect any connective tissue. B cells are thought to be activated for unknown reasons to produce autoantibodies and autoantigens,

Now that we have explored the different types of hypersensitivity, let's put that knowledge into practice. During the shift change, you receive reports on the following patients. Which patient would you see first following report?

- An 11-year-old male with a history of a peanut allergy having an anaphylactic reaction
- A 28-year-old male diagnosed with contact dermatitis secondary to poison ivy exposure
- A 67-year-old female diagnosed with severe hay fever
- A 30-year-old female with a positive tuberculin skin test

When considering these types of situations, start by considering who is at risk of dying or losing a vital function (e.g., limb or organ failure) first. If none of the conditions is life threatening, then consider which ones are acute. Acute issues always take priority over chronic conditions. Maslow's hierarchy of needs and patient safety are other important considerations.

Now let's get back to our group of patients. The anaphylactic reaction could be life threatening. It triggers a massive system inflammatory reaction, which causes fluid to leave the vascular system and move into the tissues. This systemic inflammatory reaction can cause tissue swelling that blocks the airway and significantly impairs respiratory efforts. The contact dermatitis, while quite uncomfortable, is not life threatening. The hay fever may be severe, but sneezing and watery eyes are not life threatening. The positive skin test may indicate an active tuberculosis infection, which may eventually be life threatening, but it is a chronic condition that does not require immediate life-saving measures. In this group of patients, the nurse should see the 11-year-old first because he requires immediate assessment and measures to prevent death.

which then combine to form immune complexes. These immune complexes fight against the body's own tissues (e.g., nucleic acids, red blood cells, platelets, and lymphocytes). Hyperactive helper T cells and subdued suppressor T cells are thought to create a prime environment for B cells to overproduce.

This unpredictable disorder most often harms the heart, joints, skin, lungs, blood vessels, liver, kidneys, and nervous system (TABLE 2-5). SLE occurs 9 times more often in women than in men, especially between the ages of 15 and 50, and is more common in Asians and African Americans.

Because patients with SLE can have a wide variety of symptoms and different combinations of organ involvement, no single test can definitively establish the diagnosis of this disorder. To improve the accuracy of the diagnosis of SLE, 11 criteria were established. Some patients suspected of having SLE may never develop enough of these criteria to qualify for a definite diagnosis; other patients accumulate enough criteria to merit SLE diagnosis only after months or years. When a person has four or more of these criteria, the diagnosis of SLE is strongly suggested. Nevertheless, diagnosis may be made in some settings in patients with only a few of these

TABLE 2-5	Common Manifestations of Systemic Lupus Erythematosus
Joints	Polyarthritis, with swollen, painful joints, without damage; arthralgia
Skin	Butterfly rash with erythema on cheeks and over nose, or rash on body; photosensitivity—exacerbation with sun exposure; ulcerations in oral mucosa; hair loss
Kidneys	Glomerulonephritis with antigen–antibody deposits in glomerulus, causing inflammation with marked proteinuria and progressive renal damage
Lungs	Pleurisy—inflammation of the pleural membranes, causing chest pain
Heart	Carditis—inflammation of any layer of the heart, commonly pericarditis
Blood vessels	Raynaud's phenomenon—periodic vasospasms in fingers and toes, accompanied by pain
Central nervous system	Psychoses, depression, mood changes, seizures
Bone marrow	Anemia, leukopenia, thrombocytopenia

classical criteria, and treatment may be instituted at this stage. The 11 criteria used for diagnosing systemic lupus erythematosus are organized into the SOAP BRIAN MD mnemonic:

- **S**erositis (inflammation of the serous membranes that line the lungs [pleura], heart [pericardium], and inner abdomen [peritoneum])
- **O**ral ulcers
- **A**rthritis
- **P**hotosensitivity
- **B**lood disorders (low counts of white or red blood cells, or platelets)
- **R**enal involvement (abnormal amounts of urine protein or clumps of cellular elements, called casts, which are detectable with a urinalysis)
- **I**mmunologic phenomena
- **A**ntinuclear antibodies
- **N**eurologic disorder (e.g., brain irritation manifested as seizures or psychosis)
- **M**alar rash ("butterfly" rash over the cheeks of the face)
- **D**iscoid rash (patchy redness that can cause scarring)

In addition to these 11 criteria, other tests can be helpful in evaluating patients with SLE to determine the severity of organ involvement. These tests include routine testing of the blood to detect inflammation (e.g., erythrocyte sedimentation rate and C-reactive protein), blood-chemistry testing, direct analysis of internal body fluids, and tissue biopsies. Abnormalities in body fluids and tissue samples (kidney, skin, and nerve biopsies) can further support the diagnosis of SLE (e.g., urinalysis, serum creatinine, liver function tests, echocardiography). The appropriate testing procedures are selected for the patient on an individual basis.

Treatment of SLE is directed at symptom management. General strategies include stress reduction, exercise, and sleep. Medical treatment includes nonsteroidal anti-inflammatory drugs (NSAIDs) to reduce pain and inflammation in joints, muscles, and other tissues. Corticosteroids may also be used to treat SLE. Corticosteroids are more potent than NSAIDs in reducing inflammation and restoring function when the disease is active, particularly when internal organs are affected, but they have multiple side effects (e.g., weight gain, risk for infection, hyperglycemia, and high blood pressure) that must be considered. Biologic disease-modifying antirheumatic drugs

(DMARDs) reduce pain and tissue damage as a result of inflammation. DMARDS are more potent than NSAIDs and corticosteroids, but they carry significantly more risks (e.g., risk for infection, organ damage). As the disease progresses, use of these agents may be necessary to prevent severe complications of SLE. Antimalarial drugs can treat fatigue, joint pain, rashes, and pleural inflammation by suppressing the immune system. Immunosuppressants may be used for patients with kidney and nervous system involvement. Additionally, plasmapheresis can remove antibodies and other immune substances from the blood to suppress immunity.

Immunodeficiency

A diminished or absent immune response increases susceptibility to infections. **Immunodeficiencies** may be primary (reflecting a defect with the immune system) or secondary (reflecting an underlying disease or factor that is suppressing the immune system). The most common forms of immunodeficiency are caused by viral infections or are iatrogenic reactions to therapeutic drugs (e.g., corticosteroids and chemotherapy). The problem may be either acute or chronic. **Primary deficits** involve basic developmental failures, many of which result from genetic or congenital abnormalities (e.g., hypogammaglobulinemia). **Secondary or acquired immunodeficiency** refers to a loss of immune function because of a specific cause; such causes may include infection, splenectomy, malnutrition, hepatic disease, drug therapy, or stress.

Immunodeficiency states predispose patients to opportunistic infections. **Opportunistic infections** are infections caused by pathogens that do not usually cause disease in healthy individuals (e.g., toxoplasmosis, Kaposi sarcoma, candidiasis infections). These infections often arise from a disruption of normal flora. Opportunistic infections can be difficult to treat successfully and can become life threatening. These infections need to be identified and treated early to improve the patient's prognosis.

Diagnosis of the immunodeficiency state includes the identification of recurrent or persistent infections. Diagnostic procedures involve measurements of immunoglobulin levels, white blood cells, and T-cell counts. Treatment for immunodeficiency states is individualized for the specific deficiency and may include gamma globulin, bone marrow transplants, or thymus transplants. Reverse isolation precautions (e.g.,

Twenty-eight-year-old Steve Crosby is admitted to the hospital from his healthcare provider's clinic office. This patient was diagnosed as HIV positive 4 years ago. He presented to the clinic with fatigue, a productive cough, and a 10-pound weight loss over the last month. A tuberculosis (TB) skin test was administered in the clinic. Admission orders include "Isolation precautions for possible TB."

1. Which of the following statements by this patient indicates that he understands why he is at risk for TB?

    A. "I realize my helper T cells are diminished from HIV. Those are the cells needed to fight TB."

    B. "I may get TB because my viral load count is diminished."

    C. "I am at risk for developing TB because I was born with a low number of helper T cells."

    D. "I realize I am at risk for acquiring TB because I used intravenous drugs in the past."

One of the unlicensed assistive personnel (UAP) caring for Mr. Crosby says, "Now that Mr. Crosby's condition has worsened and he is symptomatic, shouldn't added precautions be posted on his door to protect staff members?"

2. Which information should the nurse give the UAP?

    A. Reverse isolation precautions should be implemented to protect the staff.

    B. Respiratory precautions are all that are needed, and those are already posted on the door.

    C. Following standard precautions will minimize the exposure to blood and body fluids.

    D. Staff members caring for Mr. Crosby should begin prophylactic medications.

The UAP has been assigned to help Mr. Crosby with hygiene. As the UAP prepares to enter his room, the nurse observes her putting on a gown, gloves, mask, and goggles.

3. What should the nurse say to the UAP?

    A. "Wearing all that equipment is a waste of supplies, and we have already had budget cuts."

    B. "Can you tell me what you are getting ready to do?"

    C. "Don't you know all that equipment is not necessary?"

    D. "Wearing all that equipment may frighten Mr. Crosby."

It is important that Mr. Crosby understands how to prevent spreading HIV before he is discharged home. When discussing infection control practices with the nurse, Mr. Crosby says, "I have heard that condoms don't always prevent HIV."

4. How should the nurse respond?

    A. "Where do you usually get your health information?"

    B. "I will have an AIDS educator come discuss condom use with you."

    C. "I know you would feel terrible if you gave someone HIV because you didn't use a condom."

    D. "If used properly and regularly, latex condoms are highly effective in preventing HIV transmission."

hand washing, limiting visitors, and avoiding fresh flowers) can limit the person's exposure to pathogens, thereby decreasing his or her risk for infection.

AIDS

Acquired immunodeficiency syndrome (AIDS) is a deadly, sexually transmitted disease caused by the human immunodeficiency virus (HIV), a retrovirus. HIV attacks and weakens the immune system. There are two primary strains of the virus: HIV-1 is the most prevalent strain in the United States, and HIV-2 is the most prevalent strain in Africa.

According to the Centers for Disease and Control and Prevention (CDC), approximately 35 million people worldwide and 1.2 million people in the United States are living with HIV. HIV is the seventh leading cause of death in individuals 25 to 44 years of age in the United States, down from the number one cause of mortality in this age group in 1995. In 2014, African Americans made up only 12% of the U.S. population but accounted for 44% of all new cases of HIV infections. Diagnoses of new cases among women have declined 40% since 2005. In 2014, men having sex with men (MSM) accounted for 67% of all new cases of HIV infections. Cases involving female-to-female transmission (women having sex with women) are rare. In terms of regional presence of AIDS in the United States, the South accounted for most new AIDS diagnoses (54%), persons living with

AIDS diagnosis (44%), and AIDS deaths (47%) (CDC, 2014).

HIV is transmitted through direct contact with infected blood, blood products, or body fluids (e.g., human milk, vaginal secretions, semen, cerebrospinal fluid, and saliva). Even though saliva and tears can contain HIV, only very low concentrations of the virus are present in these fluids. HIV is not transmitted through saliva and kissing unless open sores are present. The risk of acquiring HIV from an accidental needle stick is minimal (1 in 300 or 0.3%), but the risk of transmission from sharing needles is significantly greater (1 in 150). There has been only one confirmed case of occupational HIV transmission to healthcare workers reported to the CDC since 1999; however, underreporting is possible because such reporting is voluntary. There is a 13% to 40% chance of an infected mother transmitting this infection to her child, but early administration of antiretroviral therapy can decrease the transmission risk by approximately 1%. The antiretroviral drug most commonly used to prevent maternal transmission is Retrovir (zidovudine), which has a high safety index. Cesarean delivery can further decrease the risk of HIV transmission to the fetus.

As a retrovirus, HIV requires a host to survive. Once it gains access to the body, the virus invades the CD4 cells. Once inside the CD4 cells, it uses an enzyme, reverse transcriptase, to convert the viral RNA to DNA. The viral DNA then becomes integrated into the CD4 cell's own DNA. As the infected CD4 cell reproduces, it inadvertently produces viral copies. Meanwhile, the virus replicates inside the CD4 cell to the point that the cell membrane is compromised, releasing millions of viral copies into the bloodstream. Each viral copy then attaches to a new CD4 cell to start the process over again.

The HIV infectious process takes three forms—immunodeficiency, autoimmunity, and neurologic dysfunction. The immunodeficiency aspect includes opportunistic infections. The autoimmunity aspect includes lymphoid interstitial pneumonitis, arthritis, and hypergammaglobulinemia. Finally, the neurologic dysfunction aspect includes the AIDS dementia complex, HIV encephalopathy, and peripheral neuropathies.

Once infected, an individual may not experience any symptoms other than a brief episode of flulike symptoms (e.g., fever, malaise, headache, and lymphopathy), referred to as acute retroviral syndrome. After this brief early infection episode, the individual may remain asymptomatic for months to years while the virus is methodically infecting and destroying CD4 cells. As more and more CD4 cells are destroyed, the individual begins to have symptoms (e.g., lymphopathy, diarrhea, weight loss, fever, cough, shortness of breath). The individual becomes more symptomatic as more CD4 cells are destroyed. Over the next 10 years, serious clinical manifestations begin appearing as the individual moves into the late phase of infections.

HIV infection in children may appear differently than the progression just described. Children who are HIV positive may experience the following manifestations:

- Difficulty gaining weight
- Difficulty growing normally
- Problems walking
- Delayed mental development
- Severe forms of common childhood illnesses such as ear infections (otitis media), pneumonia, and tonsillitis

Diagnosis is established through a set of laboratory tests as early as 1 month after exposure to the virus. In the past, enzyme-linked immunosorbent assay, in combination with the Western blot test, was used to confirm diagnosis. Now, several rapid tests are available that can give highly accurate information within as little as 20 minutes. These tests look for antibodies to the virus using blood or fluid samples collected on a treated pad that is rubbed on the upper and lower gums. The oral test is almost as sensitive as the blood test and eliminates the need for drawing blood. A positive reaction on a rapid test requires a blood test to confirm the diagnosis, however. The rapid-diagnosis tests are relatively new and were originally approved for use only in certified laboratories; they may not be widely available. The Food and Drug Administration has also approved one HIV test for home use. The Home Access HIV-1 test is as accurate as a clinical test. Unlike a home pregnancy test, however, this test is mailed in and then results are retrieved from a toll-free number in 3 to 7 business days, thereby ensuring privacy and anonymity for patients. All positive results are retested.

Once HIV/AIDS is confirmed, a test to predict the probable disease progression, or viral load, will be conducted. The plasma viral load, or number of viral particles per milliliter of blood, is an indication of clinical progression—the higher the viral load, the further the progression. The test for viral load is also known as the polymerase chain reaction. The polymerase chain reaction is the most appropriate test for infants because the mother's circulating antibodies will make the infants test positive. The aim of antiretroviral therapy is to reduce the viral load to a point that the body's immune system can keep the virus in check. Viral load can also be an indicator of treatment success, along with other indicators (e.g., CD4 count and presence of opportunistic infections).

HIV infection progression is classified based on two systems: CD4 count and symptom presentation (**TABLE 2-6**). These classifications systems are used to track progression and treatment effectiveness.

Although there is no cure for AIDS, antiretroviral therapy is used to control the reproduction of the virus and slow the progression of the disease. Highly active antiretroviral therapy (HAART)—the recommended approach—includes three or more antiretroviral medications from different classes. The approved classes include nucleoside/nucleotide reverse

TABLE 2-6	HIV/AIDS Classification Systems
CD4 Classification System	
Category 1	CD4 cell count $\geq$ 500 cells/mm^3
Category 2	CD4 cell count 200–499 cells/mm^3
Category 3	CD4 cell count < 200 cells/mm^3
Clinical Presentation Classification System	
Category A	Asymptomatic HIV infection Persistent, generalized lymph node enlargement Acute HIV infection with accompanying illness or history of acute HIV infection
Category B	Bacillary angiomatosis (skin infection) Oropharyngeal or vaginal candidiasis (yeast) infection Fever or diarrhea lasting longer than a month Idiopathic thrombocytopenic purpura (autoimmune bleeding disorder) Pelvic inflammatory disease (infection of the female reproduction organs) Peripheral neuropathy (peripheral nerve damage)
Category C	Bacterial pneumonia, recurrent ($\geq$ 2 episodes in 12 months) Candidiasis of the respiratory tract and esophagus Invasive cervical cancer Fungal infections Parasitic and protozoan infections (> 1-month duration) Cytomegalovirus disease Encephalopathy Herpes simplex: chronic ulcers (> 1-month duration) Histoplasmosis Kaposi sarcoma Lymphoma *Mycobacterium avium* complex *Mycobacterium tuberculosis* *Pneumocystis jiroveci* (formerly *carinii*) pneumonia Progressive multifocal leukoencephalopathy *Salmonella* septicemia Toxoplasmosis of the brain Wasting syndrome due to HIV (involuntary weight loss > 10% of baseline body weight) associated with either chronic diarrhea ($\geq$ 2 loose stools per day $\geq$ 1 month) or chronic weakness and documented fever $\geq$ 1 month)

transcriptase inhibitors, non-nucleoside reverse transcriptase inhibitors, protease inhibitors, integrase inhibitors, fusion inhibitors, entry inhibitors, and pharmacokinetic enhancers. HAART has been very effective in suppressing HIV replication, but resistance can occur if the patient does not strictly adhere to the prescribed regimen. Genetic tests are now available that can determine whether the patient's particular HIV strain is resistant to a particular drug, and this information can be used to ensure that the best possible combination of drugs is prescribed. Other treatment strategies may include medications to treat specific opportunistic infections as they arise, manage the numerous drug side effects (e.g., high cholesterol and blood glucose), and prevent reexposure.

Continued exposure to HIV can increase the viral load and introduce another strain—both factors that can accelerate the disease's progression. An HIV vaccine has been in development for years, but an effective and safe vaccine has yet to reach the market.

Preventing HIV transmission is a worldwide public health priority. Prevention includes the following strategies:

- Avoiding contact with bodily fluids
- Avoiding activities that increase risk of exposure to those bodily secretions (e.g., drug use and multiple sexual partners)
- Education
- Using condoms with every sexual experience
- Preexposure prophylaxis (PrEP) (daily, low-dose antiretroviral therapy for high-risk individuals)
- Male circumcision (reduces the risk of female-to-male transmission of HIV and other sexually transmitted infections)

Developing a Strong Immune System

The key to preventing infectious diseases is building a strong immune system. Many people assume that the best way to stay healthy is to avoid exposure. However, because

Myth Busters

Despite efforts to educate the public, many misconceptions persist regarding HIV/AIDS.

Myth 1: I can get HIV by being around people who are HIV positive.

Evidence has consistently demonstrated that HIV cannot be spread through touch, tears, or saliva. In addition, HIV is not stable outside the body. The virus cannot be transmitted through toilet seats, water fountains, eating utensils, exercise equipment, hugging, or kissing.

Myth 2: I can get HIV from mosquitoes.

Although HIV spreads through blood, several studies have shown that mosquitoes cannot transmit HIV even in areas with high numbers of mosquitoes and HIV cases. Mosquitoes do not inject the blood they consume into the next person they bite, and the virus lives only a short time in the insect.

Myth 3: If I'm receiving treatment, I can't spread the HIV virus.

Effective treatment can decrease the viral load in the blood, even to the point that the virus

cannot be detected by a blood test. However, the virus can hide in other areas of the body, waiting for an opportunity to increase its replication again. The risk of transmission is lower when the viral load is lower, but transmission is still possible.

Myth 4: My partner and I are both HIV positive, so there's no reason to practice safer sex.

Continued exposure to HIV can increase the viral load and introduce another strain—both factors that can accelerate the disease's progression. Practicing safer sex (e.g., wearing condoms and using other barriers) can limit exposure to HIV and other sexually transmitted infections.

Myth 5: You can't get HIV from oral sex.

It is true that the risk of transmission through oral sex is lower than with other types of sex, but HIV can be transmitted by having oral sex with either a man or woman who is HIV positive.

Let's put the things you have learned about the body's defenses into practice. Which of the following individuals would be at highest risk for impaired immune function?

- A 23-year-old female who weighs 5% more than her ideal body weight
- A 78-year-old male with poorly controlled diabetes mellitus
- An 89-year-old male with controlled hypertension
- A 45-year-old female who was recently widowed

When considering this type of question, you start by counting things that might impair the immune system. The patient with the most risk factors is at the greatest risk. Eliminate any information that does not increase risk. For instance, being male or female does not impair immune function, so eliminate that factor from your consideration.

Let's look at each of the example patients. The 23-year-old is not in an increased age range and is fairly close to her ideal body weight; she has no risk factors. The 78-year-old is assigned one risk factor for his increased age and another for his chronic disease. Go ahead and give him another risk factor because his diabetes is uncontrolled—now he has three risk factors. The 89-year-old has one risk factor for his increased age and another for having a chronic disease, but his hypertension is controlled. He has two risk factors. Finally, the 45-year-old has only one risk factor, the stress of being recently widowed. After examining all of these patients, the 78-year-old male is at the most risk for impaired immune function owing to his three risk factors.

the immune system is a memory system, it requires early exposure to antigens to operate optimally. Exposure to microbes is limited today because of small family units, good sanitation, and widespread antibiotic use. Research suggests that avoiding oversanitizing our environment can increase exposure to microbes earlier and help develop a stronger immune system.

At-risk individuals and states that specifically put individuals at risk for an impaired immune system include the following:

- The very young and the very old
- Poor nutrition
- Impaired skin integrity
- Circulatory issues
- Alterations in normal flora due to antibiotic therapy
- Chronic diseases, especially diabetes mellitus
- Corticosteroid therapy
- Chemotherapy
- Smoking
- Alcohol consumption
- Immunodeficiency states

The following strategies can be employed to build a healthy immune system:

- Increasing fluid intake
- Eating a well-balanced diet
- Increasing antioxidants and protein intake
- Getting adequate sleep
- Avoiding caffeine and refined sugar
- Spending time outdoors
- Reducing stress

CHAPTER SUMMARY

Humans are in a constant state of warfare with often unseen enemies. The body takes a multilevel approach to prevent attacks and eliminate invaders. Problems can occur at any of these levels that can lead to overreactions, underreactions, and inappropriate reactions. These altered reactions can produce disease states that negatively affect the body. Multiple conditions can impair the body's ability to battle, but when armed with the appropriate weapons, the body becomes a fighting machine that can withstand many a fierce invader.

REFERENCES

Centers for Disease Prevention and Control (CDC). (2014). HIV/AIDS. Retrieved from http://www.cdc.gov/hiv/

Chiras, D. (2011). *Human biology* (7th ed.). Burlington, MA: Jones & Bartlett.

Elling, B., Elling, K., & Rothenberg, M. (2004). *Anatomy and physiology*. Sudbury, MA: Jones and Bartlett.

Gould, B. (2015). *Pathophysiology for the health professions* (5th ed.). Philadelphia, PA: Elsevier.

Pommerville, J. C. (2013). *Alcamo's fundamentals of microbiology* (10th ed.). Burlington, MA: Jones & Bartlett.

Porth, C. (2010). *Essentials of pathophysiology* (3rd ed.). Philadelphia, PA: Lippincott Williams & Wilkins.

Professional guide to pathophysiology (3rd ed.). (2010). Philadelphia, PA: Lippincott Williams & Wilkins.

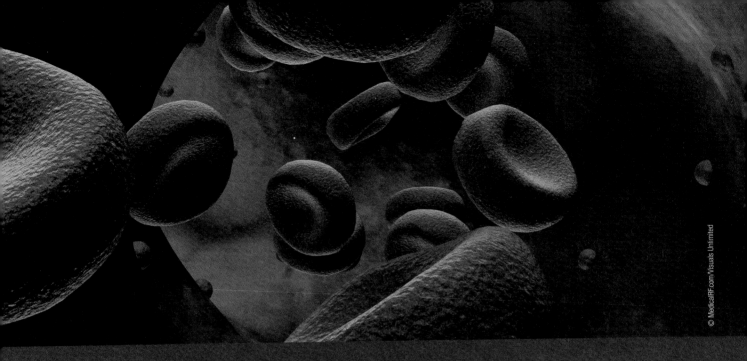

CHAPTER 3
Hematopoietic Function

LEARNING OBJECTIVES

- Discuss normal hematopoietic function.
- Describe and compare diseases of the white blood cells.
- Describe and compare diseases of the red blood cells.
- Describe and compare diseases of the platelets.

KEY TERMS

anemia
disseminated intravascular coagulation (DIC)
erythrocyte
hematocrit
hematopoiesis
hemoglobin
hemoglobin S

hemolysis
hemophilia A
idiopathic thrombocytopenic purpura (ITP)
infectious mononucleosis
leukemia
leukocyte
leukocytopenia

leukocytosis
multiple myeloma
neutropenia
neutrophil
pancytopenia
plasma
plasmin
pus

thrombocyte
thrombocytopenia
thrombocytosis
thromboplastin
thrombotic thrombocytopenic purpura (TTP)
von Willebrand's disease

Blood is the life fluid of the human body, and it is essential for health and homeostasis. The approximately 5 liters of blood continuously circulating in the human body provides nutrients and oxygen to tissues while aiding in the excretion of waste products. Blood consists of plasma, blood cells, and platelets. Disease occurs when there are too few, too many, or dysfunctional blood components. These conditions can result from congenital or genetic causes, but they can also be acquired from medical treatment. Healthcare providers, especially nurses, play a pivotal role in identifying those persons at risk and assisting in the management of these diseases.

Normal Hematopoietic Function

Blood is both a viscous fluid and a tissue. **Hematopoiesis** is the process of blood formation, and it occurs primarily in the bone marrow. Stem cells (primitive cells) differentiate the precursors for the different blood cells. Blood accomplishes its functions through its various components—the **plasma** (liquid protein), **leukocytes** (white blood cells), **erythrocytes** (red blood cells), and **thrombocytes** (platelets) (**TABLE 3-1**). Plasma is a transport medium that carries the blood cells as well as antibodies, nutrients, electrolytes, hormones, lipids, and waste products. Leukocytes are key players in the inflammatory response and infectious process (see the *Immunity* chapter).

TABLE 3-1	Summary of Blood Cells				
Name	**Light Micrograph**	**Description**	**Concentration (Number of Cells/mm³)**	**Life Span**	**Function**
Red blood cells (RBCs)		Biconcave disk; no nucleus	4 to 6 million	120 days	Transport oxygen and carbon dioxide
White blood cells (WBCs)					
Neutrophil		Approximately twice the size of RBCs; multilobed nucleus; clear-staining cytoplasm	3,000 to 7,000	6 hours to a few days	Phagocytize bacteria
Eosinophil		Approximately same size as neutrophil; large pink-staining granules; bilobed nucleus	100 to 400	8 to 12 days	Phagocytizes antigen–antibody complex; attacks parasites
Basophil		Slightly smaller than neutrophil; contains large, purple cytoplasmic granules; bilobed nucleus	20 to 50	A few hours to a few days	Releases histamine during inflammation
Monocyte		Larger than neutrophil; cytoplasm is grayish blue; no cytoplasmic granules; U- or kidney-shaped nucleus	100 to 700	Lasts many months	Phagocytizes bacteria, dead cells, and cellular debris
Lymphocyte		Slightly smaller than neutrophil; large, relatively round nucleus that fills the cell	1,500 to 3,000	Can persist for many years	Involved in immune protection, either attacking cells directly or producing antibodies
Platelets		Fragments of megakaryocytes; appear as small dark-staining granules	250,000	5 to 10 days	Play several key roles in blood clotting

Blood clot formation

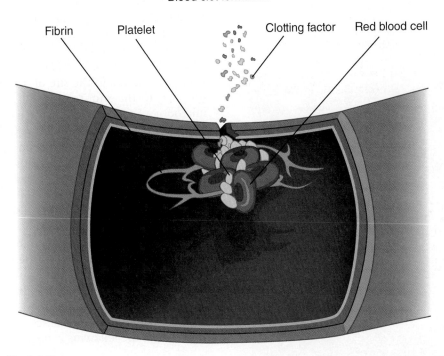

FIGURE 3-1 Blood clotting.

Erythrocytes are disk-shaped cells that carry oxygen to tissues and transport carbon dioxide out of the tissues for its subsequent removal from the body. Erythrocytes contain proteins and **hemoglobin**, which binds to oxygen, giving blood its red color. The brighter the shade of red, the more the blood is saturated with oxygen. **Hematocrit** refers to how much of the blood volume comprises erythrocytes.

Thrombocytes, along with clotting factors, control coagulation. Carried passively in the blood, thrombocytes are coated with a sticky material that causes them to adhere to irregular surfaces. Clotting is a quick chain reaction stimulated by the release of **thromboplastin** from damaged cells lining the blood vessels in the area of an injury (**FIGURE 3-1**; **FIGURE 3-2**). In conjunction with the initiation of the clotting cascade (**FIGURE 3-3**), platelets containing contractile proteins pull the edges of the wound together. Blood clots do not persist indefinitely; if they did so, they would clog up the entire circulatory system. **Plasmin** is an enzyme that dissolves clots once healing has occurred.

Diseases of the White Blood Cells

Leukocytes are a diverse group of cells that trigger the inflammatory process and combat infections. Normal white blood cell (WBC)

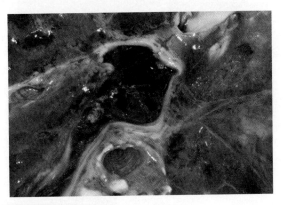

FIGURE 3-2 Blood clot.
© SPL/Science Source

levels range from 5,000 to 10,000 cells/mL^3 blood. **Leukocytosis** describes states characterized by increased WBC levels, and **leukocytopenia** refers to decreased WBC levels. Leukocytosis can indicate an active infectious process, whereas leukocytopenia can indicate an immune deficiency state (e.g., bone marrow suppression). The blood, by way of the circulatory system, transports leukocytes to the site of an infection. When the leukocytes arrive at the scene, they leak through the capillary wall to the site of trauma or invasion (**FIGURE 3-4**). Most leukocyte disorders originate from deficiencies of one or more of the varying leukocytes.

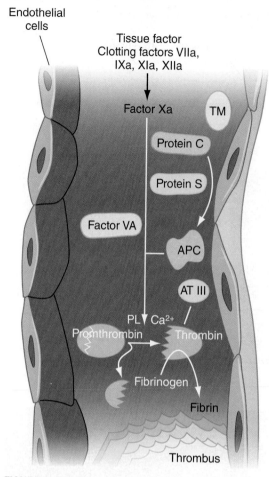

FIGURE 3-3 Clotting cascades.

Modified from Dean, L. (2000). Mutations and blood clots: How point mutations in clotting factor genes conspire to increase the risk of thrombosis. In L. Dean, J. McEntryre (Eds.), *Coffee break: Tutorials for NCBI tools*. Retrieved from http://www.ncbi.nlm.nih.gov/books/NBK2318

Neutropenia

Usually the first responders to arrive on the scene of an infection, **neutrophils** are attracted by various chemicals released by infected tissue (**FIGURE 3-5**). These cells escape from the capillary wall and migrate to the site of infection. Once they get to the site, neutrophils phagocytize microorganisms, preventing the infection from spreading. As the neutrophils are fully utilized, the infected cells die and become part of the yellowish wound drainage, or **pus**.

Neutropenia refers to a decrease in circulating neutrophils to fewer than 1,500 cells/mL (the normal range is 2,000–7,500 cells/mL). When fewer of these first responders are available, the body is poorly equipped to fight infections. The degree to which the body can fight infections, especially bacterial infections, is related to the severity of the neutropenia. In other words, the lower the neutrophil count, the less the body's ability to fight infections. Causes of neutropenia may include the following conditions:

- Increased usage (e.g., infection and inflammation)
- Drug suppression (e.g., immunosuppressants and chemotherapies)
- Radiation therapy
- Congenital conditions (e.g., periodic or cyclic)
- Bone marrow cancers (e.g., leukemias and lymphomas)

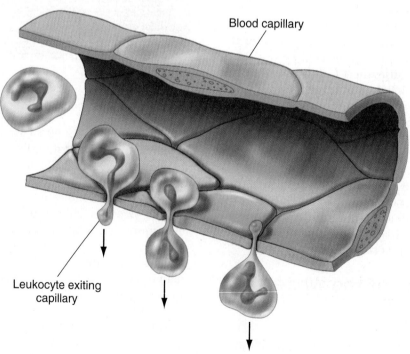

FIGURE 3-4 Leukocyte movement.

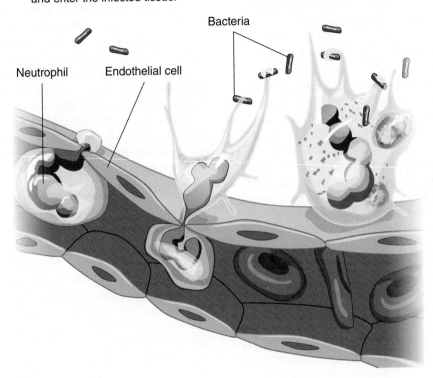

1. Foreign invaders signal nearby neutrophils to squeeze through endothelial cells that line the blood vessel and enter the infected tissue.

2. Through a cell-eating process known as phagocytosis, the neutrophil ingests the bacteria and releases toxic products that kill the bacteria.

Bacteria

Neutrophil   Endothelial cell

FIGURE 3-5 The role of neutrophils.

- Spleen destruction (e.g., Felty's syndrome)
- Vitamin deficiency (e.g., B_{12} and folate deficiency)

Clinical manifestations of neutropenia initially include signs and symptoms of bacterial and fungal infections (e.g., malaise, chills, and fever). The respiratory tract is the most common site of infection. Mouth ulcerations are also often associated with neutropenia, as are ulcerations of the skin, vagina, and gastrointestinal tract.

Diagnostic procedures center primarily on serum neutrophil levels. Additionally, a bone marrow biopsy may be performed to determine the cause of the neutropenia. Antibiotic therapy is used to treat infections as they develop. Identification and treatment of the cause of the neutropenia is crucial for positive outcomes. Hematopoietic growth factors such as granulocyte colony-stimulating factor may be used to stimulate maturation and differentiation of neutrophils.

Infectious Mononucleosis

Infectious mononucleosis, also known as "mono" and the "kissing disease," is an infection most often caused by the Epstein-Barr virus (EBV). EBV is a commonly encountered virus of the herpes family. Infectious mononucleosis is most frequently seen in adolescents and young adults. According to the Centers for Disease Control and Prevention (CDC, 2014), as many as 95% of adults ages 35–40 in the United States test positive for EBV antibodies. Most people have been exposed to the virus as children, and because of this exposure, they have developed immunity to the virus. Consequently, most people who are exposed to EBV do not develop infectious mononucleosis.

EBV infects B cells by killing the cells or being incorporated into their genome. The B cells infected with EBV produce heterophile antibodies that can be identified to diagnose the disease. Once the disease is eliminated, a few B cells remain altered, giving the individual an asymptomatic infection for life and the potential to occasionally spread EBV to others. Infectious mononucleosis is usually spread by person-to-person contact. Although saliva is the primary method of transmission, transmission can also occur through coughing or sneezing, which causes small droplets of infected saliva and/or mucus to become suspended in the air to be inhaled by others. EBV can also survive several hours outside the body, so transmission can occur through sharing utensils and glasses. The incubation period for infectious mononucleosis is between 4 and 6 weeks. During an infection, a person can transmit the virus to others for at least a few weeks.

According to the CDC (2014), depending on the method used to detect the virus, anywhere from 20% to 80% of people who have recovered from infectious mononucleosis will continue to secrete EBV in their saliva for years due to periodic reactivations of the viral infection. Because healthy people without symptoms also secrete the virus during reactivation episodes throughout their lifetime, isolation of people infected with EBV is not necessary. It is currently believed that these healthy people who secrete EBV particles are the primary reservoir for transmission of EBV among humans.

Onset of the clinical manifestations of infectious mononucleosis is usually insidious. The initial manifestations of malaise, anorexia, and chills can last 1–3 days. Following this period, the manifestations intensify and include severe sore throat, fever, and lymphopathy. The acute phase usually lasts 2–3 weeks. Some patients may not fully recover for 2–3 months, but most people recover without incident. Possible complications of infectious mononucleosis include hepatitis, ruptured spleen, and meningitis.

Diagnosis of infectious mononucleosis can be confirmed through the heterophile antibody test (Monospot test) 2–3 weeks post exposure. At that time, increased lymphocytes, increased monocytes, and atypical T lymphocytes (enlarged) in the blood will be present and can be identified by the test. Other laboratory tests can be performed to exclude other disorders that present similarly to infectious mononucleosis (e.g., streptococcal pharyngitis). Leukocyte counts may also be increased when a person has infectious mononucleosis.

Treatment of infectious mononucleosis is primarily symptomatic and supportive. Strategies may include bed rest, hydration, analgesics, corticosteroids, and antipyretics. Vigorous contact sports should be avoided in the acute illness and recovery phases to prevent rupture of the spleen.

Lymphomas

Lymphomas are cancers that develop from lymphatic cells. They are the most common blood cancers (National Cancer Institute [NCI], 2014a). According to the CDC (2013),

lymphoma is the eighth most common cancer in adults and the fifth most common cancer in children. There are several subtypes of lymphoma, but the two main types of lymphomas are Hodgkin's and non-Hodgkin's lymphoma. Non-Hodgkin's lymphoma is far more common than Hodgkin's disease. Risk factors for both types of lymphoma include infection with the human immunodeficiency virus (HIV) or EBV. Additional risk factors for non-Hodgkin's lymphoma include (1) the presence of an inherited immune or autoimmune condition, (2) infection with *Helicobacter pylori* or human T-cell leukemia/lymphoma virus type 1 (HTLV-1), and (3) exposure to pesticides.

Hodgkin's Lymphoma

Hodgkin's lymphoma can start in any lymph node of the lymphatic system, but most often arises in the lymph nodes of the upper body (e.g., the neck, chest, and upper arms). The affected lymph nodes swell and compress surrounding tissue. Systemically, the cancer cells spread from one lymph node to the next through the lymphatic vessels. In rare cases, the disease spreads into the blood vessels and other structures, in a process that continues until late in the disease. The cancer cells of Hodgkin's lymphoma are unique; they are called Reed-Sternberg cells (or Hodgkin cells) (**FIGURE 3-6**). These cells are an abnormal type of B lymphocyte that is much larger than normal lymphocytes. The T lymphocytes also appear to have defects, and the total lymphocyte number decreases.

The two main types of Hodgkin's lymphoma are classical Hodgkin's disease (which has several subtypes) and nodular lymphocyte predominance Hodgkin's disease. These types differ in the way the cancer cells appear under a

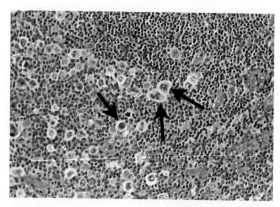

FIGURE 3-6 Reed-Sternberg cells associated with Hodgkin's lymphoma.

© Dr. E. Walker/Science Source

microscope. Identification of which type the patient is experiencing is important because these variants grow and spread in different ways, and they are often treated differently. Classical Hodgkin's disease will be discussed further here because it accounts for 95% of all Hodgkin's disease cases.

Although the incidence of this disease is on the decline, the CDC (2013) reports that Hodgkin's disease occurs primarily in adults 20–40 years of age, with equal prevalence across genders. A second peak occurrence is seen in men older than 50 years of age. Due to improvements in the treatment of Hodgkin's lymphoma, mortality has decreased by nearly 50% over the past 25 years. Over the same period, incidence has remained relatively steady. Prognosis is further improved when the disease is localized and is treated early, with many cases considered cured. Although the prognosis is excellent for patients with Hodgkin's disease, those who are treated with radiation may be at increased risk of stroke and transient ischemic attack (DeBruin et al., 2009).

Hodgkin's disease has the following clinical manifestations:

- Swollen, painless lymph nodes
- Weight loss
- Persistent fever
- Night sweats
- Generalized pruritus
- Coughing, trouble breathing, or chest pain
- Malaise
- Recurrent infections
- Splenomegaly

Diagnostic procedures primarily center on biopsy of the affected lymph node. Biopsy samples reveal the presence of Reed-Sternberg cells. Other diagnostic procedures consist of a physical examination, complete blood count, and chest X-rays.

A staging system is used to grade the severity and progression of the disease (**FIGURE 3-7**):

- **Stage I:** The lymphoma cells are in one lymph node group (such as in the neck or the underarm), or if the lymphoma cells are not in the lymph nodes, they are in only one part of a tissue or an organ (such as the lung).
- **Stage II:** The lymphoma cells are in at least two lymph node groups on the same side of (either above or below) the diaphragm, or the lymphoma cells are in one part of a tissue or an organ and the lymph nodes near that organ (on the same side of the diaphragm). Lymphoma cells may be in other lymph node groups on the same side of the diaphragm.
- **Stage III:** The lymphoma cells are in lymph nodes above and below the diaphragm. Lymphoma cells may be found in one part of a tissue or an organ (such as the liver, lung, or bone) near these lymph node groups. The cells may also be found in the spleen.
- **Stage IV:** Lymphoma cells are found in several parts of one or more organs or tissues, or the lymphoma cells are in an organ (such as the liver, lung, or bone) and in distant lymph nodes.
- **Recurrent:** The disease returns after treatment.

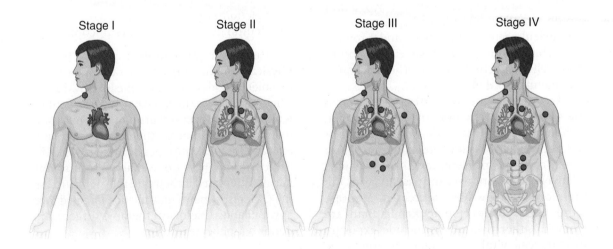

Stage I   Stage II   Stage III   Stage IV

● Site of lymphoma

FIGURE 3-7 Stages of Hodgkin's lymphoma.

Staging involves computed tomography scan, magnetic resonance imaging, positron emission tomography scan, and bone marrow biopsy. Other staging procedures may include biopsies of other lymph nodes, the liver, or other tissue. After diagnosis, the usual cancer treatment is implemented (combination of chemotherapy, radiation, and surgery).

Non-Hodgkin's Lymphoma

Non-Hodgkin's lymphoma can start at any age and in any lymph node. Non-Hodgkin's lymphoma is more common in Caucasians as compared to other ethnic groups. Many different types of this disease are possible. These types can be divided into aggressive (fast-growing) and indolent (slow-growing) types, and they can arise from either B cells (80% of cases) or T cells. Non-Hodgkin's lymphoma is similar to Hodgkin's lymphoma in its clinical manifestations, staging, and treatment; the differences lie in the spread and diagnosis of the disease. Non-Hodgkin's lymphoma involves multiple nodes scattered throughout the body and metastasizes in an unorganized manner. Metastasis is often present at diagnosis. With non-Hodgkin's lymphoma, no Reed-Sternberg cells are present. Additionally, non-Hodgkin's lymphoma is more difficult to treat. The prognosis for patients with this disease is poor, but improving.

Leukemias

Leukemia is a cancer of the leukocytes. With this disease, the bone marrow makes abnormal leukocytes, or leukemia cells. Unlike normal blood cells, leukemia cells do not die when they should, so they sometimes begin crowding normal leukocytes, erythrocytes, and thrombocytes. This crowding makes it difficult for normal blood cells to function properly. The exact cause of leukemia is unknown.

According to the NCI (2014a), leukemia is the second most common blood cancer. Although it affects 10 times as many adults as children, leukemia is the most common cancer among children. Incidence rates have remained relatively consistent over the past 20 years, but the mortality rates have decreased. Men are more likely to develop leukemia than are women. Other risk factors include exposure to chemical, viral, and radiation mutagens; smoking; use of chemotherapies; certain disease conditions (e.g., Down syndrome); and immunodeficiency disorders.

Leukemias are grouped as either acute or chronic. The four most common types of leukemia are identified here:

- **Acute lymphoblastic leukemia (ALL):** Affects primarily children (accounts for approximately 75% of all childhood leukemias); responds well to therapy, and carries a good prognosis.
- **Acute myeloid leukemia (AML):** Affects primarily adults; responds fairly well to treatment, and carries a prognosis somewhat worse than that of acute lymphoblastic leukemia.
- **Chronic lymphoid leukemia (CLL):** Affects primarily adults; responds poorly to therapy, yet most patients live many years after diagnosis.
- **Chronic myeloid leukemia (CML):** Affects primarily adults; responds poorly to chemotherapy, but the prognosis is improved with allogeneic bone marrow transplant.

Leukemia has the following clinical manifestations:

- Leukopenia (frequent infections)
- Anemia (pallor, fatigue, dyspnea, and decreased activity tolerance)
- Thrombocytopenia (petechiae, bleeding gums, hematuria, and prolonged bleeding time)
- Lymphadenopathy
- Joint swelling
- Bone pain
- Weight loss
- Anorexia
- Hepatomegaly
- Splenomegaly
- Central nervous system dysfunction

Diagnostic procedures include a history, physical examination, peripheral blood smears, complete blood count, and bone marrow biopsy. Chemotherapy is the mainstay of treatment for leukemia, and several courses may be necessary to eradicate the cancer. Chemotherapy is more effective for the acute types of leukemia than for the chronic types. Bone marrow transplants may be attempted if chemotherapy is unsuccessful. Other treatments may include targeted therapy, radiation, biological therapy, surgery, and donor lymphocyte infusion.

Multiple Myeloma

Multiple myeloma is a cancer of the plasma cells that most often affects older adults. This disease is characterized by excessive numbers of abnormal plasma cells in the bone marrow crowding the blood-forming cells and causing Bence Jones proteins to be excreted in the urine. Multiple bone tumors develop and bone destruction occurs, leading to hypercalcemia and pathologic fractures. Hypercalcemia leads to renal impairment and neuromuscular issues. Tumor cells can spread through the lymph nodes and infiltrate organs.

According to the NCI (2014b), multiple myeloma is the third most common blood cancer. Over the past 20 years, its incidence and mortality rates have remained relatively stable. This disease is more common in men than in women. Additionally, African Americans have about twice the incidence and mortality rates of Caucasians.

The onset of multiple myeloma is usually insidious, and malignancy is often well advanced upon diagnosis. Clinical manifestations of multiple myeloma include the following:

- Anemia (pallor, fatigue, dyspnea, and decreased activity tolerance)
- Thrombocytopenia (petechiae, bleeding gums, hematuria, and prolonged bleeding time)
- Leukopenia (frequent infections)
- Decreased bone density
- Bone pain
- Hypercalcemia (neuromuscular dysfunction)
- Renal impairment

The diagnosis of multiple myeloma is often made incidentally during routine blood tests for other conditions. For example, the presence of anemia and a high serum protein may suggest further testing is needed. Diagnostic procedures include serum and urine protein, calcium, renal function tests, complete blood count, biopsy, X-rays, computed tomography, and magnetic resonance imaging.

Multiple myeloma is not considered curable, but chemotherapy improves the remission rate. Additional treatments may include corticosteroids, angiogenesis inhibitors, targeted therapies, stem cell transplants, biological therapy, radiation therapy, and supportive care. The median survival time is 3 years. Analgesics are used to treat bone pain. Blood dyscrasias, hypercalcemia, and renal impairment are treated as needed.

Diseases of the Red Blood Cells

Erythrocytes are the most prevalent blood cell in the human body—millions can be found in a single drop of blood (the normal range is 4.2–5.9 million cells/µL). These cells function primarily to transport oxygen to the tissue and the waste products for excretion. Most diseases of the red blood cells (RBCs) are related to the quantity or quality of the erythrocytes.

Anemia

Anemia is a common acquired or inherited disorder of the erythrocytes that impairs the oxygen-carrying capacity of the blood. This condition can result from (1) a decrease in the number of circulating erythrocytes (e.g., blood loss or decreased production), (2) a reduction in hemoglobin content, or (3) the presence of abnormal hemoglobin. Some anemias are treated easily, whereas others can cause lifelong problems. The clinical manifestations of anemia reflect the decreased oxygen-carrying capacity, regardless of the disease's cause:

- Weakness
- Fatigue
- Pallor
- Syncope
- Dyspnea
- Tachycardia

Anemia is diagnosed when hematocrit is less than 41% in males and less than 37% in females; that is, hemoglobin concentration falls to less than 13.5 g/dL in males and less than 12 g/dL in females. Treatment depends on the specific type of anemia experienced.

Iron-Deficiency Anemia

According to the World Health Organization (2016), iron-deficiency anemia is the most widespread anemia in the world. This type of anemia is most commonly seen in women of childbearing age, children younger than 2 years of age, and the elderly. Iron-deficiency anemia occurs when the supply of iron necessary to produce hemoglobin is inadequate to meet the demand of hemoglobin production. It may be caused by decreased iron consumption, decreased iron absorption, or increased bleeding (such as occurs during menstruation and as a result of some cancers). Iron is ingested through animal and plant sources. Although the average American ingests more than 10 mg of iron each day, which is within the recommended daily allowance, only about 10% of the ingested iron is actually absorbed. When an iron deficiency exists, erythrocytes will become pale (hypochromic) and small (microcytic) (**FIGURE 3-8**).

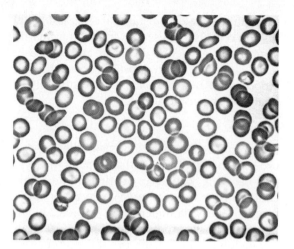

FIGURE 3-8 Iron-deficiency anemia.

In addition to the previously mentioned anemia signs and symptoms, the following clinical manifestations may be associated with iron-deficiency anemia:

- Cyanosis (blue coloration) to sclera of the eyes
- Brittle nails
- Decreased appetite (especially in children)
- Headache
- Irritability
- Stomatitis
- Unusual food cravings (pica)
- Delayed healing

Diagnostic procedures for iron-deficiency anemia include a complete blood count, serum ferritin, serum iron, and transferring saturation. Additional tests may be performed to determine the cause (e.g., fecal occult blood test) (see **FIGURE 3-9**).

Treatment includes the identification and resolution of the underlying cause of the iron-deficiency anemia. Other strategies to increase iron levels include increasing consumption of iron-rich foods (e.g., liver, red meat, fish, beans, raisins, and green leafy vegetables) or administering iron supplements. Additionally, foods or supplements high in vitamin C should be increased because vitamin C increases the absorption of iron.

Pernicious Anemia

Pernicious anemia is also known as vitamin B_{12} deficiency and megaloblastic anemia. This type of anemia is characterized by large (macrocytic), immature erythrocytes (**FIGURE 3-10**). Pernicious anemia most often results from cyanocobalamin (vitamin B_{12}) deficiency. This deficiency usually occurs gradually and from a lack of intrinsic factor. Intrinsic factor is a protein produced by the stomach that is necessary for vitamin B_{12} to be absorbed in the stomach. The lack of intrinsic factor arises because of the actions of autoantibodies, with the subsequent immune reaction leading to atrophy of the gastric mucosa and glands.

Vitamin B_{12} is necessary for DNA synthesis, and a deficiency of this nutrient leads to decreased cell division and cell maturation. Too little vitamin B_{12} gradually causes neurologic

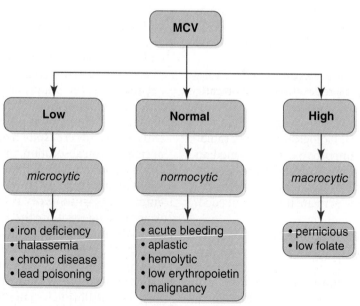

FIGURE 3-9 Mean Corpuscular Volume Changes with Anemia.

Mrs. Williams is a 45-year-old Caucasian woman who sought medical attention for fatigue that developed during the previous month. She reported no chest pain, but did feel mildly short of breath with exertion such as after walking up a flight of stairs. She denied any rectal bleeding, but she had heavy menstrual periods for about a year. Her past medical history included being treated for anemia following her third pregnancy 10 years earlier. She was not taking any prescribed medications. Her family history revealed that her parents were born in Italy and died when she was in grade school. She did not know their medical history.

A physical examination revealed that Mrs. Williams's general appearance was pale but with no acute distress. Her vital signs were blood pressure 125/90 mm Hg, heart rate 118 beats/min regular, and respirations 26 breaths/min. No significant changes in the blood pressure and heart rate were noted between the supine and upright positions. Other findings included pale conjunctiva and moist mucous membranes without lesions. No adenopathy or hepatosplenomegaly was noted. Breath sounds were clear to auscultation, and the heart had a regular rate and rhythm with a murmur. The abdomen was soft, nontender, and nondistended. A rectal examination revealed no masses, and heme-negative brown stool was present. Additionally, Mrs. Williams reported that she was taking aspirin 81 mg daily, she is a vegetarian who eats a lot of cereal, and she did not have an urge to eat ice.

Mrs. Williams's laboratory tests revealed the following results:

CBC	Result	Normal Range
WBC	8.2×10^3/mL	4.8–10.8×10^3/mL
Hgb	8.0 g/dL	12–15.6 g/dL
Hct	24%	35–46%
RBC	4.0×10^6/mL	3.8–5×10^6/mL
MCV	60 µL/red cell	80–96.1 µL/red cell
MCH	20 pg/red cell	27.5–33.2 pg/red cell
MCHC	33 g/L	33.4–35.5 g/L
RDW	16.5	11.5–14.5
platelets	500,000/mL	150–400,000/mL
reticulocyte count	3%	0.5–1.7%
absolute reticulocyte count	40,000/mL	25,000–75,000/mL
LDH	210 U/L	0–304 U/L

CBC = complete blood count; WBC = white blood cells; Hgb = hemoglobin; Hct = hematocrit; RBC = red blood cells; MCV = mean corpuscular volume; MCH = mean corpuscular hemoglobin; MCHC = mean corpuscular hemoglobin concentration; RDW = red cell distribution width; LDH = lactate dehydrogenase.

1. Which type of hematologic disorder would you suspect based on Mrs. Williams's history, physical examination, and laboratory values?

    A. Infectious mononucleosis
    B. Iron-deficiency anemia
    C. Pernicious anemia
    D. Thalassemia

2. Which of Mrs. Williams clinical signs are reflective of the body's effort to compensate for her red blood cells' decreased oxygen-carrying capacity?

    A. Heart rate 118 beats/min and respiration rate 26 breaths/min
    B. Hematocrit 24% and hemoglobin 8 g/dL
    C. Blood pressure 125/90
    D. Persistent fatigue

Mrs. Williams was placed on iron supplements. Her hemoglobin (Hgb) was expected to be normal after approximately 8 weeks of iron therapy, which was anticipated to raise the Hgb about 1 g/dL per week. However, her Hgb was 9.5 g/dL after 8 weeks.

Following those results, Mrs. Williams was asked whether she had been taking the iron supplements as ordered and whether she had been tolerating the medication. Additionally, she was asked whether she was having dark, tarry stools, which would indicate gastrointestinal bleeding. Mrs. Williams reported that she had taken the iron supplement for only 2 weeks because it made her nauseated and constipated. Mrs. Williams was instructed to take the iron supplement with a light carbohydrate such as crackers or toast to minimize the nausea and to take measures to prevent constipation (e.g., increasing fiber and water intake). After implementing these measures and taking the iron supplement as ordered for 8 weeks, Mrs. Williams's Hgb returned to normal.

3. In addition to iron supplements, which kinds of food would be recommended for Mrs. Williams to consume?

   A. Milk, cheese, soybeans, broccoli, and almonds

   B. Green leafy vegetables and avocados

   C. Orange juice, raisins, bananas, cantaloupe, and fish

   D. Liver, red meat, eggs, dark green leafy vegetables, nuts, and legumes

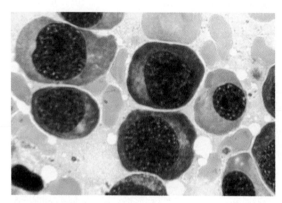

FIGURE 3-10 Pernicious anemia.
© Michael Abbey/Science Source

problems because of a breakdown in myelin. The neurologic effects may be seen before anemia is diagnosed. In addition to the usual signs and symptoms of anemia, pernicious anemia is associated with the following clinical manifestations:

- Bleeding gums
- Diarrhea
- Impaired sense of smell
- Loss of deep tendon reflexes
- Anorexia
- Personality or memory changes
- Positive Babinski's sign (a pathological reflex in which the first toe extends and flexes toward the top of the foot and the other toes fan out when the sole of the foot is firmly stroked)
- Stomatitis
- Paresthesia of the hands and feet
- Unsteady gait, especially in the dark

Diagnostic tests for pernicious anemia include serum vitamin B_{12} levels, Schilling's test (measures vitamin B_{12} absorption), complete blood count, gastric analysis, and bone marrow biopsy. Treatment of pernicious anemia includes vitamin B_{12} injections if no intrinsic factor is being produced; oral vitamin B_{12} can be administered for those individuals who are producing intrinsic factor.

Aplastic Anemia

Aplastic anemia is a rare but serious type of anemia that is a result of the bone marrow failing to make enough blood cells. This lack of erythrocytes, leukocytes, and platelets is referred to as **pancytopenia**. A lack of these blood cells leads to a series of complications (e.g., infections, bleeding, hypoxia, fatty replacement of marrow, and death). Aplastic anemia may be temporary or permanent. Causes of aplastic anemia include the following:

- Idiopathic causes
- Autoimmune causes (e.g., systemic lupus erythematosus and rheumatoid arthritis)
- Medications and treatments (e.g., chemotherapy and radiation)
- Viruses
- Toxins (e.g., pesticides, arsenic, and benzene)
- Genetic abnormalities (e.g., myelodysplastic syndrome)
- Infectious diseases (e.g., EBV, cytomegalovirus, parvovirus, and HIV)
- Pregnancy (often resolves after delivery)
- Cancer

Clinical manifestations include signs and symptoms of general anemia (e.g., weakness, pallor, and dyspnea), leukocytopenia (e.g., recurrent infections), and thrombocytopenia (e.g., bleeding). As blood cell levels decline, clinical manifestations worsen.

Diagnostic tests for aplastic anemia include complete blood count and bone marrow biopsy. Prompt treatment of the underlying causes and any complications as they arise is crucial for positive outcomes. Treatment of underlying causes may include discontinuation of medications or treatments. Treatment of complications may include the following measures:

- Oxygen therapy
- Infection control measures (e.g., hand washing, avoiding groups, and avoiding fresh flowers)
- Infection treatment (e.g., antibiotics)
- Bleeding precautions (e.g., electric razors, soft-bristle toothbrushes, and injury prevention)
- Hematopoietic stimulants (e.g., erythropoietin and colony-stimulating factors)
- Immunosuppressant therapy (e.g., cyclosporine and methylprednisolone)
- Anti-infectives (e.g., antibiotics and antiviral medications)
- Blood transfusions
- Bone marrow transplants

Hemolytic Anemia

Hemolytic anemia results from excessive destruction, or **hemolysis**, of erythrocytes. Causes of hemolytic anemia include idiopathic causes, autoimmune causes, genetics, infections (e.g., malaria), blood transfusion reactions, and blood incompatibility in the neonate. Several types of hemolytic anemia exist, including sickle cell anemia, thalassemia, and erythroblastosis fetalis. Specifics in regard to pathogenesis, clinical manifestations, diagnosis, and treatment vary based on type.

Sickle Cell Anemia

Sickle cell anemia is a genetic type of hemolytic anemia in which the erythrocytes have an abnormal crescent or sickle shape (**FIGURE 3-11**). It is caused by an abnormal type of hemoglobin called **hemoglobin S**. Hemoglobin S distorts the shape of erythrocytes, especially when the body's supply of oxygen is low. These fragile, sickle-shaped cells deliver less oxygen to the body's tissues. These cells also can clog easily in small blood vessels and break into pieces that disrupt blood flow.

Sickle cell anemia is an inherited disorder that is neither recessive nor dominant (see the *Cellular Function* chapter). The allele for the sickle cell gene is co-dominant—meaning that if a person inherits the sickle cell gene from one

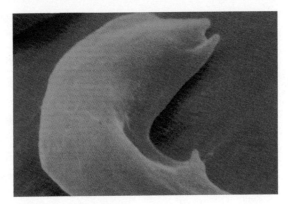

FIGURE 3-11 Sickle cell anemia.
© Dr. Stanley Flegler/Visuals Unlimited, Inc.

parent and the normal erythrocyte gene from the other parent, both genes will be expressed. Someone who inherits the hemoglobin S gene from one parent and a normal hemoglobin gene (A) from the other parent, meaning a heterozygous pair of alleles, will have sickle cell trait. Persons with sickle cell trait do not have the symptoms of true sickle cell anemia because fewer than half of their erythrocytes are sickled. Those persons who inherit the hemoglobin S gene from both parents, creating a homozygous allele pair, have sickle cell disease. Sickle cell disease is more severe because almost all of the individual's erythrocytes are abnormal. Sickle cell disease is much more common in people of African (1 out of every 500 births) and Mediterranean descent. Sickle cell disease is also seen in people from South and Central America, the Caribbean, and the Middle East.

Clinical manifestations usually do not appear in newborns because fetal hemoglobin protects the red blood cells from sickling. The fetal hemoglobin is replaced by adult hemoglobin, however, when a child reaches 4 to 5 months of age. Swelling in the hands and feet, often in conjunction with a fever, is usually the first symptom. The swelling results from the sickled cells occluding the blood vessels and blocking blood flow in and out of the hands and feet. Most patients will experience painful episodes, or crises, that can last for hours to days. Pain is caused by obstruction of small blood vessels as the sickled cells clog up the vessels, leading to ischemia and necrosis. Complications of these blood vessel occlusions depend on their location (**TABLE 3-2**). The number and severity of these crises vary among patients, but episodes can be triggered by dehydration, stress, high altitudes, fever, and extreme temperatures. Because of improved disease understanding and management,

TABLE 3-2 | **Complications of Blood Vessel Occlusions in Sickle Cell Anemia**

Area of Occlusion	Result
Bone	Susceptibility to osteomyelitis due to *Staphylococcus* infection
Papillae of renal medulla	Gross hematuria Renal tubular concentrating defects
Eye	Retinopathy Blindness
Sinus	Stroke
Spleen	Hyposplenism Susceptibility to infection
Liver	Jaundice Hepatomegaly
Miscellaneous	Cardiomegaly Slow-healing leg ulcers

most patients with sickle cell anemia now live into their 50s.

The clinical manifestations of sickle cell anemia reflect the hypoxia and tissue ischemia that occurs in the disease, and the complications that can result from them:

- Abdominal pain
- Bone pain
- Dyspnea
- Delayed growth and development
- Fatigue
- Fever
- Jaundice (yellowish skin)
- Pallor
- Tachycardia
- Skin ulcers on the lower legs
- Angina
- Excessive thirst
- Frequent urination
- Painful and prolonged erection (priapism)
- Vision impairment
- Frequent infections
- Acute chest syndrome (a potentially life-threatening condition that causes chest pain, coughing, difficulty breathing, and fever)
- Splenic sequestration (a potentially life-threatening condition that causes sudden weakness, pale lips, tachypnea, extreme thirst, left quadrant abdominal pain, and tachycardia)
- Leg ulcers
- Stroke

Carriers of the defective gene can be detected by hemoglobin electrophoresis, a simple blood test. Additionally, the sickle cell test can determine whether the hemoglobin is normal or sickled. A complete blood count and bilirubin test are useful in determining diagnosis and progression.

There is no single best treatment for all people with sickle cell disease. Stem cell transplants are the option for a cure. Medications (e.g., Hydrea [hydroxyurea]) are available to reduce the frequency of crises. Avoidance of sickling triggers is also helpful. Other strategies include the following measures:

- Oxygen therapy
- Hydration
- Pain management (e.g., opioids, relaxation techniques, distraction)
- Infection control measures
- Vaccinations
- Blood transfusions
- Bone marrow transplants
- Genetic counseling for those persons with sickle cell trait

Thalassemia

Thalassemia is another genetic type of anemia, which results in abnormal hemoglobin. This disease follows an autosomal dominant inheritance pattern (see the *Cellular Function* chapter). The abnormal hemoglobin is a result of a lack of one of the two proteins that collectively make up hemoglobin (alpha and beta globin). Thalassemia occurs most frequently in persons of Mediterranean descent. Other ethnic groups affected by thalassemia include those of Asian, Indian, and African descent. Severe cases can lead to death in childhood. Patients with moderate cases and those treated effectively can survive into their 30s.

Thalassemia has the following clinical manifestations:

- Abortion
- Delayed growth and development
- Fatigue
- Dyspnea
- Heart failure
- Hepatomegaly
- Splenomegaly
- Bone deformities
- Jaundice

Upon examination, erythrocytes will appear microcytic and hypochromic, and they vary in size. Iron levels may be increased. A complete blood count is also useful in diagnosis (low mean corpuscular volume [MCV] and mean corpuscular hemoglobin concentration [MCHC]). Treatment may not be necessary in mild cases. Severe cases, however, can cause early death due to heart failure, usually between the ages of 20 and 30. If treatment is warranted, it includes blood transfusion, chelation therapy, bone marrow transplants, and splenectomy.

Polycythemia Vera

Polycythemia vera is a disorder in which the bone marrow produces too many blood cells. This rare condition is considered a neoplastic disease because of the uncontrolled proliferation of cells. The exact cause of this disease, which occurs most frequently in men, is unknown. As blood cell numbers increase, so does the blood volume and viscosity. Blood vessels become distended and blood flow is sluggish. The following complications are possible:

- Tissue ischemia and necrosis
- Thrombosis
- Hypertension
- Heart failure
- Hemorrhage
- Splenomegaly
- Hepatomegaly
- Acute myeloblastic leukemia

Clinical manifestations of polycythemia vera include the following:

- Cyanotic or plethoric (reddish) skin
- High blood pressure
- Tachycardia
- Dyspnea
- Headaches
- Visual abnormalities

Diagnostic procedures for polycythemia vera include complete blood counts, bone marrow biopsy, and uric acid levels. Treatment strategies include chemotherapy (specifically hydroxyurea), radiation, and phlebotomy (removal of blood). Management of clotting and bleeding disorders us employed as needed.

Diseases of the Platelets

Platelets are vital components of the coagulation process. Normal platelet levels range from 150,000 to 350,000 cells/mL^3. **Thrombocytosis** refers to increased platelet levels, and **thrombocytopenia** describes the condition of decreased platelet levels. Thrombocytosis increases the risk of thrombus formation, while thrombocytopenia increases the risk of bleeding and infection.

Capillaries are relatively delicate structures that can leak from even minor injuries. Fortunately, the platelets, along with the coagulation process, quickly halt any such leaking. Diseases of the platelets include issues in quantity and quality of platelets.

Hemophilia A

Hemophilia A, or classic hemophilia, is an X-linked recessive bleeding disorder (see the *Cellular Function* chapter). This condition involves a deficiency or abnormality of clotting factor VIII. The severity of the disorder varies depending on the amount of factor VIII present in the blood.

Severe forms of hemophilia A become apparent early on. Bleeding is the main symptom of the disease and sometimes, though not always, occurs if an infant is circumcised. Additional bleeding problems may be seen when the infant starts crawling and walking. Mild cases may go unnoticed until later in life, when they are detected during surgery or trauma. Internal bleeding may happen anywhere, and bleeding into joints, or hemarthrosis, is common. Other manifestations include petechiae, bruising, gastrointestinal bleeding, and hematuria.

Diagnosis of hemophilia A includes the examination of bleeding studies. Bleeding time and prothrombin time are usually normal, but partial prothromboplastin time, activated partial prothromboplastin time, and coagulation time are prolonged. Serum levels of factor VIII are low.

Treatment strategies include replacing clotting factors through transfusions and Advate (antihemophilic factor, a recombinant DNA product). To prevent a bleeding crisis, patients can be taught to give factor VIII concentrates at home at the first signs of bleeding. People with severe forms of the disease may need regular preventive treatment. Mild hemophilia may be treated with desmopressin (DDAVP), which helps the body release factor VIII that is stored within the lining of blood vessels. Additionally, bleeding precautions should be employed (e.g., electric razors, soft-bristle toothbrush, and injury prevention).

Von Willebrand's Disease

Von Willebrand's disease is the most common hereditary bleeding disorder. It results from a deficit of von Willebrand factor, which ordinarily causes platelets to come together (aggregate) and stick (adhere) to the vessel wall in times of injury. Several forms of von Willebrand's disease are distinguished:

- **Type 1** is the most common (70–80%) and mildest form. It follows an autosomal dominant inheritance pattern (see the *Cellular Function* chapter). The level of von Willebrand factor in the blood is reduced. Because this form is often very mild, most cases go undiagnosed. Type 1 does not usually cause spontaneous bleeding, but significant bleeding can occur with trauma or surgery.
- **Type 2** occurs in 15–20% of cases. It can be either autosomal dominant or recessive, and five subtypes exist. In type 2, the building blocks (multimers) that make up the von Willebrand factor are smaller than usual or break down easily.
- **Type 3** follows an autosomal recessive inheritance pattern. Severe bleeding problems are seen with this type due to the lack of measurable von Willebrand factor or factor VIII.
- **Acquired type** occurs in persons with Wilms' tumor, congenital heart disease, systemic lupus erythematosus, and hypothyroidism.

Clinical manifestations of von Willebrand's disease include abnormal bleeding. Diagnosis requires bleeding studies (e.g., bleeding time, prothrombin time, and partial prothromboplastin time) and factor VIII levels. Treatment, if needed, includes infusions of cryoprecipitate or administration of desmopressin (DDVAP); DDVAP increases the release of von Willebrand factor and factor VII. Additionally, measures are used to control bleeding and prevent injury (e.g., pressure dressings).

Disseminated Intravascular Coagulation

Disseminated intravascular coagulation (DIC) is a life-threatening disorder that occurs as a complication of other diseases and conditions (e.g., serious acute infections). Normally, during injury, clotting factors (Figure 3-3) become activated and travel to the injury site to help stop bleeding. However, in persons with DIC, these factors become abnormally active. In fact, they may become active as an inappropriate immune reaction. Consequently, small blood clots form within the blood vessels, and some of these clots can occlude blood supply to tissue and organs. Over time, the clotting factors become used up. When this happens, the person is at risk for serious bleeding from even a minor injury.

Learning Points

In DIC, hypercoagulation uses up all the available clotting factors. Once available clotting factors are utilized, the patient begins excessively bleeding. In other words, the individual clots, clots, clots, and then bleeds, bleeds, bleeds!

It is not clear why certain disorders lead to DIC, but typical triggers include the following conditions:

- Blood transfusion reaction
- Cancer (e.g., leukemia, aplastic anemia, and metastatic carcinoma)
- Infection in the blood by bacteria or fungus
- Pregnancy complications (e.g., retained placenta after delivery, abruptio placentae, and eclampsia)
- Recent surgery or anesthesia
- Sepsis (an overwhelming infection)
- Severe liver disease
- Severe tissue injury (e.g., burns and head injury)
- Cardiac arrest
- Poisonous snake bites

Clinical manifestations of DIC include signs and symptoms of tissue and organ ischemia (e.g., angina, confusion, and dyspnea) and abnormal bleeding (e.g., petechiae, epistaxis, and hematuria). Additionally, indicators of complications such as shock and multiple organ failure will appear.

Diagnostic procedures for DIC consist of complete blood counts and bleeding studies (e.g., fibrinogen levels, prothrombin time, partial prothromboplastin time, and fibrinogen degradation products). Management of DIC is complicated but starts with the identification and treatment of the underlying cause. The treatment of the DIC disorder itself is a delicate balance between preventing clots and treating bleeding (**FIGURE 3-12**).

Idiopathic Thrombocytopenic Purpura

Idiopathic thrombocytopenic purpura (ITP) is a hypocoagulopathy state resulting from the immune system destroying its own platelets. Circulating immunoglobulin G reacts with the platelets, which are then destroyed in the spleen and liver.

ITP can be either acute or chronic. Acute ITP is more common in children. This form of the disease typically has a sudden onset and is self-limiting. Chronic ITP is more common in adults aged 20–50 and in women. Prognosis is usually good for both acute and chronic ITP.

Causes of ITP include the following:

- Idiopathic causes
- Autoimmune diseases
- Immunizations with a live vaccine
- Immunodeficiency disorders (e.g., AIDS)
- Viral infections

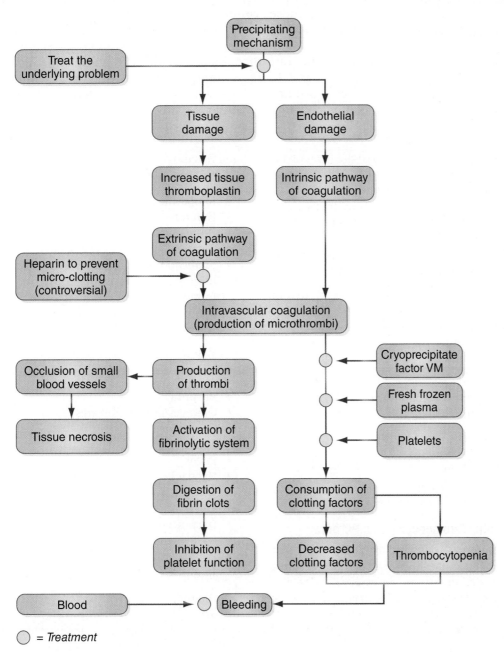

FIGURE 3-12 Understanding DIC and its treatment.

Now that we have learned about the various blood dyscrasias, let's put that knowledge into practice. During shift change, you receive reports on the following patients. Who would you see first following report?

- A 32-year-old with pernicious anemia who needs to receive a vitamin B$_{12}$ injection
- A 40-year-old with iron-deficiency anemia who needs an iron injection
- A 67-year-old with acute myelocytic leukemia (AML) who has petechiae on the legs
- An 81-year-old with thrombocytopenia and an increased abdominal girth

Remember to go through the usual thought process—who would die first, acute versus chronic conditions, Maslow's hierarchy of needs, and patient safety. Starting with the patient with the pernicious anemia, vitamin B$_{12}$ is the mainstay of treatment, but the therapy is not a matter of life or death. The same is true for the patient with iron-deficiency anemia. Additionally, both of these conditions are chronic. The patient with AML and petechiae warrants consideration because that condition is acute and there is some mild bleeding—but hold off on making the decision until you look at all the patients. Finally, consider the thrombocytopenia patient experiencing increased abdominal girth. What would cause the increased abdominal girth? You must consider that this patient may be bleeding into the peritoneal cavity. This active bleeding would be worse than the mild bleeding in the patient with AML. You should see the 81-year-old patient to assess for other manifestations of internal hemorrhage (e.g., hypotension and tachycardia) so that measures could be implemented immediately (e.g., notifying the healthcare provider and administering blood products).

Clinical manifestations take the form of abnormal bleeding (e.g., petechiae, epistaxis, and hematuria). Diagnostic procedures include complete blood counts, bone marrow biopsy, and humoral studies. Thrombocyte counts will often be less than 20,000/mL.

The following treatment strategies may be employed for acute ITP:

- Glucocorticoid steroids (prevent further platelet immune destruction)
- Immunoglobulins (prevent further platelet destruction)
- Plasmapheresis
- Platelet pheresis

Treatment strategies for chronic ITP include these measures:

- Glucocorticoid steroids
- Immunoglobulins
- Splenectomy
- Blood transfusions
- Immunosuppressant therapy

Thrombotic Thrombocytopenic Purpura

Thrombotic thrombocytopenic purpura (TTP) is a coagulation disorder resulting from a deficiency of an enzyme necessary for cleaving von Willebrand factor. This enzyme deficiency leads to increased clotting, which in turn decreases available platelets. Fewer platelets can lead to bleeding under the skin and purple-colored spots called purpura; therefore, TTP is characterized by thrombi, thrombocytopenia, and bleeding. TTP may be caused by any of the following conditions:

- Idiopathic causes
- Heredity
- Bone marrow transplants
- Cancer
- Medications (e.g., platelet aggregation inhibitors, immunosuppressants, and hormone replacement)
- Pregnancy
- HIV

TTP is characterized by these clinical manifestations:

- Purpura
- Changes in consciousness
- Confusion
- Fatigue
- Fever
- Headache
- Tachycardia
- Pallor
- Dyspnea on exertion
- Speech changes
- Weakness
- Jaundice

Diagnostic procedures for TTP include a history, physical examination, complete blood counts, blood smears, and lactate dehydrogenase levels. Plasmapheresis is the centerpiece of TTP treatment. Additionally, a splenectomy and glucocorticoid steroids may be necessary.

CHAPTER SUMMARY

Blood serves many purposes in the body. If this life fluid does not function properly, the body cannot maintain health and homeostasis; therefore, problems with any types of blood cells can lead to widespread and life-threatening problems. Hematologic problems can result from a variety of origins but usually lead to abnormal cell numbers or function. Timely identification and treatment of these disorders is vital for positive health-care outcomes.

REFERENCES

Centers for Disease Control and Prevention (CDC). (2013). United States cancer statistics. Retrieved from https://nccd.cdc.gov/uscs/toptencancers.aspx

Centers for Disease Control and Prevention (CDC). (2014). Epstein-Barr virus and infectious mononucleosis. Retrieved from http://www.cdc.gov/epstein-barr/

Chiras, D. (2011). *Human biology* (7th ed.). Burlington, MA: Jones & Bartlett Learning.

Copstead, L., & Banasik, J. (2014). *Pathophysiology* (5th ed.). St. Louis, MO: Elsevier.

Dean, L. (2006, April 26). Mutations and blood clots: How point mutations in clotting factor genes conspire to increase the risk of thrombosis. In L. Dean & J. McEntryre (Eds.), *Coffee break: Tutorials for NCBI tools.* Retrieved from http://www.ncbi.nlm.nih.gov/books/NBK2318

DeBruin, M., Dorresteijn, L., van't Veer, M., van der Pal, H., Kappelle, A., Alman, B., & van Leeuwen, F. (2009). Increased risk of stroke and transient ischemic attack in 5-year survivors of Hodgkin lymphoma. *Journal of National Cancer Institute, 101*(13), 928–937.

Elling, B., Elling, K., & Rothenberg, M. (2004). *Anatomy and physiology.* Sudbury, MA: Jones and Bartlett.

National Cancer Institute (NCI). (2014a). A snapshot of leukemia. Retrieved from http://www.cancer.gov/researchandfunding/snapshots/leukemia

National Cancer Institute (NCI). (2014b). A snapshot of myeloma. Retrieved from http://www.cancer.gov/researchandfunding/snapshots/myeloma

Porth, C. (2011). *Essentials of pathophysiology* (6th ed.). Philadelphia, PA: Lippincott Williams & Wilkins.

Professional guide to pathophysiology (3rd ed.). (2010). Philadelphia, PA: Lippincott Williams & Wilkins.

Schick, P. K. (2006). Anemia. Retrieved from http://teachingcases.hematology.org/schick06/index.cfm

World Health Organization. (2016). Micronutrient deficiencies. Retrieved from http://www.who.int/nutrition/topics/ida/en/index.html

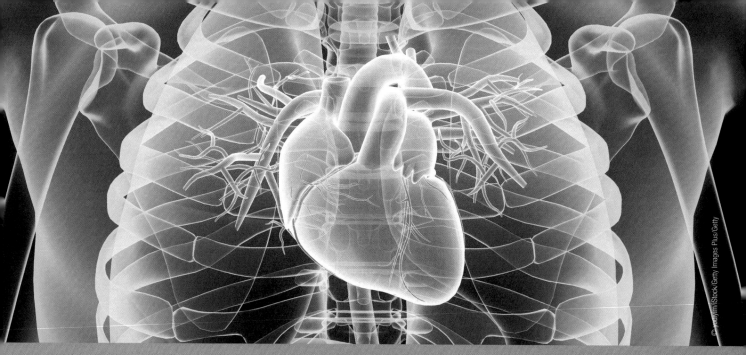

CHAPTER 4
Cardiovascular Function

LEARNING OBJECTIVES

- Discuss normal cardiovascular anatomy and physiology.
- Describe and compare cardiovascular alterations resulting in decreased cardiac output.

- Describe and compare cardiovascular alterations resulting in altered tissue perfusion.
- Explore cardiovascular alterations resulting in both decreased cardiac output and altered tissue perfusion.

KEY TERMS

afterload
aldosterone
anaphylactic shock
aneurysm
angina
antidiuretic hormone
aorta
aortic valve
arrhythmia
arteriole
artery
atherosclerosis
atresia
atrioventricular (AV) node
automaticity
baroreceptor
bundle branches
bundle of His
capillary
cardiac output
cardiac tamponade
cardiogenic shock

cardiomyopathy
chemoreceptor
chronotropic
compensatory mechanism
conductivity
constrictive pericarditis
coronary artery disease (CAD)
depolarization
diastole
diastolic dysfunction
dilated cardiomyopathy
dissecting aneurysm
distributive shock
dromotropic
dyslipidemia
dysrhythmia
eclampsia
edema
embolus
endocardium
essential hypertension
excitability

exsanguination
fatty streaks
fibrous plaque
fusiform aneurysm
heart failure
high-density lipoproteins (HDLs)
hypertension
hypertrophic cardiomyopathy
hypovolemic shock
infarction
infective endocarditis
inferior vena cava
inotropic
left atrium
left-sided heart failure
left ventricle
lipid
low-density lipoproteins (LDLs)
lung
lymph

lymphatic system
lymphedema
malignant hypertension
mitral valve
mixed dysfunction
myocardial infarction (MI)
myocarditis
myocardium
neurogenic shock
pacemaker
pericardial effusion
pericarditis
pericardium
peripheral vascular disease (PVD)
peripheral vascular resistance (PVR)
pregnancy-induced hypertension (PIH)
preload
primary hypertension
progressive stage

pulmonary artery	repolarization	stable angina pectoris	tunica adventitia
pulmonary circulation	restrictive cardiomyopathy	stenosis	tunica intima
pulmonary vein	right atrium	stroke volume	tunica media
pulmonic valve	right-sided heart failure	superior vena cava	unstable angina
pulse pressure	right ventricle	systemic circulation	varicose vein
Purkinje network of fibers	saccular aneurysm	systole	vein
Raynaud's disease	secondary hypertension	systolic dysfunction	venule
regurgitation	septic shock	thromboangiitis obliterans	
renin–angiotensin–	shock	thrombus	
aldosterone system	sinoatrial (SA) node	tricuspid valve	

The cardiovascular system is composed of the heart, blood vessels, lymphatic system, and blood (see the *Hematopoietic Function* chapter). This chapter focuses on normal and abnormal states of the heart and blood vessels. The components of the cardiovascular system work together to maintain life. Additionally, these components play a crucial role in the functioning of other systems. This pivotal role begins early in life, when the fetus is about 4 weeks old, and lasts until the end of life. Disorders of the cardiovascular system are common and complex, as they often affect other systems. Nurses in all areas of practice will likely encounter patients with problems in this system and will need to be equipped to respond to their intricate needs.

Anatomy and Physiology

The cardiovascular system is similar to the plumbing in a house. Both have a pump (the heart), a network of pipes (the blood vessels), and fluid (blood). The cardiovascular system delivers vital oxygen and nutrients to cells, removes waste products, and transports hormones. Circulation is divided into two branches—pulmonary and systemic (FIGURE 4-1). In the

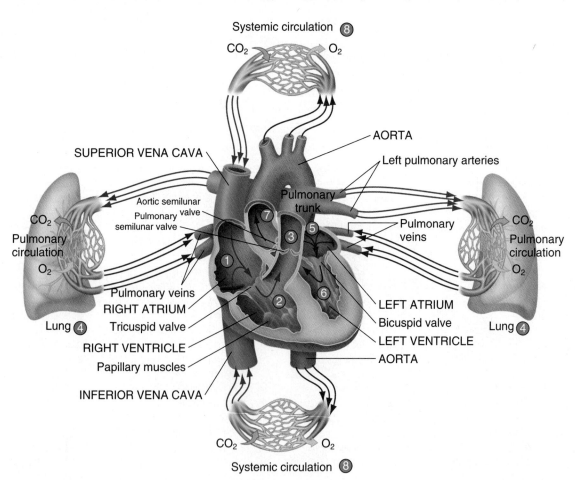

FIGURE 4-1 The cardiovascular system.

pulmonary circulation, the waste product—carbon dioxide—is exchanged for oxygen in the **lungs** through diffusion (FIGURE 4-2). In the **systemic circulation**, blood carries oxygen and nutrients to all cells and waste products to the kidneys, liver, and skin for excretion. To accomplish these transportation functions, the cardiovascular system requires a properly functioning heart to propel the blood by rhythmic contractions. The blood circulates through three types of vessels—arteries, capillaries, and veins. The lymphatic system assists in maintaining homeostasis by returning excess fluid from the body's tissues back to the circulatory system as well as by playing a vital role in the immune system (see the *Immunity* chapter). The following sections review the basic anatomy and physiology of the cardiovascular system.

Heart

Roughly the size of a closed fist, the heart is a muscular organ that pumps blood throughout the body (FIGURE 4-3). It is the workhorse of the cardiovascular system, pumping blood through the body's 50,000 miles of blood vessels and beating approximately 100,000 times per day. If you had a dollar for every heartbeat, you would be a millionaire in just 10 days. The heart can quickly adjust its rate to meet the ever-changing needs of the body.

The heart is located in the thoracic cavity between the lungs and behind the sternum. The pericardial sac, or **pericardium**, encloses the heart to provide protection and support. This sac contains approximately 50 mL of fluid and protects the heart against trauma from surrounding structures, invasions of foreign organisms, and friction from the constant movement. The pericardium provides support in terms of anchoring the heart and prevents overdistention.

The **myocardium**, the middle layer of the heart, is the muscle portion of the organ. The walls of the ventricles, especially the left ventricle, are thicker than the atrium because of the distance to which those chambers must pump blood. The atria are receiving chambers that

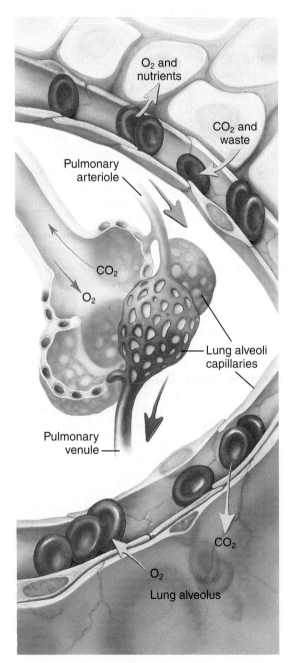

FIGURE 4-2 Pulmonary gas exchange.

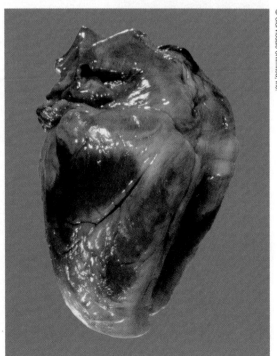

FIGURE 4-3 A normal heart.

pump blood to their respective ventricles. The ventricles pump blood outside the heart to the lungs and the systemic circulation.

The **endocardium** is the inner epithelial layer of the heart that makes up the cardiac valves; these valves function to ensure one-way flow of blood through the heart (FIGURE 4-4).

Understanding the blood flow through the heart is essential to understanding structural alterations and appreciating how they result in decreased cardiac output and/or altered tissue perfusion (FIGURE 4-5). As illustrated in blue in Figure 4-5, blood low in oxygen and rich in carbon dioxide enters the right side of the heart from the systemic circulation through the **superior vena cava** and the **inferior vena cava**. These veins empty blood directly into the **right atrium**. The right atrium pumps the blood through the **tricuspid valve** to the **right ventricle**. The right ventricle pumps the blood through the **pulmonic valve** to the pulmonary arteries. The pulmonary arteries then carry the blood to the lungs for oxygenation.

The newly oxygenated blood returns from the lungs to the heart through the pulmonary veins. From the pulmonary veins, blood enters the **left atrium**. The left atrium pumps blood through the **mitral valve** to the **left ventricle**. The left ventricle then pumps blood through the **aortic valve** to the **aorta**. At this point, the

blood is transported to the body, beginning with the coronary arteries (if the heart's needs are not met first, no other needs will be met) and the carotid arteries (the brain controls the vital bodily functions). Both atria fill and contract simultaneously; likewise, both ventricles fill and contract simultaneously (FIGURE 4-6). This coordinated contraction occurs due to the internal timing device, or **pacemaker**, of the conduction system.

Conduction System

Left to their own devices, cardiac muscle cells would contract individually, which would create a disorderly and ineffective contraction. The muscle cells are able to contract in an organized manner, however, due to the internal electrical stimulus initiated by a pacemaker. The brain controls the heart rate and contractility through sympathetic and parasympathetic stimulation of the autonomic nervous system. Basically, the heart's pacemaker acts like a generator creating an impulse for every heartbeat. **Conductivity** is the ability of cells to conduct electrical impulses. The ability of the cells to respond to electrical impulses is referred to as **excitability**. Cardiac cells are able to generate an impulse to contract even with no external nerve stimulus, a process called **automaticity**.

All cardiac muscle cells can initiate impulses, but normally the conduction pathway originates in the **sinoatrial (SA) node** located high in the right atrium (FIGURE 4-7). Impulses originating in the SA node travel through the right and left atria, resulting in atrial contraction. The SA node automatically generates impulses ranging from 60 to 100 beats per minute (sinus rhythm). The impulse then travels to the **atrioventricular (AV) node**, which is located in the right atrium adjacent to the septum. Although it does not usually initiate impulses unless the SA node begins failing, the intrinsic rate of impulses in the AV node is 40–60 beats per minute. The impulses are delayed, or move slowly, through the AV node to allow for complete ventricular filling.

Next, the impulses move in rapid succession through the **bundle of His**, right and left **bundle branches**, and **Purkinje network of fibers**, which stimulates ventricular contraction. If the impulses fail to fire from the SA or AV node, the ventricles will attempt to pace themselves. The ventricles can generate impulses at 20–40 beats per minute, which may not result in adequate cardiac output because the ventricles may beat before they have a

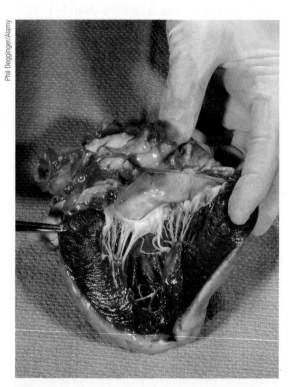

Phil Degginger/Alamy

FIGURE 4-4 Heart valves.

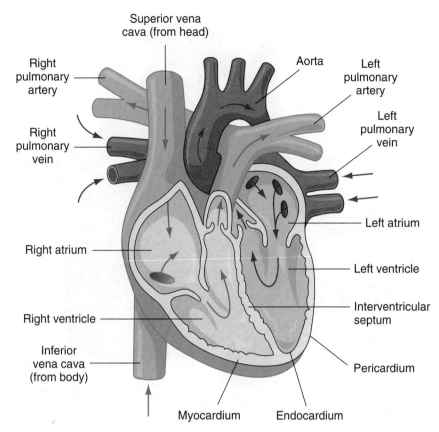

Superior vena
cava (from head)

Aorta

Right
pulmonary
artery

Left
pulmonary
artery

Left
pulmonary
vein

Right
pulmonary
vein

Left atrium

Right atrium

Left ventricle

Interventricular
septum

Right ventricle

Inferior
vena cava
(from body)

Pericardium

Myocardium   Endocardium

FIGURE 4-5 Blood flow through the heart.

chance to fill with blood. These optional pacemakers in the heart function as a fail-safe mechanism to sustain life.

The cardiac impulse conduction produces an electric current that can be read by electrodes attached to the skin at various points of the body, producing an electrocardiogram (EKG)

(**FIGURE 4-8**). Organized **depolarization** (an increase in electrical charge through the exchange of ions across the cell membrane) of the cardiac cells generates cardiac muscle contraction. On the EKG reading, atrial contraction is represented by depolarization in the P wave, and ventricular contraction is represented by

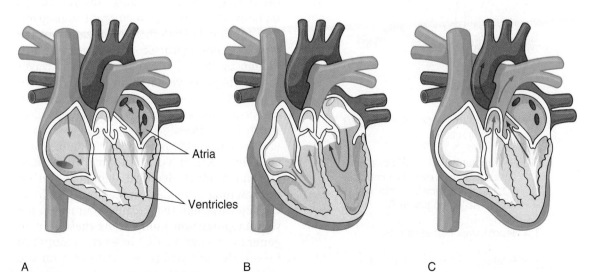

Atria

Ventricles

A   B   C

FIGURE 4-6 Blood flow through the heart. (a) Blood enters both atria simultaneously from the systemic and pulmonary circuits. (b) When full, the atria pump their blood into the ventricles. (c) When the ventricles are full, they contract simultaneously, delivering the blood to the pulmonary and systemic circuits.

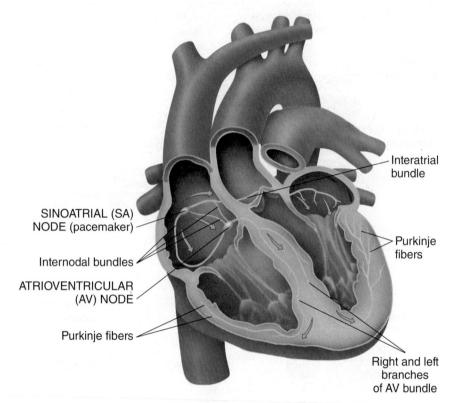

FIGURE 4-7 Electrical conduction through the heart.

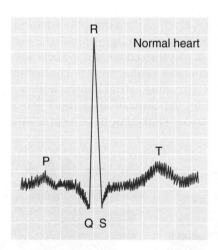

P = Atrial depolarization, which triggers atrial contraction.

QRS = Depolarization of AV node and conduction of electrical impulse through ventricles. Ventricular contraction begins at R.

T = Repolarization of ventricles.

P to R interval = Time required for impulses to travel from SA node to ventricles.

FIGURE 4-8 Characteristic features of a normal electrocardiogram.

depolarization in the large QRS complex. The more intense the contraction, the higher the wave or complex. Because the force required for the atria to pump blood into the ventricles is minimal compared to the force required for the ventricles to pump blood to the entire body, the P wave is smaller than the QRS complex. The T wave represents **repolarization**, or recovery, of the ventricles. In repolarization, the ions line up on both sides of the cell membrane in preparation for depolarization. Repolarization of the atria does not appear on an EKG because it is hidden by the other, more prominent waveforms. Abnormal variations in the EKG, known as **arrhythmias** or **dysrhythmias**, may indicate acute problems, such as **infarction** or electrolyte imbalances.

Cardiac muscle cells require sodium (Na^+), potassium (K^+), and calcium (Ca^+) ions to initiate and conduct electrical signals as well as the resulting muscular contraction. To initiate the depolarization that creates contraction, the sodium–potassium pump shifts these ions to generate a charge. Ca^+ balance is required for muscle contractility, especially in a muscle that contracts many times each minute. Additionally, the neurologic system controls cardiac function, and it requires Na^+ balance to function properly.

The brain (specifically the medulla) monitors and controls cardiac function through the autonomic nervous system, endocrine system, and cardiac tissue. These functions include the rate of contraction (**chronotropic** effect), rate of electrical conduction (**dromotropic** effect), and strength of contraction (**inotropic** effect). Receptors in the brain, heart, blood vessels, and kidneys continuously monitor body functions to maintain homeostasis. **Chemoreceptors** detect chemical changes in the blood, and **baroreceptors**, located in the carotid arteries, detect pressure in the heart and arteries. If homeostasis is interrupted, receptors begin to fire and neurotransmitters or hormones that activate either the sympathetic nervous system (SNS) or the parasympathetic nervous system (PNS) are released. Stimulating the SNS will increase heart rate and blood pressure, whereas PNS stimulation will decrease heart rate and blood pressure.

Blood Pressure

Blood pressure refers to the force that blood exerts on the walls of blood vessels. This pressure is described as a fraction with the **systole** (work) measurement as the top number and the **diastole** (rest) measurement as the bottom number. According to the American Heart Association, a normal blood pressure reading should be in the range of 120/80 mm Hg to maintain health and limit chronic disease risk. The systolic pressure is the force the blood exerts on the arteries when ejected from the left ventricle. The diastolic pressure is the force in the arteries when the ventricles are relaxed. Blood pressure is commonly measured using a sphygmomanometer and the brachial artery. **Pulse pressure** is the difference between the systolic and diastolic pressures and represents the force the heart generates each time it contracts.

Blood pressure changes in response to the individual's activity and stress level, and it also varies at different points of the body. Cardiac output and peripheral vascular resistance significantly affect blood pressure ($BP = CO \times PVR$, where BP is blood pressure, CO is cardiac output, and PVR is peripheral vascular resistance). Other variables that influence blood pressure include blood volume and viscosity, venous return, heart rate, cardiac contractility, and arterial elasticity. Typically, increases in these variables will increase blood pressure—with the exception of arterial elasticity. **Cardiac output** refers to the amount of blood the heart pumps in one minute. This amount is determined by stroke volume and heart rate ($CO = SV \times HR$, where CO is cardiac output, SV is stroke volume,

and HR is heart rate). **Stroke volume** is the amount of blood ejected from the heart with each contraction. **Peripheral vascular resistance (PVR)** is the force opposing the blood in the peripheral circulation; it increases as the diameter of the blood vessels decreases. Stimulation of the SNS can initiate systemic vasoconstriction to raise blood pressure. This vasoconstriction is helpful in times of hypotension, such as with shock. PVR affects **afterload**, the pressure that the left ventricle must exert to get the blood out of the heart and into the aorta. The higher the afterload, the harder it is for the heart to eject the blood, thus lowering stroke volume. In addition to afterload, stroke volume is affected by **preload**, the amount of blood returning to the heart that the heart must then manage. Additionally, both afterload and preload can affect blood pressure. As afterload and preload increase, blood pressure increases.

Hormones also influence blood pressure. **Antidiuretic hormone** increases water reabsorption in the kidney, which increases blood volume and blood pressure. Additionally, antidiuretic hormone is a vasoconstrictor, which increases PVR. **Aldosterone** increases blood volume by increasing the reabsorption of Na^+ in the kidneys; Na^+ attracts water. Increasing renal water reabsorption increases blood volume.

The **renin–angiotensin–aldosterone system** in the kidneys is another vital control and compensatory mechanism that becomes activated when renal blood flow is decreased, as is often the case in hypotensive states (FIGURE 4-9). When renal blood flow decreases, renin is released from the kidneys, activating angiotensin I, which is then converted to angiotensin II (a vasoconstrictor), and stimulating aldosterone

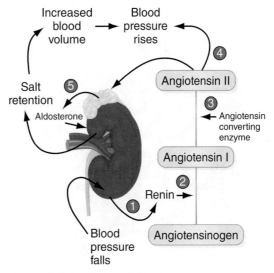

FIGURE 4-9 Role of kidneys in blood pressure.

secretion. In hypotensive states, this mechanism raises blood pressure and maintains the blood supply to vital organs. In chronic disease states such as hypertension, this mechanism is inappropriately activated because of vasoconstriction to the kidneys, further contributing to the hypertension.

Blood Vessels

Blood vessels are the intricate highway system along which the blood travels. **Arteries** carry blood away from the heart, while **veins** carry blood back to the heart. Left ventricular contractions project blood through the arteries, while valves in the veins assist in moving the blood back to the heart against gravity. Once arteries leave the heart, they begin branching into smaller vessels called **arterioles** (FIGURE 4-10). These vessels continue branching into even smaller, thin-walled vessels called **capillaries**. Their thin walls allow oxygen and nutrients to shift out of the capillaries into the cells. Additionally, carbon dioxide and waste products shift from the cells into the capillaries. This exchange occurs through diffusion (see the *Cellular Function* chapter). Once blood is utilized at the cellular level, the blood moves through the capillaries and transitions into larger vessels known as **venules**. The venules continue to merge into larger vessels until they become veins, much as small streams unite to form a river.

Generally, arteries carry blood rich in oxygen and nutrients, while veins carry blood saturated with carbon dioxide and metabolic waste. One exception to this pattern occurs in the pulmonary arteries and veins. The **pulmonary arteries** carry oxygen-depleted blood away from the right side of the heart to the lungs for gas exchange (Figure 4-2). Following gas exchange in the lungs,

the oxygen-saturated blood returns to the left side of the heart through the **pulmonary veins**.

The walls of the blood vessels consist of three layers (FIGURE 4-11). The **tunica intima** is the smooth, thin, inner layer of the blood vessels. The **tunica media**, the middle layer, is composed of elastic tissue and smooth muscle that is responsible for the vessel's ability to change diameter. The outer layer, the **tunica adventitia**, consists of elastic and fibrous connective tissues that

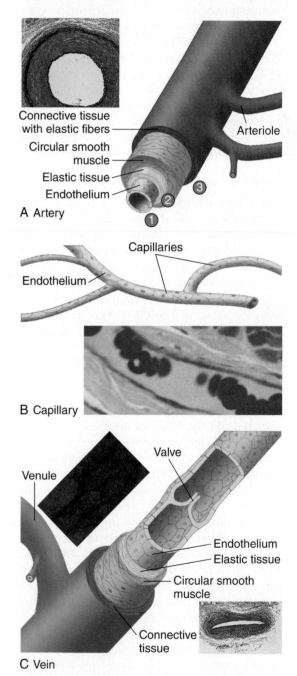

FIGURE 4-11 The walls of the blood vessels are composed of three layers of tissue: the endothelium, elastic tissue, and the connective tissue. (a) Artery; (b) capillary; (c) vein.

Artery photo: © Cabisco/Visuals Unlimited, Inc.; Capillary photo: © Ed Reschke/ Photolibrary/Getty Images; Vein photos: © Cabisco/Visuals Unlimited, Inc. and © Dr. John D. Cunningham/Visuals Unlimited, Inc.

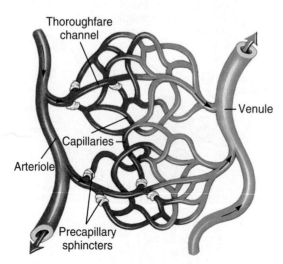

FIGURE 4-10 The circulatory system.

provide the necessary "give" to accommodate the rush of blood with each cardiac contraction.

Lymphatic System

The **lymphatic system** is an extensive network of vessels and glands that returns excess fluid in body tissue to the circulatory system and works with the immune system (see the *Immunity* chapter). Interstitial fluid surrounds cells and provides a medium through which nutrients, gases, and wastes can diffuse between the capillaries and the cells. Capillaries are continuously replenishing this fluid. Normally, the fluid outflow from the capillaries exceeds the fluid returned. Lymph capillaries absorb the excess fluid (**FIGURE 4-12**). This fluid, or **lymph**, drains from these capillaries into larger vessels and ducts that empty into large veins at the base of the neck. The movement of lymph occurs in much the same way that blood travels through the veins, with the assistance of valves and body movement.

The lymphatic system also includes several organs—lymph nodes, the spleen, the thymus, and the tonsils. These organs primarily function in the immune response (see the *Immunity* chapter). Located in clusters throughout the body, lymph nodes are a network of fibers and irregular channels that slow down the lymph flow. As the lymph passes through the nodes, the fibers filter out bacteria, viruses, and cellular debris. Numerous macrophages line the channels to phagocytize microorganisms and other material.

Normally, the rate at which lymph is produced equals the rate at which it is removed. In some body states, however, the amount of lymph produced exceeds the capacity of the system. For example, burns can cause extensive damage to capillaries, causing them to leak fluid into the tissues. This flooding results in excessive fluid in the tissue, or **edema**. In contrast, lymphatic vessels may sometimes become occluded, often because of infection.

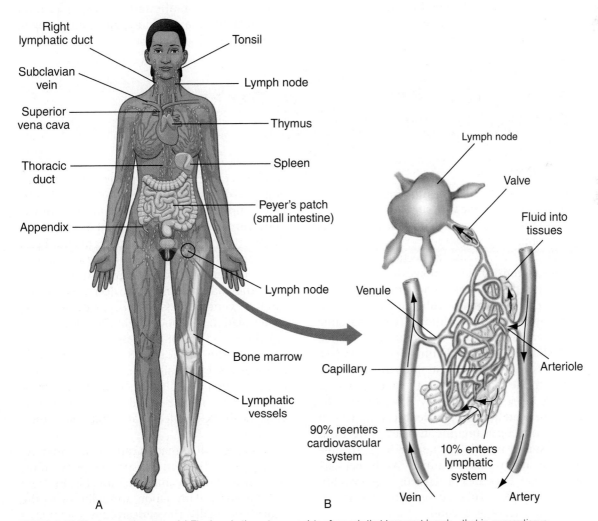

FIGURE 4-12 The lymphatic system. (a) The lymphatic system consists of vessels that transport lymph—that is, excess tissue fluid—back to the circulatory system. (b) Lymph is picked up by lymphatic capillaries that drain into larger vessels. Like the veins, the lymphatic vessels contain valves that prohibit backflow. Lymph nodes are interspersed along the vessels and serve to filter the lymph.

UNDERSTANDING CONDITIONS THAT AFFECT THE CARDIOVASCULAR SYSTEM

When considering alterations in the cardiovascular system, organizing them based on their basic underlying pathophysiology can increase understanding. These concepts are based on the two major cardiac-related nursing diagnoses—decreased cardiac output and altered tissue perfusion. Understanding what each of those diagnoses means facilitates understanding of the conditions that lead to their development.

Decreased cardiac output refers to states in which the amount of blood being pumped by the heart is less than normal. Decreased cardiac output can be associated with changes in preload, afterload, contractility, or dysrhythmias. Typical manifestations reflect the inability to meet the body's needs and may include fatigue, oliguria, cyanosis, fluid accumulation, and decreased peripheral pulses.

Altered tissue perfusion refers to a state in which there is a decrease in nutrition and oxygenation at the cellular level due to a deficit in capillary blood flow supply. Altered tissue perfusion can be associated with an interruption of blood flow, decreased cellular exchange, or fluid shifts. Typical manifestations reflect cellular ischemia and may include pain, skin changes, and signs of organ necrosis.

ALTERATIONS RESULTING IN DECREASED CARDIAC OUTPUT

Pericarditis

Pericarditis refers to an inflammation of the pericardium—the sac that surrounds, protects, and supports the heart. This inflammation is most commonly triggered by viral infections (usually after a respiratory infection), but it may also result from other infections, thoracic trauma (e.g., surgery, radiation, accidents), myocardial infarction, malignancy, tuberculosis, uremia, and autoimmune conditions (e.g., systemic lupus erythematosus, rheumatoid arthritis, scleroderma). In this inflammatory process (see the *Immunity* chapter), fluid shifts from the capillaries to the space between the pericardial sac and the heart. This fluid may be serous (resulting from heart failure), purulent (resulting from infections), serosanguineous (resulting from neoplasms or uremia), or hemorrhagic (resulting from aneurysms or trauma). As the pericardial tissue becomes inflamed, the swollen pericardial tissue rubs against the swollen cardiac tissue, creating friction.

Fluid can accumulate in the pericardial cavity, creating a **pericardial effusion**. This condition can eventually progress to life-threatening **cardiac tamponade** (FIGURE 4-13). In cardiac tamponade, the fluid accumulates in the pericardial cavity to the point that it compresses the heart. This compression prevents the heart from stretching and filling during diastole, resulting in decreased cardiac output. Arterial pressures then fall (because of the decreased cardiac output), venous pressures rise (because of the accumulation of blood within the systemic circulation), and the pulse pressure narrows (because of the arterial and venous pressure changes). Additionally, the heart sounds are muffled upon auscultation because the excess fluid drowns out the sound. Heart failure, cardiogenic shock, and death can result from cardiac tamponade.

Chronic inflammation can lead to **constrictive pericarditis**. In constrictive pericarditis, the pericardium becomes thick and fibrous from the chronic inflammation and adheres to the heart. Essentially, the pericardium resembles a restrictive rubber band that has lost its elasticity. The loss of elasticity restricts cardiac filling,

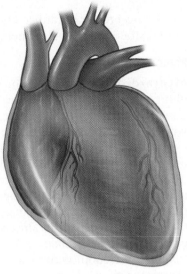
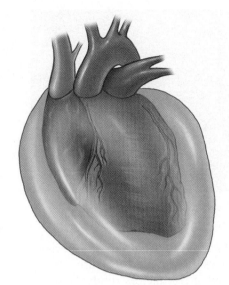

Normal heart   Cardiac tamponade

FIGURE 4-13 Cardiac tamponade.

decreasing cardiac output and causing systemic congestion.

Clinical manifestations of pericarditis include the following signs and symptoms:

- Pericardial friction rub (a grating sound heard when the breath is held)
- Sharp, sudden, severe chest pain that increases with deep inspiration and decreases when the patient sits up and leans forward
- Dyspnea
- Tachycardia
- Palpitations
- Edema
- Flulike symptoms (e.g., fever, chills, and myalgia)

Diagnosis of pericarditis is accomplished through a history, physical examination, complete blood count (CBC), EKG, chest X-ray, echocardiogram, computed tomography (CT), and magnetic resonance imaging (MRI). Treatment focuses on treating the underlying cause (e.g., antibiotics) and reducing the inflammation (e.g., nonsteroidal and steroidal anti-inflammatory drugs). Analgesics may be administered to manage pain. Additionally, bed rest is important to reduce metabolic needs and cardiac workload. Oxygen therapy can increase available oxygen. A pericardiocentesis may be performed to withdraw excess fluid from pericardium, or a pericardiectomy (a surgical procedure in which a window is created in the pericardium) may be performed to release constriction and allow excess fluid to drain into the pleural cavity.

Infective Endocarditis

Infective endocarditis (previously called bacterial endocarditis) is an infection of the endocardium (inner layers of the heart) or heart valves. *Streptococcus viridans*, commonly found in the mouth, accounts for 50% of all infective endocarditis cases (National Institutes of Health [NIH], 2010). This bacterium can gain access to the bloodstream during dental procedures. *Staphylococcus aureus* and *S. enterococcus*—bacteria commonly found on the skin and in the gastrointestinal tract—are also frequent causative agents.

The pathogenesis of this condition involves endothelial damage, which attracts platelets and stimulates thrombus formation. Vegetation (including platelets, fibrin, microorganisms, inflammatory cells, and granulomatous tissue) collects on the internal structures because of damage from the infection, much like the process that occurs when a boat's anchor is placed in a body of water for an extended length of time. With each heart contraction, some of this vegetation is dislodged and ejected from the heart. These small thrombi move throughout the body, collecting in the microcirculation and creating microhemorrhages (e.g., petechiae and hematuria). The thrombi can also travel to other locations, in which case they are known as embolisms, and become lodged there. These emboli can cause serious and often life-threatening complications such as myocardial infarction, stroke, seizures, and pulmonary embolism. In addition, the heart valves can become scarred and perforated (**FIGURE 4-14**). If untreated,

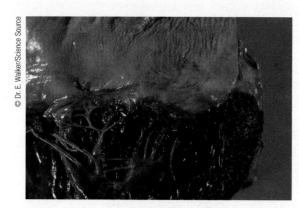

FIGURE 4-14 Infective endocarditis.

infective endocarditis is usually fatal, especially when it involves the valvular structures.

The following risk factors render patients more vulnerable to development of infective endocarditis:

- Intravenous drug use or presence of an intravenous catheter for an extended period
- Valvular disorders
- Prosthetic heart valves
- Implanted cardiac devices (e.g., pacemaker, internal cardioverter)
- Rheumatic heart disease
- Coarctation of the aorta
- Congenital heart defects (e.g., tetralogy of Fallot)
- Marfan syndrome

Clinical manifestations of infective endocarditis include the following:

- Flulike symptoms (e.g., fever, chills, myalgia)
- Embolization (e.g., myocardial infarction, pulmonary embolism, stroke, splenic infarction)
- Heart murmur
- Petechiae
- Splinter hemorrhages under the nails
- Hematuria
- Osler's nodes (tender, raised, subcutaneous lesions on the fingers and toes)
- Edema

Diagnostic procedures for infective endocarditis include a history, physical examination, blood cultures, CBC, urinalysis, serum rheumatoid factor, erythrocyte sedimentation rate, EKG, and echocardiogram. Treatment focuses on the causative agent (e.g., antibiotics or antifungals). Infective endocarditis often requires long-term anti-infective therapy (a minimum of 4 weeks). Other treatments are initiated to maintain cardiac function and treat other symptoms:

- Bed rest
- Oxygen therapy

- Antipyretics
- Surgical repair of cardiac valves
- Prosthetic valve replacement

Myocarditis

Myocarditis is an inflammation of the myocardium, or heart muscle. This uncommon condition is poorly understood because at least several weeks (in some cases a decade) elapse between exposure of the causative agent and the development of symptoms. Myocarditis is usually caused by viral (e.g., influenza, coxsackie, cytomegalovirus, adenovirus, hepatitis C, herpes, HIV, or parvovirus), bacterial (e.g., Lyme disease, *Chlamydia*, *Mycoplasma*, or *Streptococcus*), or fungal (e.g., *Aspergillus*, *Candida*, *Cryptococcus*, or *Histoplasma*) infection. Other causes may include allergic reactions, chemical exposure, radiation, or inflammatory disorders (e.g., rheumatoid arthritis or sarcoidosis). Penetration of organisms, blood cells, toxins, and immune substances into the myocardium can result in muscle fiber dysfunction and degeneration that can impair contractility and conduction. Most cases of myocarditis are benign, but some result in heart failure, cardiomyopathy, dysrhythmias, and thrombi development.

The patient may be asymptomatic, but when present, clinical manifestations of myocarditis include the following:

- Flulike symptoms (e.g., fever, chills, myalgia)
- Dyspnea
- Dysrhythmias
- Tachycardia
- Heart murmurs
- Chest discomfort
- Cardiac enlargement
- Pale, cool extremities
- Syncope
- Decreased urine output
- Joint pain and swelling

Diagnosis of myocarditis is accomplished through a history, physical examination, blood cultures, EKG, cardiac enzymes (e.g., troponin and creatinine kinase), CBC, erythrocyte sedimentation rate, chest X-rays, echocardiogram, and myocardium biopsy. Management centers on treating the causative agent (e.g., antibiotics and antifungals). Antipyretics, anticoagulants, antidysrhythmics, diuretics, and immunosuppressants (e.g., corticosteroids or nonsteroidal anti-inflammatory drugs) may be used to treat symptoms or complications. Increasing bed rest, restricting activity, and limiting fluids can reduce cardiac workload.

Mrs. Fulcher is a 58-year-old married homemaker who was recently discharged from the hospital because of recurrent infective endocarditis. Her most recent episodes were a *Staphylococcus aureus* infection of the mitral valve 12 months ago and a *Streptococcus mutans* infection of the aortic valve 1 month ago. During her most recent hospitalization, an echocardiogram showed aortic stenosis, moderate aortic insufficiency, chronic valvular vegetation, and moderate atrial enlargement. In addition, Mrs. Fulcher has a history of chronic joint pain.

After being home for 1 week, Mrs. Fulcher was readmitted to your telemetry floor with endocarditis. She reports chills, fever, fatigue, joint pain, malaise, and a headache for the last 24 hours. Upon admission, IV infusion of normal saline at 125 mL/hr and vancomycin IV every 8 hours was ordered to be continued over the next 4 weeks. Other routine medications ordered included furosemide (Lasix), amlodipine (Norvasc), and metoprolol (Lopressor). At admission, Mrs. Fulcher's blood pressure was 172/48 mm Hg (supine) and 100/40 mm Hg (sitting), her pulse was 116, respirations were 20, and her temperature was 101.9°F. Additional assessment findings included a murmur; 2+ pitting tibial edema; no peripheral cyanosis; lungs sounds clear bilateral; orientation to person, place, and time but drowsiness; hematuria; and multiple petechiae on the skin of her arms, legs, and chest.

1. What is the significance of the orthostatic hypotension, the wide pulse pressure, and tachycardia?
2. What is the significance of the hematuria, joint pain, and petechiae?
3. For which complications of embolization should Mrs. Fulcher be assessed?

Valvular Disorders

Valvular disorders cause disruption of normal blood flow through the heart. These disorders are distinguished based one the valve affected and the type of alteration. Two types of alterations can occur—stenosis or regurgitation.

Stenosis is a narrowing of a tubular structure—in this case, heart valves. When the valves are stenosed, blood moving through the valve is reduced, causing blood to back up in the chamber just before the valve. **Atresia** refers to a lack of the valve opening that would otherwise allow blood flow. Pressures in the overfilled chambers increase to pump against the resistance of the stenosed valve. Because the heart (specifically the chamber) is working harder, hypertrophy of the chambers develops. Hypertrophy and increased workload escalate the heart's oxygen demands, but the decreased cardiac output resulting from the stenosis makes it difficult to meet these increased demands. Decreased cardiac output diminishes blood delivery to the coronary arteries that supply the heart. Without adequate blood flow, the heart deteriorates.

Regurgitation, also called insufficiency or incompetence, occurs when the valve leaflets do not completely close. Normally, heart valves allow blood to flow in one direction; incompetent valves, however, allow blood to flow in both directions. This regurgitation of blood increases the amount of blood that must be pumped and, in turn, the cardiac workload. The increased workload contributes to hypertrophy developing in the affected chambers. Additionally, the increased blood volume in the heart causes the chambers to dilate to accommodate the larger volume.

Valvular disorders may have a number of causes:

- Congenital defects
- Infective endocarditis
- Rheumatic fever
- Hypertension
- Myocardial infarction
- Cardiomyopathy
- Heart failure

The clinical manifestations of valvular disorders depend on the valve involved and the nature of the alteration (**TABLE 4-1**). Diagnostic procedures for valvular heart disease consist of a history, physical examination, heart catheterization, chest X-rays, echocardiogram, EKG, or MRI. Medications often used to treat valvular disorders include diuretics, antidysrhythmics, vasodilators, angiotensin-converting enzyme (ACE) inhibitors, beta-adrenergic blockers, and anticoagulants that decrease the workload on the heart. Additional strategies may include the following measures:

- Oxygen therapy
- Low-sodium diet
- Surgical valve repair (e.g., balloon valvuloplasty)
- Prosthetic valve replacement (e.g., mechanical or biological pig, cow, or human valve)

TABLE 4-1   Clinical Manifestations of Valvular Stenosis and Regurgitation

Manifestation	Aortic Stenosis	Aortic Regurgitation	Mitral Stenosis	Mitral Regurgitation	Tricuspid Regurgitation
Cardiovascular effects	Left ventricular hypertrophy, angina	Left heart hypertrophy, angina	Right ventricular hypertrophy, angina	Left heart hypertrophy, angina	Right heart hypertrophy, angina
General symptoms	Fatigue	Fatigue	Fatigue, edema	Fatigue, dizziness, peripheral edema	Peripheral edema
Respiratory effects	Dyspnea on exertion	Dyspnea on exertion	Dyspnea on exertion, orthopnea, paroxysmal, nocturnal dyspnea, predisposition to respiratory infections, hemoptysis, pulmonary hypertension	Dyspnea; occasional hemoptysis	Dyspnea
Central nervous system effects	Syncope, especially on exertion	Syncope	Neural deficits only associated with emboli	None	None
Gastrointestinal effects	None	None	Ascites; hepatic angina with hepatomegaly	None	Ascites, hepatomegaly (with heart failure)
Heart rate, rhythm	Bradycardia, variety of dysrhythmias	Palpitations, water hammer pulse	Palpitations	Palpitations	Atrial fibrillation
Heart sounds	Systolic murmur	Diastolic and systolic murmurs	Diastolic murmur, accentuated first heart sound	Murmur throughout systole	Murmur throughout systole
Most common cause	Congenital, rheumatic fever	Bacterial endocarditis; aortic root disease	Rheumatic fever	Insufficient valve; coronary artery disease	Congenital

Modified from Huether, S., & McCance, K. (2000). *Understanding pathophysiology* (2nd ed.). St. Louis, MO: C. V. Mosby.

Cardiomyopathy

Cardiomyopathy generally refers to a group of conditions that weaken and enlarge the myocardium. These conditions may be acquired or inherited. Most cardiomyopathies are classified into three groups—dilated, hypertrophic, and restrictive (FIGURE 4-15).

Dilated cardiomyopathy develops when the ventricles become enlarged and weakened. Usually this condition starts in the left ventricle and eventually affects the right ventricle. Risk for developing dilated cardiomyopathy increases with age, and this condition is more common in African American men. Most cases are idiopathic. Dilated cardiomyopathy can be inherited, but secondary causes include the following:

- Chemotherapy (specifically doxorubicin and daunorubicin)
- Alcoholism
- Cocaine and amphetamine abuse
- Pregnancy
- Infections
- Thyrotoxicosis (hypermetabolic syndrome resulting from increased levels of thyroid hormones)
- Diabetes mellitus

Normal heart

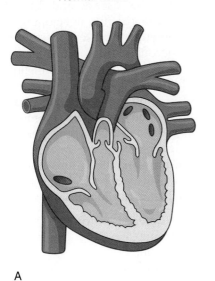

A

Dilated cardiomyopathy

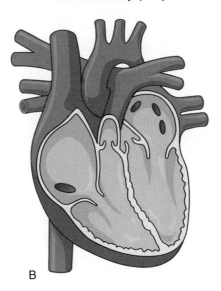

B

Hypertrophic cardiomyopathy

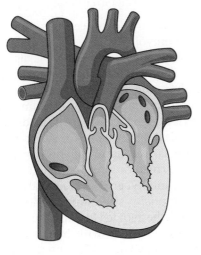

C

Restrictive cardiomyopathy

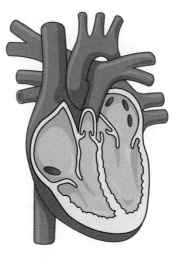

D

FIGURE 4-15 Comparing cardiomyopathies.

- Neuromuscular diseases (e.g., muscular dystrophy)
- Hypertension
- Coronary artery disease
- Hypersensitivity to medications

Dilated cardiomyopathy occurs when myocardium muscle fibers are extensively damaged by cardiomegaly and ventricular dilation. Consequently, myocardial contractility is decreased, resulting in impaired systolic function and decreased cardiac output. Blood can stagnate in the heart, causing thrombi to develop. The SNS and the kidneys attempt to compensate for the falling cardiac output by increasing the heart rate and the blood volume. Symptoms develop as these compensatory mechanisms begin failing. Deterioration is rapid once symptoms appear.

The following clinical manifestations of dilated cardiomyopathy often develop insidiously:

- Dyspnea
- Fatigue
- Nonproductive cough
- Orthopnea (difficulty breathing while lying down)
- Paroxysmal nocturnal dyspnea (difficulty breathing at night)
- Dysrhythmias
- Angina (cardiac chest pain that often occurs with exertion)
- Dizziness
- Activity intolerance
- Blood pressure changes
- Tachycardia
- Murmurs
- Abnormal lung sounds (e.g., crackles and wheezes)
- Tachypnea
- Peripheral edema
- Ascites (fluid in the peritoneal cavity)
- Weak pedal pulses
- Cool, pale extremities
- Poor capillary refill
- Hepatomegaly
- Jugular vein distension

Diagnostic procedures for dilated cardiomyopathy include an echocardiogram, EKG, chest X-ray, heart catheterization, and nuclear studies. Treatment is mainly supportive, focusing on relieving heart failure symptoms by decreasing afterload and enhancing contractility. Pharmacologic treatments usually include ACE inhibitors, diuretics, digoxin (Lanoxin), beta-adrenergic blockers, and antidysrhythmics to decrease the cardiac workload. Other management strategies include an implantable cardiac defibrillator, cardioversion, pacemaker, valvular repair, and heart transplant. Additionally, lifestyle modification includes a low-fat, low-sodium diet, tobacco cessation, physical activity, and abstinence from alcohol.

Unlike dilated cardiomyopathy, which affects only systolic function, **hypertrophic cardiomyopathy** affects both systolic and diastolic function. Hypertrophic cardiomyopathy is very common, affecting 1 out of 500 people (NIH, 2016). This condition is more common in those persons who have a more sedentary lifestyle, and it appears to have an autosomal dominant genetic base. Hypertension, obstructive valvular disease, and thyroid disease increase the risk for developing hypertrophic cardiomyopathy. The hypertrophied ventricle wall becomes stiff and unable to relax during ventricular filling. With a reduction in ventricular filling, cardiac output decreases while atrial and pulmonary pressures increase. Hypertrophic cardiomyopathy is a common cause of sudden cardiac death in young people, especially young athletes.

Clinical manifestations of hypertrophic cardiomyopathy are similar to those associated with dilated cardiomyopathy:

- Dyspnea on exertion
- Fatigue
- Syncope
- Orthopnea
- Angina
- Activity intolerance
- Dysrhythmias
- Left ventricular failure
- Myocardial infarction

Diagnostic procedures for hypertrophic cardiomyopathy are similar to those for dilated cardiomyopathy. Treatment goals include reducing ventricular stiffness, improving ventricular filling, and enhancing cardiac output. Beta-adrenergic blockers and calcium-channel blockers are often included in the medication regimen. Surgical removal of excess myocardium may be necessary for those patients who do not respond well to medications. Treatment of any dysrhythmias and hypertension may also be warranted. Additionally, strenuous activity (e.g., running) should be avoided because most cases of sudden death associated with hypertrophic cardiomyopathy have occurred with this type of activity.

Restrictive cardiomyopathy is the least common of the cardiomyopathies, but it is endemic in parts of South and Central America, India, Asia, and Africa. This type of cardiomyopathy is characterized by rigidity of the ventricles, leading to diastolic dysfunction. Causes of restrictive cardiomyopathy include the following conditions:

- Amyloidosis (buildup of fat and proteins in the heart muscle)
- Hemochromatosis (excessive amounts of iron in the heart)
- Radiation exposure to the chest
- Connective tissue diseases
- Buildup of scar tissue after a myocardial infarction
- Sarcoidosis (cellular growths on various organs)
- Cardiac neoplasms

Many cases are asymptomatic, but the following clinical manifestations may also appear with restrictive cardiomyopathy:

- Fatigue
- Dyspnea
- Orthopnea
- Abnormal lung sounds
- Angina
- Hepatomegaly
- Jugular vein distension
- Ascites
- Murmurs
- Peripheral cyanosis
- Pallor

Diagnostic procedures include those for the two previously discussed cardiomyopathies. Management focuses on treating the underlying cause, dysrhythmias, and heart failure. A heart transplant may be necessary when the heart can no longer meet the body's demands. The prognosis with restrictive cardiomyopathy is generally poor, with death often occurring from heart failure.

Electrical Alterations

As previously mentioned, normal myocardial contraction is accomplished by electrical impulses originating in the SA node, the natural pacemaker of the heart. Normal electric conduction is referred to as sinus rhythm, whereas deviations from normal are referred to as dysrhythmias or arrhythmias. Dysrhythmias vary in severity and are classified according to their origin (FIGURE 4-16). Their effects on cardiac output and blood pressure are partially influenced by their site of origin, which also determines the dysrhythmias' clinical significance. Causes of dysrhythmias include the following conditions:

- Acid–base imbalances
- Hypoxia
- Congenital heart defects
- Connective tissue disorders
- Degeneration of conductive tissues (usually as a result of aging)
- Drug toxicity
- Electrolyte imbalances (especially potassium and calcium)
- Stress
- Myocardial hypertrophy
- Myocardial ischemia or infarction

Clinical manifestations may vary according to the specific dysrhythmia (Figure 4-16). Some dysrhythmias may be asymptomatic, whereas others can cause sudden death. The danger and symptoms depend on the extent they reduce cardiac output. Some general manifestations of dysrhythmias include the following signs and symptoms:

- Palpitations
- Fluttering sensation
- Skipped beats
- Fatigue
- Confusion
- Syncope
- Dyspnea
- Abnormal heart rate

Diagnostic procedures for dysrhythmias include a history, physical examination, EKG, and invasive electrophysiologic studies. Additional tests may be performed to identify the underlying cause. Pharmacology is the mainstay of treatment (Figure 4-16). Other interventions may include an internal cardiac defibrillator, pacemaker, cardioversion, defibrillation, and ablation. Avoiding triggers such as caffeine, tobacco, and stress can decrease the occurrence and severity of some dysrhythmias.

Heart Failure

Heart failure, often referred to as heart failure, is a condition in which the heart is unable to pump an adequate amount of blood to meet the body's metabolic needs. This pump inadequacy epitomizes the nursing diagnosis of decreased cardiac output, and it leads to decreased cardiac output, increased preload, and increased afterload. These three events, in turn, result in decreased contractility and stroke volume. Some general causes of heart failure include congenital heart defects, myocardial

Dysrhythmia	Features	Causes

Supraventricular Rhythms

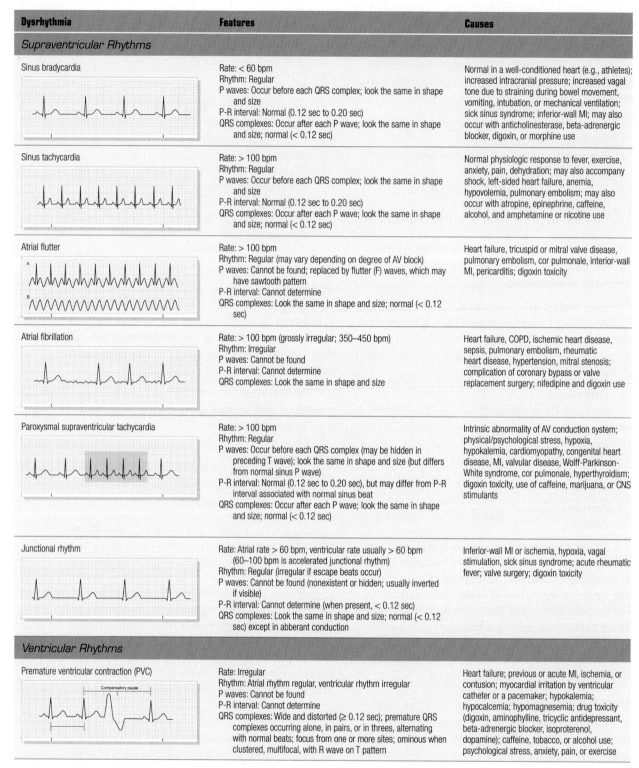

Sinus bradycardia	Rate: < 60 bpm Rhythm: Regular P waves: Occur before each QRS complex; look the same in shape and size P-R interval: Normal (0.12 sec to 0.20 sec) QRS complexes: Occur after each P wave; look the same in shape and size; normal (< 0.12 sec)	Normal in a well-conditioned heart (e.g., athletes); increased intracranial pressure; increased vagal tone due to straining during bowel movement, vomiting, intubation, or mechanical ventilation; sick sinus syndrome; inferior-wall MI; may also occur with anticholinesterase, beta-adrenergic blocker, digoxin, or morphine use
Sinus tachycardia	Rate: > 100 bpm Rhythm: Regular P waves: Occur before each QRS complex; look the same in shape and size P-R interval: Normal (0.12 sec to 0.20 sec) QRS complexes: Occur after each P wave; look the same in shape and size; normal (< 0.12 sec)	Normal physiologic response to fever, exercise, anxiety, pain, dehydration; may also accompany shock, left-sided heart failure, anemia, hypovolemia, pulmonary embolism; may also occur with atropine, epinephrine, caffeine, alcohol, and amphetamine or nicotine use
Atrial flutter	Rate: > 100 bpm Rhythm: Regular (may vary depending on degree of AV block) P waves: Cannot be found; replaced by flutter (F) waves, which may have sawtooth pattern P-R interval: Cannot determine QRS complexes: Look the same in shape and size; normal (< 0.12 sec)	Heart failure, tricuspid or mitral valve disease, pulmonary embolism, cor pulmonale, interior-wall MI, pericarditis; digoxin toxicity
Atrial fibrillation	Rate: > 100 bpm (grossly irregular; 350–450 bpm) Rhythm: Irregular P waves: Cannot be found P-R interval: Cannot determine QRS complexes: Look the same in shape and size	Heart failure, COPD, ischemic heart disease, sepsis, pulmonary embolism, rheumatic heart disease, hypertension, mitral stenosis; complication of coronary bypass or valve replacement surgery; nifedipine and digoxin use
Paroxysmal supraventricular tachycardia	Rate: > 100 bpm Rhythm: Regular P waves: Occur before each QRS complex (may be hidden in preceding T wave); look the same in shape and size (but differs from normal sinus P wave) P-R interval: Normal (0.12 sec to 0.20 sec), but may differ from P-R interval associated with normal sinus beat QRS complexes: Occur after each P wave; look the same in shape and size; normal (< 0.12 sec)	Intrinsic abnormality of AV conduction system; physical/psychological stress, hypoxia, hypokalemia, cardiomyopathy, congenital heart disease, MI, valvular disease, Wolff-Parkinson-White syndrome, cor pulmonale, hyperthyroidism; digoxin toxicity, use of caffeine, marijuana, or CNS stimulants
Junctional rhythm	Rate: Atrial rate > 60 bpm, ventricular rate usually > 60 bpm (60–100 bpm is accelerated junctional rhythm) Rhythm: Regular (irregular if escape beats occur) P waves: Cannot be found (nonexistent or hidden; usually inverted if visible) P-R interval: Cannot determine (when present, < 0.12 sec) QRS complexes: Look the same in shape and size; normal (< 0.12 sec) except in abberant conduction	Inferior-wall MI or ischemia, hypoxia, vagal stimulation, sick sinus syndrome; acute rheumatic fever; valve surgery; digoxin toxicity

Ventricular Rhythms

Premature ventricular contraction (PVC)	Rate: Irregular Rhythm: Atrial rhythm regular, ventricular rhythm irregular P waves: Cannot be found P-R interval: Cannot determine QRS complexes: Wide and distorted (≥ 0.12 sec); premature QRS complexes occurring alone, in pairs, or in threes, alternating with normal beats; focus from one or more sites; ominous when clustered, multifocal, with R wave on T pattern	Heart failure; previous or acute MI, ischemia, or contusion; myocardial irritation by ventricular catheter or a pacemaker; hypokalemia; hypocalcemia; hypomagnesemia; drug toxicity (digoxin, aminophylline, tricyclic antidepressant, beta-adrenergic blocker, isoproterenol, dopamine); caffeine, tobacco, or alcohol use; psychological stress, anxiety, pain, or exercise

FIGURE 4-16 Types of cardiac dysrhythmias.

Reproduced from *Arrhythmia recognition: The art of interpretation,* courtesy of Tomas B. Garcia, MD.

Dysrhythmia	Features	Causes
Ventricular tachycardia 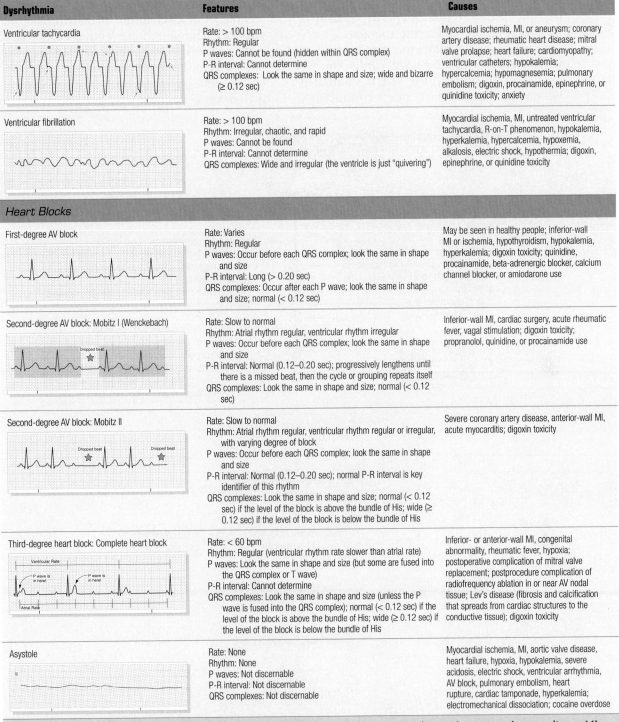	Rate: > 100 bpm Rhythm: Regular P waves: Cannot be found (hidden within QRS complex) P-R interval: Cannot determine QRS complexes: Look the same in shape and size; wide and bizarre (≥ 0.12 sec)	Myocardial ischemia, MI, or aneurysm; coronary artery disease; rheumatic heart disease; mitral valve prolapse; heart failure; cardiomyopathy; ventricular catheters; hypokalemia; hypercalcemia; hypomagnesemia; pulmonary embolism; digoxin, procainamide, epinephrine, or quinidine toxicity; anxiety
Ventricular fibrillation	Rate: > 100 bpm Rhythm: Irregular, chaotic, and rapid P waves: Cannot be found P-R interval: Cannot determine QRS complexes: Wide and irregular (the ventricle is just "quivering")	Myocardial ischemia, MI, untreated ventricular tachycardia, R-on-T phenomenon, hypokalemia, hyperkalemia, hypercalcemia, hypoxemia, alkalosis, electric shock, hypothermia; digoxin, epinephrine, or quinidine toxicity

Heart Blocks

First-degree AV block	Rate: Varies Rhythm: Regular P waves: Occur before each QRS complex; look the same in shape and size P-R interval: Long (> 0.20 sec) QRS complexes: Occur after each P wave; look the same in shape and size; normal (< 0.12 sec)	May be seen in healthy people; inferior-wall MI or ischemia, hypothyroidism, hypokalemia, hyperkalemia; digoxin toxicity; quinidine, procainamide, beta-adrenergic blocker, calcium channel blocker, or amiodarone use
Second-degree AV block: Mobitz I (Wenckebach)	Rate: Slow to normal Rhythm: Atrial rhythm regular, ventricular rhythm irregular P waves: Occur before each QRS complex; look the same in shape and size P-R interval: Normal (0.12–0.20 sec); progressively lengthens until there is a missed beat, then the cycle or grouping repeats itself QRS complexes: Look the same in shape and size; normal (< 0.12 sec)	Inferior-wall MI, cardiac surgery, acute rheumatic fever, vagal stimulation; digoxin toxicity; propranolol, quinidine, or procainamide use
Second-degree AV block: Mobitz II	Rate: Slow to normal Rhythm: Atrial rhythm regular, ventricular rhythm regular or irregular, with varying degree of block P waves: Occur before each QRS complex; look the same in shape and size P-R interval: Normal (0.12–0.20 sec); normal P-R interval is key identifier of this rhythm QRS complexes: Look the same in shape and size; normal (< 0.12 sec) if the level of the block is above the bundle of His; wide (≥ 0.12 sec) if the level of the block is below the bundle of His	Severe coronary artery disease, anterior-wall MI, acute myocarditis; digoxin toxicity
Third-degree heart block: Complete heart block	Rate: < 60 bpm Rhythm: Regular (ventricular rhythm rate slower than atrial rate) P waves: Look the same in shape and size (but some are fused into the QRS complex or T wave) P-R interval: Cannot determine QRS complexes: Look the same in shape and size (unless the P wave is fused into the QRS complex); normal (< 0.12 sec) if the level of the block is above the bundle of His; wide (≥ 0.12 sec) if the level of the block is below the bundle of His	Inferior- or anterior-wall MI, congenital abnormality, rheumatic fever, hypoxia; postoperative complication of mitral valve replacement; postprocedure complication of radiofrequency ablation in or near AV nodal tissue; Lev's disease (fibrosis and calcification that spreads from cardiac structures to the conductive tissue); digoxin toxicity
Asystole	Rate: None Rhythm: None P waves: Not discernable P-R interval: Not discernable QRS complexes: Not discernable	Myocardial ischemia, MI, aortic valve disease, heart failure, hypoxia, hypokalemia, severe acidosis, electric shock, ventricular arrhythmia, AV block, pulmonary embolism, heart rupture, cardiac tamponade, hyperkalemia; electromechanical dissociation; cocaine overdose

Notes: AV = atrioventricular; bpm = beats per minute; CNS = central nervous system; COPD = chronic obstructive pulmonary disease; MI = myocardial infarction.

FIGURE 4-16 (*continued*)

infarction, heart valve disease, dysrhythmias, thyroid disease (either hyperthyroidism or hypothyroidism), and severe anemia.

Several compensatory mechanisms are activated in times of decreased cardiac output (FIGURE 4-17). Initially, the SNS is stimulated, which increases heart rate, contractility, vasoconstriction, and antidiuretic hormone secretion. These mechanisms increase cardiac output in the beginning, but eventually they lead to excessive preload and afterload. The compensatory mechanisms continue to struggle to meet the body's metabolic needs until excessive myocardial oxygen demand and preload result in

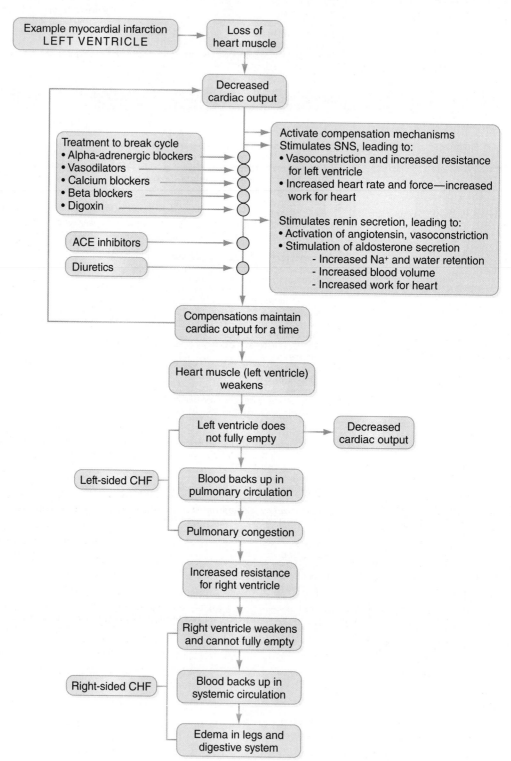

FIGURE 4-17 Course of heart failure.

decreased contractility and decompensation. This cycle becomes much like trying to bail water out of a sinking ship. Initially, the efforts to bail the water are able to keep the ship afloat, but eventually the flood of incoming water is more than can be removed. Declining cardiac output also leads to decreased renal perfusion, which activates the renin–angiotensin–aldosterone system. This activation further contributes to the vasoconstriction and fluid retention. Ventricular hypertrophy is another compensatory mechanism, but the enlarged myocardium eventually exceeds the oxygen supply and decreases contractility. All of these compensatory mechanisms are helpful at first, but in the end they create a vicious cycle that perpetuates the heart failure.

Heart failure can be categorized in several ways—systolic dysfunction, diastolic dysfunction, and mixed. **Systolic dysfunction** is characterized by decreased cardiac output due to decreased contractility. The causes of this decreased contractility include chronic ischemia from coronary artery disease (most common), dysrhythmias, dilated cardiomyopathy, chronic alcohol abuse, and myocarditis. **Diastolic dysfunction** is characterized by decreased ventricular filling from abnormal myocardial relaxation and increased left ventricular pressure. This type of heart failure is caused by conditions that stiffen the myocardium, such as coronary artery disease, hypertrophic and restrictive cardiomyopathy, and pericardial disease. Most patients have a combination of systolic and diastolic dysfunction, known as **mixed dysfunction**.

Heart failure can be classified as left- or right-sided heart failure (FIGURE 4-18). **Left-sided heart failure** is a result of ineffective left ventricular contractility. As cardiac output falls, blood that is not being pumped out into the body backs up first in the left atrium and then in the pulmonary circulation. Pulmonary congestion, dyspnea, and activity intolerance develop as blood backs up in the lungs. If blood continues to accumulate, pulmonary edema and right-sided heart failure will develop. Common causes of left-sided heart failure include left ventricular infarction, hypertension, and aortic and mitral valve stenosis. **Right-sided heart failure** is a result of ineffective right ventricular contractility. As a consequence of this condition, blood does not move appropriately out of the right ventricle. Blood backs up first in the right atrium and then in the peripheral circulation, causing increased pressures in the peripheral capillary bed. The patient begins to gain weight, as fluid

is not excreted by the kidneys. Tissue becomes edematous, as pressures in the capillaries push fluid out of the circulatory system. The most frequent cause of right-sided failure is increased pulmonary resistance because of respiratory disease (also known as cor pulmonale). Additionally, pulmonic and tricuspid valve stenosis can strain the right side of the heart. Most patients have a combination of left- and right-sided heart failure.

Heart failure can present as an acute or chronic problem. Acute heart failure may be related to a temporary condition and resolve with treatment of that condition. Chronic heart failure, in contrast, is a progressive condition that may have exacerbations, or an acute worsening, which will require additional treatment measures.

The clinical manifestations of heart failure depend on the side affected and on the severity. The manifestations of right-sided failure reflect systemic fluid accumulation, while left-sided failure is characterized by pulmonary fluid accumulation (**TABLE 4-2**).

A grading system is used to classify the severity of heart failure (I–IV, with IV being the most severe). Diagnosis and grading of heart failure are based on the following measures:

- History
- Physical examination
- Chest X-ray
- Arterial blood gases
- Echocardiogram
- EKG
- Brain natriuretic peptide (a hormone released by the ventricles in response to overstretching)

Management of heart failure begins with identifying and treating the underlying causes. Additional strategies include lifestyle modification (e.g., weight reduction, tobacco cessation, reduced salt consumption, fluid restriction, and exercise), ACE inhibitors (to stop the renin–angiotensin–aldosterone cycle), diuretics (to remove excess fluid), inotropics (to increase myocardial contractility), beta-adrenergic blockers (to slow the heart rate and thereby increase diastolic filling), calcium-channel blockers (to slow the heart rate and thereby increase diastolic filling), biventricular pacemaker, intra-aortic balloon pump, and heart transplant.

Congenital Heart Defects

Congenital heart defects include a number of structural issues that may be present at birth,

Left-sided heart failure

1. Left ventricle weakens and cannot empty

2. Decreased cardiac output to system

3. Decreased renal blood flow stimulates renin-angiotensin and aldosterone secretion

4. Backup of blood into pulmonary vein

5. High pressure in pulmonary capillaries leads to pulmonary congestion or edema

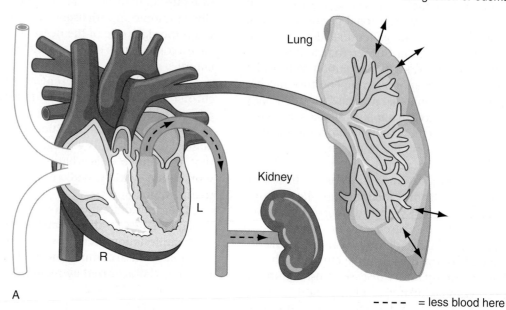

A

- - - - = less blood here

Right-sided heart failure

1. Right ventricle weakens and cannot empty

2. Decreased cardiac output to system

3. Decreased renal blood flow stimulates renin-angiotensin and aldosterone secretion

4. Backup of blood into systemic vein (venae cavae)

5. Increased venous pressure results in edema in legs and liver and abdominal organs

6. Very high venous pressure causes distended neck vein and cerebral edema

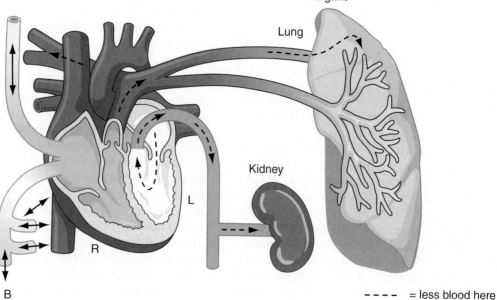

B

- - - - = less blood here

FIGURE 4-18 Effects of left- and right-sided heart failure.

TABLE 4-2   Clinical Manifestations of Left- and Right-Sided Heart Failure

	Left-Sided Heart Failure	Right-Sided Heart Failure
Causes	Infarction of left ventricle, aortic valve stenosis, hypertension, and hyperthyroidism	Infarction of right ventricle, pulmonary valve stenosis, and pulmonary disease (cor pulmonale)
Basic effects	Decreased cardiac output and pulmonary congestion	Decreased cardiac output and systemic congestion
Manifestations	Pulmonary congestion, dyspnea, and activity intolerance	Edema and weight gain
Forward effects (decreased output)	Fatigue, weakness, dyspnea, exercise intolerance, and cold intolerance	Fatigue, weakness, dyspnea, exercise intolerance, and cold intolerance
Compensations	Tachycardia, pallor, secondary polycythemia, and daytime oliguria	Tachycardia, pallor, secondary polycythemia, and daytime oliguria
Backup effects	Orthopnea, cough, shortness of breath, paroxysmal nocturnal dyspnea, hemoptysis, and rales	Dependent edema in feet, hepatomegaly, splenomegaly, ascites, distended neck veins, headache, and flushed face

affecting 8 out of 1,000 births (NIH, 2011). Such heart defects are the most common type of birth defects. They can vary from simple to complex and involve the myocardium, heart valves, and vessels near the heart. Examples of congenital heart defects include the following conditions:

- Septal defects (holes in the wall that separates the heart chambers)
- Patent ductus arteriosus (failure of the ductus arteriosus [the vessel between the aorta and the pulmonary artery] to close after birth)
- Valve disorders (e.g., stenosis, atresia, regurgitation)
- Coarctation of the aorta (narrowing of the aorta)
- Dextro-transposition of the great arteries (the aorta and the pulmonary artery are switched in position)
- Tetralogy of Fallot (combination of pulmonary valve stenosis, a large ventricular septal defect, misplacement of the aorta directly over the ventricular septal defect, and right ventricular hypertrophy)

Heredity may play a role in some heart defects. In addition, some genetic disorders (e.g., Down syndrome), fetal exposure to tobacco and certain medications, and maternal health status (e.g., preexisting diabetes, obesity) can increase the risk of these defects.

Depending on the defect, few or no manifestations may be present. When present, manifestations may include the following symptoms:

- Heart murmur
- Dyspnea
- Tachypnea
- Cyanosis
- Fatigue
- Chest pain or discomfort
- Difficulty gaining weight

In addition, heart failure may develop due to the increased cardiac workload as a result of the defect.

Diagnostic procedures for congenital heart defects include a history (including the mother's history), physical examination, fetal ultrasound, echocardiogram, EKG, chest X-ray, and cardiac catheterization. Treatment depends on the type and severity of the defect. Strategies may include repair with a heart catheterization or surgery, heart transplant, and medications to manage symptoms and complications (e.g., diuretics, antidysrhythmics, antihypertensives).

CONDITIONS RESULTING IN ALTERED TISSUE PERFUSION

Aneurysms

Walls of arteries can weaken because of high pressures, plaque, and infections. These weakened areas balloon outward, a condition known as **aneurysm** (FIGURE 4-19). This weakening happens much like a worn spot on a tire or a bulge in an old balloon. Just like the tire and the balloon, an aneurysm can rupture when the pressure builds inside the wall or when the wall becomes too thin. When it ruptures, blood spills out of the circulatory system, also known as **exsanguination**. Aneurysms may also develop slow leaks as opposed to rupturing.

The following factors increase the risk of developing aneurysm:

- Congenital weakening of the arterial wall
- Atherosclerosis
- Hypertension
- Dyslipidemia
- Diabetes mellitus
- Tobacco usage
- Advanced age
- Trauma
- Infection (e.g., syphilis)

True aneurysms are those that affect all three layers of the vessel. Two major types of true aneurysms exist—saccular and fusiform (FIGURE 4-20). A **saccular aneurysm** is a bulge on the side of the vessel. With a **fusiform aneurysm**, the aneurysm affects the entire circumference of the vessel. A false aneurysm, in contrast, does not affect all three layers of the vessel; an example of this type is a **dissecting aneurysm**. With dissecting aneurysms, the weakening occurs in the inner layers (Figure 4-20; FIGURE 4-21).

Clinical manifestations of aneurysms may vary based on their location. Some common locations for these defective areas include the abdominal aorta, the thoracic aorta, and the cerebral, femoral, and popliteal arteries. Most aneurysms are asymptomatic until they rupture. If present, symptoms may include a pulsating mass, pain, respiratory difficulty (e.g., dyspnea and cough), and neurologic decline (e.g., confusion or lethargy).

Diagnosis of aneurysms often occurs incidentally during a routine physical examination or X-ray. Other diagnostic procedures include echocardiogram, CT, MRI, and arteriograph. The goal of treatment is to prevent rupture by eliminating or treating causes (e.g., control blood pressure). Surgical intervention is the only effective treatment; it is performed if symptoms are present or if the aneurysm's diameter is more than 5 cm in an asymptomatic patient. If rupture occurs, immediate surgery is required.

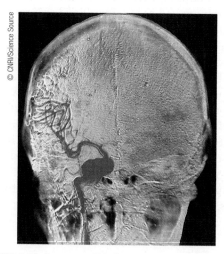

© CNRI/Science Source

FIGURE 4-19 Aneurysm. This X-ray shows a ballooning of one of the arteries in the brain. If untreated, an aneurysm can rupture, causing a stroke.

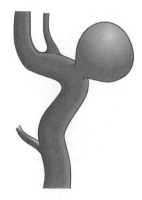 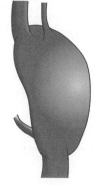

Saccular aneurysm

Fusiform aneurysm

FIGURE 4-20 Types of aneurysms.

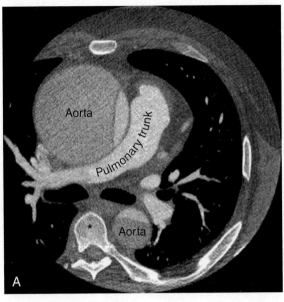 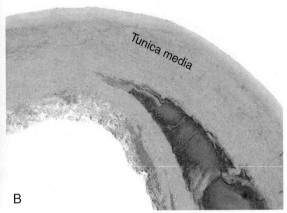

FIGURE 4-21 Aortic dissection.

Courtesy of Dr. Donald Yandow, Department of Radiology, University of Wisconsin School of Medicine and Public Health.

Dyslipidemia

Dyslipidemia, or hyperlipidemia, refers to an elevated level of **lipids** in the blood. These lipids include cholesterol and triglycerides, which are necessary for cellular membrane formation (see the *Cellular Function* chapter). Increased lipid levels have been linked to multiple disease conditions, including atherosclerosis, peripheral vascular disease, coronary artery disease, hypertension, and stroke.

Lipids are introduced into the bloodstream in two ways—diet and liver production (**FIGURE 4-22**). Dietary cholesterol is found in animal products, and dietary triglycerides are found in saturated fats (e.g., fried foods and cakes). The human liver makes more cholesterol than the body could possibly use, so even though cholesterol is necessary for survival, it is not necessary to eat it. Familial dyslipidemia usually results from an increase in liver production of cholesterol. Additional risk factors for dyslipidemia include excessive alcohol consumption, smoking, sedentary lifestyle, obesity, diabetes mellitus, hypothyroidism, and renal disease.

When cholesterol is present, it moves through the bloodstream in large molecules much like cooking lard. When triglycerides are present, they move through the bloodstream in large sticky molecules, much like gum. These sticky, fatty molecules travel through the circulatory system clogging small vessels and coating

Learning Points

Dietary cholesterol comes from animal products. To keep this origin in mind, remember that this lipid *must come from something with a face*. To gauge the amount of cholesterol in the product, think of how many legs the animal has. For example, a cow with four legs has more cholesterol than a chicken with two legs, which has more cholesterol than a fish with no legs. An exception to this rule is deer. A deer has four legs but is a very lean animal; therefore, it has less cholesterol than a cow. When considering pork, the amount of cholesterol depends on the cut of meat. Bacon has cholesterol content more like beef, whereas pork chops are more like chicken in terms of their cholesterol content. Finally, an egg may not have any legs yet, but one yolk contains more cholesterol than you need all day (the recommended daily allowance is less than 200 mg/day). These points create an image that not only helps you remember the cholesterol in foods but also is great to use with patients because it is easy to remember.

larger ones, much like what happens when oils and grease are poured down a drain.

Lipids, or lipoproteins, are classified according to their density. This density is based on the amount of triglycerides, which are low in density, versus the amount of proteins, which are highly dense. The main classes of lipoproteins are chylomicrons: very-low-density lipoproteins, **low-density lipoproteins (LDLs)**, and **high-density lipoproteins (HDLs)**. The most significant of these lipoproteins are LDL and HDL.

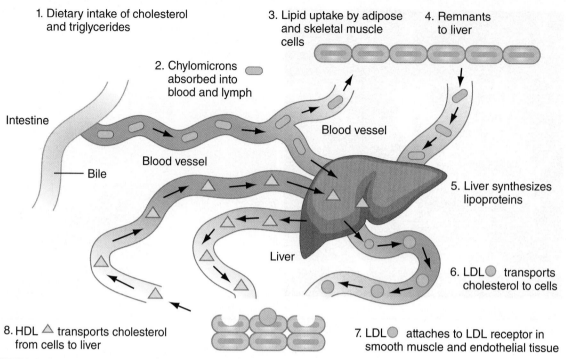

1. Dietary intake of cholesterol and triglycerides

2. Chylomicrons absorbed into blood and lymph

3. Lipid uptake by adipose and skeletal muscle cells

4. Remnants to liver

Intestine

Blood vessel

Bile

Blood vessel

Liver

5. Liver synthesizes lipoproteins

6. LDL○ transports cholesterol to cells

7. LDL○ attaches to LDL receptor in smooth muscle and endothelial tissue

8. HDL △ transports cholesterol from cells to liver

FIGURE 4-22 Transportation of lipids in the blood.

Learning Points

LDL is known as the bad cholesterol because most serum cholesterol is made up of LDL. The small, dense molecules of LDL are more invasive than the other lipoproteins. You can remember this point by considering it the "**l**ow-**d**own **l**ousy" cholesterol. Because it is the bad cholesterol, you want the LDL level as low as you can get it. Ways to decrease LDL through lifestyle modifications include dietary changes such as avoiding high-cholesterol, high-fat foods.

HDL is known as the good cholesterol because it assists in removing some of the cholesterol from the bloodstream. You can remember this point by considering it the "**h**appy" cholesterol. Because it is the good cholesterol, you want the HDL level as high as you can get it. Ways to increase HDL through lifestyle modifications include tobacco cessation and exercise.

Dyslipidemia is often asymptomatic until it develops into other diseases (e.g., atherosclerosis, coronary artery disease, or stroke). At that point, the symptoms are related to those diseases. Cholesterol screening and lipid profiles can identify specific lipid abnormalities (**TABLE 4-3**). Further testing (e.g., angiography, ultrasound, and nuclear scanning) can be conducted to determine the development of complications.

The goal of treatment is to normalize lipid levels and prevent complications. Initially,

treatment regimens to lower lipid levels include lifestyle modifications:

- Consumption of low-cholesterol, low-fat foods
- Routine exercise
- Moderate alcohol consumption
- Weight reduction (if applicable)
- Tobacco cessation (if applicable)

Other treatment approaches are implemented if these lifestyle modifications are unsuccessful. While a wide range of lipid-lowering pharmacologic agents exist, pharmacologic treatment primarily focuses on HMG-CoA reductase inhibitors (also known as "statins") (American College of Cardiology & American Heart Association, 2013). Other pharmacologic agents (e.g., anticoagulants and antiplatelet agents) may be added as necessary to prevent or treat complications.

Atherosclerosis

If lipid levels are not normalized in dyslipidemia, atherosclerosis often develops. **Atherosclerosis** is a chronic inflammatory disease characterized by thickening and hardening of the arterial wall. Lesions (or plaques) composed of lipids develop on the vessel wall and calcify over time. Development of these lesions causes vessel

TABLE 4-3   Adult Treatment Panel (ATP) III Classification of LDL, Total, and HDL Cholesterol (mg/dL)

LDL Cholesterol: Primary Target of Therapy

< 100	Optimal
100–129	Near optimal/above optimal
130–159	Borderline high
160–189	High
≥ 190	Very high

Total Cholesterol

< 200	Desirable
200–239	Borderline high
≥ 240	High

HDL Cholesterol

< 40	Low
≥ 60	High

Triglycerides

< 150	Normal
150–199	Borderline high
200–499	High
≥ 500	Very high

Modified from Third report of the National Cholesterol Education Program (NCEP) Expert Panel on detection, evaluation, and treatment of high blood cholesterol in adults (Adult Treatment Panel III) final report. (2002). NIH Publication No. 02-5215. Retrieved from https://www.nhlbi.nih.gov/health-pro/guidelines/current/cholesterol-guidelines/final-report

obstruction, platelet aggregation (collection), and vasoconstriction. Atherosclerosis can lead to peripheral vascular disease, coronary artery disease, thrombi, hypertension, renal disease, and stroke (FIGURE 4-23). When arteries are narrowed and hardened, the heart must work harder to pump the blood through them. In addition to dyslipidemia, other factors contributing to the development of atherosclerosis include diabetes mellitus, hypertension, stress, and tobacco use.

Atherosclerosis development is initiated by endothelial injury to the vessel wall (FIGURE 4-24). Dyslipidemia, hypertension, tobacco, diabetes mellitus, elevated C-reactive protein levels (released as a result of inflammation), elevated homocysteine levels, autoimmune processes, and some bacterial infections can cause this injury. The injured cells become more permeable, suffer from free radical damage, and become inflamed. Leukocytes, macrophages, and cytokines are activated with the initiation of the inflammatory process, which creates more damage. The LDL becomes oxidized and permeates the vessel wall, exacerbating the injury and creating **fatty streaks**. Fibrous tissue and smooth muscle cells migrate to the site, increasing the size of the lesion and transforming it into **fibrous plaque**.

Much like dyslipidemia, atherosclerosis is often asymptomatic until complications develop. At that point, clinical manifestations will be related to those specific diseases. Diagnostic procedures for atherosclerosis include those that identify contributing factors (e.g., lipid, C-reactive protein, and homocysteine levels). Increased C-reactive protein levels indicate the presence of inflammation and are considered a risk factor for atherosclerosis. Other diagnostic procedures are used to determine whether complications have developed (e.g., angiography, ultrasound, and nuclear scanning).

Treatment for atherosclerosis is similar to that for dyslipidemia, but with the addition of angioplasty to open occluded arteries (FIGURE 4-25), bypass procedures to detour blood around the occlusions, laser procedures to disintegrate the plaque, and atherectomy to

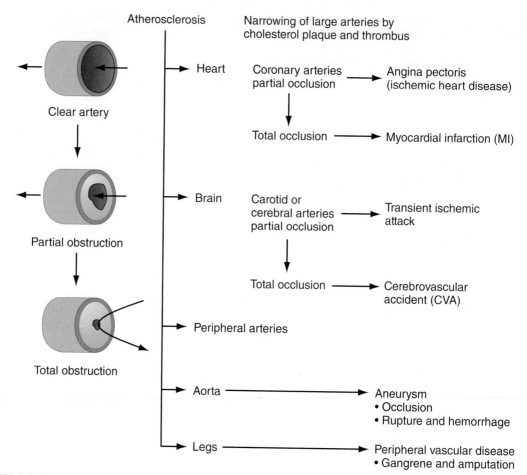

FIGURE 4-23 Possible complications of atherosclerosis.

remove the plaque. B-complex vitamins can help lower homocysteine levels.

Peripheral Vascular Disease

Peripheral vascular disease (PVD) refers to a narrowing of the peripheral vessels (arteries or veins). Most often this condition is caused by atherosclerosis, but it can also be caused by a thrombus, inflammation (e.g., thromboangiitis obliterans), or vasospasm (e.g., Raynaud's disease and Raynaud's phenomenon). **Thrombo-angiitis obliterans**, or Buerger's disease, is an inflammatory condition of the arteries (**FIGURE 4-26**). **Raynaud's disease** is a result of vasospasm of the arteries, most often of the hands, that occurs because of sympathetic stimulation (**FIGURE 4-27**). Raynaud's phenomenon describes the situation in which such vasospasm occurs in association with an autoimmune disease (e.g., systemic lupus erythematosus and scleroderma). As vessel occlusion increases, the ischemia to the affected tissue worsens. Risk factors for developing PVD are similar to those

for developing atherosclerosis, but with the addition of autoimmune disease.

Clinical manifestations of PVD are related to the local tissue ischemia and appear in the extremities. Most symptoms occur during activity, when the oxygen demand exceeds the oxygen supply. The presence of symptoms at rest is an indicator of worsening disease. Manifestations include the following:

- Pain
- Intermittent claudication (pain that occurs in the lower legs during activity)
- Numbness
- Burning
- Wounds that do not heal
- Changes in skin color (pallor, cyanosis, rubor)
- Hair loss, especially in areas farthest from the heart, such as the toes
- Impotency

Diagnostic procedures for PVD include a history, physical examination, ankle/brachial

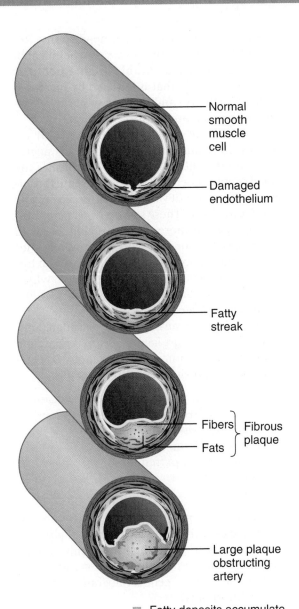

FIGURE 4-24 Development of atherosclerosis.

- Normal smooth muscle cell
- Damaged endothelium
- Fatty streak
- Fibers ⎫ Fibrous
- Fats ⎬ plaque
- Large plaque obstructing artery

▣ Fatty deposits accumulate in the wall of the artery

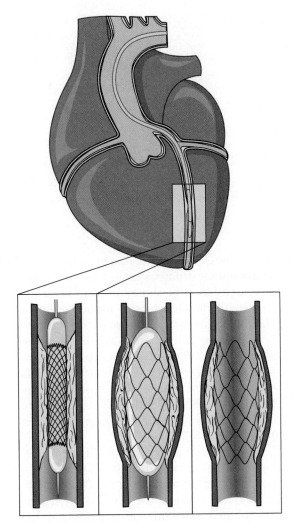

FIGURE 4-25 Principles of angioplasty.

Coronary Artery Disease

When atherosclerosis develops in the arteries supplying the myocardium, **coronary artery disease (CAD)** develops. In CAD, blood flow temporarily diminishes in the coronary arteries, causing subsequent oxygen reduction to the

index (which compares blood pressure in the arms and the legs), treadmill exercise test, angiography, ultrasounds, and MRI. Treatment strategies for PVD include controlling or reducing contributing factors (e.g., by making dietary changes or by tobacco cessation, physical activity, weight reduction, stress reduction, diabetes management, and hypertension control), in addition to direct intervention aimed at the occlusion (e.g., angioplasty, bypass procedures, laser procedures, and atherectomy). Pharmacologic management includes antiplatelet agents, anticoagulants, thrombolytics, and lipid-lowering medications.

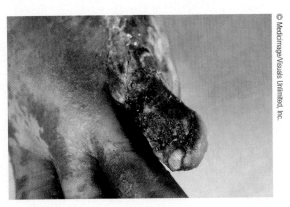

FIGURE 4-26 Thromboangiitis obliterans.

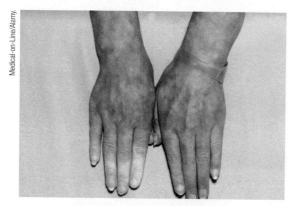

Medical-on-Line/Alamy.

FIGURE 4-27 Raynaud's phenomenon.

cardiac muscle. This reduction in oxygen to the cardiac muscle produces chest pain, or **angina**. Decreased blood flow may or may not cause permanent damage to the myocardium, or infarction. Along with atherosclerosis (the most common cause), vasospasm is another prevalent cause of CAD. Other causes of CAD include cardiomyopathy and thrombi. Additional contributing factors for CAD—some modifiable and some not—are similar to those for atherosclerosis (e.g., diabetes mellitus, hypertension, stress, and tobacco) (**TABLE 4-4**).

Despite great advancements in treatment, cardiovascular disease (including CAD) remains the leading cause of death in the United States for men and women. CAD is also the leading cause of myocardial infarction (Centers for Disease Control and Prevention [CDC], 2015).

The left ventricle is the most susceptible to ischemic damage because more arteries supply it to meet its increased needs for oxygen. With CAD, oxygen supply is insufficient to meet this demand. As ischemia develops, lactic acid and metabolic wastes accumulate, causing angina. This accumulation can stimulate other nerves, causing the pain to radiate to other parts of the body. Additionally, chronic ischemia causes EKG

changes (usually ST-segment depression). Reducing oxygen demand reverses ischemia and, in turn, reduces pain. **Stable angina pectoris** refers to ischemia that is initiated by increased demand (activity) and relieved with the reduction of that demand (rest).

The cascade of events in which plaque ulcerates, inflammation occurs, platelets aggregate, and thrombi form further diminishes the blood supply. As a result, platelets release thromboxane A_2, a potent vasoconstrictor, causing the arteries to spasm. These spasms trigger an unrelenting cycle of more platelet aggregation and more spasms. Chest pain eventually becomes unpredictable, occurs at rest, or increases in frequency or intensity. This change in pain, which is known as **unstable angina**, is considered a preinfarction state.

In addition to causing myocardial infarctions, CAD can cause heart failure, dysrhythmias, and sudden death. Clinical manifestations of CAD include the following signs and symptoms:

- Angina that can radiate to other locations (e.g., jaw, neck, arm, or back)
- Indigestion-like sensation
- Nausea and vomiting
- Cool, clammy extremities
- Diaphoresis
- Fatigue

Diagnostic procedures for CAD involve identifying contributing factors (e.g., lipid profile, angiography, and nuclear imaging). Additionally, a history, physical examination, exercise stress test, echocardiogram, and EKG will be informative.

Treatment focuses on preventing myocardial infarction by reducing modifiable risk factors through the same strategies used to treat dyslipidemia and atherosclerosis (e.g., dietary changes, tobacco cessation, physical activity, weight reduction, stress reduction,

TABLE 4-4	Risk Factors for Coronary Artery Disease			
Nonmodifiable Risk Factors	**Modifiable Risk Factors**	**Negative Risk Factors**	**Emerging Risk Factors**
Age: men > 45 years; women > 55 years or premature menopause Family history: history of premature coronary artery disease in first-degree male relatives > 55 years or first-degree female relatives > 65 years	Tobacco use Obesity Physical inactivity Stress Diabetes mellitus Hyperlipidemia Hypertension	High HDL cholesterol	Elevated C-reactive protein and homocysteine levels

diabetes management, hypertension control, angioplasty, bypass procedures, laser procedures, antiplatelet agents, anticoagulants, thrombolytics, and lipid-lowering medications). Additional medications that may be added to the regimen include nitrates, beta-adrenergic blockers, and calcium-channel blockers to vasodilate the coronary arteries and increase the oxygen supply. Oxygen therapy may also be used to increase oxygen supply.

Thrombi and Emboli

A **thrombus** is a blood clot that consists of platelets, fibrin, erythrocytes, and leukocytes. Such clots can form anywhere in the circulatory system (**TABLE 4-5**). Three conditions—endothelial injury, sluggish blood flow, and increased coagulopathy (collectively referred to as Virchow's triad)—promote thrombus formation (**FIGURE 4-28**). When a vessel wall is injured, the endothelial damage attracts platelets and inflammatory mediators to the site, thereby stimulating clot formation. Stagnant blood flow allows platelets and clotting factors to accumulate and adhere to the vessel wall. Hypercoagulopathy states promote clot formation inappropriately.

The consequences of thrombus formation may include occlusion of a blood vessel or embolus development. An **embolus** occurs when a portion or all of the thrombus breaks loose and travels through the circulatory system, eventually becoming embedded in a smaller vessel. In addition to thrombi, any other bodies (e.g., air, fat, tissue, bacteria, amniotic fluid, tumor cells, and foreign substances) traveling through the circulatory system can become emboli.

Emboli that originate in the venous circulation, such as with deep vein thrombus (**FIGURE 4-29**), travel to the right side of the heart and then on to the pulmonary circulation, creating a pulmonary embolism (**FIGURE 4-30**). Most emboli in the arterial system originate in the left side of the heart and travel to other organs such as the brain and heart, causing an infarction.

TABLE 4-5	Comparison of Venous and Arterial Thrombi	
Manifestation	**Venous Thrombus**	**Arterial Thrombus**
Pulse	Present	Weak or absent
Skin color	Rubor	Cyanotic
Skin temperature	Cool	Warm
Edema	Present	Minimal or absent
	Venous Thrombus	**Arterial Thrombus**

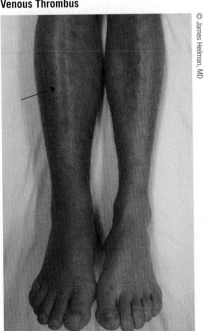

© James Heilman, MD

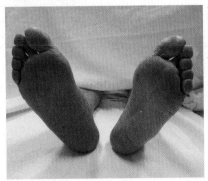

© James Heilman, MD

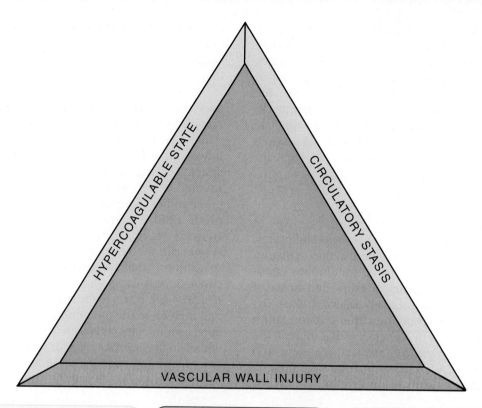

FIGURE 4-28 Virchow's triad.

Clinical manifestations of thrombi and emboli depend on whether they are arterial or venous, as well as their location. Diagnostic procedures include arteriography, ultrasound, echocardiogram, and MRI.

Treatment of thrombi and emboli centers on prevention and includes increasing mobility, hydration, antiembolism hosiery, sequential compression devices, and medications (e.g., antiplatelet agents and anticoagulants). In the presence of active thrombi, these prevention strategies may be dangerous and should be avoided. For example, mobility and sequential compression devices may dislodge a stationary clot. Treatment of active thrombi may include thrombolytic agents or embolectomy.

Varicose Veins

Varicose veins, or varicosities, are dilated, tortuous, engorged veins that develop because of improper venous valve function (**FIGURE 4-31**). The location where they are most commonly found is the legs, but they can also occur in the esophagus (esophageal varices) and the rectum (hemorrhoids). Increased venous pressure and blood pooling cause the veins to enlarge, stretching the valves. The valves become incompetent, blood flow is reversed, and venous pressure and distension are further increased. Capillary pressure increases, causing fluid and pigment to leak out, leading to edema and skin discoloration. As a result, stasis pigmentation (brown skin discoloration), subcutaneous induration (thick, hardened skin), dermatitis (skin inflammation), and thrombophlebitis (vein inflammation resulting from a thrombus) can occur. The pressure caused by the edema can decrease circulation, resulting in metabolic needs not being met. Failure to meet cellular oxygen and nutrient needs can, in turn, lead to necrosis and venous stasis ulcers.

The following factors increase a person's risk for developing varicosities:

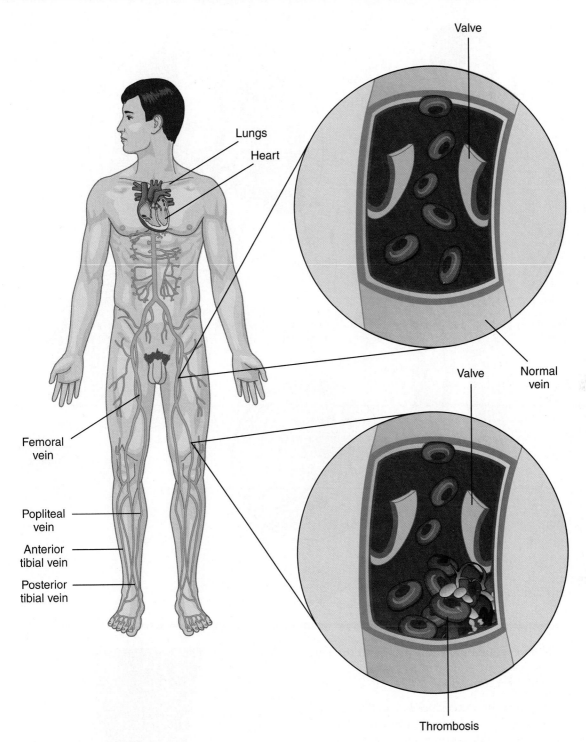

FIGURE 4-29 Deep vein thrombosis.

- Genetic predisposition
- Pregnancy
- Obesity
- Prolonged sitting or standing
- Alcohol abuse and liver disorders (esophageal varices)
- Constipation (hemorrhoids)

Clinical manifestations are usually minor and include the following signs and symptoms:

- Irregular, purplish, bulging veins
- Pedal edema
- Fatigue
- Aching in the legs

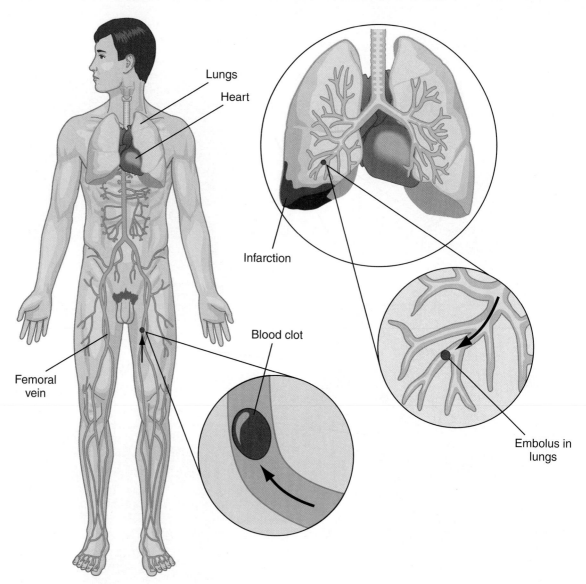

FIGURE 4-30 Pulmonary embolism.

- Shiny, pigmented, hairless skin on the legs and feet
- Skin ulcer formation

Diagnosis of varicosities is usually accomplished through visualization during physical examination. Additional tests may include Doppler ultrasound and venogram. Treatment ranges from conservative to invasive and includes the following measures:

- Rest with the affected leg elevated
- Compression stockings
- Avoiding prolonged standing or sitting
- Exercise
- Sclerotherapy (injection of a sclerosing agent that produces fibrosis inside the vessel)
- Surgical removal

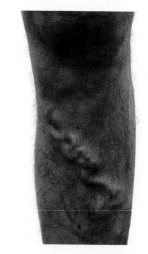

FIGURE 4-31 Varicose vein.

© Audie/Shutterstock

Lymphedema

Lymphedema refers to swelling, usually in the arms and legs, because of lymph obstruction (FIGURE 4-32). This swelling can occur on its own (primary) or because of another disease or condition (secondary). Primary lymphedema is rare and related to a congenital absence or decreased number of lymphatics. Secondary lymphedema is usually related to one of the following events:

- Surgery (when lymph nodes and lymph vessels are removed or severed, as with a mastectomy)
- Radiation (causes scarring and inflammation of lymph nodes or lymph vessels, restricting the flow of lymph fluid)
- Cancer (occludes lymphatic vessels)
- Infection (can infiltrate lymph vessels and lymph nodes, restricting the flow of lymph fluid)
- Injury (damages lymph nodes or lymph vessels)

Clinical manifestations of lymphedema include edema and skin changes. The edema may be unilateral or bilateral, and it usually occurs in the extremities. Skin changes include hyperpigmentation, ulceration, and thickening (referred to as brawny edema). The skin begins to appear like elephant skin, thick and rough.

Diagnostic procedures consist of a physical examination, MRI, CT, Doppler ultrasound, and nuclear imaging. Treatment of lymphedema includes the following measures:

- Sequential compression devices
- Compression stockings
- Exercise
- Massage therapy (complex decongestive physiotherapy)

- Antibiotics (to treat existing infections)
- Benzopyrone agents (to increase lymphatic flow)
- Diuretics (to remove excess fluid as it returns to the circulatory system)
- Surgery (to remove excess skin)

Myocardial Infarction

Myocardial infarction (MI) is death of the myocardium from a sudden blockage of coronary artery blood flow (FIGURE 4-33; FIGURE 4-34). This blockage exemplifies the nursing diagnosis of altered tissue perfusion and may be caused by atherosclerosis, thrombus, or vasospasm. In most cases, tears in the plaque buildup associated with atherosclerosis trigger platelet aggregation and cause a thrombus to form. As a result of the occlusion, the myocardial oxygen supply cannot meet the body's demand for oxygen. An MI occurs in progressive stages as the blood flow to the myocardium decreases. Cells die as their coronary blood and oxygen supplies dwindle. This death may occur gradually or suddenly, depending on the time frame in which the occlusion develops. The trigger for the MI is not always known, but such events may occur after physical exertion, while sleeping or resting, during outside activity in cold weather, and with severe emotional stress.

Other names for MI include heart attack and acute coronary syndrome. Risk factors for such an event include those for atherosclerosis (e.g., dyslipidemia, diabetes mellitus, hypertension, stress, and tobacco). Cardiovascular disease (including CAD) is the leading cause of death in the United States, and death usually results from

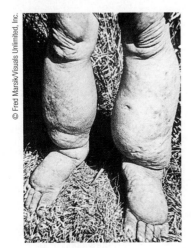

© Fred Marsik/Visuals Unlimited, Inc.

FIGURE 4-32 Lymphedema.

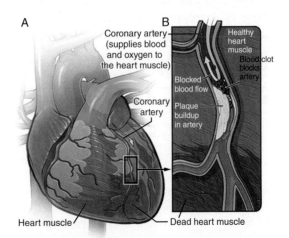

FIGURE 4-33 Myocardial infarction. (a) An overview of a heart and coronary artery showing damage (dead heart muscle) caused by a heart attack. (b) A cross section of the coronary artery with plaque buildup and a blood clot.

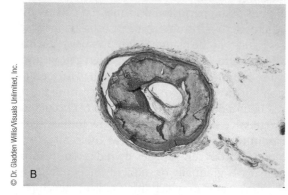

© SIU/Visuals Unlimited, Inc.

© Dr. Gladden Willis/Visuals Unlimited, Inc.

FIGURE 4-34 Myocardial infarction. (a) Sectioned heart showing myocardial infarction of the posterior left ventricle. (b) Severely occluded coronary artery with calcification from an elderly woman with a fatal myocardial infarction.

cardiac damage after an MI. Prognosis improves with early and aggressive treatment.

Some people do not experience symptoms of MI. Such an asymptomatic MI is known as a silent MI. Silent MIs generally occur in persons who have diabetes mellitus, neurologic dysfunction (e.g., neuropathy), or history of an MI because of decreased pain innervations. When

clinical manifestations are present, they include the following signs and symptoms:

- Unstable angina (typically described as a pressure or tightness in the arms, shoulder, neck, teeth, jaw, abdomen, or back that may radiate to other locations)
- Fatigue
- Nausea and vomiting
- Shortness of breath
- Coughing
- Diaphoresis
- Indigestion
- Elevation in cardiac biomarkers (**TABLE 4-6**)
- EKG changes (**FIGURE 4-35**)
- Dysrhythmias (e.g., ventricular tachycardia, ventricular fibrillation, and asystole)
- Anxiety
- Syncope
- Dizziness

Complications are more likely to occur when MIs are not treated early and aggressively. Those complications may include heart failure, dysrhythmias, cardiac shock, thrombosis, and death.

Diagnostic procedures for MIs consist of a history, physical examination, EKG, cardiac

Learning Points

Initial treatment of an MI can be remembered using the acronym MONA:

- **M**orphine
- **O**xygen
- **N**itroglycerin
- **A**spirin

Initiating these strategies during the triage and assessment period is critical to achieve optimal patient outcomes.

TABLE 4-6	**Cardiac Biomarkers**		
Biomarker	**Onset**	**Advantages**	**Disadvantages**
CK-MB	4–6 hours	Rapid Cost-effective Detected early in infarction	Loss of specificity with skeletal muscle damage Detected after 6 hours of myocardial necrosis
Myoglobin	1 hour	Highly sensitive Early detection of MI, within 2 hours Detects reperfusion Most useful in ruling out MI	Low specificity with skeletal muscle injury Rapid return to normal
Troponins	2–6 hours	Powerful tool for risk stratification Greater sensitivity and specificity than CK-MB Detects recent MI, up to 2 weeks prior to testing Helpful to determine therapy Detection of reperfusion	Low sensitivity to MI of less than 6 hours Require repeat measures at 8–12 hours if first result is negative Less able to detect late, minor MIs

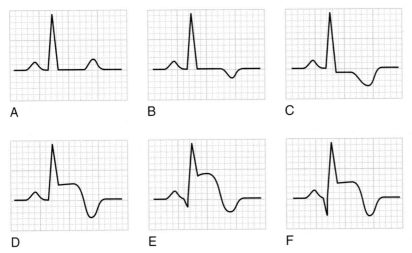

FIGURE 4-35 EKG ischemia and infarction patterns. (a) Normal EKG for comparison. (b) Mild ischemia demonstrated by inverted T wave. (c) Moderate ischemia demonstrated by slight ST-segment depression and inverted T wave. (d) and (e) ST-segment elevation myocardial infarction. (f) ST-segment myocardial infarction with prominent Q wave indicating more severe myocardial damage.

Modified from *Introduction to 12-Lead ECG: The Art of Interpretation*, courtesy of Tomas B. Garcia, MD.

biomarkers, stress testing, nuclear imaging, and angiography. Treatment is complex and depends on when the individual sought treatment (FIGURE 4-36). Prognosis hinges on initiating treatment early—ideally within 90 minutes of symptom onset. After that point, treatment options and ability to reverse damage become limited. If a patient survives the MI, it is vital that the individual takes steps to prevent another MI through lifestyle modifications and other measures (e.g., dietary changes, tobacco cessation, physical activity, weight reduction, stress reduction, diabetes management, hypertension control, angioplasty, bypass procedures, laser procedures, antiplatelet agents, anticoagulants, thrombolytics, and lipid-lowering medications) to treat atherosclerosis.

CONDITIONS RESULTING IN DECREASED CARDIAC OUTPUT AND ALTERED PERFUSION

Hypertension

Hypertension is a prolonged elevation in blood pressure. It is one of the most prevalent chronic health conditions in the United States, affecting approximately 70 million Americans (CDC, 2016). Hypertension is the leading risk factor for cardiovascular disease (e.g., coronary artery disease, myocardial infarction, heart failure, and stroke). In hypertension, the heart must work harder than normal to pump the blood to all the parts of the body, in part due to vasoconstriction that increases afterload. Because of this vasoconstriction, renal blood flow decreases, resulting in an inappropriate activation of the renin–angiotensin–aldosterone system (FIGURE 4-37).

A classification scheme for blood pressure has been developed by the Joint National Committee on Prevention, Detection, Evaluation, and Treatment of High Blood Pressure (JNC 8) (James et al., 2014). JNC 8 provides guidelines for classifying blood pressure levels in children, adolescents, and adults, as well as treatment based on those classifications (FIGURE 4-38).

Risk factors for developing hypertension include the following:

- Age: Vessel compliance decreases with aging. Through early middle age, high blood pressure is more common in men, whereas women are more likely to develop high blood pressure after menopause.
- Race: Hypertension is more prevalent in African Americans.
- Family history.
- Overweight or obesity: Excessive weight amplifies oxygen and nutrient needs; when the circulating blood volume increases to meet these greater needs, the increased volume exerts greater pressure on the artery walls.
- Physical inactivity: Increases heart rate, which increases cardiac workload.

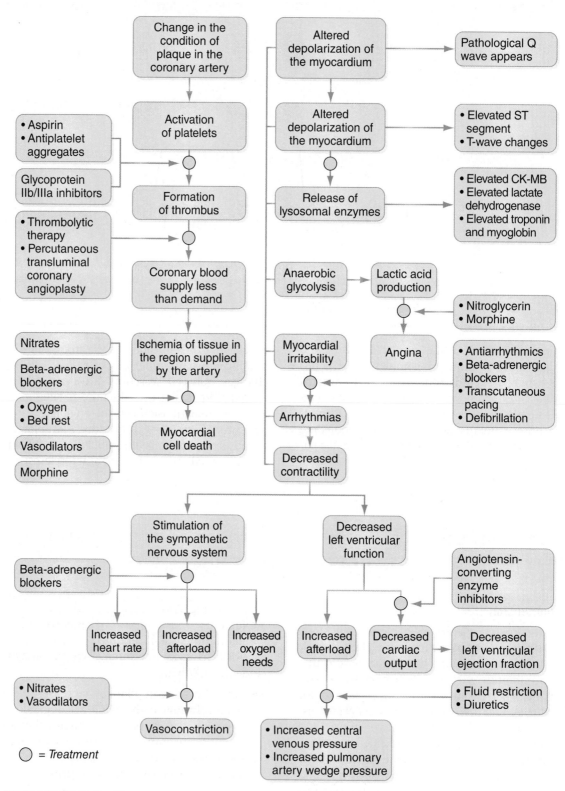

FIGURE 4-36 Treating an MI.

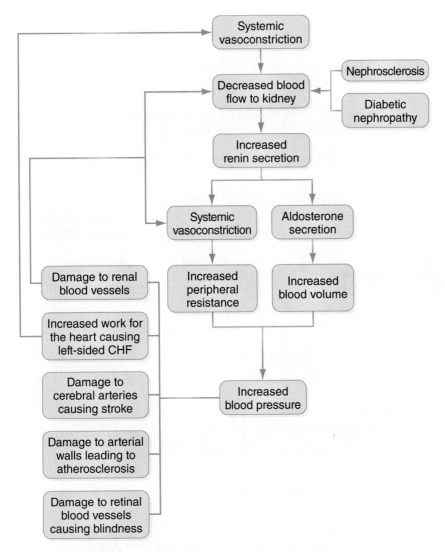

FIGURE 4-37 Development of hypertension.

- Tobacco use: Nicotine immediately raises blood pressure temporarily, and the chemicals in tobacco can damage artery walls over time.
- High-sodium diet: Too much sodium causes fluid retention, which increases blood pressure.
- Low-potassium diet: Potassium helps balance the amount of sodium in cells; without enough potassium, too much sodium accumulates in the blood.
- High vitamin D intake: This factor has an uncertain effect, though vitamin D may affect the renin–angiotensin–aldosterone system.
- Excessive alcohol consumption: Over time, heavy drinking—that is, more than two to three drinks in one sitting—can damage the heart.
- Stress: High levels of stress can lead to a temporary, but dramatic, increase in blood pressure.

Hypertension is divided into two major forms—primary and secondary. In most hypertension cases in adults, there is no identifiable cause. This type of hypertension, called **primary hypertension** or **essential hypertension**, tends to develop gradually over many years. The other cases of hypertension are caused by an underlying condition. This type of hypertension, called **secondary hypertension**, tends to appear suddenly and cause higher blood pressure than does primary hypertension. A variety of conditions and medications can lead to secondary hypertension:

- Renal disease (e.g., renal artery stenosis, polycystic kidney disease, and diabetic nephropathy)
- Adrenal gland tumors
- Certain congenital heart defects (e.g., coarctation of the aorta)

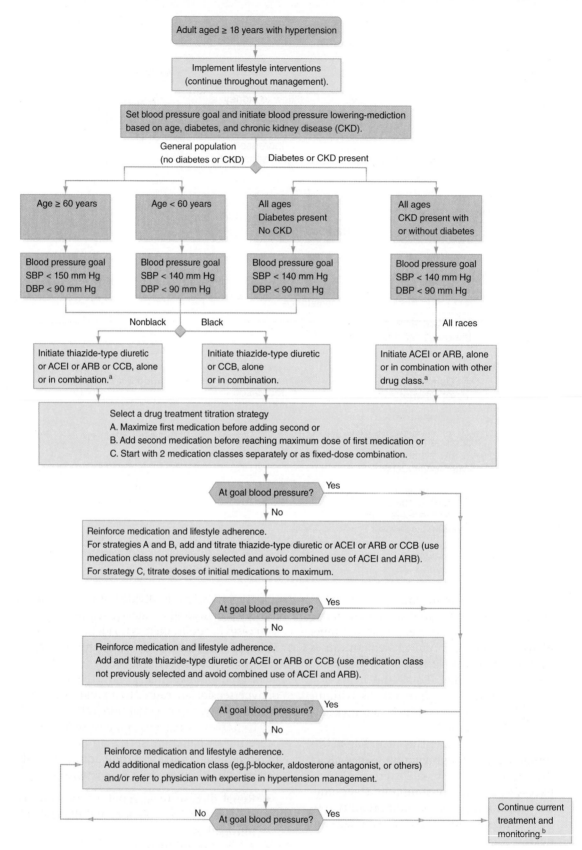

FIGURE 4-38 JNC 8 hypertension guideline management algorithm.

- Certain medications (e.g., birth control pills, hormone replacement therapy, antihistamines, decongestants, and glucocorticoid steroids)
- Illegal drugs (e.g., cocaine and amphetamines)

Another form of this disease is malignant hypertension. **Malignant hypertension** is an especially intense form of hypertension that may not respond well to treatment efforts.

Occasionally, hypertension is classified as systolic or diastolic, depending which measurement is elevated. Often, elderly persons have higher systolic readings and lower diastolic readings because of aging changes.

Hypertension can also occur during pregnancy, referred to as **pregnancy-induced hypertension (PIH)**. Other names for PIH include toxemia and preeclampsia. Indicators of PIH include high blood pressure, proteinuria, and edema. PIH can worsen, leading to **eclampsia**. In eclampsia, seizures often occur because of the PIH. Risk factors for developing PIH include a history of PIH, renal disease, diabetes mellitus, multiple fetuses, and maternal age younger than 20 years or older than 40 years. PIH can lead to multiple problems, including miscarriages, poor fetal development, and placental abruption. Management focuses on prevention and nonpharmacologic measures to protect the fetus. Treatment measures include bed rest and magnesium sulfate (to prevent seizures).

As noted earlier, hypertension is called the silent killer because many people do not have symptoms. Often by the time symptoms become evident, the hypertension is advanced or the blood pressure is remarkably high. When present, clinical manifestations include fatigue, headache, malaise, and dizziness.

Hypertension causes excessive pressure on artery walls, which damages blood vessels and organs. The higher the blood pressure and the longer it goes uncontrolled, the greater the damage. Uncontrolled high blood pressure can lead to numerous complications:

- Atherosclerosis
- Aneurysms
- Heart failure
- Stroke
- Hypertensive crisis (a severe increase in blood pressure that is a medical emergency)
- Renal damage
- Vision loss
- Metabolic syndrome (a cluster of disorders of metabolism—including increased waist circumference, high triglycerides, low HDL, high blood pressure, high blood glucose levels, and insulin resistance)
- Problems with memory or understanding

The prognosis for persons with hypertension depends on treating any underlying causes and maintaining blood pressure control. Early detection and treatment are crucial to prevent or minimize complications. Measures to diagnose hypertension include a history, physical examination, multiple blood pressure readings at varying times of the day, EKG, and laboratory tests (e.g., urinalysis, CBC, lipid panel, and a creatinine test) to determine the presence of complications.

Treatment of hypertension is based on JNC 8 standards (Figure 4-38), and adhering to the protocol will increase the likelihood of successful blood pressure control. Lifestyle changes are the mainstay of prevention and treatment. These changes can be implemented in those individuals at risk for developing hypertension. Dietary changes are the cornerstone to these lifestyle changes and include the Dietary Approaches to Stop Hypertension (DASH) diet (NIH, 2015). The research-driven DASH diet includes the following recommendations:

- Limiting saturated fat, cholesterol, total fat, and salt
- Focusing on fruits, vegetables, and fat-free or low-fat dairy products
- Increasing whole grains, fish, poultry, beans, seeds, and nuts
- Minimizing sweets, added sugar and sugary beverages, and red meats

Limiting salt consumption to 2,300 mg (less than a teaspoon) per day has been shown to lower blood pressure. Further restricting salt intake to 1,500 mg per day can lower blood pressure to an even greater extent. The 1,500 mg restriction is advised for individuals diagnosed with hypertension, diabetes, and chronic kidney disease as well as African Americans, middle-aged individuals, and older adults. Following these guidelines, particularly the salt recommendations, can significantly decrease the risk for developing hypertension.

Other lifestyle changes that can help prevent or treat hypertension include being active, maintaining a healthy weight, smoking cessation, stress management, and alcohol consumption (if used) in moderation. Additionally, individuals should have their blood pressure measured regularly with a home monitor and by healthcare professionals. These readings should be documented in a blood pressure journal (including the blood pressure reading, date, time of day, activities just before the reading, and any symptoms) and brought to visits with the healthcare provider.

Shock

Shock is a clinical syndrome resulting from inadequate tissue and organ perfusion because of decreased blood volume or circulatory stagnation. Shock can be classified into three categories based on its precipitating factors: distributive (neurogenic, septic, and anaphylactic), cardiogenic, and hypovolemic.

Shock progresses through three stages that are common to all types of shock—compensatory, progressive, and irreversible. **Compensatory mechanisms** are bodily responses that become activated when arterial pressure and tissue perfusion decrease, and that represent an effort to maintain cardiac and cerebral function. These compensatory mechanisms include the activation of the SNS and renin–angiotensin–aldosterone system. The **progressive stage** of shock begins when these compensatory mechanisms fail to maintain cardiac output. Tissues become hypoxic, cells switch to anaerobic metabolism, lactic acid builds up, and metabolic acidosis develops. This acidotic state further impairs cardiac functioning, causing sluggish blood flow, and increases the risk for disseminated intravascular coagulation (see the *Hematopoietic Function* chapter). Irreversible organ damage occurs as the shock progresses, leading to respiratory and cardiac failure (FIGURE 4-39).

In **distributive shock**, vasodilation causes hypovolemia. Three types of distributive shock are distinguished—neurogenic, septic, and anaphylactic. A loss of sympathetic tone in vascular smooth muscle and autonomic function lead to massive vasodilation in **neurogenic shock**. Blood pools in the venous system, leading to decreased venous return, cardiac output, and blood pressure. In **septic shock**, a bacterium's endotoxins activate an immune reaction. Inflammatory mediators are triggered, increasing capillary permeability and causing fluid shifts from the vascular compartment to the tissue. Falling cardiac output then leads to multisystem organ failure. **Anaphylactic shock** is a consequence of an allergic reaction. The allergic reaction leads to a cascade of events similar to that of septic shock, except that the mediators differ (see the *Immunity* chapter). Additionally, bronchospasm and laryngeal edema occur that can impair respiratory status.

Cardiogenic shock results when the left ventricle cannot maintain adequate cardiac output. Compensatory mechanisms of heart failure are triggered, but these mechanisms

Learning Points

Cutting back on salt intake can be challenging on many levels. First, eating increased amounts of salt over time decreases taste sensation on the tongue, such that foods without it will lack flavor initially. Those taste buds will wake up again with a little time. Gradually decreasing salt intake may help with this transition. For instance, have patients start by not adding salt to food once it is prepared, and then begin changing how food is prepared.

Second, salt is used in many foods of convenience as a preservative. In today's fast-paced society, these foods have become commonplace and almost a necessity. Unfortunately, processed foods (e.g., canned food, boxed meals, frozen dinners, and sandwich meats) usually contain large amounts of salt. Additionally, salt is often added to meats to preserve them, even when those meats are already naturally high in salt (e.g., pork).

Third, the practice of eating outside the home in a wide range of restaurants has increased. Salt content is difficult to control when others are preparing the food.

Finally, salt is hidden in many seasonings and condiments. As people attempt to move away from salt, they may turn to these seasonings and condiments to enhance flavor—but these items may be just as bad as using salt. Seasonings that have "salt" in their name have salt in their contents (e.g., season salt, garlic salt, and onion salt). Condiments such as hot sauce and mustard also have high salt content.

The following recommendations can help people cut back on salt and avoid foods with hidden salt content:

- Eat at home using fresh foods as much as possible.
- Attempt to purchase foods on the perimeter of the grocery store (where the fresh foods can be found) and avoid items in the center (where most of the processed foods can be found).
- Limit consumption of pork and cured meats.
- Use seasonings that are salt free or MSG free (e.g., garlic powder, onion powder).
- Read the labels of all products, paying attention to the sodium (salt) content and serving sizes.

increase cardiac workload and oxygen consumption, resulting in decreased contractility. Consequently, tissue and organ perfusion decreases, leading to multisystem organ failure.

In **hypovolemic shock**, venous return declines because of external blood volume losses (e.g., hemorrhage and dehydration). Preload drops, decreasing ventricular filling and stroke volume. As cardiac output falls, tissue and organ perfusion decreases.

Clinical manifestations of shock reflect the decreased cardiac output and impaired tissue perfusion and may vary depending on the type of shock. General manifestations include the following signs and symptoms:

- Thirst
- Tachycardia
- Restlessness and irritability
- Tachypnea progressing to Cheyne-Stokes respirations

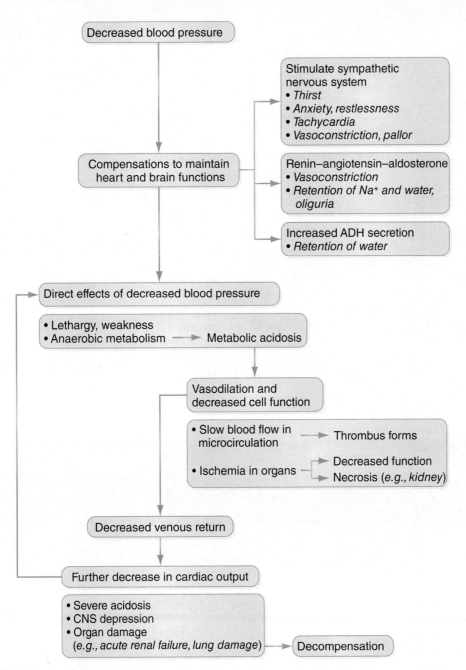

FIGURE 4-39 Progression of shock.

- Cool, pale skin
- Hypotension
- Cyanosis
- Decreased urinary output

Complications of shock can be serious:

- Acute respiratory distress syndrome (see the *Respiratory Function* chapter)
- Renal disease (see the *Urinary Function* chapter)
- Disseminated intravascular coagulation (see the *Hematopoietic Function* chapter)

- Cerebral hypoxia
- Death

Diagnostic procedures for shock consist of a CBC, cultures, coagulation studies, cardiac biomarkers, arterial blood gases, chest X-ray, hemodynamic monitoring, EKG, and echocardiogram. Prompt treatment is crucial for positive patient outcomes. Management of shock includes the identification and treatment of underlying cause, maintaining respiratory status, cardiac monitoring, and rapid fluid replacement.

Mr. Jones, a 50-year-old professor, is 5 hours post laparoscopic cholecystectomy. He is alert and oriented. His physical assessment is within normal limits, including active bowel sounds and a soft, slightly tender abdomen. He is sipping on clear liquids and conversant. The nurse is performing the final assessment and providing discharge patient education. Mr. Jones states he feels a little tired because of all the excitement about going home and feeling so good after surgery. While checking his vital signs for the discharge form, you notice that his pulse is 110 beats/min and irregular compared to the 86–90 beats/min regular pulse that he had been having since surgery. Mr. Jones states his higher pulse just reflects his excitement; he feels great, and his wife is waiting in the car at the patient discharge area for him.

1. What should you do?
2. Is there any significance in an irregular pulse? If yes, describe it.

The healthcare provider returns to the unit to assess the patient's current condition. The healthcare provider orders a stat EKG and chest X-ray, and cancels the prior written discharge order. The EKG shows atrial fibrillation with a ventricular rate of 118, with QRS and ST patterns suggesting an old anterior-wall MI. Mr. Jones continues to rest in semi-Fowler's position in bed. His wife has returned to his bedside. Upon auscultation, you note that Mr. Jones has fine crackles in bilateral lung bases, an occasional dry nonproductive cough, and hiccups, but he denies difficulty in breathing. As you turn to leave the room, you observe Mr. Jones getting out of bed and walking toward the restroom. He is holding onto the footboard stating, "I don't know. I feel sort of weak." He appears slightly tachypneic.

3. Why does Mr. Jones have crackles and cough at rest and tachypnea when walking?
4. Which diagnostic tests would commonly be prescribed for a patient such as Mr. Jones?

Now that we have learned about conditions affecting the cardiovascular system, let's put that knowledge into practice. While you are working in the emergency department, the following patients come in seeking care. Which patient is the highest priority?

- A 75-year-old female with a history of heart failure complaining of increased pedal edema over the past 3 days
- A 67-year-old male with a history of diabetes mellitus complaining of severe indigestion for the past 2 weeks
- A 52-year-old male complaining of "not feeling right," weakness, and severe nausea while working out in his garden an hour ago
- A 28-year-old female with a history of mitral valve prolapse complaining of palpitations

Remember to go through the usual thought process—who would die first, acute versus chronic conditions, Maslow's hierarchy of needs, and patient safety. Starting with the 75-year-old patient, heart failure is a chronic condition and the pedal edema has been going on for 3 days. This patient may be having an exacerbation of her heart failure, but nothing gives you any indication she is in distress. Next, you should definitely be concerned that the diabetic patient with severe indigestion for 2 weeks may have had or be having an MI. As we learned, individuals with diabetes are at increased risk for developing MIs because they typically also have high cholesterol and triglyceride levels, which can lead to atherosclerosis. Such patients do not typically have the classic chest pain associated with MI, and it is concerning that the 67-year-old patient's symptoms have been going on for 2 weeks. With the 52-year-old male who has no notable history, his symptoms could be caused by many things, ranging from dehydration to an active MI. Many times patients will present with a feeling of "impending doom" or that they are "going to die" while having an MI. This man's cardiac needs may have suddenly exceeded his blood supply while gardening. This patient should definitely stay on our radar. Finally, consider the patient having the palpitations. Mitral valve prolapse is a chronic condition that often causes dysrhythmias, most of which are not life threatening.

Although both of the male patients take high priority, the onset of the diabetic patient's symptoms was 2 weeks ago. His myocardium may be permanently damaged, and treatment options may be limited. The 52-year-old may be having an active MI, and the onset seems to be within the optimal 90 minutes for treatment. This patient should be placed on oxygen and an EKG monitor; other steps include administering nitroglycerin, having him chew an aspirin, establishing intravenous access, drawing blood for cardiac biomarkers and other tests, and administering morphine. If it is determined that the patient is having an active MI, then treatment options may include thrombolytics, angioplasty, or surgery. If MI is ruled out, then diagnosis efforts can change to identify other causes. A very close runner-up in terms of priority is the diabetic patient. In the real world, other staff would likely be available to assist with attending to his needs simultaneously, but in NCLEX questions you are typically not given those options.

CHAPTER SUMMARY

The cardiovascular system is responsible for transporting the body's life fluids to maintain a delicate internal balance. This system has a reciprocal relationship with all the other systems—one in which problems in one system create problems in another system. Problems in the cardiovascular system are highly prevalent, and understanding these issues is vital for nurses to provide appropriate care. Prevention of cardiovascular issues often includes lifestyle changes. Early identification and treatment of these conditions are crucial to improve outcomes.

REFERENCES

AAOS. (2004). *Paramedic: Anatomy and physiology*. Sudbury, MA: Jones and Bartlett.

American College of Cardiology & American Heart Association. (2013). Guideline on the treatment of blood cholesterol to reduce atherosclerotic cardiovascular risk in adults. *Journal of the American College of Cardiology*. doi: http://dx.doi.org/10.1161/CIRCULATIONAHA.116.023042

American Heart Association. (n.d.). Normal blood pressure. Retrieved from http://www.heart.org/HEARTORG/Encyclopedia/Heart-Encyclopedia_UCM_445084_Encyclopedia.jsp?levelSelected=26&title=normal%20blood%20pressure

Centers for Disease Control and Prevention (CDC). (2015). Deaths: Final data for 2013. *National Vital Statistics Report*. Retrieved from http://www.cdc.gov/nchs/data/nvsr/nvsr64/nvsr64_02.pdf

Centers for Disease Control and Prevention (CDC). (2016). High blood pressure. Retrieved from http://www.cdc.gov/bloodpressure/

Chiras, D. (2011). *Human biology* (7th ed.). Burlington, MA: Jones & Bartlett Learning.

Crowley, L. V. (2016). *An introduction to human disease* (10th ed.). Burlington, MA: Jones & Bartlett.

Elling, B., Elling, K., & Rothenberg, M. (2004). *Anatomy and physiology*. Sudbury, MA: Jones & Bartlett.

Garcia, T. B., & Holtz, N. E. (2003). *Introduction to 12-lead ECG*. Burlington, MA: Jones & Bartlett.

James, P. A., Oparil, S., Carter, B. L., Cushman, W. C., Dennison-Himmelfarb, C., Handler, J., ... Ortiz, E. (2014). 2014 Evidence-based guidelines for the management of high blood pressure in adults: Report from the panel members appointed to the Eight Joint National Committee (JNC 8). *Journal of the American Medical Association, 311*(5), 507–520.

Madara, B., & Pomarico-Denino, V. (2008). *Pathophysiology* (2nd ed.). Sudbury, MA: Jones and Bartlett.

National Institutes of Health (NIH). (2010). What is endocarditis? Retrieved from https://www.nhlbi.nih.gov/health/health-topics/topics/endo

National Institutes of Health (NIH). (2011). What are congenital heart defects? Retrieved from https://www.nhlbi.nih.gov/health/health-topics/topics/chd

National Institutes of Health (NIH). (2015). What is the DASH eating plan? Retrieved from http://www.nhlbi.nih.gov/health/health-topics/topics/dash/

National Institutes of Health (NIH). (2016). What is cardiomyopathy? Retrieved from http://www.nhlbi.nih.gov/health/health-topics/topics/cm/

Professional guide to pathophysiology (3rd ed.). (2010). Philadelphia, PA: Lippincott Williams & Wilkins.

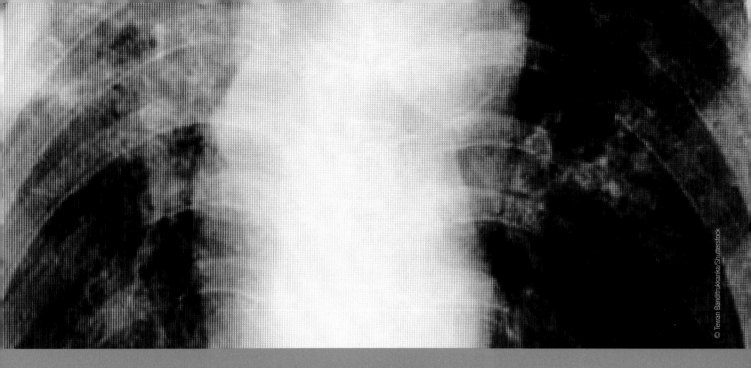

CHAPTER 5
Respiratory Function

LEARNING OBJECTIVES

- Discuss normal respiratory anatomy and physiology.
- Describe and compare infectious disorders of the respiratory system.
- Describe and compare respiratory alterations that impair ventilation.
- Describe and compare respiratory alterations that impair perfusion.

KEY TERMS

active infection
acute bronchitis
acute lung injury (ALI)
acute respiratory distress syndrome (ARDS)
acute respiratory failure (ARF)
alveoli
aspiration pneumonia
asthma
atelectasis
bacterial pneumonia
blue bloaters
bronchi
bronchiole
bronchiolitis
bronchopneumonia
bronchus
chronic bronchitis
chronic obstructive pulmonary disease (COPD)
cilium
community-acquired pneumonia

cystic fibrosis
diaphragm
drug-induced asthma
emphysema
epiglottis
epiglottitis
exercise-induced asthma
expiration
expiratory reserve volume
extrinsic asthma
forced expiratory volume in 1 second
forced vital capacity
infectious rhinitis
influenza
inspiration
inspiratory reserve volume
interstitial pneumonia
intrinsic asthma
laryngitis
laryngotracheobronchitis
larynx
Legionnaires' disease

lobar pneumonia
lung cancer
Middle East respiratory syndrome
minute respiratory volume
mucus
Mycoplasma pneumoniae
nocturnal asthma
non-small-cell carcinoma
nosocomial pneumonia
occupational asthma
perfusion
pharynx
pink puffers
pleural effusion
pleurisy
Pneumocystis jiroveci pneumonia
pneumonia
pneumothorax
primary TB infection
residual volume
rhinosinusitis

secondary TB infection
severe acute respiratory syndrome (SARS)
sinusitis
small-cell carcinoma
spontaneous pneumothorax
status asthmaticus
surfactant
tension pneumothorax
tidal volume
trachea
traumatic pneumothorax
tuberculosis (TB)
type A influenza
type B influenza
type C influenza
ventilation
ventilation/perfusion ratio (VQ ratio)
viral pneumonia
vital capacity

The respiratory system includes the organs and structures associated with breathing and gas exchange. The structures of the respiratory system are grouped into two branches—the upper respiratory tract (mouth, nasal cavity, pharynx, and larynx) (**FIGURE 5-1**) and the lower respiratory tract (trachea, bronchi, bronchioles, and alveoli). This chapter focuses on normal and abnormal states of the lungs. The respiratory tract functions automatically to provide cells with oxygen and to remove carbon dioxide waste. Disorders of the respiratory tract can become serious quickly because of the body's critical need for oxygen. Patients with these disorders will need astute nurses who respond quickly yet thoughtfully.

Anatomy and Physiology

The respiratory system provides vital oxygen and removes toxic carbon dioxide through the act of breathing. The respiratory tract allows a person to breathe in and out approximately 23,000 times each day. In fact, if you had a dollar for each breath, you would be a millionaire in a month and a half. The act of breathing allows for gas exchange of oxygen and carbon dioxide. Oxygen is necessary for cells to produce energy through cellular metabolism; carbon dioxide is the waste product of this process. Through its gas exchange functions, the respiratory system plays a pivotal role in maintaining homeostasis.

The respiratory system consists of two basic functional divisions—an air-conducting portion and a gas-exchanging portion (**TABLE 5-1**). The air-conducting portion delivers air to the lungs, while the gas-exchanging portion allows gas exchange to occur between the air and the blood (Figure 5-1). The gas-exchanging portion of the respiratory tract includes the lungs with their millions of **alveoli** and capillaries (**FIGURE 5-2**).

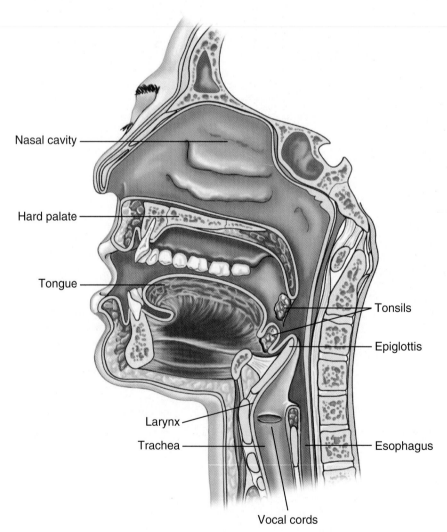

FIGURE 5-1 The upper respiratory tract.

Nasal cavity

Hard palate

Tongue

Tonsils

Epiglottis

Larynx

Trachea

Esophagus

Vocal cords

TABLE 5-1	Summary of the Respiratory System

Organ	Function
Air Conducting	
Nasal cavity	Filters, warms, and moistens air; also transports air to pharynx
Oral cavity	Transports air to pharynx; warms and moistens air; helps produce sounds
Pharynx	Transports air to larynx
Epiglottis	Covers the opening to the trachea during swallowing
Larynx	Produces sounds; transports air to trachea; helps filter incoming air; warms and moistens incoming air
Trachea and bronchi	Warm and moisten air; transport air to lungs; filter incoming air
Bronchioles	Control air flow in the lungs; transport air to alveoli
Gas Exchange	
Alveoli	Provide area for exchange of oxygen and carbon dioxide

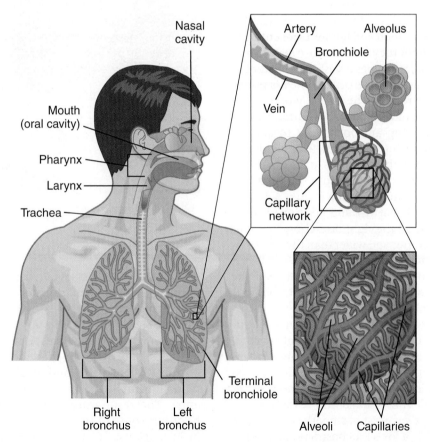

FIGURE 5-2 The respiratory system. This illustration shows the air-conducting portion and the gas-exchange portion of the human respiratory system. The insert shows a higher magnification of the alveoli where oxygen and carbon dioxide exchange occurs.

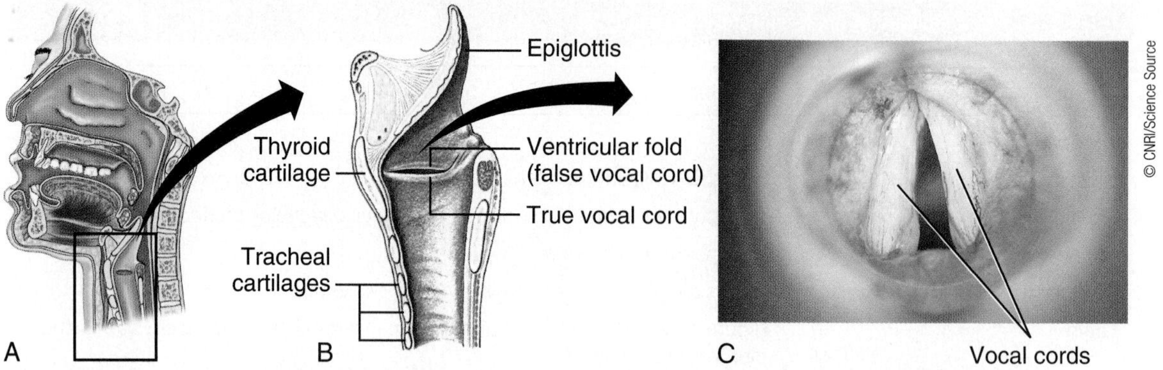

Epiglottis

Thyroid cartilage

Ventricular fold (false vocal cord)

True vocal cord

Tracheal cartilages

Vocal cords

A   B   C

© CNRI/Science Source

FIGURE 5-3 The vocal cords. (a) Uppermost portion of the respiratory system, showing the location of the vocal cords. (b) Longitudinal section of the larynx showing the location of the vocal cords. Note the presence of the false vocal cord, so named because it does not function in phonation. (c) View into the larynx of a patient showing the true vocal cords from above.

Air enters the respiratory system through the nose and mouth, then travels to the **pharynx**. The pharynx joins the **larynx**, or voice box (**FIGURE 5-3**). The larynx is made of cartilage and plays a central role in swallowing and talking. When food is swallowed, the larynx rises so that it is closed by the **epiglottis**. This process prevents food and liquids from entering the lungs, where they would cause severe irritation. Even so, food does occasionally enter the lungs, often triggering the cough reflex (a primitive protective reflex). The larynx works much like the strings of a guitar or violin to produce sound—tightening and loosening to change pitch. It opens up into the **trachea**, or windpipe. From the trachea, the air travels to the mainstem **bronchi**, where it branches into the right and left bronchi, one for each lung (**FIGURE 5-4**). The left **bronchus** is narrow and positioned more horizontally than the right bronchus; the right bronchus is shorter and wider than the left bronchus and extends downward more vertically. Because of the difference in size between the two, objects are more easily inhaled (aspirated) into the right bronchus.

Inside the lungs, the bronchi branch extensively into a series of smaller and smaller tubes, or **bronchioles**, until they reach the alveoli. This branching from larger to smaller mimics the vessels in the cardiovascular system. The walls of the bronchioles are also like the vessel walls in that they mostly consist of smooth muscle. The smooth muscle allows for constriction and dilation of the bronchioles to control air flow. When oxygen needs are higher (e.g., during exercise or stress), the airways open more (dilate) to allow more air to enter the lungs. In times of normal or decreased oxygen needs (e.g., during sleep), the airways may narrow (constrict)

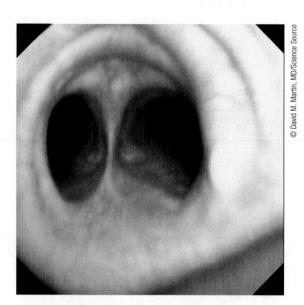

© David M. Martin, MD/Science Source

FIGURE 5-4 The bifurcation of the trachea at the carina into the right and left mainstem bronchi.

slightly. Disease processes may cause constriction to the point of impeding air flow—a dangerous development.

The air entering the respiratory tract often contains particles that can be harmful. These particles may include infectious organisms (e.g., bacteria, viruses, and fungi) and environmental agents (e.g., dust, pollen, and pollutants). The respiratory system is equipped to filter out some of these particles as well as to protect against the body those that gain entry. The air-conducting portion of the respiratory tract filters many particles by trapping them in the mucus layer (**FIGURE 5-5**). **Mucus** is a thick, sticky substance produced by the goblet cells in the epithelial lining of the nose, trachea, and bronchi. This epithelial lining also contains

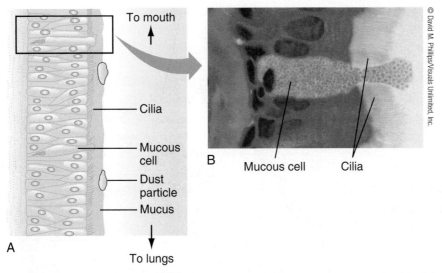

FIGURE 5-5 Mucous trap. (a) Drawing of the lining of the trachea. Mucus produced by the mucous cells of the lining of much of the respiratory system traps organisms and other particulates in the air. The cilia transport the mucus toward the mouth. (b) Higher magnification of the lining showing a mucous cell and ciliated epithelial cells.

many **cilia**, or hair-like projections, that move in a wavelike motion to propel the mucus and trapped particles upward to the mouth, where they can be expectorated (spit out). Cigarette smoking and air pollution can decrease mucus production and destroy cilia, increasing the risk of respiratory infections. Alcohol consumption can paralyze cilia, also increasing infection risk.

Additionally, the immune system is outfitted with immunoglobulin A (IgA) cells that prevent the attachment and invasion of bacteria and viruses on mucous membranes (see the *Immunity* chapter). Macrophages are also present around the alveoli in the lungs; they keep the lungs clean by phagocytizing particles that gain access to this area (**FIGURE 5-6**). Once the macrophages fill with particulates, they move into the surrounding connective tissue. When an unusually large number of particulates are present (e.g., with cigarette and marijuana smoking and when breathing in heavy pollution), the lungs become blackened by the accumulation of the particles.

The air-conducting portion of the respiratory system also moistens and warms incoming air. An extensive network of capillaries lies beneath the epithelium of the respiratory tract. These capillaries release moisture into the incoming air, humidifying it to prevent drying of the respiratory tract. The warm blood circulating through the capillaries heats this air prior to entering the lungs, protecting the lungs from cold temperatures. As the air leaves the respiratory tract, much of the water that has been added to the air condenses onto the slightly cooler lining of the nasal passages. The condensation is recycled for the next inhalation to conserve water, and contributes to runny noses on cold days.

Alveoli are the site for gas exchange with the bloodstream (**FIGURE 5-7**). Oxygen is delivered to the alveoli by the air-conducting portion of the respiratory system, and carbon dioxide is brought to the lungs by the circulatory system. Each human lung contains approximately 150 million alveoli, which collectively create a surface area approximately the size of a tennis court for gas exchange. The alveoli and capillaries are often a single cell layer thick, which further facilitates gas exchange. The amount of gas exchanged depends on the total surface area available and the thickness of the alveoli and capillary walls. The more surface area and the thinner the layers, the more rapidly gas diffuses.

Gas exchange in the alveoli requires adequate **ventilation** of air and **perfusion** of blood flow. The **ventilation/perfusion ratio**, or **VQ ratio**, is a measurement of the efficacy and adequacy of these two processes. In the ideal lung, inspired air reaches all the alveoli and all the alveoli have the same blood supply. In the real world, however, neither alveolar ventilation nor capillary blood flow is uniform. The supply of air and blood never match perfectly, even in healthy persons. Because of gravity, the lower parts of the lungs have greater blood flow than the upper parts. Distribution

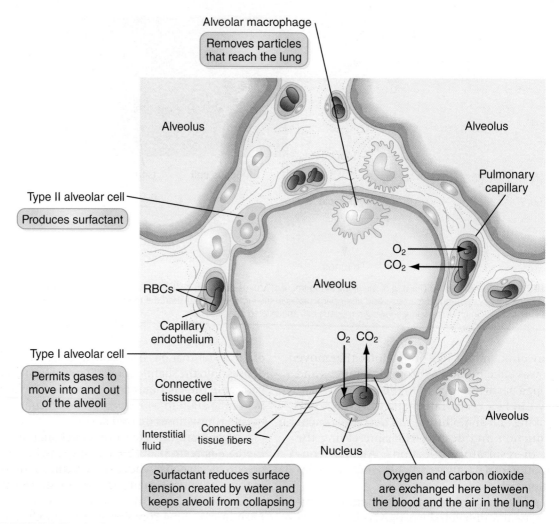

Alveolar macrophage
Removes particles that reach the lung

Alveolus

Alveolus

Pulmonary capillary

Type II alveolar cell
Produces surfactant

O_2
CO_2

RBCs

Alveolus

Capillary endothelium

O_2 CO_2

Type I alveolar cell
Permits gases to move into and out of the alveoli

Connective tissue cell

Alveolus

Interstitial fluid

Connective tissue fibers

Nucleus

Surfactant reduces surface tension created by water and keeps alveoli from collapsing

Oxygen and carbon dioxide are exchanged here between the blood and the air in the lung

FIGURE 5-6 The alveolar macrophages.

of alveolar ventilation from the top to the bottom of the lungs is also uneven. Normal ventilation is 4 liters of air per minute, and normal perfusion is 5 liters of blood per minute. This difference makes the expected VQ ratio 4/5, or 0.8. A VQ ratio higher than 0.8 indicates that ventilation exceeds perfusion, and a VQ ratio less than 0.8 indicates poor ventilation. Some respiratory disorders involve ventilation problems, whereas others result from perfusion issues. In any event, the result is impaired gas exchange.

When air is inhaled, gases are exchanged between the alveoli and the capillaries; carbon dioxide is removed through expiration, and oxygen is delivered to cells by the cardiovascular system (**FIGURE 5-8**). Hemoglobin carries oxygen to the cells, then releases it there. The rate at which hemoglobin binds and releases oxygen is affected by several factors, including temperature and pH, among other things (**FIGURE 5-9**).

The surface of the alveoli contains a substance called **surfactant**. Surfactant is a lipoprotein produced by alveoli cells that has a detergent-like quality. This watery substance produces surface tension on the alveoli, which enhances pulmonary compliance (elasticity) and prevents the alveoli from collapsing. Because the pressure in the lungs is negative compared with the atmospheric pressure, the walls of the alveoli tend to draw inward, making them collapse. This pressure is much like that seen with a vacuum-sealed pack of coffee. The pressure and, therefore, the risk of collapse further increase at the end of expiration. Surfactant promotes reinflation of the alveoli during inspiration. Disease states and other conditions can decrease surfactant, leading to the collapse of the alveoli (a condition called atelectasis). For example, premature infants lack surfactant, and smoking alters surfactant production. Synthetic surfactant may be administered to overcome any inadequacies in production.

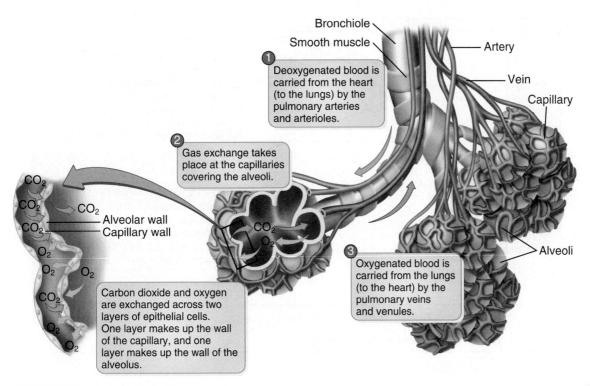

Bronchiole

Smooth muscle

Artery

Vein

Capillary

1 Deoxygenated blood is carried from the heart (to the lungs) by the pulmonary arteries and arterioles.

2 Gas exchange takes place at the capillaries covering the alveoli.

CO_2
CO_2
CO_2
CO_2

Alveolar wall
Capillary wall

CO_2
O_2

O_2
O_2

CO_2

O_2

O_2

CO_2
O_2

Carbon dioxide and oxygen are exchanged across two layers of epithelial cells. One layer makes up the wall of the capillary, and one layer makes up the wall of the alveolus.

Alveoli

3 Oxygenated blood is carried from the lungs (to the heart) by the pulmonary veins and venules.

FIGURE 5-7 Gas exchange in the lungs.

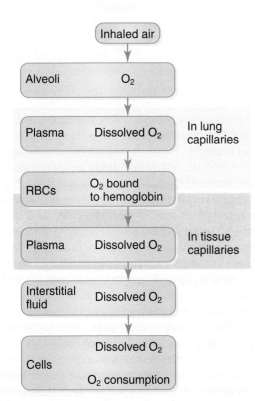

Inhaled air

Alveoli → O_2

Plasma → Dissolved O_2 — In lung capillaries

RBCs → O_2 bound to hemoglobin

Plasma → Dissolved O_2 — In tissue capillaries

Interstitial fluid → Dissolved O_2

Cells → Dissolved O_2 → O_2 consumption

FIGURE 5-8 Oxygen diffusion. Oxygen travels from the alveoli first into the blood plasma, and then into the red blood cells (RBCs), where much of it binds to hemoglobin. When the oxygenated blood reaches the tissues, oxygen is released from the RBCs and diffuses first into the plasma, then into the interstitial fluid and body cells.

The process of breathing is largely involuntary and controlled by the medulla oblongata in the brain. This center is located in the brain stem, which controls many vital functions in the body (e.g., heart rate, blood pressure, and temperature). Breathing includes two phases: **inspiration** (inhalation—moving air in) and **expiration** (exhalation—moving air out).

Inspiration is an active neural process that begins when nerve impulses travel from the brain to the **diaphragm**, the dome-shaped muscle that separates the thoracic and abdominal cavities (**FIGURE 5-10**). These impulses cause the diaphragm to contract, lower, and flatten, which draws air into the lungs. Inspiration also involves the intercostal muscles between the ribs. Nerve impulses cause the intercostal muscles to contract, lifting the ribs up and out. Contraction of the diaphragm and intercostal muscles changes the intrapulmonary pressure, causing air to naturally flow into the lungs.

In contrast, expiration is passive—it does not require muscle contraction. As the lungs fill with air, the diaphragm and intercostal muscles relax, returning to their previous position. Returning to their natural position decreases thoracic volume and increases intrapulmonary

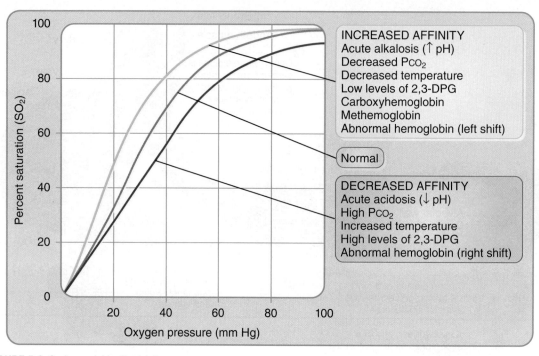

FIGURE 5-9 Oxyhemoglobin dissociation curve.

pressure. This greater pressure forces air out of the lungs. Elastic fibers in the lungs aid in passive expiration by causing the lungs to recoil. Expiration can also be active—that is, created by contracting the chest and abdominal muscles.

Air flow, both inspiratory and expiratory, can be measured to aid in diagnosis of respiratory disorders (**FIGURE 5-11**). Pulmonary function tests evaluate lung volumes and capacities. **Tidal volume** is the amount of air involved in one normal inhalation and exhalation. The average tidal volume is 500 mL, but is smaller in shallow breathing. **Minute respiratory volume** is the amount inhaled and exhaled in 1 minute. This volume is calculated by multiplying the tidal volume by the number of respirations per minute; the average is 6 liters per minute. **Inspiratory reserve volume** is the amount of air beyond the tidal volume that can be taken in with the deepest inhalation. Inspiratory reserve volume averages 2–3 liters. **Expiratory reserve volume** is the amount of air beyond tidal volume that can be forcibly exhaled beyond the normal passive exhalation. The average expiratory reserve volume is 1–1.5 liters. **Vital capacity** is the sum of the tidal volume and reserves. Some air is always present in the lungs, and this amount is called **residual volume**. Even after the most forceful exhalation,

1–1.5 liters of air remains in the lungs, which ensures efficient and consistent gas exchange. **Forced expiratory volume in 1 second** is compared to **forced vital capacity** to diagnose pulmonary disease.

The medulla controls breathing through nerve cells that generate nerve impulses to the respiratory muscles. When the lungs are full, these impulses cease, allowing the muscles to relax. Chemoreceptors inside the brain and arteries also regulate breathing. These receptors detect carbon dioxide levels and send messages to the medulla. Carbon dioxide levels normally drive breathing (**FIGURE 5-12**). When these levels go up, respiration depth and rate increase to excrete the excess carbon dioxide, and vice versa. In some disease states, this drive becomes altered, and oxygen levels drive breathing. Additionally, stretch receptors in the lungs aid in breathing by detecting when the lungs are full. In such a case, the stretch receptors in the lungs send a message to the medulla to cease firing. This effect, which is called the Hering-Breuer reflex, prevents overinflation of the lungs. The body also has oxygen receptors, but they are not very sensitive. These receptors do not generate impulses until oxygen levels fall to a critical point.

In addition to regulating oxygen and carbon dioxide levels, the lungs aid in regulating pH by altering breathing rate and depth.

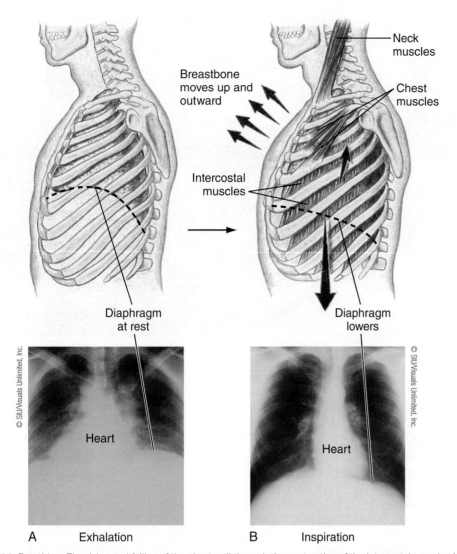

Neck muscles

Breastbone moves up and outward

Chest muscles

Intercostal muscles

Diaphragm at rest

Diaphragm lowers

Heart

Heart

© SIU/Visuals Unlimited, Inc.

© SIU/Visuals Unlimited, Inc.

A   Exhalation

B   Inspiration

FIGURE 5-10 Breathing. The rising and falling of the chest wall through the contraction of the intercostal muscles (muscles between the ribs) is shown in the diagram, illustrating the bellows effect. Inspiration is assisted by the diaphragm, which assumes a lower position in the chest. Like pulling a plunger back on a syringe, the rising of the chest wall and the lowering of the diaphragm draw air into the lungs. Illustrations and X-rays showing the lungs in full exhalation (a) and full inspiration (b).

Carbon dioxide is a source of acid in the body. Increasing the respiratory rate and depth will lead to excretion of more carbon dioxide, making the blood less acidic. Conversely, decreasing the respiratory rate and depth will cause retention of more carbon dioxide, making the blood more acidic. This compensatory mechanism allows for a quick fix of pH imbalances to reestablish homeostasis (also see the *Fluid, Electrolyte, and Acid–Base Homeostasis* chapter).

Learning Points

Carbon dioxide is the normal driving force for breathing. In other words, breathing is controlled by carbon dioxide levels. How does this translate into action? As carbon dioxide levels rise, the lungs will exhale to expel the excess carbon dioxide. To understand how strong this drive is, consider holding your breath. If you take a deep breath and try to hold it, eventually you have to let the air out. No matter how hard you try, you cannot hold your breath past a certain point. The body can be trained to hold a breath longer and longer (as swimmers and divers do), but no matter the training, you will eventually have to let it out.

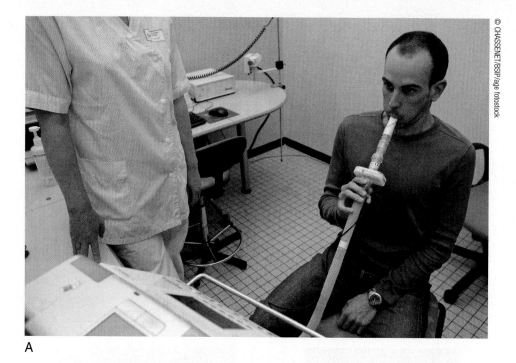

A

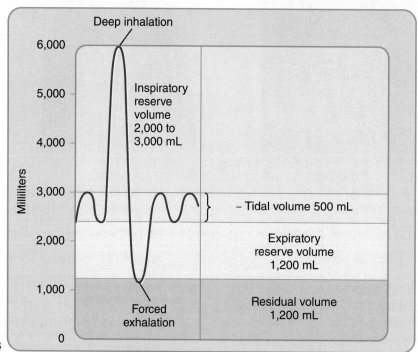

B

FIGURE 5-11 Measuring air flow. (a) This machine allows healthcare workers to determine tidal volume, inspiratory reserve volume, and other lung-capacity measurements to determine the health of an individual's lung. (b) This graph shows several common measurements.

Normal cycle

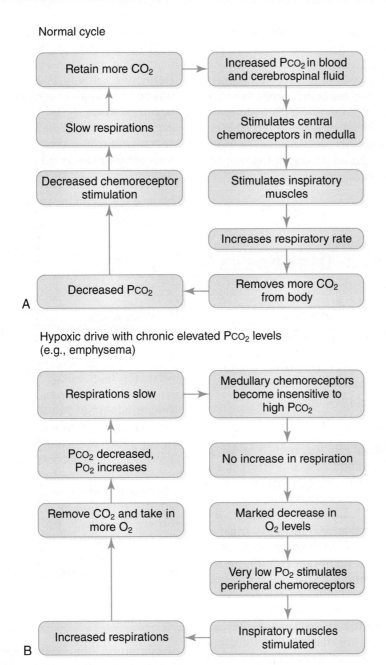

FIGURE 5-12 Normal respiratory control and hypoxic drive.

UNDERSTANDING CONDITIONS THAT AFFECT THE RESPIRATORY SYSTEM

When considering alterations in the respiratory system, it is best to organize them based on their basic underlying pathophysiology to increase understanding.

Those pathophysiological concepts include conditions that are infectious in nature, problems with ventilation, and issues with perfusion. Infectious conditions may involve either the upper respiratory tract or the lower respiratory tract. The respiratory system requires both ventilation and perfusion to function properly. Problems in either of these areas will impair the respiratory system's ability to meet the body's needs. Ventilation conditions result from problems with moving air in or out of the lungs. Perfusion conditions result from problems that prevent gas exchange; many of these conditions are cardiovascular in nature (e.g., pulmonary embolism).

When considering these conditions, also determine which respiratory-related nursing diagnosis is in play—altered gas exchange or ineffective airway clearance. Altered gas exchange includes conditions that decrease gas exchange in the lungs (e.g., asthma, emphysema, and chronic bronchitis). Impaired airway clearance includes conditions in which secretions are stagnant (e.g., pneumonia and cystic fibrosis).

INFECTIOUS DISORDERS

Upper Respiratory Tract Infections

The upper respiratory tract includes the mouth, nasal cavity, pharynx, and larynx. Infections of these structures trigger the inflammatory response, which explains many of the symptoms associated with these conditions.

Infectious Rhinitis

Infectious rhinitis, also referred to as viral rhinitis and the common cold, is a viral upper respiratory infection. The most frequent culprit is a rhinovirus, but many viruses (e.g., adenovirus and coronavirus) can cause this illness. In fact, there are more than 100 causative organisms, making it difficult to develop immunity. Infectious rhinitis is a significant contributor to work and school absences, with adults averaging 2–3 colds per year and children having even more such infections (Centers for Disease Control and Prevention [CDC], 2016b).

In infectious rhinitis, the infectious organism invades the epithelial lining of the nasal mucosa. Mild cellular inflammation leads to nasal discharge, mucus production, and shedding of the epithelial cells. This breach in the physical and chemical barriers of the respiratory tract increases vulnerability to bacterial invasions. As a consequence, secondary bacterial infections (e.g., otitis media, rhinosinusitis, bronchitis, and pneumonia) are commonly associated with viral infections (FIGURE 5-13). The risk for secondary bacterial infections is further increased in individuals who smoke because of the chronic damage done by smoke to the mucosa and cilia. Despite popular misconceptions, wet and cold conditions do not cause or increase occurrences of infectious rhinitis. Close physical contact with

the virus transmits the infection through exchanges with other humans (e.g., shaking hands) and surfaces (e.g., doorknobs and telephones). Transmission may occur through both inhalation and contact (e.g., hand to hand or hand to mucous membrane). Hands are virally contaminated 60% of the time. The apparent increase in occurrence of the infectious rhinitis during rainy and cold weather is due to increased congregation in confined spaces. Those persons in more frequent, closer contact with other people will be at higher risk for developing the infection (e.g., children in daycare centers, healthcare providers, and teachers). The virus is highly contagious because it is shed in large numbers from the nasal mucosa, and the virus can survive for several hours outside the body.

An individual who contracts infectious rhinitis usually experiences an incubation period between the invasion of the virus and the onset of symptoms that lasts approximately 2–3 days, but can be as long as 7 days. Clinical manifestations include the following signs and symptoms:

- Sneezing
- Nasal congestion or stuffiness
- Clear nasal discharge
- Sore throat
- Lacrimation (eye tearing)
- Nonproductive cough
- Malaise (generalized discomfort)
- Myalgia (muscle aches and pains)
- Low-grade fever
- Hoarseness
- Headache
- Chills

Myth Busters

A common misconception is that you get colds from being cold or wet. The fuel for this myth is the increased occurrence of colds during cold and wet weather. In fact, the weather conditions themselves do not make you sick—but the weather *does* increase congregation of people indoors to avoid those weather conditions. The congregation of people in close, closed spaces is responsible for the spread of the cold. The infectious rhinitis virus is virulent and highly contagious through close contact.

Misconceptions are hard to change; it usually takes multiple efforts. So do your part to educate the public about the truth of cold transmission and prevention!

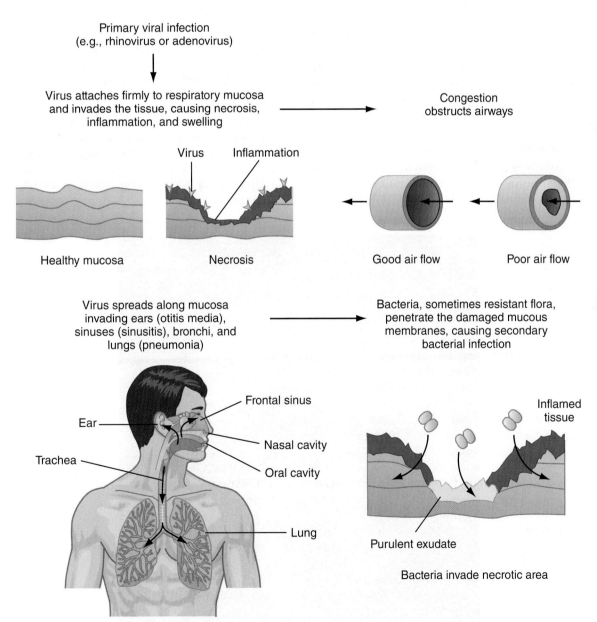

FIGURE 5-13 Complications of viral respiratory infections.

Diagnosis of infectious rhinitis is primarily made based on the presence of symptoms. Treatment is symptomatic. Most over-the-counter cold preparations are ineffective in shortening the course of the infection, and they should be avoided in children younger than 4 years. Pharmacologic therapies that may be used include antipyretics (for fever), analgesics (for discomfort), decongestants (for nasal symptoms), cough suppressants or expectorants, and antibiotics (only if a bacterial infection is present). Humidifiers can liquefy secretions to aid in expectoration. Maintaining adequate hydration can also liquefy secretions and help manage fevers. Nasal saline can ease nasal discomfort. The benefit of vitamin C in prevention and treatment remains controversial.

Proper hand washing remains the long-standing cornerstone of prevention because the hands are a significant source of transmission. Additional prevention measures include covering one's mouth when coughing and sneezing, using tissue or the upper sleeve of one's shirt, and disposing of tissue immediately after use.

Rhinosinusitis

Sinusitis is an inflammation of the sinus cavities. Sinusitis rarely occurs without concurrent rhinitis; therefore, **rhinosinusitis** is now the preferred term for sinusitis. Rhinosinusitis is most often caused by a viral infection (e.g., rhinovirus, influenza, or adenovirus). Other causative agents include bacteria (e.g., *Streptococcus pneumoniae* or *Haemophilus influenzae*) and fungi (e.g., *Aspergillus* or mucormycosis). Environmental irritants (e.g., smoke exposure and air pollutants), immunocompromised status (e.g., HIV infection), conditions that increase mucus production (e.g., cystic fibrosis or asthma), and nasal structural abnormalities (e.g., nasal polyps) can further increase risk. Rhinosinusitis can be a result of a secondary bacterial infection associated with infectious rhinitis or allergic rhinitis in which the drainage from the sinus cavity has become blocked (**FIGURE 5-14**). The drainage accumulation provides a supportive medium for bacterial growth. *Streptococcus pneumoniae* and *Haemophilus influenzae* are commonly found in the upper airways of healthy people.

Sinusitis can present as several different types:

- Acute, which lasts up to 4 weeks
- Subacute, which lasts 4–12 weeks
- Chronic, which lasts more than 12 weeks and can continue for months or even years
- Recurrent, with several attacks occurring within a year

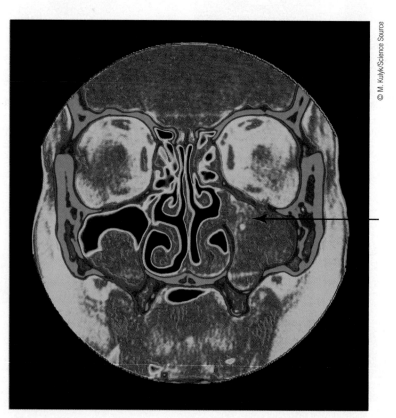

© M. Kulyk/Science Source

FIGURE 5-14 Blocked sinus.

As exudate accumulates, pressure builds in the sinus cavity, which causes facial bone pain and headache. The location of pain can indicate which sinus is affected. Other clinical manifestations of rhinosinusitis include nasal congestion, purulent nasal discharge, hyposmia (reduced ability to smell), halitosis (foul-smelling breath), mouth breathing, fever, sore throat, and malaise. Complications can include orbital cellulitis, meningitis, osteomyelitis, and abscess.

Diagnostic procedures for rhinosinusitis include a history, physical examination, nasal cultures, sinus X-ray, sinus computerized tomography (CT), and sinus transillumination (FIGURE 5-15). Treatment usually includes decongestants (to shrink swollen nasal membranes), analgesics, and nasal corticosteroid spray (to shrink swollen nasal membranes) until the sinuses begin draining. Bacterial infections require antibiotic therapy to resolve. Other measures may include humidifiers (to liquefy secretions and aid in drainage), warm compresses, adequate hydration, and avoidance of irritants (e.g., smoke, chemicals, and other allergens). In children with recurrent sinusitis and other upper respiratory infections, removing the adenoids may resolve the issue.

Epiglottitis

Epiglottitis is a life-threatening condition of the epiglottis, the protective cartilage lid covering the trachea opening. In the past, *Haemophilus influenzae* type b (Hib) was the most common cause in the United States, but widespread use of the Hib vaccine has dramatically decreased the rate of *H. influenzae* infections in recent years. With the Hib vaccine, epiglottitis is now very uncommon except in adults, who are less likely than children to receive the vaccine. Common culprits now include Group A beta-hemolytic *Streptococcus*, *Streptococcus pneumoniae*, and *Staphylococcus aureus*. Other causes include throat trauma from events such as drinking hot liquids, swallowing a foreign object, a direct blow to the throat, or smoking crack or heroin. The inflammatory response that is triggered by these events causes the epiglottis to quickly swell and block the air entering the trachea, leading to respiratory failure. The bacteria can also travel to the bloodstream, leading to sepsis, which is also life threatening because it activates a massive immune response.

The onset of clinical manifestations is typically rapid in children, developing in a matter of hours, but occurs more slowly in adults, over a few days. These manifestations include the following signs and symptoms:

- High fever
- Chills and shaking
- Sore throat and hoarseness
- Dysphagia (difficulty swallowing)
- Drooling with the mouth open
- Mild inspiratory stridor (a harsh, high-pitched sound made as a result of air movement restriction)
- Respiratory distress

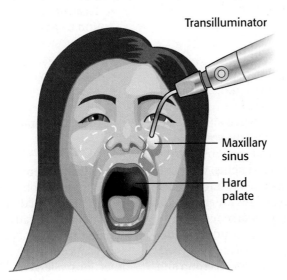

Transilluminator

Maxillary sinus

Hard palate

FIGURE 5-15 Transillumination of the sinuses.

- Central cyanosis (blue discoloration of the mouth and lips)
- Anxiety, irritability, or restlessness (a result of hypoxia)
- Pallor
- Assuming a sitting tripod position, often leaning slightly forward (a subconscious attempt to facilitate breathing)

If epiglottitis is suspected, maintaining the airway and stabilizing respiratory status is the priority before diagnostic procedures are performed. Efforts to preserve respiratory function include humidified oxygen therapy (likely delivered via mask), endotracheal intubation with mechanical ventilation, and tracheotomy. Additional efforts to minimize oxygen consumption should include keeping the patient calm and controlling fever (e.g., with antipyretics and hydration). Aerosolized epinephrine and systemic steroids (often treatments for croup) should be avoided because they may worsen the condition. Additionally, a tongue depressor should not be used to examine the patient because it can further traumatize the tissue. Once the patient is stabilized, diagnostic procedures include visualization of the epiglottis through a fiber-optic camera, X-rays (throat and chest), cultures (throat and blood), arterial blood gases (ABGs), and a complete blood count (CBC).

Intravenous antibiotics will be used to treat infections quickly. Hib vaccinations should be encouraged for children, the elderly, and immunocompromised persons so transmission rates will continue to be low. Other prevention strategies include proper hand washing, avoiding crowds, cleaning objects (e.g., toys), and not sharing objects (e.g., pacifiers and bottles).

Laryngitis

Laryngitis is an inflammation of the larynx that is usually a result of an infection, increased upper respiratory exudate, irritants (e.g., stomach acid, inhaled smoke, excessive alcohol use, or chemicals), or overuse. Viral infections (e.g., influenza, rhinovirous, and adenovirus) are the most common cause. With laryngitis, the vocal cords become irritated and edematous because of the inflammatory process. This inflammation distorts sounds, leading to hoarseness and in some cases making the voice undetectable. Occasionally, the airway can become blocked. Laryngitis can also be associated with croup and epiglottitis.

Learning Points

Epiglottitis is often misdiagnosed as croup. One distinct difference in manifestations can assist healthcare providers in moving to appropriate life-saving treatment more quickly. With epiglottitis, patients "look worse than they sound." With croup, they "sound worse than they look" due to the seal-like barking cough. Additionally, cough is not generally seen with epiglottitis. Although severe croup can cause complete airway obstruction, it is rarely life threatening. Picking up on this significant manifestation can save the patient's life!

Clinical manifestations of laryngitis usually last less than a week and include the following signs and symptoms:

- Hoarseness
- Weak voice or voice loss
- Tickling sensation and raw feeling in the throat
- Sore, dry throat
- Dry cough
- Swollen nodes of the neck
- Leukocytosis (if bacterial)
- Difficulty breathing (in children)

Diagnostic procedures for laryngitis include a history, physical examination, CBC, and laryngoscopy. A biopsy may be conducted if symptoms persist, because throat cancer can mimic acute laryngitis. Treatment depends on the cause, and many times the laryngitis will improve without treatment. Treatment strategies aim to increase comfort or decrease the duration of the inflammation:

- Warm humidity
- Resting the voice
- Increasing fluid intake
- Treating the underlying cause (e.g., infection or gastric reflux)
- Analgesics
- Throat lozenges
- Gargling with salt water
- Avoidance of decongestants, antihistamines, and corticosteroids (they dry out the mucous membranes)

Laryngotracheobronchitis

Laryngotracheobronchitis, or croup, is a common viral infection in children 3 months to 3 years of age. Other children and adults may also contract it. Routine causative agents include parainfluenza viruses, adenoviruses, and respiratory syncytial virus. Additional causes include bacterial infections, allergens, and irritants (e.g., stomach acid, inhaled smoke, or chemicals). Outbreaks and epidemics occur in autumn to early winter, but cases can occur sporadically year-round. Croup was once a deadly disease caused by diphtheria bacteria, but the introduction of antibiotics and immunizations have improved its prevention and treatment. Today, most cases of croup are mild. Nevertheless, this disease can still be dangerous.

Croup generally affects the larynx and trachea, but it may sometimes extend to the bronchi. This condition usually begins as an upper respiratory infection with nasal congestion and cough. The larynx and surrounding area swell, leading to airway narrowing and obstruction. This swelling can lead to respiratory failure. Clinical manifestations worsen at night and usually resolve in about a week. These manifestations include the following signs and symptoms:

- Low-grade fever
- Nasal congestion
- Seal-like barking cough (because of laryngeal swelling)
- Hoarseness
- Inspiratory stridor
- Mild expiratory wheezing
- Dyspnea
- Anxiety
- Central cyanosis

Diagnostic procedures for croup consist of a history, physical examination, X-rays (throat), throat cultures, ABGs, and CBC. A throat X-ray will reveal a narrowing of the trachea (often referred to as the steeple sign) in 50% of cases (**FIGURE 5-16**).

Croup is usually self-limiting but can be life threatening without supportive therapy. Treatment strategies include cool humidity, corticosteroids (to decrease edema), humidified oxygen (e.g., an oxygen tent over an infant's crib), bronchodilators (to open the airway), hydration (to combat fever, moisten the airway, and liquefy secretions), and aerosolized epinephrine (in severe respiratory distress). Cool humidity may decrease edema, but no studies have supported this treatment. This intervention should be avoided in patients with asthma because it may trigger bronchial constriction. Cool humidity can be accomplished with a cool-mist humidifier, exposure to cool outside air especially at night, and exposure to cold shower mist in a closed bathroom. Strategies to decrease oxygen consumption include keeping the patient calm and avoiding unnecessary procedures. Additionally, educating the public regarding diphtheria vaccination compliance is critical to manage this once life-threatening condition.

Acute Bronchitis

Acute bronchitis is an inflammation of the tracheobronchial tree or large bronchi. This inflammation is most commonly caused by a wide range of viruses (e.g., influenza, rhinovirus, respiratory syncytial virus, and adenovirus). Bacterial invasions (e.g., *Streptococcus pneumoniae* and *Haemophilus influenzae*), irritant inhalation (e.g., smoke, marijuana, pollution, and ammonia), and allergic reactions are less frequent causes. Young children, the elderly, and smokers are at the highest risk for developing acute bronchitis.

In acute bronchitis, the bronchial lining becomes irritated and the airways become narrowed due to the results of the inflammatory process (e.g., capillary dilation, edema, and exudate). Clinical manifestations of acute bronchitis are usually mild and resolve in 7–10 days, but coughing may linger for several weeks after the infection is resolved. These manifestations include the following:

- Productive or nonproductive cough
- Dyspnea
- Wheezing

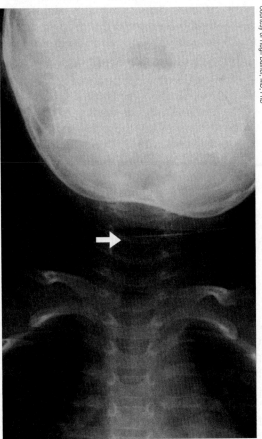

Courtesy of Hugh Dainer, MD, PhD

FIGURE 5-16 Steeple sign.

- Abnormal lung sounds (usually rales or rhonchi)
- Low-grade fever
- Pharyngitis
- Malaise
- Myalgia
- Chest discomfort

Diagnosis of acute bronchitis is usually based on symptoms. Additionally, a CBC, cultures (e.g., nasal secretions, sputum, blood), and chest X-ray may be performed for differential diagnosis purposes.

Acute bronchitis is generally self-limiting; therefore, treatment is often supportive. Pharmacologic treatment may include antipyretics, analgesics, antihistamines, decongestants, cough suppressants, bronchodilators, and antibiotics (in case of bacterial infection). Use cough suppressants cautiously, as coughing mobilizes secretions and can prevent pneumonia. Other strategies include increasing fluid intake, avoiding smoke, and humidifying air.

Influenza

Influenza, or flu, is a viral infection that may affect the upper and lower respiratory tract. Three types are distinguished—A, B, and C. These influenza viruses are highly adaptive and constantly mutate, which in turn prevents the development of any long-term immune defense.

- **Type A influenza**, which includes several subtypes, is the most common type of influenza virus. This type is usually responsible for the most serious epidemics and global pandemics, such as those that occurred in the United States in 1918, 1957, 1968, and 2009. A subgroup of type A is H1N1, colloquially referred to as the swine flu, which was responsible for a serious pandemic that started in the United States and Mexico in 2009.
- **Type B influenza** outbreaks can also cause regional epidemics, but the disease is generally milder than that caused by type A.
- **Type C influenza** causes sporadic cases and minor, local outbreaks. Type C has never been connected with a large epidemic.

Type A influenza viruses are found in humans and many animals (e.g., ducks, chickens, pigs, and whales). Type B is isolated primarily in humans, whereas Type C is found in humans, pigs, and dogs.

Type A influenza has been found in aquatic birds for years without causing harm to them, but recently this frequently mutating flu virus has shown that it can jump the species barrier from wild birds to domesticated poultry and swine. Pigs can be infected by avian and human flu, especially in areas where human contact is frequent. If a pig becomes infected with the avian and human flu simultaneously, the two types may exchange genes. This "reassorted" flu can sometimes spread from pigs to humans and may cause a more or less severe strain. In 1997, for the first time, scientists found that a form of avian H5N1 flu skipped the pig step and infected humans directly. Alarmed health officials feared a worldwide epidemic (a pandemic). Fortunately, the virus could not pass from person to person, so it did not spark an epidemic. As of July 2016, there had been 854 confirmed human cases of this avian flu virus worldwide, which resulted in 450 deaths (World Health Organization [WHO], 2016a).

Millions of Americans contract the flu each year. The flu season (i.e., when the incidence is the highest) in the United States is typically between October and March. The virus is transmitted through the inhalation or contact with respiratory droplets. Children are two to three times more likely than adults to contract the flu, and children frequently spread the virus to others. The 2015–2016 U.S. flu season saw mostly influenza type A (H1N1 and H3N2) (CDC, 2016a). This flu season was less severe, as compared to the moderately severe 2014–2015 season, and did not reach the pandemic levels of the 2009–2010 season. The 2015–2016 flu season saw fewer outpatient visits for influenza-like illness, rates of hospitalization, and reported deaths attributed to pneumonia and influenza compared with recent years. Persons at greater risk for having negative outcomes because of the flu include children, elderly, individuals who are immunocompromised, pregnant women, those who are severely obese (with a body mass index of 40 or higher) and individuals with preexisting chronic diseases (e.g., asthma, cardiovascular disease, diabetes mellitus, kidney disease). Often deaths associated with the flu are a result of secondary bacterial pneumonia.

The influenza virus has an incubation period of 1–4 days, with peak transmission risk starting at approximately 1 day before onset of symptoms and lasting 4–7 days afterward in adults. Children can be infectious for more than 10 days, and young children can spread the virus for 6 days before the onset of symptoms occurs. Severely immunocompromised persons can spread the virus for weeks or months. Flu differs from the common cold in that the flu usually has a sudden onset of symptoms (**TABLE 5-2**).

TABLE 5-2	Comparison of Infectious Rhinitis and Influenza Manifestations	
Symptoms	**Infectious Rhinitis**	**Influenza**
Fever	Rarely	Usual; high (100°F to 102°F, but occasionally higher, especially in young children); lasts 3–4 days
Headache	Rare	Common
Myalgia	Slight	Usual; often severe
Malaise	Sometimes	Usual; can last up to 2–3 weeks
Exhaustion	Never	Usual; at the beginning of the illness
Stuffy nose	Common	Sometimes
Sneezing	Usual	Sometimes
Sore throat	Common	Sometimes
Chest discomfort, cough	Mild to moderate, nonproductive cough	Common; can be severe

Modified from National Institutes of Allergy and Infectious Disease. (2008). Is it the cold or the flu? Retrieved from http://www.niaid.nih.gov/topics/Flu/Documents/sick.pdf

Clinical manifestations of the flu include the following signs and symptoms:

- Fever
- Headache
- Chills
- Dry cough
- Body aches
- Nasal congestion
- Sore throat
- Sweating
- Malaise
- Vomiting and diarrhea (more common in children than in adults)

Typically, fever and body aches last 3–5 days, while cough and fatigue may last for 2 or more weeks.

Diagnostic procedures for influenza consist of a history, physical examination, rapid flu screen, and flu culture (a nasal culture that tests for the presence of the virus). Treatment is symptomatic and supportive unless a secondary bacterial infection is present. Antiviral medications can reduce the severity and the duration of the symptoms. These antivirals can also be given on a postexposure basis to decrease the likelihood of developing the flu. Other strategies include increased fluid intake, adequate rest, antipyretics, and analgesics. Prevention strategies are similar to those used to prevent the common cold (e.g., hand washing and avoiding crowds), but also include vaccinations.

Currently, vaccinations exist for the seasonal flu and H1N1 flu (if warranted). Four types of seasonal flu vaccinations are produced—regular seasonal flu vaccine (the form most commonly administered to people 6 months and older), high-dose vaccine (for people age 65 and older), intradermal vaccine (for people age 18–64), and intranasal flu vaccine (produced from a live, weakened virus, unlike the other vaccines that are produced from a killed virus; approved for healthy, nonpregnant people age 2–49). Prior to each flu season (usually before the previous season is over), the CDC develops a seasonal flu vaccine based on predictions of the likely strain to be encountered. In the United States, the seasonal flu vaccine should be administered each year in October and is recommended to everyone age 6 months and older, especially those in high-risk groups (e.g., persons with a chronic medical condition, age 65 or older, pregnant, living in a community setting, healthcare providers, and household contacts). When outbreaks of other types of the flu occur, as with the H1N1 influenza in 2009, the CDC develops vaccinations specific for those strains.

Vaccine development can be a lengthy process. In many cases, the vaccines are grown in fertilized chicken eggs for approximately 10 months. Therefore, flu vaccines should not be administered to persons with egg allergies. Additionally, children younger than 6 months and people with a history of Guillain-Barré syndrome should not be vaccinated. People with an active febrile illness should wait to be vaccinated until after the illness resolves.

Myth Busters

A common misconception is that you can get the flu from the flu vaccine. What fuels this myth is that some people may experience very mild flulike symptoms (e.g., low-grade fever, aches, malaise) after receiving the vaccination. These symptoms do not occur because the individual has a mild case of the flu; rather, they are due to the process through which the immune system develops antibodies against the virus. An additional factor fueling this myth is the possibility that people may still have the flu even after receiving the vaccination. This infection is not caused by the flu vaccine; rather, it occurs because the person encountered a strain of the flu that was not covered by the vaccination. Remember, the vaccination is based on predictions. Negative outcomes from the flu vaccine are rare and minimal. So get vaccinated and encourage others to do the same!

Lower Respiratory Tract Infections

The lower respiratory tract includes the trachea, bronchi, bronchioles, and alveoli.

Bronchiolitis

Bronchiolitis refers to a common acute inflammation of the bronchioles that usually results from a viral infection frequently caused by the respiratory syncytial virus (RSV). This infection most often occurs in children younger than 1 year of age, and incidence increases in the fall and winter months. According to the CDC (2014a), 2.1 million children younger than the age of 5 years seek medical attention annually for RSV infection, and nearly all children will have an RSV infection by the time they are 2 years old. Bronchiolitis can also be caused by parainfluenza, influenza, adenoviruses, and metapneumoviruses (an emerging paramyxovirus).

When the virus infects the bronchioles, these small airways become inflamed and swollen. As a result of the inflammatory process, mucus collects in these airways. The combination of edema and mucus prevents air flow into the alveoli. Transmission of RSV occurs through contact with or inhalation of infected respiratory droplets. Factors contributing to the development of bronchiolitis include neonatal prematurity, asthma family history, and cigarette smoke exposure.

Clinical manifestations of bronchiolitis vary in severity but include the following signs and symptoms:

- Nasal drainage
- Nasal congestion
- Cough
- Wheezing
- Abnormal lung sounds (e.g., rhonchi or rales)
- Rapid, shallow respirations
- Labored breathing (e.g., chest retractions, nasal flaring, and grunting)
- Dyspnea or tachypnea
- Fever
- Tachycardia
- Malaise

Diagnostic procedures include a history, physical examination, CBC, and ABGs. Since bronchiolitis may be caused by many viruses, mucus swab to identify the virus is not necessary (Ralston et al., 2014). Routine chest X-ray is also not necessary unless complications are suspected. Bronchiolitis can progress to atelectasis (collapse of the alveoli) and respiratory failure without aggressive and early treatment; therefore, airway management and respiratory stability are the treatment foci. Hospitalization is often required, and intubation may be necessary if the child decompensates or respiratory failure occurs. Other treatment strategies include oxygen therapy, cool humidity, suctioning secretions, increased fluids (either by mouth or intravenously), keeping the child calm, bronchodilators, and corticosteroids. No specific treatment for RSV infection is available.

Prevention strategies are the same as those previously discussed for other infectious respiratory conditions (e.g., hand washing and avoiding crowds). Palivizumab (Synagis) can be given to at-risk infants during RSV season to prevent and minimize infection. A vaccine for RSV is in development but is not yet commercially available.

Pneumonia

Pneumonia is an inflammatory process caused by numerous infectious agents (e.g., bacteria, viruses, and fungi) and injurious agents or events (e.g., aspiration and smoke). According to the CDC (2015b), pneumonia accounts for 1.1 million hospitalizations and more than 53,000 deaths in the United States annually. *Streptococcus pneumoniae* is responsible for 75% of all cases of pneumonia, and the most common viral causes are

TABLE 5-3   Comparison of Viral and Bacterial Pneumonia

	Viral	Bacterial
Cough	Nonproductive	Productive
Fever	Low grade	Higher
WBC	Normal (low)	Elevated
X-ray	Minimal change	Infiltrates
Severity	Less	More
Antibiotics	No	Yes

influenza, parainfluenza, and RSV. **Viral pneumonia** and **bacterial pneumonia** have some notable differences (**TABLE 5-3**). Viral pneumonia is usually mild and heals without intervention, but it can lead to virulent bacterial pneumonia.

Irritating agents or events can also lead to pneumonia—for example, aspiration of gastric contents, endotracheal intubation, respiratory suctioning, and inhalation of smoke or chemicals. **Aspiration pneumonia** frequently occurs when the gag reflex is impaired because of a brain injury or anesthesia. Aspiration can also occur because of impaired lower esophageal sphincter closure secondary to nasogastric tube placement or disease (e.g., gastroesophageal reflux disease). Additionally, inappropriate gastric tube placement can lead to tube-feeding formulas entering the lungs rather than the stomach. Gastric contents and tube-feeding formulas irritate the lung tissue, triggering the inflammatory response. The inflammatory response increases mucus production, which can in turn lead to atelectasis and pneumonia. Tube-feeding formulas also contain sugar and protein, creating a superior medium in which bacteria can grow and flourish. Finally, pneumonia can develop from stasis of pulmonary secretions. Activities such as movement, talking, and coughing normally keep pulmonary secretions moving, and adequate hydrations keep secretions thin. When these secretions become thick and stagnate, ciliary action cannot remove the bacteria-laden mucus, leading to pneumonia.

Pneumonia is classified based on the causative agents or events previously discussed and its location in the lung (**TABLE 5-4**). **Lobar pneumonia** is confined to a single lobe and is described based on the affected lobe (e.g., right upper lobe). **Bronchopneumonia** is the most frequent type and is a patchy pneumonia spread throughout several lobes. **Interstitial pneumonia**, or atypical pneumonia, occurs in the areas between the

TABLE 5-4   Types of Pneumonia

	Lobar Pneumonia	Bronchopneumonia	Interstitial Pneumonia
Distribution	All of one or two lobes	Scattered small patches	Scattered small patches
Cause	*Streptococcus pneumoniae*	Multiple bacteria	Influenza virus; *Mycoplasma*
Pathophysiology	Inflammation of the alveolar wall and leakage of cells, fibrin, and fluid into alveoli, causing consolidation	Inflammation and purulent exudates in alveoli, often developing from pooled secretions or irritation	Interstitial inflammation around alveoli Necrosis of bronchial epithelium
Onset	Sudden and acute	Insidious	Variable
Signs	High fever Chills Productive cough of rusty sputum Rales progressing to absent breath sounds in affected lobes	Mild fever Productive cough of yellow-green sputum Dyspnea	Variable fever Nonproductive hacking cough Headache Myalgia

alveoli. Interstitial pneumonia is routinely caused by viruses (e.g., influenza type A and B) or by uncommon bacteria (e.g., *Legionella pneumophilia* and *Mycoplasma pneumoniae*).

Legionnaires' disease is a specific type of pneumonia that is caused by *Legionella pneumophilia*. These bacteria thrive in warm, moist environments (e.g., air-conditioning systems, standing freshwater, respiratory therapy equipment, and whirlpools). Legionnaires' disease is not contagious. Instead, most people acquire this type of pneumonia from inhaling the bacteria as they are spread by an air-conditioning system or spa. Persons with a weakened immune system are at highest risk for developing Legionnaires' disease. Although most people with this type of pneumonia recover without incident, the disease can be fatal if untreated. Symptoms are similar to other types of pneumonia and usually appear 10–14 days post exposure. Additional symptoms may include nausea, vomiting, and diarrhea. In addition to the usual pneumonia diagnostic procedures, a urine test can be performed to identify the presence of *Legionella* antigens. Treatment of Legionnaires' disease follows the usual pneumonia treatment protocol.

Mycoplasma pneumoniae causes a common type of pneumonia that usually affects people younger than 40 years of age. People who live or work in crowded places such as schools, homeless, and prisons are at higher risk of developing this type of pneumonia. *Mycoplasma* infection is usually mild and responds well to antibiotics, but it can be serious. Skin rash, arthralgia, and hemolysis may also be present.

Severe acute respiratory syndrome (SARS) is a respiratory illness that presents similarly to atypical pneumonia. First identified in China, its prevalence rates remain higher in Asian countries. SARS is caused by a coronavirus, SARS-CoV. Transmission occurs through inhalation of respiratory droplets or close contact, although oral–fecal contact may also be a mechanism of transmission. SARS has high mortality and morbidity rates. The incubation period for this disease is 2–7 days. The first stage presents as a flulike syndrome (e.g., fever, chills, headache, myalgia, anorexia, and diarrhea) that lasts 3–7 days. Several days later, a dry cough and dyspnea develop as the lungs become damaged and the patient moves into the second stage of the disease. Interstitial congestion and hypoxia progress rapidly. Additionally, liver damage can occur. If the patient continues to the third stage, severe and sometimes fatal respiratory distress can develop. Diagnostic procedures for SARS consist of a history, physical examination, and chest X-ray. Treatment focuses on maintaining oxygenation and respiratory status, with strategies including oxygen therapy, bronchodilators, and antiviral drugs. Endotracheal intubation with mechanical ventilation support may be required as hypoxia worsens.

An emerging illness in the same coronavirus family is **Middle East respiratory syndrome** (MERS-CoV). It was first reported in Saudi Arabia in 2012 and has since spread to several other countries, including the United States (CDC, 2016c). Between its discovery in April 2012 and July 2013, 1,800 cases and 640 deaths from this disease were reported worldwide (WHO, 2016b). The virus is currently isolated to four countries in the Arabian Peninsula. It seems to spread through close contact, but the CDC is still working on better understanding the virus (CDC, 2016c).

Pneumonia is also classified according to where it is acquired. **Nosocomial pneumonia** refers to pneumonia that develops more than 48 hours after a hospital admission. Ventilator-associated pneumonia (VAP) is an example of nosocomial pneumonia. With this disease, the endotracheal tube provides a portal of entry for bacteria. In contrast, **community-acquired pneumonia** is acquired outside the hospital or healthcare setting.

Most healthy people do not develop pneumonia from fungal exposure. Instead, many of these illnesses occur as opportunistic infections, which can be fatal in immunocompromised individuals (e.g., children and persons with AIDS or cancer). *Pneumocystis jiroveci* **pneumonia**, formerly known as *Pneumocystis carinii* pneumonia, is a specific type of pneumonia that is caused by yeastlike fungus. Its diagnosis is accomplished through identification of the fungus through a sputum culture. Aggressive and early treatment will improve outcomes in these vulnerable patients. Other fungal-related pneumonias include histoplasmosis, coccidiomycosis, and cryptococcal pneumonia. In addition to previously discussed risk factors, persons at risk for developing pneumonia and having serious complications include children, the elderly, immunocompromised individuals, those with existing chronic disease conditions, smokers, and alcoholics. Otherwise-healthy patients usually recover completely from pneumonia when treated properly. By comparison, high-risk persons are more likely to develop complications including septicemia, pulmonary edema, lung abscess, pleural effusion, and acute respiratory distress syndrome.

Clinical manifestations of pneumonia may vary depending on type and include the following signs and symptoms:

- Productive or nonproductive cough
- Fatigue
- Pleuritic pain
- Dyspnea
- Fever
- Chills
- Abnormal lung sounds (e.g., crackles or rales)
- Pleural rub
- Tachypnea
- Mental status changes (especially in the elderly)
- Leukocytosis

Early diagnosis and treatment of pneumonia are paramount to have positive outcomes. Diagnostic procedures may include a history, physical examination, chest X-ray, sputum cultures, CBC, ABGs, and bronchoscopy. Endotracheal intubation may be necessary to provide ventilation support and maintain oxygenation. Additional treatment strategies include antibiotics (if bacterial infection is present), bronchodilators, corticosteroids, antipyretics, analgesics, humidified oxygen therapy, chest physiotherapy, increased fluids (either by mouth or intravenously), and rest. If aspiration is the cause of the pneumonia, additional treatment includes eliminating the causes and not giving the patient anything by mouth until swallowing studies can be performed. Pneumonia prevention strategies include hand washing, avoiding crowds, vaccinations (e.g., for pneumococcus, influenza, and Hib), mobilizing secretions (e.g., turning, coughing, deep breathing), and smoking cessation.

Tuberculosis

Tuberculosis (TB), an ancient disease, is one of the world's deadliest conditions. Although on the decline, TB remains a major cause of illness, with one-third of the world's population being infected. According to the World Health Organization, TB was responsible for approximately 1.5 million deaths worldwide in 2014, and it is the leading cause of death for persons infected with HIV (WHO, 2016c). In the United States, TB rates are higher among Asians, Native Hawaiians, and other Pacific Islanders (CDC, 2014b).

TB is caused by *Mycobacterium tuberculosis*, a slow-growing aerobic (requires oxygen) bacillus that is somewhat resistant to the body's immune efforts. Person-to-person transmission occurs through the inhalation of tiny infected aerosol droplets (**FIGURE 5-17**). Only people with active TB can spread the disease to others. The bacillus is capable of surviving in dried sputum for weeks, but ultraviolet light, heat, alcohol, glutaraldehyde, and formaldehyde destroy it. Many people contract TB but do not develop the disease because of an intact, healthy immune system or early treatment. Multidrug-resistant TB strains are relatively rare in the United States but account for 1 in 30 new TB cases and 1 in 5 previously diagnosed cases worldwide. Extensively drug-resistant TB is very rare in the United States, with only 2 known cases of occurring in 2014; in contrast, this global threat has been linked to cases in more than 100 countries.

Although TB most frequently involves the lungs, it can also affect other organs and tissues (e.g., liver, brain, and bone marrow). TB is often considered an opportunistic infection because it is more likely to become active in someone with a weakened immune system. At-risk persons, then, include those with immune deficiency (e.g., AIDS and cancer), malnutrition, diabetes mellitus, and alcoholism. Poverty, overcrowding, homelessness, and drug abuse also increase the risk for acquiring TB.

There are two stages of TB pathogenesis—primary and secondary infection. **Primary TB infection** occurs when the bacillus first enters the body. In this phase, macrophages engulf the microbe, causing a local inflammatory response. Some bacilli travel to the lymph nodes, activating the type IV hypersensitivity reaction (see the *Immunity* chapter). Lymphocytes and macrophages congregate to form a granuloma (an epithelial nodule). The granuloma contains some live bacilli, forming a tubercle. Caseous necrosis, a cottage cheese–like material, develops in the center of the tubercle (see the *Cellular Function* chapter). An intact immune system can resist this development, so the lesions—referred to as Ghon complexes (**FIGURE 5-18**)—remain small, become walled off by fibrous tissue, and calcify. The bacilli can remain dormant and viable in the tubercle for years as long as the immune system is intact. In this phase, the individual has been infected by the bacilli and remains asymptomatic.

When the primary infection can no longer be controlled, the infection progresses to the **secondary infection (active infection)** phase. During this phase, TB can spread throughout the lungs and to other organs. Clinical

Tuberculosis

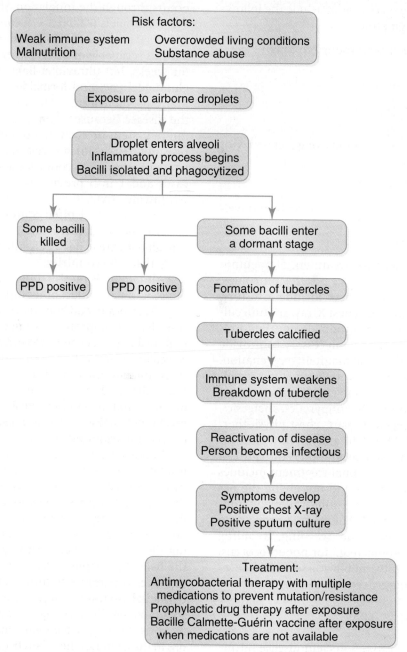

FIGURE 5-17 Tuberculosis.

TB skin testing is only useful as a screening tool to identify new TB exposure cases. Once a person's immune system has developed antibodies against TB, the person tests positive. This immunity reaction happens after the first exposure and vaccination administration. A person can be treated for TB, and he or she will continue to test positive because the antibodies are still present. Chest X-rays and sputum cultures are better diagnostic procedures once someone has tested positive. So remember … once positive, always positive!

manifestations begin to appear in the secondary infection phase:

- Productive cough
- Hemoptysis (coughing up blood or bloody sputum)
- Night sweats
- Fever
- Chills
- Fatigue
- Unexplained weight loss

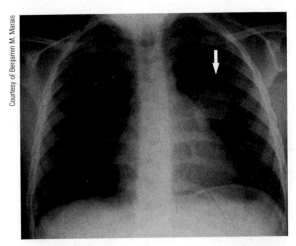

FIGURE 5-18 Ghon complexes.

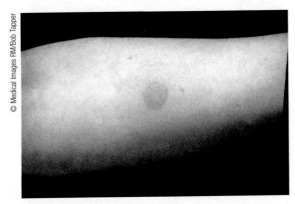

FIGURE 5-19 Positive TB skin test.

- Anorexia
- Miscellaneous symptoms depending on other organ involvement

Diagnostic procedures for TB are multifaceted, usually beginning with a TB skin test (Mantoux test). For the TB skin test, a small amount of a purified protein derivative tuberculin is injected just below the dermis. If the person has been infected by the bacilli, a local reaction (e.g., redness and induration) will occur (FIGURE 5-19). Persons will test positive once the bacilli trigger the inflammatory response (Figure 5-18). A history of bacillus Calmette-Guérin (BCG) vaccination will produce a false-positive reaction. Additionally,

previously treated TB will generate a false-positive reaction. Conversely, persons with immature (e.g., children) or compromised (e.g., AIDS or cancer) immune systems may not generate enough of a response to test positive. Because of the uncertainty that the TB skin test creates, chest X-rays and sputum cultures (most definitive) are used after a positive TB skin test is noted (either to confirm an original case or to assess reinfection). A computed tomography (CT) scan can also be used to visualize TB lesions, because this imaging modality is more sensitive than an X-ray. Nucleic acid amplification may be performed on the sputum to detect the presence of resistant strains.

TB is often successfully treated in the home setting; however, it takes diligence to eradicate the disease. Treatment requires an average of 6–9 months of antimicrobial therapy. Combination therapy (consisting of two or more drugs) is recommended to prevent the emergence of resistant strains. The slow-growing bacilli have a high mutation rate, with those mutations often appearing when the pathogen is exposed to monotherapy. Because TB is a public health risk, antituberculin medications are provided free of charge by the U.S. Public Health Service. In some states, therapy noncompliance is unlawful, and imprisonment may be used to ensure adherence when other measures fail (e.g., direct observed therapy). Compliance is a common problem in treating TB because of the length of therapy and the medication side effects (e.g., nausea, paresthesias, and discolored bodily secretions). Patient education, including an emphasis on taking the entire regimen of drugs as ordered, is crucial to maximize therapy success and prevent resistance.

Strategies to prevent the transmission of TB include respiratory precautions (e.g., TB-approved masks, covering one's mouth when coughing, and disposing of tissues), adequate ventilation (if the patient is at home), and placing the patient in a negative-pressure isolation room (if he or she is hospitalized). The bacillus Calmette-Guérin vaccination is primarily used in children and in developing countries.

ALTERATIONS IN VENTILATION

Asthma

Asthma is a chronic pulmonary disease that produces intermittent, reversible airway obstruction. It is characterized by acute airway inflammation, bronchoconstriction, bronchospasm, bronchiole edema, and mucus production (FIGURE 5-20).

Asthma is one of the most common chronic illness in children in the United States, affecting 26 million people. Prevalence rates

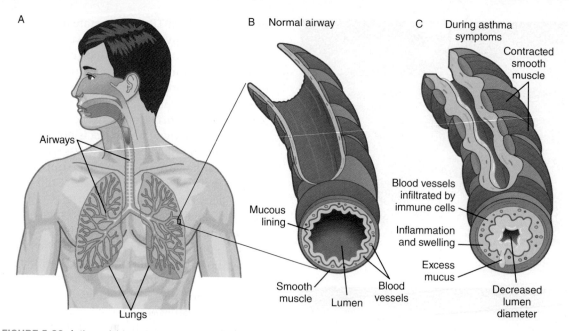

FIGURE 5-20 Asthma. (a) Location of the lungs and airways in the body. (b) Cross section of a normal airway. (c) Cross section of an airway during asthma symptoms.

associated with asthma increased from 2001 to 2010, while death rates decreased over the same period (CDC, 2015c). The prevalence rate increase may be a result of surging urbanization and pollution. Another theory, referred to as the hygiene hypothesis, suggests that the modern Western lifestyle's focus on hygiene and sanitation limits early childhood allergen and infection exposure, thereby rendering individuals more vulnerable when they do finally encounter allergens and infectious agents. Women are more likely to have asthma than men, but in children, boys are more likely to have asthma than girls. Persons of multiple races and African American adults and children are more likely to have asthma than Caucasian adults and children. Other risk factors include lower socioeconomic status, obesity, smoke exposure, and family history.

Asthma is usually classified according to its cause (extrinsic, intrinsic, nocturnal, exercise-induced, occupational, or drug-induced) and by its severity (mild intermittent, mild persistent, moderate persistent, and severe persistent) (**TABLE 5-5**). **Extrinsic asthma** is a result of increased immunoglobulin E (IgE) synthesis and airway inflammation, which leads to mast cell destruction and inflammatory mediator release. Extrinsic triggers include allergens such as food, pollen, dust, and medications. The release of the inflammatory mediators in response to these triggers causes bronchoconstriction, increased capillary permeability, and mucus production. Extrinsic asthma generally presents in childhood or adolescence. **Intrinsic asthma** is not an allergic reaction and usually presents after age 35 years. Intrinsic triggers include upper respiratory infections, air pollution, emotional stress, smoke, exercise, and cold exposure.

Nocturnal asthma usually occurs between 3:00 and 7:00 a.m. and is thought to be related to circadian rhythms. At night, cortisol and epinephrine levels decrease, while histamine levels increase. Changes in these naturally occurring substances lead to bronchoconstriction.

Exercise-induced asthma is common and usually occurs 10–15 minutes after physical activity ends. Symptoms can linger for an hour with this type of asthma. The airways can become cool and dry during exercise, and asthmatic symptoms may be a compensatory mechanism to warm and moisten the airways. Following each episode of exercise-induced asthma, a refractory (symptom-free) period begins within 30 minutes and can last 90 minutes. During this time, little or no bronchospasm can be induced even if the person is rechallenged with vigorous exercise. Athletes often take advantage of this fact by warming up vigorously to induce a refractory period prior to competition.

TABLE 5-5	Classification of Asthma Severity				
Step/Classification*	**Daytime Symptoms**	**Nighttime Symptoms**	**PEF or FEV$_1$†**	**PEF Variability**
Step 1: Mild intermittent	≤ 2/week	≤ 2/week	≥ 80%	< 20%
Step 2: Mild persistent	> 2/week, but < daily	> 2 nights/month	> 80%	20–30%
Step 3: Moderate persistent	Daily	> 1 night/week	60–80%	> 30%
Step 4: Severe persistent	Continual	Frequent	≤ 60%	> 30%

* Classification is based on symptoms and lung function before treatment. Patients should be assigned to the most severe step in which any feature occurs.

† Percentage of predicted function.

PEF = peak expiratory flow (rate); FEV$_1$ = forced expiratory volume in 1 second.

Data from National Heart, Lung, and Blood Institute. (2007). National Asthma Education and Prevention Program, Expert Panel Report 3: Guidelines for the diagnosis and management of asthma. NIH Publication Number 08-5846. Retrieved from https://www.nhlbi.nih.gov/files/docs/guidelines/asthsumm.pdf

Occupational asthma is caused by a reaction to substances encountered at work (e.g., plastic or formaldehyde). Symptoms develop over time, worsening with each exposure and improving when away from work (e.g., on weekends or during vacations).

Drug-induced asthma is frequently caused by aspirin and can be fatal. Reactions can be delayed up to 12 hours after drug ingestion. Aspirin and other drugs (e.g., nonsteroidal anti-inflammatory drugs) prevent the conversion of prostaglandins, which stimulate leukotriene release—a powerful bronchoconstrictor.

Regardless of the classification system used, asthma attacks are the body's response to bronchial inflammation. Stage 1 of an acute asthma attack is primarily related to bronchospasm, and is usually signaled by coughing. Peaking within 15 to 30 minutes, the inflammatory mediators responsible for this stage include leukotrienes, histamine, and some interleukins. Stage 2 of an asthma attack peaks within 6 hours of symptom onset. This stage is a result of airway edema and mucus production. The alveolar hyperinflation causes air trapping. Bronchospasm, smooth muscle contraction, inflammation, and mucus production combine to narrow the airways.

Clinical manifestations of asthma include the following:

- Wheezing
- Shortness of breath
- Dyspnea
- Chest tightness
- Cough
- Tachypnea
- Anxiety

Status asthmaticus is a life-threatening, prolonged asthma attack that does not respond to usual treatment. Maintaining a patent airway is critical in such cases, and endotracheal intubation with ventilation support may be necessary. In addition, acid–base imbalances—specifically respiratory alkalosis (from expelling too much carbon dioxide because of tachypnea)—can develop. Treatment of these conditions is crucial to improve outcomes.

Diagnostic procedures can be used to identify those persons with asthma as well as to track progression of the disease. These diagnostic procedures include a history, physical examination, pulmonary function tests (Figure 5-11), chest X-ray, ABGs, CBC, challenge testing, and allergen testing.

Asthma cannot be cured, but its symptoms can be controlled. Unless treated promptly, asthma attacks can lead to impaired gas exchange and death. Left untreated, long-term asthma can result in bronchial damage and scarring. The goals of treatment are to minimize the occurrence and severity of asthma attacks. Pharmacologic treatment includes inhaled and systemic corticosteroids, bronchodilators, beta agonists, nebulizer treatments, leukotriene mediators, mast cell stabilizers, and anticholinergics. Additional strategies include the following measures:

- Develop an asthma plan (FIGURE 5-21) and teach it to all caregivers
- Avoid triggers
- Keep the environment clean
- Limit environmental fabrics
- Filter indoor air
- Maintain a healthy immune system (e.g., exercise, get adequate nutrition)

Asthma Action Plan

For: _____   Doctor: _____   Date: _____
Doctor's Phone Number_____   Hospital/Emergency Department Phone Number _____

GREEN ZONE

Doing Well

- No cough, wheeze, chest tightness, or shortness of breath during the day or night
- Can do usual activities

And, if a peak flow meter is used,

Peak flow: more than _____
(80 percent or more of my best peak flow)

My best peak flow is: _____

Before exercise

Take these long-term control medicines each day (include an anti-inflammatory).

Medicine	How much to take	When to take it
_____	_____	_____
_____	_____	_____
_____	_____	_____
_____	_____	_____
□ _____	□ 2 or □ 4 puffs _____	5 to 60 minutes before exercise

YELLOW ZONE

Asthma Is Getting Worse

- Cough, wheeze, chest tightness, or shortness of breath, or
- Waking at night due to asthma, or
- Can do some, but not all, usual activities

-Or-

Peak flow: _____ to _____
(50 to 79 percent of my best peak flow)

First Add: quick-relief medicine—and keep taking your GREEN ZONE medicine.

_____   □ 2 or □ 4 puffs, every 20 minutes for up to 1 hour
(short-acting beta₂-agonist)   □ Nebulizer, once

Second **If your symptoms (and peak flow, if used) return to GREEN ZONE after 1 hour of above treatment:**
□ Continue monitoring to be sure you stay in the green zone.
-Or- _____
If your symptoms (and peak flow, if used) do not return to GREEN ZONE after 1 hour of above treatment:
□ Take: _____   □ 2 or □ 4 puffs or □ Nebulizer
(short-acting beta₂-agonist)
□ Add: _____   mg per day For _____ (3–10) days
(oral steroid)
□ Call the doctor □ before/ □ within _____ hours after taking the oral steroid.

RED ZONE

Medical Alert!

- Very short of breath, or
- Quick-relief medicines have not helped, or
- Cannot do usual activities, or
- Symptoms are same or get worse after 24 hours in Yellow Zone

-Or-

Peak flow: less than _____
(50 percent of my best peak flow)

Take this medicine:

□ _____   □ 4 or □ 6 puffs or □ Nebulizer
(short-acting beta₂-agonist)
□ _____   mg
(oral steroid)

Then call your doctor NOW. Go to the hospital or call an ambulance if:
- You are still in the red zone after 15 minutes AND
- You have not reached your doctor.

DANGER SIGNS ■ **Trouble walking and talking due to shortness of breath**   ■ Take □ 4 or □ 6 puffs of your quick-relief medicine AND
■ **Lips or fingernails are blue**   ■ Go to the hospital or call for an ambulance _____ NOW!
(phone)

FIGURE 5-21 Example of asthma action plan.

Chronic Obstructive Pulmonary Disease

Chronic obstructive pulmonary disease (COPD) describes a group of chronic respiratory disorders characterized by irreversible, progressive tissue degeneration and airway obstruction. These debilitating conditions can impair an individual's ability to work and function independently. Severe hypoxia and hypercapnia can lead to respiratory failure. The chronic hypercapnia shifts the normal breathing drive from the need to expel excess carbon dioxide to the need to raise oxygen levels (Figure 5-12). Additionally, COPD can lead to cor pulmonale, a type of right-sided heart failure due to lung disease (see the *Cardiovascular Function* chapter).

The most significant contributing factor to developing COPD is cigarette smoking. Other contributing factors include the inhalation of pollution and chemical irritants. Groups at higher risk of developing COPD also include Caucasians, women, individuals of lower socioeconomic status, and persons with a history of asthma.

Prevalence rates for COPD are likely underestimated because this disease is often asymptomatic in its early stages or is masked by smoking symptoms. According to the CDC (2015a), COPD was the third leading cause of death in the United States in 2011. Fifteen million Americans are currently diagnosed with COPD. Symptoms usually present around 60 years of age. A rare familial type of COPD (emphysema only), alpha-1 antitrypsin deficiency, presents much earlier—in the 30s or 40s.

COPD is often one of or a mixture of two diseases—chronic bronchitis and emphysema (FIGURE 5-22). These two diseases are discussed next.

Chronic Bronchitis

Chronic bronchitis is an obstructive respiratory disorder characterized by inflammation of the bronchi, a productive cough, and excessive mucus production. This disorder differs from acute bronchitis in that the chronic type is not necessarily caused by an infection and symptoms persist longer. As previously mentioned, cigarette smoking is the greatest contributing factor for chronic bronchitis. The

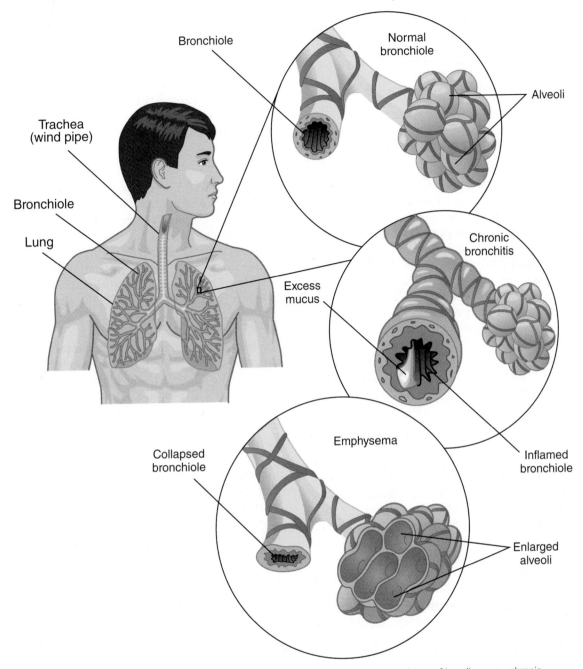

FIGURE 5-22 Chronic obstructive pulmonary disease (COPD) is often one disease or a mixture of two diseases—chronic bronchitis and emphysema.

inflammatory response results in mucous gland hyperplasia, edema, excessive mucus production, bronchoconstriction, and cough in defense against inhaled irritants. Airway resistance affects inspiratory and expiratory air flow. Impaired pulmonary defenses (e.g., cilia damage and decreased phagocytic activity) result in frequent respiratory infections and, in some cases, respiratory failure.

Airway resistance results in hypoventilation, hypoxemia, cyanosis, hypercapnia, polycythemia,

clubbing of fingers, and dyspnea at rest. Additional clinical manifestations include the following signs and symptoms:

- Abnormal lung sounds (e.g., wheezing and rhonchi)
- Edema
- Weight gain
- Malaise
- Chest pain
- Fever

Diagnostic procedures for chronic bronchitis consist of a history (persistent, productive cough for at least 3 months in a year for 2 consecutive years), physical examination, chest X-ray, pulmonary function tests (Figure 5-11), ABGs, and CBC. The goal of treatment is to maintain airway patency. Treatment strategies include oxygen therapy (in limited amounts, because too much will knock out the newly oxygen-centered drive for breathing), bronchodilators, corticosteroids, antibiotics (if bacterial infection is present), postural drainage, chest physiotherapy, and increased hydration.

Emphysema

Emphysema is an obstructive respiratory disorder that results in the destruction of the alveolar walls, leading to large, permanently inflated alveoli. Lung tissue normally remodels during periods of growth and repair related to infections and inflammation. Enzymes are involved in this process to prevent excessive tissue damage. Enzyme deficiency, however, may result from genetic predisposition (fewer than 2% of cases) and smoking. Smoking triggers inflammation, causing changes in these enzyme levels and leading to structural changes. Emphysema gradually turns the alveoli into large, irregular pockets with gaping holes, which in turn limits the amount of oxygen entering the bloodstream. The elastic fibers and surfactant that normally keep the alveoli open are slowly destroyed, so the alveoli collapse during expiration, trapping air in the lungs. The loss of elastic recoil and hyperinflation of the alveoli narrow the terminal bronchioles, but inspiration is not affected.

Coughing is usually not a symptom. Instead, emphysema is characterized by the following clinical manifestations:

- Dyspnea upon exertion
- Diminished breath sounds
- Wheezing
- Chest tightness
- Tachypnea
- Hypoxia
- Hypercapnia
- Increased anterior–posterior thoracic diameter (from 1:2 to 1:1), giving the chest a "barrel" appearance
- Activity intolerance
- Anorexia
- Malaise

Diagnosis and progress monitoring are accomplished through the same procedures that are used for chronic bronchitis. Treatment strategies include those identified for chronic bronchitis, plus pursed-lip breathing and lung reduction surgery. Pursed-lip breathing increases expiratory resistance and produces airway backpressure, preventing collapse of the alveoli.

Cystic Fibrosis

Cystic fibrosis is a common inherited respiratory disorder (approximately 1,000 new patients are diagnosed each year in the United States) that presents at birth (Cystic Fibrosis Foundation, n.d.). Caucasians are more likely to develop cystic fibrosis than other ethnic groups, followed by Latinos and American Indians. This life-threatening condition causes severe lung damage and nutrition deficits. Cystic fibrosis changes the cells that produce mucus, sweat, saliva, and digestive secretions. As a result, these normally thin secretions become thick and tenacious. Instead of lubricating the respiratory tract, the secretions occlude airways, ducts, and passageways.

The genetic defect that leads to cystic fibrosis has been isolated to chromosome 7, and transmission follows an autosomal recessive pattern (see the *Cellular Function* chapter). More than 10 million Americans are carriers of this faulty gene, and many do not know they are carriers. The genetic deficit is related to a protein involved in sodium, chloride, and water cellular transport. The lungs and pancreas are primarily affected, but other organs can also be involved (e.g., liver, intestines, sinuses, and reproductive organs).

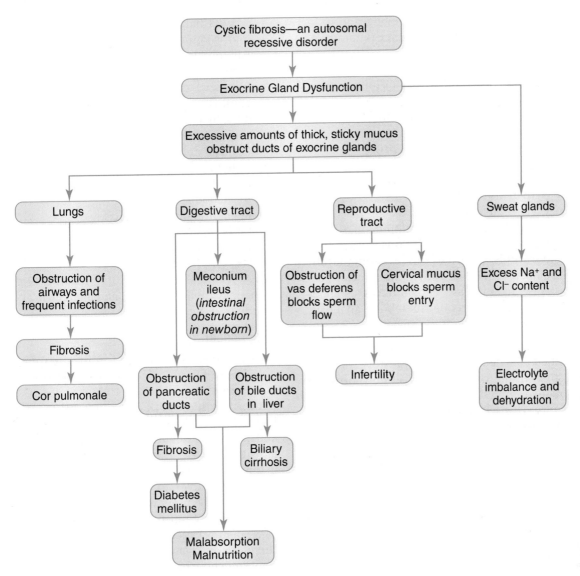

FIGURE 5-23 Cystic fibrosis.

Atelectasis develops as airways are obstructed, leading to permanent damage (**FIGURE 5-23**). Mucus stagnates, becoming a prime medium for bacterial growth. Infections are recurrent and contribute to the progressive lung destruction. Bronchiectasis and emphysema-like changes are common as fibrosis and obstructions advance. Respiratory failure is the most common cause of death in people who have cystic fibrosis. Ultimately, cor pulmonale (right-sided heart failure) or respiratory failure occurs.

In the digestive tract, the mucus blocks the intestines, producing a meconium ileus in the newborn. It also blocks pancreas ducts, leading to a pancreatic enzyme excretion deficit. Without these digestive enzymes, malabsorption and malnutrition develop. The trapped digestive enzymes damage pancreatic tissue, contributing to the development of diabetes mellitus and

osteoporosis. Blocked bile ducts add to the malabsorption issues and increase risk for developing cirrhosis.

Salivary glands are only mildly affected by blockages. Sweat glands produce sweat high in sodium chloride, which can cause electrolyte imbalances in times of excessive loss (e.g., during exercise or hot weather). Obstructions in the reproductive system can lead to sterility and infertility.

Clinical manifestations of cystic fibrosis may appear at birth and progressively worsen throughout the life span. Lung function often starts declining in early childhood. These manifestations, which vary in severity, include the following signs and symptoms:

- Meconium ileus
- Salty skin (parents may notice that their baby's skin tastes salty when they kiss the child)

- Steatorrhea (fatty, foul-smelling stools)
- Fat-soluble vitamin deficiency (vitamins A, D, E, and K)
- Voracious appetite
- Chronic cough with tenacious sputum (may include hemoptysis)
- Frequent respiratory infections
- Hypoxia
- Audible rhonchi and wheezing
- Dyspnea
- Fatigue
- Activity intolerance
- Digital clubbing
- Delayed growth and development
- Development of complications (e.g., chronic bronchitis, failure to thrive, cardiomegaly, diabetes mellitus, pancreatitis, rectal prolapse, liver disease, cholelithiasis, osteoporosis, hyponatremia, metabolic alkalosis, and infertility)

Diagnosis of cystic fibrosis can be accomplished prenatally when family history warrants testing. In the United States, all newborns are screened for cystic fibrosis regardless of family history. This screening involves analysis of the newborn's blood for higher than normal levels of immunoreactive trypsinogen (IRT), a chemical released by the pancreas. IRT level may be elevated because of prematurity or a stressful delivery; therefore, other tests are used to confirm the diagnosis. Sweat analysis can be conducted at about 2–3 weeks of age to detect electrolyte abnormalities (particularly high levels of chloride). The Delta F508 test can identify the chromosome 7 mutation, and it is often used if a false-negative sweat test is suspected or to identify carrier status of siblings. In addition, stool can be evaluated for the presence of pancreatic content. Other tests that assess lung function include chest X-rays, pulmonary function tests, and ABGs.

Cystic fibrosis treatment requires diligent family involvement and an interdisciplinary approach because of the progressive, multisystem nature of the disease. Improved treatment regimens have improved the life expectancy for patients who have cystic fibrosis, with some people living into their 40s or 50s. Treatment often requires a multidisciplinary team including cystic fibrosis specialists, respiratory therapists, dietitians, and psychological counselors. Strategies include the following measures:

- Pancreatic enzyme replacement
- Bile salt replacement

- A well-balanced, high-protein, low-fat, high-sodium diet
- Fat-soluble vitamin replacement
- Increased fluid intake
- Intensive chest physiotherapy (includes chest clapping or percussion, which can be done by hand or with a mechanical percussor)
- Postural drainage
- Coughing exercises
- Humidified air
- Bronchodilators
- Regular, moderate exercise
- Early, aggressive treatment of infections with antibiotics
- Oxygen therapy
- Avoidance of respiratory irritants (e.g., smoke, pollution, dust, and allergens)
- Heart–lung transplant

Lung Cancer

Lung cancer is the second most often diagnosed cancer in men and women and the leading cause of cancer in the United States (U.S. Cancer Statistics Working Group, 2012). After increasing for decades, lung cancer incidence and mortality rates are now decreasing in parallel with decreases in rates of cigarette smoking in this country. Frequently, other cancers—such as breast and liver, to name a few—metastasize (spread) to the lung tissue.

Smoking contributes to the majority (80–90%) of lung cancer cases. The more than 4,000 chemicals in cigarette smoke include carcinogens and chemicals that paralyze cilia. The risk for developing lung cancer is directly related to the length of time a person smokes and the number of cigarettes smoked. Secondhand smoke can also be a significant contributing factor, and in fact, some research has indicated that it may be worse than firsthand smoking. Smoking cessation or removing the smoke exposure will gradually decrease risk. Inhalation of other chemicals (e.g., asbestos, radon gas, tar, and pollution) and chronic lung disease can also increase risk (FIGURE 5-24).

The lungs provide an optimal environment for tumor development and growth. Carcinogens can seek refuge in the many nooks and crannies of the air passages, having an opportunity to cause cellular changes (usually metaplasia) there. The scores of blood vessels supplying the lungs serve as entrance points for distant cancer cells to gain access, and those vessels furnish the cancer with a rich blood source to facilitate its growth.

Lung Cancer

Smoking
Secondhand smoke
Air pollution
Chronic lung injury

↓

Initial phase:
Epithelial cell damage
Deoxyribonucleic acid (DNA)
mutation p53 gene mutation

If exposure is
stopped, the effects
are reversed

If exposure
continues:

↓

Phase 2:
Cancer develops
Metastasis

↓

Treatment:
Smoking cessation
Chemotherapy
Radiation therapy
Surgical resection
Scan for and treat
metastasis

FIGURE 5-24 Lung cancer.

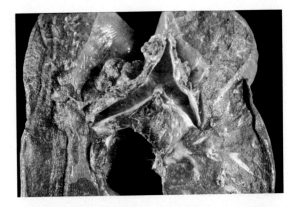

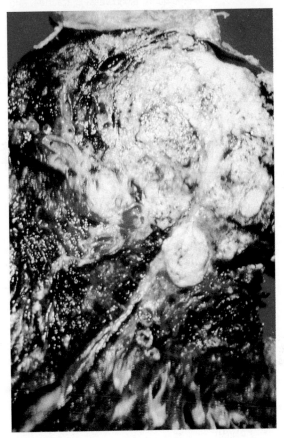

FIGURE 5-25 The normal (top) and cancerous (bottom) lung.

Top photo: © University of Alabama at Birmingham Department
of Pathology PEIR Digital Library (http://peir.net)

Bottom photo: Courtesy of National Cancer Institute

Lung cancers are divided into two types—small cell and non–small cell. **Small-cell carcinoma**, often referred to as oat-cell carcinoma, occurs almost exclusively in heavy smokers and is less frequent than non-small-cell cancers. **Non-small-cell carcinoma**, often referred to as bronchogenic carcinoma, is the most common type of malignant lung cancer, accounting for 85% of all cases of lung cancer. This very aggressive lung cancer is classified into several subgroups—squamous cell carcinoma, adenocarcinoma, and bronchioalveolar carcinoma.

Upon exposure to the carcinogen, irreversible oncogene DNA mutations and inactivation of tumor suppressor genes occur. If carcinogen exposure continues, cancer develops (**FIGURE 5-25**).

Tumors in the lungs lead to several issues, including the following:

- Airway obstruction
- Inflammation of lung tissue, eliciting coughing and contributing to infections
- Fluid accumulation in the pleural space (e.g., pleural effusion, hemothorax, and pneumothorax)
- Paraneoplastic syndrome (endocrine dysfunction associated with hormone secretion from the tumor)

Clinical manifestations of lung cancer are insidious because they mimic signs of smoking:

- Persistent cough or a change in usual cough
- Dyspnea

TABLE 5-6	Staging and Treatment of Non-Small-Cell Lung Cancer	
Stage	**Description**	**Usual Treatment Plan**
Stage I	Cancer has invaded the underlying lung tissue but has not spread to the lymph nodes.	Surgery
Stage II	Cancer has spread to neighboring lymph nodes or invaded the chest wall.	Surgery, radiation, and chemotherapy
Stage IIIA	Cancer has spread from the lung to lymph nodes in the center of the chest.	Combined chemotherapy and radiation, sometimes surgery based on results of treatment
Stage IIIB	Cancer has spread locally to areas such as the heart, blood vessels, trachea, and esophagus—all within the chest—or to lymph nodes in the area of the collarbone or to the tissue that surrounds the lungs within the rib cage (pleura).	Chemotherapy, sometimes radiation
Stage IV	Cancer has spread to other parts of the body, such as the liver, bones, or brain.	Chemotherapy, targeted drug therapy, clinical trials, supportive care

TABLE 5-7	Staging and Treatment of Small-Cell Lung Cancer	
Stage	**Description**	**Usual Treatment Plan**
Limited	Cancer is confined to one lung and to its neighboring lymph nodes.	Combined chemotherapy and radiation, sometimes surgery
Extensive	Cancer has spread beyond one lung and nearby lymph nodes, and may have invaded both lungs, more remote lymph nodes, or other organs.	Chemotherapy, clinical trials, supportive care

- Hemoptysis
- Frequent respiratory infections
- Chest pain
- Hoarseness
- Weight loss
- Anorexia
- Anemia
- Fatigue
- Other symptoms specific to the site(s) of metastasis

Diagnostic procedures for lung cancer include a history, physical examination, chest X-ray, CT, MRI, bronchoscopy, sputum studies, biopsy, positron emission tomography, bone scans, and pulmonary function tests. Treatment is based on staging and follows the usual pattern for cancer treatment—that is, chemotherapy, surgery, and radiation (**TABLE 5-6**; **TABLE 5-7**). The treatment is generally palliative because the tumor rarely responds favorably to treatment. Early diagnosis and treatment, however, may improve this prognosis. Other strategies include those to maintain optimal respiratory function—oxygen therapy, bronchodilators, and antibiotics (if bacterial infections are present).

Pleural Effusion

A **pleural effusion** is the accumulation of excess fluid in the pleural cavity. Normally, a very small amount of fluid drained from the lymphatic system is present in this space to lubricate the constantly moving lungs. Excessive fluid in the pleural cavity can compress the lung and limit expansion during inhalation. Effusions vary in nature and may affect both lungs or one lung. Fluid that can accumulate to create the effusion includes exudates (due to inflammation), transudates (due to increased hydrostatic pressure), blood (due to trauma), and pus (due to infection). The consequence of this effusion depends on its type, location, amount, and fluid accumulation rate. Large amounts of fluids can cause the pleural membranes to separate, preventing their cohesion during inhalation (**FIGURE 5-26**; **FIGURE 5-27**). This lack of cohesion

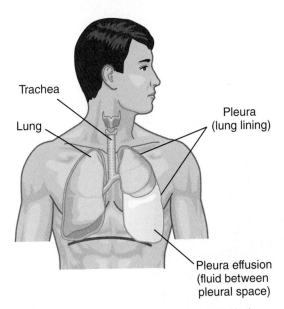

Trachea

Lung

Pleura (lung lining)

Pleura effusion (fluid between pleural space)

FIGURE 5-26 Pleural effusion is a buildup of fluid in the lining of the lungs.

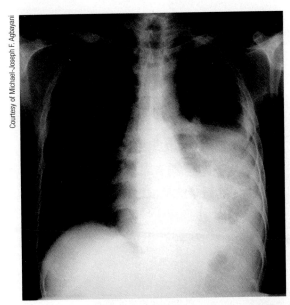

FIGURE 5-27 X-ray of pleural effusion.

impedes full expansion, leading to atelectasis and a pneumothorax. Large effusions can also impair venous return in the inferior vena cava and cardiac filling by putting pressure on those structures.

Pleurisy, or pleuritis, can precede or follow the effusion, or it may occur independently. Pleurisy comprises inflammation of the pleural membranes, which leads to swollen and irregular tissue. This inflammation is often associated with pneumonia and creates friction in the pleural membranes.

Clinical manifestations of pleural effusion include the following signs and symptoms:

- Dyspnea
- Chest pain (usually sharp and worsening with inhalation)
- Tachypnea
- Tracheal deviation (toward the unaffected side)
- Diminished or absent lung sounds over the affected area
- Dullness to percussion over the affected area
- Tachycardia
- Pleural friction rub (pleurisy)

Diagnostic procedures for pleural effusion include a history, physical examination, chest X-ray, CT, ABGs, CBC, and thoracentesis (needle aspiration of fluid) with subsequent examination of fluid. Treatment focuses on addressing the underlying cause. Regardless of etiology, removal of the fluid is necessary to promote full expansion of the lungs. Strategies to do so may include thoracentesis, placement of a chest drainage tube, and antibiotics.

Pneumothorax

Pneumothorax refers to air in the pleural cavity. The presence of atmospheric air in the pleural cavity and the separation of pleural membranes can lead to atelectasis. The resulting pressure can cause a partial or complete collapse of a lung (**FIGURE 5-28**; **FIGURE 5-29**). A small pneumothorax causes mild symptoms and may heal on its own. A larger pneumothorax generally requires aggressive treatment to remove the air and reestablish pulmonary negative pressure. Risk factors for developing pneumothorax include smoking, tall stature, and history of lung disease or previous pneumothorax.

Several types of pneumothorax are distinguished, based on their cause. A **spontaneous pneumothorax** develops when air enters the pleural cavity from an opening in the internal airways. Primary spontaneous pneumothorax occurs when a small air blister (bleb) on the top of the lung ruptures. Blebs are caused by a weakness in the lung tissue and can rupture from changes in air pressure, such as occur when scuba diving, flying, mountain climbing, or listening to extremely loud music. Additionally, a primary spontaneous pneumothorax may happen while smoking marijuana—a deep inhalation, followed by slow breathing out against partially closed lips, forces the smoke deeper into the lungs. Most commonly, these blebs rupture for no obvious

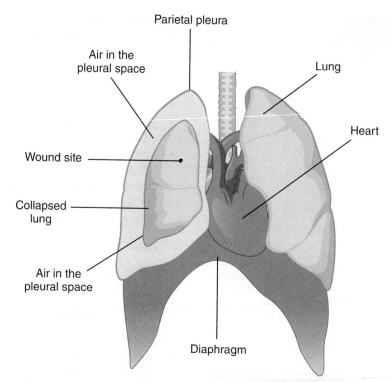

FIGURE 5-28 A pneumothorax occurs when air leaks into the pleural space between the parietal and visceral pleura. The lung collapses as air fills the pleural space and the two pleural membranes are no longer in contact with each other.

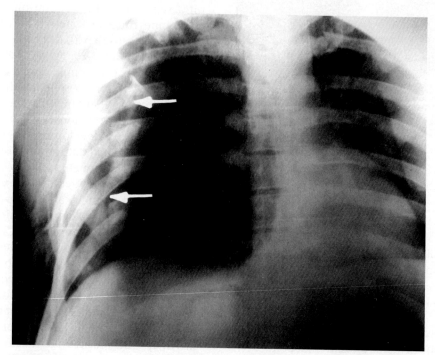

FIGURE 5-29 X-ray of pneumothorax.

Courtesy of Leonard V. Crowley, MD, Century College.

reason, although genetic factors may play a role. A primary spontaneous pneumothorax is usually mild because pressure from the collapsed portion of the lung may, in turn, collapse the bleb.

A secondary spontaneous pneumothorax develops in people with preexisting lung disease (e.g., emphysema, pneumonia, cystic fibrosis, or lung cancer). In these cases, the pneumothorax occurs because the diseased lung tissue is weakened. Secondary spontaneous pneumothorax can be more severe and even life threatening because diseased tissue can create a larger opening, allowing more air to enter the pleural space. Additionally, pulmonary disease reduces lung reserves, making any further reduction in lung function more serious.

A **traumatic pneumothorax** stems from a blunt trauma (e.g., vehicle air bag deployment) or penetrating injury (e.g., knife or gunshot wounds) to the chest. These injuries can inadvertently occur during certain medical procedures, such as chest tube insertion, cardiopulmonary resuscitation, and lung or liver biopsy.

A **tension pneumothorax** is the most serious type of pneumothorax; it occurs when the pressure in the pleural space is greater than the atmospheric pressure. This increased pressure arises due to trapped air in the pleural space or entering air from a positive-pressure mechanical ventilator. The force of the air can cause the affected lung to collapse completely and shift the heart toward the uncollapsed lung (called a mediastinal shift), compressing the unaffected lung and

the heart (**FIGURE 5-30**). Tension pneumothorax progresses rapidly and is fatal if not treated quickly.

Clinical manifestations vary in severity depending on the type of pneumothorax. These manifestations include the following signs and symptoms:

- Sudden chest pain over the affected lung
- Chest tightness
- Dyspnea
- Tachypnea
- Decreased breath sounds over the affected area
- Asymmetrical chest movement
- Trachea and mediastinum deviation toward the unaffected side
- Anxiety
- Tachycardia
- Pallor
- Hypotension

Diagnostic procedures for pneumothorax consist of a history, physical examination, chest X-ray, CT, and ABGs. Treatment usually involves removal of the air and reestablishment of negative pressure, allowing for full expansion of the lungs. Such strategies may include thoracentesis and placement of a chest drainage tube with suction (which removes fluid and reestablishes negative pressure). Surgery may be required in some cases to correct and prevent future episodes. During surgery, the leak is repaired and a chemical may be used to scar the area (pleurodesis).

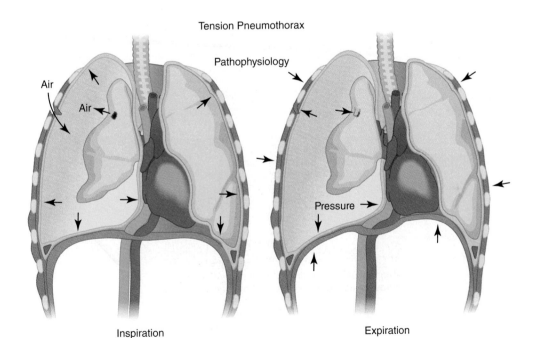

FIGURE 5-30 Tension pneumothorax. A one-way valve allows air into the pleural space during inspiration, but not out during expiration.

Acute Respiratory Distress Syndrome

Acute respiratory distress syndrome (ARDS) is a sudden failure of the respiratory system, often as a result of fluid accumulation in the alveoli. ARDS has many other names, such as shock lung, wet lung, and stiff lung. **Acute lung injury (ALI)** refers to a slightly less severe form of ARDS. Multiple conditions can precipitate ARDS, including prolonged shock, burns, aspiration, and smoke inhalation. This condition involves an acute hypoxemia resulting from a systemic event (e.g., trauma, septicemia, acute pancreatitis, drug overdose, cardiopulmonary bypass, or transfusion reaction) or a pulmonary event (e.g., illicit drug and toxic gas inhalation, pneumonia, RSV infection, gastric acid aspiration, near drowning, and fat embolism) that is not

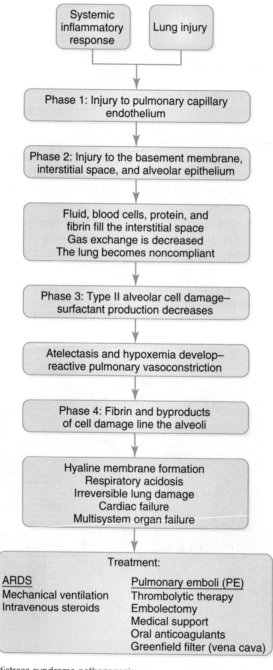

FIGURE 5-31 Acute respiratory distress syndrome pathogenesis.

cardiac in origin. ARDS develops rapidly, often within 90 minutes of a systemic inflammatory response or within 48 hours of a lung injury. Other risk factors include the presence of a chronic lung disease (e.g., emphysema, chronic bronchitis, and asthma), alcoholism, age greater than 65 years, and mechanical ventilation. ARDS is fatal in one-third of cases. Individuals who survive will fully recover, but it may take as long as a year for them to regain complete lung function.

In ARDS, injury to the alveoli and the capillary membranes leads to the release of chemical inflammatory mediators (FIGURE 5-31; FIGURE 5-32). These mediators increase capillary permeability, promote fluid and protein accumulation in the alveoli, and damage surfactant-producing cells. These events result in decreased gas exchange, reduced pulmonary blood flow, and limited lung expansion. Diffuse atelectasis and reduced lung capacity ensue. Lung damage progresses as neutrophils migrate to the site, releasing proteases and other mediators once there. A hyaline membrane—a thin layer of tissue—forms in the alveoli and causes them to become stiff. Additionally, increased platelet aggregation promotes microemboli development. If the patient survives, scattered necrosis and fibrosis are apparent throughout the lungs. ARDS is similar in pathogenesis to disseminated intravascular coagulation (see the *Hematopoietic Function* chapter).

ARDS is a serious condition that can lead to several complications:

- Respiratory failure
- Respiratory and metabolic acidosis
- Pulmonary fibrosis
- Pneumothorax
- Bacterial lung infections (e.g., stasis pneumonia and VAP)
- Decreased lung function
- Renal failure
- Stress ulcer
- Thromboembolism
- Muscle wasting
- Memory, cognitive, and emotional issues (due to brain damage as a result of the hypoxia)

Clinical manifestations of ARDS can develop suddenly and include the following signs and symptoms:

- Dyspnea
- Labored (requiring the use of accessory muscles), shallow respirations
- Abnormal lung sounds (e.g., rales and rhonchi)
- Productive cough with frothy sputum
- Hypoxia

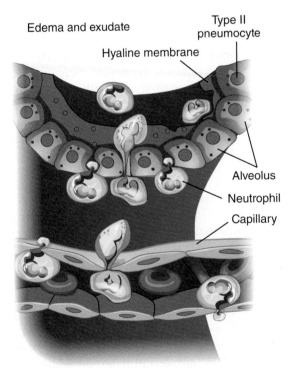

Edema and exudate

Hyaline membrane

Type II pneumocyte

Alveolus

Neutrophil

Capillary

Acute respiratory distress syndrome:

In ARDS, type I cells die as a result of diffuse alveolar damage.

Intra-alveolar edema follows, after which there is formation of hyaline membrane composed of proteinaceous axudate and cell debris.

In the acute phase, the lungs are markedly congested and heavy.

Type II cells multiply to line the alveolar surface.

Interstitial inflammation is characteristic.

The lesion may heal completely or progress to interstitial fibrosis.

FIGURE 5-32 Acute respiratory distress syndrome.

- Cyanosis
- Fever
- Hypotension
- Tachycardia
- Restlessness
- Confusion
- Lethargy
- Anxiety

Diagnostic procedures for ARDS consist of a history, physical examination, ABGs, chest X-ray, CT, and CBC. The main goal of treatment is to maintain adequate oxygenation and respiratory status. Such strategies include endotracheal intubation with a mechanical ventilator (including positive end-expiratory pressure [PEEP]), high-dose oxygen therapy, corticosteroids, inhaled beta agonists, and antibiotics (if bacterial infections are present), as well as prevention and treatment of emboli (e.g., embolectomy, anticoagulants, and antiplatelet agents). Other strategies include nutritional support (e.g., enteral feedings), conservative fluid therapy, sedation, and stress ulcer prophylaxis.

ALTERATIONS IN VENTILATION AND PERFUSION

Atelectasis

Atelectasis refers to incomplete alveolar expansion or collapse of the alveoli. It occurs when the walls of the alveoli stick together. Atelectasis may be caused by the following conditions:

- Surfactant deficiencies (surfactant is the lipoprotein that coats the inside of the alveoli, allowing them to remain open at the end of expiration)
- Bronchus obstruction (e.g., foreign objects, mucus plugs, and tumors)
- Lung tissue compression (e.g., tumor, pneumothorax, and pleural effusion)
- Increased surface tension (e.g., pulmonary edema)
- Lung fibrosis (e.g., emphysema)

When alveoli are not filled with air, they shrivel much like raisins. This ventilation issue can, in turn, impair blood flow through the lung. The ineffective ventilation and perfusion then impair gas exchange. Surgery and immobility increase the risk for developing atelectasis for this reason.

Atelectasis can occur in either small or large areas. If only a small area is affected, the respiratory rate will increase in an attempt to control carbon dioxide levels (increasing the respiratory rate will increase the excretion of carbon dioxide). The larger the area affected, the more severe the symptoms experienced. Necrosis, infection (e.g., pneumonia), and permanent lung damage can occur if the alveoli are not reinflated quickly.

The clinical manifestations of atelectasis are due to impaired ventilation and perfusion:

- Diminished breath sounds
- Dyspnea
- Tachypnea
- Asymmetrical lung movement
- Anxiety
- Restlessness
- Tracheal deviation
- Tachycardia

Diagnostic procedures for atelectasis include a history, physical examination, chest X-ray (FIGURE 5-33), CT, bronchoscopy, ABGs, and CBC. Treatment focuses on remedying the underlying causes (e.g., antibiotics, thoracentesis) and reinflating the alveoli. Incentive spirometry (a device to promote ventilation) is effective in reinflating the alveoli. For more severe cases, continuous positive airway pressure or endotracheal intubation may be necessary for ventilation support. Prevention strategies include increasing mobility (e.g., turning and ambulating), coughing, and deep breathing exercises (e.g., incentive spirometry) every 1–2 hours. Effective pain management and postoperative incisional splinting increase the likelihood that these interventions will be performed adequately.

Acute Respiratory Failure

Acute respiratory failure (ARF) is a life-threatening condition that can result from a variety of disorders (e.g., COPD, asthma, ARDS, amyotrophic lateral sclerosis, alcohol

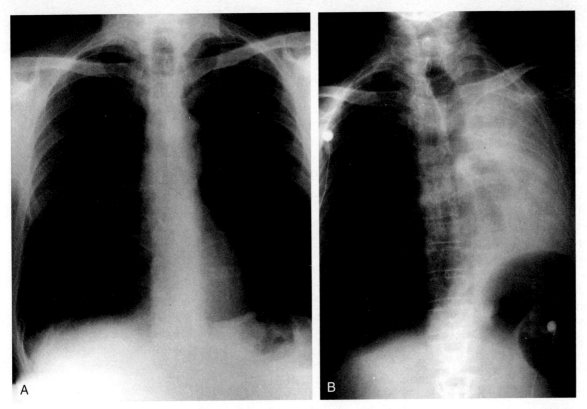

FIGURE 5-33 X-ray of atelectasis. (a) Normal lung. (b) Lung with atelectasis.
Courtesy of Leonard V. Crowley, MD, Century College.

or drug overdose, and spinal cord injury). In ARF, oxygen levels become dangerously low (less than 50 mm Hg) or carbon dioxide levels become dangerously high (greater than 50 mm Hg). Normally, oxygen levels are in the range of 80–100 mm Hg and carbon dioxide levels are in the range of 35–45 mm Hg. The low oxygen levels observed in ARF are not sufficient to meet the body's metabolic needs, and the nervous system quickly becomes affected by the shortage of oxygen. This gas level becomes progressively worse as the patient's condition worsens. Respiratory acidosis develops as the carbon dioxide levels rise (see the *Fluid, Electrolyte, and Acid–Base Homeostasis* chapter). The hypoxia and acidosis trigger a reflex pulmonary vasoconstriction, further impairing gas exchange and increasing cardiac workload. The heart decompensates from the lack of oxygen, which could lead to cardiac arrest. Respiratory arrest may occur as the respiratory system ceases all activity from the strain.

Clinical manifestations are usually evident and result from the impaired gas exchange:

* Shallow respirations
* Headache
* Tachycardia
* Dysrhythmias
* Lethargy
* Confusion

Diagnostic procedures for ARF consist of a history, physical examination, ABGs, chest X-ray, electrocardiogram (EKG), and CBC. Treatment focuses on resolving the cause and maintaining adequate respiratory status. Strategies include oxygen therapy, endotracheal intubation with ventilation support (some patients may require a tracheostomy), bronchodilators, antibiotics (if bacterial infection is present), corticosteroids, and treatment of emboli (e.g., embolectomy and anticoagulants). Cardiac support is usually inevitable as the heart arrests under the strain (e.g., cardiopulmonary resuscitation, sympathomimetic medications, and inotropic agents).

Now that we have learned what can go wrong in the respiratory system, let's put that knowledge into practice. While working in the emergency department, the following patients need to be triaged. Which patient would have the highest priority?

- A 6-month-old female with fever, audible inspiratory stridor, and restlessness
- A 25-year-old male with nasal drainage and hoarseness
- A 40-year-old female with fever, severe body aches, and nasal congestion
- A 59-year-old male with stage III bronchiogenic carcinoma who reports nausea and pain that measures a 6 on a 0–10 scale

Once again, you go through the usual thought process—who would die first, acute versus chronic conditions, Maslow's hierarchy of needs, and patient safety. Starting with the 6-month-old, the combination of manifestations reflects the possibility of epiglottitis or some other acute infectious respiratory process. Inspiratory stridor indicates that the child may have limited air entering the lungs due to an obstruction. The restlessness could be an indication of hypoxia. Additionally, the patient's young age increases the likelihood of her decompensating quickly. This patient definitely needs to stay on your radar. The 25-year-old is exhibiting manifestations likely due to laryngitis, which is not usually life threatening. Additionally, there is no indication that this patient is in any respiratory distress. The 40-year-old likely has the flu. Although extremely uncomfortable, the flu is not usually life threatening in otherwise healthy adults. Also, this patient is not displaying any respiratory distress. Finally, consider the 59-year-old with lung cancer. Lung cancer is often life threatening, but this patient was admitted with pain and nausea. Although nausea and pain are uncomfortable, they are not life-threatening conditions. Furthermore, this patient is not exhibiting any manifestations indicating respiratory distress. After considering all the patients to be triaged, it becomes clear that the 6-month-old should take priority and be seen first because she is exhibiting signs of respiratory distress.

Mr. Dan Griffith is a 65-year-old male who presented to the emergency department with shortness of breath and chest tightness of recent onset. He has a 7-year history of chronic obstructive pulmonary disease and is on oxygen at home. Physical assessment reveals a respiratory rate of 32 and slightly labored, temperature of 98.9°F, and SpO$_2$ of 86% while on oxygen via nasal cannula at 2 L/min.

1. Which of the following additional manifestations would be expected with a patient with emphysema?

    A. Productive cough with thick sputum

    B. A-P thoracic diameter of 1:1
    C. Cyanosis
    D. Edema

2. Mr. Griffith is admitted to the pulmonary unit with acute exacerbation of emphysema. Six hours after arriving to the floor, you notice that his respiration rate has dropped from 28 to 8 breaths/min. The nurse notes that Mr. Griffith's oxygen is set at 8 L/min via nasal cannula. Which action should the nurse take next?

    A. Call respiratory therapy to administer an albuterol treatment

    B. Auscultate the patient's breath sounds
    C. Change the nasal cannula to a mask
    D. Decrease the rate of oxygen flow

3. Which of the following nursing diagnoses would be the highest priority for Mr. Griffith?

    A. Ineffective airway clearance
    B. Impaired gas exchange
    C. Activity intolerance
    D. Self-care deficit

4. On his second day in the hospital, Mr. Griffith's morning weight indicates a 5-pound weight gain

since admission. The client's weight gain may reflect which associated complication of emphysema?

A. Metabolic acidosis
B. Respiratory alkalosis
C. Cor pulmonale
D. Pneumonia

5. With treatment, Mr. Griffith's condition is improving. The nurse is teaching him how to perform pursed-lip breathing for when he goes home. He asks the nurse to describe the purpose of this breathing technique. The nurse explains that:

A. It prolongs expiration, thereby decreasing the amount of air trapped in the alveoli.
B. It prolongs inspiration, thereby increasing oxygenation.
C. It strengthens the accessory muscles.
D. It decreases the use of accessory muscles.

CHAPTER SUMMARY

The respiratory system plays a crucial role by supplying the oxygen essential for cellular metabolism and excreting the carbon dioxide waste product of that metabolism. Because of this vital function, respiratory disorders can cause extensive and devastating problems throughout the body. Often the healthcare team has a limited amount of time to identify and respond to some of these respiratory disorders so as to control their negative consequences. Additionally, many of these diseases are preventable; therefore, identifying those persons at increased risk and implementing prevention strategies can limit the severity or halt the development of these debilitating conditions. Prevention, early detection, and prompt treatment will improve outcomes of patients with these conditions, and nurses are uniquely positioned to have a positive influence on their health.

REFERENCES

Centers for Disease Control and Prevention (CDC). (2014a). Respiratory syncytial virus infection. Retrieved from http://www.cdc.gov/rsv/research/us-surveillance.html

Centers for Disease Control and Prevention (CDC). (2014b). Tuberculosis. Retrieved from http://www.cdc.gov/tb/publications/factsheets/statistics/tbtrends.htm.cdc.gov/nchs/data/databriefs/db94.htm#x2013;2010

Centers for Disease Control and Prevention (CDC). (2015a). Chronic obstructive pulmonary disease. Retrieved from http://www.cdc.gov/copd/index.html

Centers for Disease Control and Prevention (CDC). (2015b). Pneumonia. Retrieved from http://www.cdc.gov/nchs/fastats/pneumonia.htm

Centers for Disease Control and Prevention (CDC). (2015c). Trends in asthma prevalence, health care use, and mortality in the United States, 2001–2010. Retrieved from http://www

Centers for Disease Control and Prevention (CDC). (2016a). 2015–2016 influenza season week 39 ending October 1, 2016. Retrieved from https://www.cdc.gov/flu/weekly/pdf/External_F1641.pdf

Centers for Disease Control and Prevention (CDC). (2016b). Common cold. Retrieved from http://www.cdc.gov/dotw/common-cold/index.html

Centers for Disease Control and Prevention (CDC). (2016c). Middle East respiratory syndrome. Retrieved from http://www.cdc.gov/coronavirus/mers/index.html

Chiras, D. (2011). *Human biology* (7th ed.). Burlington, MA: Jones & Bartlett Learning.

Crowley, L. V. (2016). *An introduction to human disease* (10th ed.). Burlington, MA: Jones & Bartlett Learning.

Cystic Fibrosis Foundation. (n.d.). About cystic fibrosis. Retrieved from http://www.cff.org/AboutCF/

Elling, B., Elling, K., & Rothenberg, M. (2004). *Anatomy and physiology*. Sudbury, MA: Jones and Bartlett.

Gould, B. (2015). *Pathophysiology for the health professions* (5th ed.). Philadelphia, PA: Elsevier.

Madara, B., & Pomarico-Denino, V. (2008). *Pathophysiology* (2nd ed.). Sudbury, MA: Jones and Bartlett.

National Institutes of Allergy and Infectious Disease. (2016). Cold versus flu. Retrieved from http://www.cdc.gov/flu/about/qa/coldflu.htm

Professional guide to pathophysiology (3rd ed.). (2010). Philadelphia, PA: Lippincott Williams & Wilkins.

Ralston, S., Lieberthal, A., Meissner, H., Alverson, B., Baley, J., Gadomski, A., Hernandez-Cancio, S. (2014). Clinical practice guideline: The diagnosis, management, and prevention of bronchiolitis. *Pediatrics, 134*(5), e1474–e1502.

U.S. Cancer Statistics Working Group. (2012). *United States cancer statistics: 1999–2008 incidence and mortality web-based report*. Atlanta, GA: Department of Health and Human Services, Centers for Disease Control and Prevention, and National Cancer Institute.

World Health Organization (WHO). (2016a, July). Influenza at the human–animal interface. Retrieved from http://www.who.int/influenza/human_animal_interface/Influenza_Summary_IRA_HA_interface_07_19_2016.pdf?ua=1

World Health Organization (WHO). (2016b). Middle East respiratory syndrome coronavirus. Retrieved from http://www.who.int/emergencies/mers-cov/en/

World Health Organization (WHO). (2016c). Tuberculosis. Retrieved from http://www.who.int/mediacentre/factsheets/fs104/en/

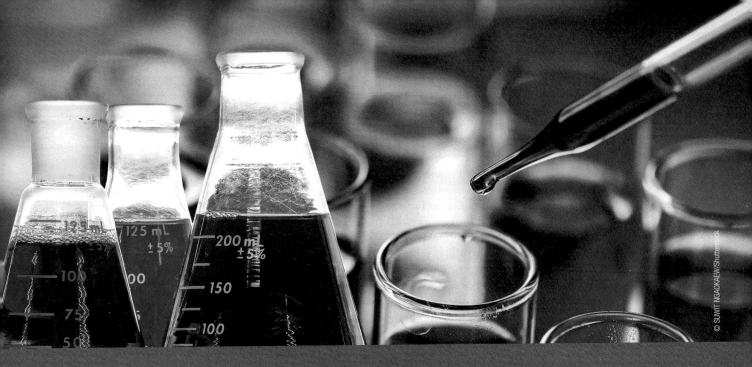

CHAPTER 6
Fluid, Electrolyte, and Acid–Base Homeostasis

LEARNING OBJECTIVES

- Explain fluid distribution and movement in the body.
- Describe and compare fluid imbalance disorders.
- Explain normal electrolyte functions in the body.
- Describe and compare electrolyte disorders.
- Explain normal pH regulation.
- Describe and compare acid–base disorders.
- Analyze arterial blood gases.

KEY TERMS

aldosterone
anasarca
anion
anion gap
antidiuretic hormone (ADH)
arterial blood gas (ABG)
atrial natriuretic peptide
bicarbonate–carbonic acid
  system
calcium
cation
chloride
Chvostek's sign
dehydration
depolarization
edema
extracellular fluid

fluid deficit
fluid excess
fluid volume deficit
fluid volume excess
fully compensated
hemoglobin system
hypercalcemia
hyperchloremia
hyperkalemia
hypermagnesemia
hypernatremia
hyperphosphatemia
hypertonic solution
hypervolemia
hypocalcemia
hypochloremia
hypokalemia

hypomagnesemia
hyponatremia
hypophosphatemia
hypotonic solution
hypovolemia
interstitial
intracellular fluid
intravascular
isotonic solution
magnesium
metabolic acidosis
metabolic alkalosis
nonvolatile acid
osmolarity
partially compensated
pH
phosphate system

phosphorus
potassium
protein system
repolarization
respiratory acidosis
respiratory alkalosis
sodium
third spacing
tonicity
transcellular
Trousseau's sign
uncompensated
volatile acid
volatile gas
water intoxication

The human body requires a delicate balance, or homeostasis, to function optimally (see *Introduction to Pathophysiology*). The body continuously employs strategies to maintain this balance. Fluids, electrolytes, and pH all play critical roles in sustaining homeostasis. Fluids are distributed in various body compartments and move among these compartments to preserve equilibrium. Electrolytes are vital for cellular function, and they work with the various fluids to maintain stability. Acid–base balance is critical for health and is achieved through a complex buffer system. Fluids, electrolytes, and pH have a dynamic relationship in which imbalances in one area can cause imbalances in the other two. Additionally, the other areas can serve to compensate for those imbalances. When compensatory mechanisms fail to reestablish homeostasis, many bodily functions are impaired, and serious consequences can result. In such a case, medical interventions will be necessary to reestablish stability.

Fluid Balance

Distribution

Body fluid is made of water and solutes. Water is the medium within which metabolic reactions and other processes occur. Water carries nutrients into the cells, waste products out of the cells, enzymes in digestive secretions, and blood cells around the body. Fluid also facilitates movement of body parts (e.g., the joints, lungs, and heart). Fluid found inside the cells is referred to as **intracellular fluid**, and fluid found outside the cells is referred to as **extracellular fluid**. Extracellular fluid is further divided into **interstitial** (between the cells) and **intravascular** (inside the blood vessels) compartments. The cell membrane serves as a barrier that substances and water must pass through to move to or from the intracellular compartment. A third compartment in which fluid is found is the **transcellular** compartment, which includes the following types of fluids:

- Fluid in the peritoneal, pleural, and pericardial cavities
- Cerebrospinal fluid
- Fluid in the joint spaces, lymph system, eyes, and gastrointestinal tract

Collectively, the intracellular fluid accounts for approximately two-thirds of the body's water. This intracellular fluid is rich in potassium, magnesium, phosphates, and proteins. The remaining one-third of the body fluid makes up the extracellular fluid. Approximately 80% of the extracellular fluid is found in the interstitial compartment, and the remaining 20% is found in the intravascular compartment. The extracellular fluid is rich in sodium, chloride, and bicarbonate. Blood (serum) electrolyte tests examine only intravascular electrolytes, but inferences from these tests can be made as to what is occurring in the other compartments. Transcellular fluid accounts for approximately 1% of the body's fluid.

Fluid Movement

Fluids are constantly circulating throughout the body and moving among compartments to maintain homeostasis. To preserve its stability, the body exchanges solutes and water between compartments to compensate for conditions that increase or decrease losses. This movement between compartments is primarily accomplished through osmosis, the movement of fluid (specifically water) across a semipermeable membrane from an area of lower concentration to an area of higher concentration (see the *Cellular Function* chapter). Often water is overlooked as a solvent, but it also has a concentration in any solution. Consequently, water moves across the semipermeable membranes to an area of lower water concentration until equilibrium is achieved.

Because water moves freely across cell membranes, equilibrium is usually easy to achieve. The movement of water depends on hydrostatic (push) and osmotic (pull) pressures (**FIGURE 6-1**). Proteins and electrolytes contribute to the osmotic pressure of a fluid (**FIGURE 6-2**). At the arteriolar end of the capillary, the blood hydrostatic pressure (blood pressure) exceeds the opposing interstitial hydrostatic pressure, thereby moving (pushing) fluid out of the intravascular compartment and into the interstitial compartment to meet cellular needs. At the venous end of the capillary, the blood hydrostatic pressure is decreased and the osmotic pressure is increased, thereby moving (pulling) fluid from the interstitial compartment to the intravascular compartment to aid in the exchange of waste products to be excreted. To be an effective osmole, the solute must not be able to pass passively through a semipermeable membrane (e.g., protein).

Tonicity is the osmotic pressure of two solutions separated by a semipermeable membrane. This characteristic is often used to describe the cell's response to an external solution (**FIGURE 6-3**). Much like osmotic pressure, tonicity is influenced by solutes that cannot cross the

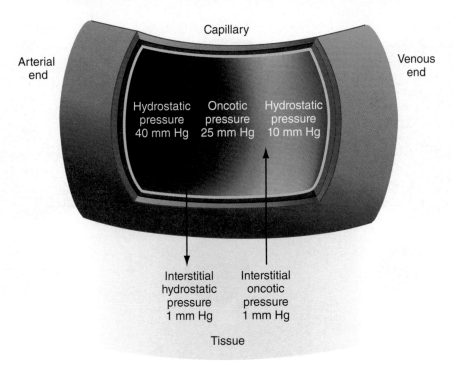

FIGURE 6-1 Pressures that control fluid balance.

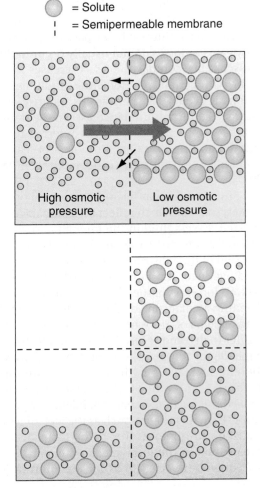

○ = Solvent
◯ = Solute
⌇ = Semipermeable membrane

High osmotic
pressure

Low osmotic
pressure

FIGURE 6-2 Osmotic pressure.

membrane. In health care, the external solution described in relation to tonicity consists of intravenous solutions, specifically those containing electrolytes (crystalloids) that are used to treat a variety of patient conditions (e.g., dehydration and shock). These solutions are defined in terms of three classifications of tonicity—isotonic, hypotonic, and hypertonic. **Isotonic solutions** (e.g., 0.9% saline and lactated Ringer's solution) have concentrations of solutes equal to those in the intravascular compartment. As a result of these equivalent solute concentrations, isotonic solutions allow fluid to move equally between compartments and do not cause notable shifts in fluid volume. **Hypotonic solutions** (e.g., 0.45% saline) have a lower concentration of solutes than those in the intravascular compartment. Hypotonic solutions cause fluid to shift from the intravascular compartment to the intracellular space. **Hypertonic solutions** (e.g., 5% dextrose in 0.9% saline, 3% saline) have a higher concentration of solutes than those in the intravascular compartment. Hypertonic solutions cause fluid to shift from the intracellular compartment to the intravascular space.

Additionally, fluid is added to the body through the ingestion of food and fluids and as a cellular by-product. Approximately 100 mL of water is needed per 100 calories ingested to help with metabolism and waste elimination. Fluid is primarily lost in the urine and feces, but

Hypertonic   Isotonic   Hypotonic

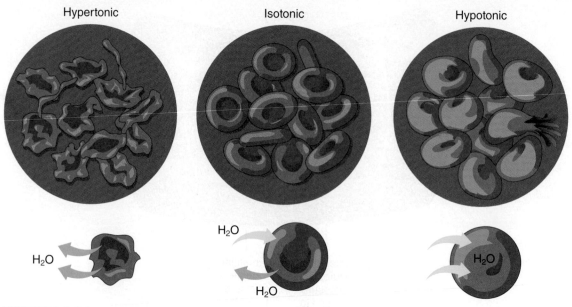

FIGURE 6-3 Cellular response to tonicity.
Courtesy of Mariana Ruiz Villarreal

additional insensible (immeasurable) losses occur through the skin (e.g., perspiration) and the respiratory tract (e.g., breathing, coughing, talking, and mechanical ventilation).

Body fluid intake and output balance is maintained through several mechanisms. The osmoreceptor cells, for example, sense intravascular fluid volume. Decreased fluid volume or increased **osmolarity** (solute concentration) triggers the thirst mechanism in the hypothalamus to increase oral intake. The thirst sensation occurs with even the smallest water losses and is one of the best regulators of water balance. This thirst sensation can decrease with aging (a phenomenon called hypodipsia). **Antidiuretic hormone (ADH)** regulates fluid volume by controlling water losses in the urine. Released from the pituitary gland in times of decreased fluid volume and increased osmolarity, ADH promotes reabsorption of water into the blood from the renal tubules. The hormone known as **aldosterone** is released to conserve more water when necessary (e.g., when a person has low blood pressure) by increasing reabsorption of sodium and water in the renal tubules. Finally, another hormone, **atrial natriuretic peptide**, is released when the atria of the myocardium becomes overstretched, indicating increased fluid volume. This peptide stimulates renal vasodilation, thereby increasing urinary output. Additionally, atrial natriuretic peptide suppresses aldosterone secretion, further increasing urinary output.

Fluid Excess

Ideally, daily fluid intake should equal the amount of fluid lost. Most significant increases in fluid accumulation occur in the interstitial, intravascular, or intracellular spaces; significant daily gains or losses do not usually occur in the transcellular compartments. Increases may occur with certain physiological conditions or traumatic events (e.g., pericarditis, pleurisy, and ascites). Significant fluid increases in the transcellular compartment are often referred to as **third spacing** because fluid is not easily exchanged among the other extracellular fluids.

Fluid excess has been given several other names, some of which reflect the compartment affected. Excess fluid in the interstitial space is generally referred to as **edema**. Edema is a problem of fluid distribution, not necessarily of fluid overload. It occurs when hydrostatic and osmotic forces favor the movement of fluid from the intravascular compartment to the interstitial space. Edema occurs when hydrostatic forces are greater than osmotic forces. For example, blood stagnates in the periphery with heart failure, thereby increasing hydrostatic pressure and pushing fluid out of the vessel (see the *Cardiovascular Function* chapter). Edema may also be localized to one area, such as the feet, or generalized throughout the body (**anasarca**). Excess fluid in the intravascular compartment is frequently referred to as **hypervolemia** or

Tonicity reflects the relationship certain nutrients and electrolytes have with water. Both sodium and glucose attract water—water will go wherever the higher concentrations of sodium and glucose are. In the case of intravenous (IV) fluids, the concentration of sodium and glucose in the intravascular compartment is adjusted to attract or repel water. For example, 0.9% (isotonic) saline has a sodium concentration similar to that found in the intravascular space, so no fluid shifts between compartments when it is administered to patients. Instead, fluid is just replaced in the intravascular compartment. Hypotonic (0.45%) saline has a lower concentration of sodium than that usually found in the intravascular space, so its administration causes water to move out of the intravascular compartment and into the intracellular compartment. The same phenomenon occurs when patients receive glucose or dextrose in a solution. Finally, hypertonic (3%) saline has a higher concentration of sodium than that usually found in the intravascular space, so water moves from the intracellular compartment to the intravascular compartment when patients receive it as an IV formulation. Remember: Wherever sodium and glucose are, water will follow!

fluid volume excess. Often hypervolemia results from excessive sodium or water intake or insufficient losses. In such a case, the intake becomes greater than the body's compensatory mechanisms can manage. The excess fluid volume strains the left ventricle, which can cause left-sided heart failure over time (see the *Cardiovascular Function* chapter). Fluid excess can also occur in the intracellular space, a condition known as **water intoxication**. Intracellular fluid excess can lead to the rupture, or lysis, of the cells. Cerebral cells are the most sensitive to lysis.

Fluid excess may result from the following conditions:

- Excessive sodium or water intake, including that caused by the following:
  - High-sodium diet (e.g., processed foods, sodas, and certain seasonings)
  - Psychogenic polydipsia (excessive water ingestion)
  - Hypertonic fluid administration
  - Free water
  - Enteral feedings
- Inadequate sodium or water elimination, including that caused by the following:
  - Hyperaldosteronism (which increases sodium retention and, in turn, water retention)
  - Cushing's syndrome (a condition of excessive corticosteroid, which contains

high levels of sodium; see the *Endocrine Function* chapter)
  - Syndrome of inappropriate antidiuretic hormone (excessive ADH levels, which increases fluid retention)
  - Renal failure (the kidneys are unable to eliminate fluid or waste products; see the *Urinary Function* chapter)
  - Liver failure (the liver is unable to synthesize protein, impairing colloidal pressures; see the *Gastrointestinal Function* chapter)
  - Heart failure (the heart is unable to pump blood effectively, leading to decreased blood flow to the kidneys and fluid shifts; see the *Cardiovascular Function* chapter)

Clinical manifestations of fluid excess include the following signs and symptoms:

- Peripheral edema (the skin usually indents with pressure, a condition referred to as pitting; FIGURE 6-4)
- Periorbital edema (swelling around the eyes)
- Anasarca (generalized edema; the skin may begin to weep fluid)
- Cerebral edema, which causes headache, confusion, irritability, anxiety, nausea, and vomiting
- Dyspnea
- Bounding pulse
- Tachycardia
- Jugular vein distension
- Hypertension
- Polyuria (large amounts of pale yellow urine)
- Rapid weight gain (3 pounds in a week or 1–2 pounds in a day; 1 pound approximately equals 500 mL of fluid)
- Crackles (abnormal lung sound)
- Bulging fontanelles (in infants)

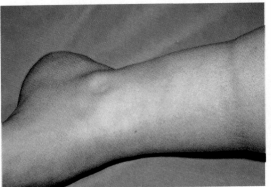

FIGURE 6-4 Pitting edema.

A demonstration of the severity of water intoxication can be seen in a story familiar to many. A radio station was having a contest. The contestant who could drink the most water without voiding would win the contest. Because water is limited in electrolytes such as sodium, excessive water intake in a short period can cause the sodium concentration in the vascular space to drop in relationship to the water. The sodium concentration in the tissue is then higher than that in the blood, which causes water to move out of the vascular space and into the interstitial space. This fluid quickly caused cerebral edema (see the *Neural Function* chapter), decreased neurologic functioning, and death in the individual who consumed the most water in the contest. The sad thing is that a nurse called into the radio station to warn station officials that this contest was dangerous, yet the station went ahead with it. This seemingly harmless act had grave consequences.

The main diagnostic procedure for fluid excess is the complete blood count (CBC). When excess fluid is present, urine and blood specific gravity and osmolality will be decreased due to solute dilution. Blood cells—especially the red blood cells and platelets—may be decreased because of the high ratio of fluid.

Management of fluid excess focuses on identifying and treating the underlying cause. Strategies may consist of wearing compression stockings, administering diuretics, restricting sodium and fluids, and maintaining the patient in high Fowler's position. In severe cases of intracellular and interstitial fluid excess, hypertonic solutions may be given to shift the excess fluid from these spaces to the intravascular space, where it can be excreted. To aid in excretion, a diuretic may be administered.

Fluid Deficit

Fluid deficit occurs when total body fluid levels are insufficient to meet the body's needs. Such a fluid deficit may be referred to as **dehydration**. Fluid deficit of the intravascular compartment is often referred to as **fluid volume deficit** or **hypovolemia**. Fluid deficit can occur independently or with electrolyte deficits, such as a sodium deficit. As fluid levels decrease, sodium levels, along with levels of other blood solutes (e.g., blood cells and electrolytes), increase because of hemoconcentration. Climbing sodium levels trigger fluid shifts from other compartments as the body attempts to maintain homeostasis. When losses are greater than these shifts can accommodate, the cells shrink. Fluid volume levels decrease, causing hypotension.

Causes of fluid deficits include the following:

- Inadequate fluid intake, such as that caused by the following:
  - Poor oral intake (such as occurs in the event of stroke or dementia)
  - Inadequate IV fluid replacement
- Excessive fluid or sodium losses, such as those caused by the following:
  - Gastrointestinal losses (vomiting, diarrhea, and nasogastric suctioning)
  - Excessive diaphoresis (sweating)
  - Prolonged hyperventilation
  - Hemorrhage
  - Nephrosis (also called nephrotic syndrome; a degenerative renal disease that causes excessive protein losses, leading to fluid movement out of the intravascular compartment)
  - Diabetes mellitus (which causes renal glucose excretion and, in turn, results in water losses)
  - Diabetes insipidus (an inability to concentrate urine, leading to excessive water losses)
  - Burns (heat denatures proteins, which disrupts colloidal pressure)
  - Open wounds (increased drainage)
  - Ascites
  - Effusions
  - Excessive use of diuretics
  - Osmotic diuresis that can occur with hypertonic tube feedings or administering parenteral feedings too quickly

Clinical manifestations of fluid deficits include the following signs and symptoms:

- Thirst
- Altered level of consciousness
- Hypotension
- Tachycardia
- Weak, thready pulse
- Flat jugular veins
- Dry mucous membranes
- Decreased skin turgor
- Oliguria
- Weight loss
- Sunken fontanelles (in infants)

An example of osmotic diuresis can be seen in a tragic case in which a newborn was fed concentrated formula by mistake. Often, tube feeding and baby formulas are high in glucose and other electrolytes. Many times these formulas come concentrated for shipping purposes. The newborn's father was unaware that the formula required dilution prior to feeding it to his child. The high concentrations of glucose caused excessive urination, and the baby died because of hypertonic dehydration.

Diagnostic procedures for fluid deficit consist of a history, physical examination, measurements of intake and output, daily weights, blood chemistry, urine analysis, and CBC. Urine and blood specific gravity and osmolality will be increased, indicating a high concentration of solutes. Blood cells—especially red blood cells and platelets—may be increased because of the low ratio of fluid.

Management focuses on identifying and treating the underlying cause of the fluid deficit. Strategies include fluid replacement—oral fluids for mild losses and intravenous fluids for greater losses (either isotonic or hypotonic).

Electrolyte Balance

Electrolytes play a crucial role in homeostasis. Electrolytes are minerals with electrical charges found in the blood, urine, and other body fluids. Electrolytes in the body include sodium, chloride, potassium, calcium, magnesium, and phosphorus (**TABLE 6-1**). **Cations** are positively charged, whereas **anions** are negatively charged. Electrolytes are important in muscle and neural activity and in acid–base and fluid balance.

Sodium

Sodium is considered the most significant cation. The most prevalent electrolyte within the extracellular fluid, sodium's primary function is to control serum osmolality and water balance. Sodium also has an affinity for chloride and helps maintain acid–base balance when combined with bicarbonate (HCO_3).

Sodium is regulated by the kidneys as well as aldosterone produced by the adrenal cortex. In times of high serum osmolality or low blood volume, aldosterone is released and the kidneys retain sodium. The opposite is true when serum osmolality decreases and fluid volume increases. The sympathetic nervous system assists the kidneys in sodium regulation by changing the glomerular filtration rate, which is a reflection of renal blood flow. Increasing the glomerular filtration rate increases sodium excretion; decreasing the glomerular filtration rate decreases sodium excretion. The renin–angiotensin–aldosterone mechanism (see the *Cardiovascular Function* chapter) also manipulates sodium in the kidneys; this mechanism is triggered in times of decreased renal perfusion (e.g., hypovolemia and hypotension). Renin, a protein, converts angiotensinogen to angiotensin I; subsequently, angiotensin I is converted to angiotensin II in the lungs. Angiotensin II causes the kidneys to retain sodium and, in turn, water.

The cellular membrane is permeable to sodium, but it is dependent on the sodium–potassium pump to transport these ions (see the *Cellular Function* chapter). Sodium facilitates muscle and nerve impulses through the pump. As sodium moves into the cell, potassium shifts out of the cell, resulting in **depolarization** (increasing the membrane potential or excitability) of the cell membrane. When sodium shifts out of the cell, potassium moves back into the cell, resulting in **repolarization** (restoring the resting potential) of the cell membrane.

Sodium is primarily brought into the body through dietary intake. The recommended dietary allowance (RDA) of sodium is 2–4 grams. This electrolyte can be found in many sources, such as table salt (1 teaspoon contains more than 2 grams of sodium), processed or prepackaged foods (e.g., canned foods and deli meats), snack foods (e.g., chips), condiments (e.g., ketchup

TABLE 6-1	Normal Serum Values of the Major Electrolytes*	
Electrolyte	**Normal Range**
Sodium (Na$^+$)	135–145 mEq/L
Chloride (Cl$^-$)	98–108 mEq/L
Potassium (K$^+$)	3.5–5 mEq/L
Calcium (Ca^{++})	4–5 mEq/ L
Phosphorus (P)	2.5–4.5 mg/dL
Magnesium (Mg^{++})	1.8–2.4 mEq/L

*Values may vary slightly.

and hot sauce), and certain cooking seasonings (e.g., garlic salt and season salt).

Normally, sodium losses occur in the kidneys. Excessive losses can occur through the gastrointestinal tract through vomiting, diarrhea, and nasogastric suctioning. Extensive burns can also cause sodium losses through the skin. Finally, sodium losses can occur with excessive sweating (e.g., fever and strenuous exercise).

Hypernatremia

Hypernatremia results from high serum sodium levels (greater than 145 mEq/L). The excessive sodium levels generally lead to high serum osmolality (greater than 295 mOsm/kg) because of the imbalance between sodium and water. As sodium levels rise, water shifts out of the intracellular and interstitial spaces and into the intravascular compartment.

Hypernatremia usually results from ingesting excessive sodium without consuming a proportionate amount of water or through water losses that exceed the amount of sodium being lost. Hypernatremia may be caused by a variety of conditions:

- Excessive sodium, such as that caused by the following:
  - Excessive sodium ingestion
  - Hypertonic IV saline (3% saline) administration
  - Cushing's syndrome (a condition associated with excessive corticosteroids, which contain high levels of sodium)
  - Corticosteroid use
- Deficient water, such as that caused by the following:
  - Decreased water ingestion
  - Loss of thirst sensation
  - Inability to drink water (which might occur if a person is unconscious or confused)
  - Third spacing
  - Vomiting
  - Diarrhea
  - Excessive sweating
  - Prolonged episode of hyperventilation (increases insensible water losses)
  - Diuretic use
  - Diabetes insipidus (excessive water loss as a result of insufficient ADH levels)

Clinical manifestations of hypernatremia can range from subtle to serious, depending on the severity of the hypernatremia itself, and include the following signs and symptoms:

- Increased temperature
- Warm, flushed skin
- Dry and sticky mucous membranes
- Dysphagia (difficulty swallowing)
- Increased thirst
- Irritability and agitation
- Weakness
- Headache
- Seizures
- Lethargy
- Coma
- Blood pressure changes
- Tachycardia
- Weak, thready pulse
- Edema
- Decreased urine output (can be high with diabetes insipidus)

Diagnostic procedures for hypernatremia include a history, physical examination, blood chemistry, and urine analysis. Other procedures (e.g., computed tomography [CT] and magnetic resonance imaging [MRI]) may be conducted to identify causation.

Management of hypernatremia focuses on treating the underlying cause. If the cause is related to water loss, treatment begins with replacing water and remedying any electrolyte deficits. Glucose-electrolyte solutions (e.g., sports drinks) are given orally for less severe cases. More severe cases can be corrected with intravenous hypotonic (e.g., 5% dextrose in water or 0.45% saline) solutions. The healthcare professional must use caution to avoid correcting the hypernatremia too rapidly. The brain can become accustomed to the high levels of sodium; as the levels drop with the treatment of hypernatremia, water moves into cerebral cells, causing cerebral edema. Generally, one should not correct hypernatremia by administering water and electrolyte solutions faster than 1 mEq/L per hour. Diuretics may be necessary if the patient is hypervolemic. Additionally, seizure precautions (e.g., low lighting and decreased stimuli) and neurologic checks should be added to the patient's plan of care.

Hyponatremia

Hyponatremia results from low serum sodium levels (less than 135 mEq/L). Serum osmolality levels also fall below 275 mOsm. As sodium levels decrease, water shifts into brain cells, causing cerebral edema. Additionally, nerve conduction becomes impaired as the sodium levels fall.

Hyponatremia results from excessive sodium losses or increased water gains (referred to as dilutional hyponatremia):

- Deficient sodium, including that caused by the following:
  - Diuretic use
  - Gastrointestinal losses (e.g., vomiting and diarrhea)
  - Excessive sweating
  - Insufficient aldosterone levels (Addison's disease)
  - Adrenal insufficiency
  - Dietary sodium restrictions
- Excessive water, including that caused by the following:
  - Hypotonic intravenous saline (0.45% saline)
  - Hyperglycemia (excess glucose in the blood attracts water from the intracellular and interstitial spaces)
  - Excessive water ingestion
  - Renal failure
  - Syndrome of inappropriate antidiuretic hormone
  - Heart failure (circulation stagnation leads to decreased renal excretion)

Clinical manifestations of hyponatremia may vary in severity depending on the sodium level:

- Anorexia
- Gastrointestinal upset (e.g., abdominal cramps, nausea, vomiting, and diarrhea)
- Poor skin turgor
- Dry mucous membranes
- Blood pressure changes (decreased with hypovolemia and increased with hypervolemia)
- Pulse changes (weak with hypovolemia and bounding with hypervolemia)
- Edema
- Headache
- Lethargy
- Confusion
- Diminished deep tendon reflexes
- Muscle weakness
- Seizures
- Coma

Diagnostic procedures for hyponatremia are similar to those for hypernatremia. Management focuses on treating the underlying cause (e.g., administering corticosteroids for Addison's disease). In cases caused by excessive water, oral intake may be limited. In cases caused by deficient sodium, oral intake may be increased. Correction of sodium levels should be done slowly so as not to overload the heart from fluid shifting into the intravascular space. Additionally, seizure precautions (e.g., low lighting and decreased stimuli) and neurologic checks should be added to the patient's plan of care.

Chloride

Chloride is a mineral electrolyte and the major extracellular anion. Chloride assists in fluid distribution by attaching to sodium or water. Because of its negative charge, chloride can bind and travel with positively charged ions (e.g., sodium, potassium, calcium). This electrolyte is found in gastric secretions, pancreatic juices, and bile. In the stomach, it unites with hydrogen to form hydrochloric acid. Chloride is abundant in cerebrospinal fluid, where it binds with sodium. When bound to sodium, it behaves just like sodium in regard to water balance. When bound to hydrogen, chloride plays an important role in acid–base balance. The kidneys are primarily responsible for chloride excretion, but some chloride is also lost through sweating.

Diet is the main source of chloride. The chloride RDA is 3–9 grams. Chloride is easily obtained through consumption of a balanced diet. Common sources of chloride include table salt, fruits, vegetables, cheese, milk, eggs, fish, canned foods, and processed meats. Chloride is primarily excreted in the kidneys.

Hyperchloremia

Hyperchloremia is an excess amount of chloride in the blood (greater than 108 mEq/L). Hyperchloremia is usually a result of an underlying condition; it does not have its own clinical manifestations, but the companion condition may cause signs and symptoms. Some causes of hyperchloridemia include:

- Increased chloride intake or exchange, including that caused by the following:
  - Hypernatremia
  - Hypertonic intravenous solution
  - Metabolic acidosis
  - Hyperkalemia
- Decreased chloride excretion, including that caused by the following:
  - Hyperparathyroidism (increases calcium levels, which attracts chloride)
  - Hyperaldosteronism (increases sodium levels, which attracts chloride)
  - Renal failure (decreased chloride excretion)

Diagnostic procedures include a history, physical examination, blood chemistry, urine analysis, and measurement of arterial blood gases (ABGs). Management of hyperchloremia focuses on treating the underlying cause. Administering diuretics to assist in eliminating sodium will, in turn, assist in the removal of chloride. Administering bicarbonate can correct acidosis if present.

Hypochloremia

Hypochloremia occurs when chloride levels fall below 98 mEq/L. Hypochloremia rarely occurs in the absence of other abnormalities; therefore, like hyperchloremia, it does not have its own set of clinical manifestations. Causative conditions include the following:

- Decreased chloride intake or exchange, such as that accompanied by the following:
  - Hyponatremia
  - Administration of 5% dextrose in water intravenous solution
  - Water intoxication
  - Hypokalemia
- Increased chloride excretion, such as that which occurs with the following:
  - Diuretics (sodium loss, which in turn increases chloride excretion)
  - Vomiting (excessive loss of hydrochloric acid)
  - Metabolic alkalosis
  - Other gastrointestinal losses (such as those that occur with fistula, ileostomy, nasogastric suction, and diarrhea)

Diagnostic procedures for hypochloremia are similar to those for hyperchloremia. Treatment focuses on correcting the underlying cause. Some of those strategies include increasing oral sodium intake and administering sodium-containing intravenous solutions. Additionally, ammonium chloride can be given with caution to raise chloride levels. Saline solutions can also be used to irrigate gastric tubes.

Potassium

Potassium is the primary intracellular cation. It plays a crucial role in electrical conduction, acid–base balance, and metabolism (carbohydrate, protein, and glucose). Potassium is present in huge quantities in the intracellular space—a store that can be utilized if serum levels drop. However, certain circumstances (e.g., lysis) cause excessive amounts of potassium to shift to the intravascular space, which can be dangerous (especially within the heart). Serum potassium cannot fluctuate very much—either up or down—without causing serious issues. The sodium–potassium pump and the kidneys regulate potassium. The diet

(e.g., cantaloupes, raisins, bananas, oranges, green leafy vegetables, and lentils) is the primary source of potassium. The RDA for potassium is 40–60 mEq. In addition to potassium being excreted in the kidneys, it is lost through the gastrointestinal tract.

Hyperkalemia

Hyperkalemia refers to serum potassium levels greater than 5 mEq/L. Hyperkalemia is unusual in the healthy individual and may be a medical emergency. Generally, this imbalance is caused by conditions that impair excretion, increase intake, or release potassium out of the cells:

- Deficient excretion, such as occurs with the following:
  - Renal failure
  - Addison's disease (decreased levels of aldosterone decrease potassium secretion)
  - Certain medications (e.g., potassium-sparing diuretics, nonsteroidal anti-inflammatory drugs, and angiotensin-converting enzyme inhibitors), which can also alter aldosterone levels
  - Gordon's syndrome (a rare genetic disorder in which the kidneys are unable to respond to aldosterone)
- Excessive intake, such as occurs with the following:
  - Oral potassium supplements
  - Salt substitutes (many contain large amounts of potassium to create a "salty" taste)
  - Rapid intravenous administration of diluted potassium (administering potassium undiluted can be lethal)
- Increased release from cells, including that associated with the following:
  - Acidosis (increased serum hydrogen levels cause potassium to shift out of the cells; lack of insulin in diabetic ketoacidosis impairs the transportation of potassium in the cell)
  - Blood transfusions (can cause blood cell lysis, which releases intracellular potassium)
  - Burns or any other cellular injuries (can cause cell lysis, which releases intracellular potassium)

Hyperkalemia can affect several body systems in which potassium plays key functions, including the nervous, cardiac, respiratory, and gastrointestinal systems. The severity of these effects depends on the extent of the hyperkalemia. Clinical manifestations of hyperkalemia include the following signs and symptoms:

- Muscle weakness
- Paresthesia (numbness or tingling)
- Flaccid paralysis
- Bradycardia
- Dysrhythmias (some of which can be fatal)
- Electrocardiogram (EKG) changes (long PR interval, wide QRS, peaked T wave, and depressed ST segment [FIGURE 6-5; see the *Cardiovascular Function* chapter])
- Cardiac arrest
- Respiratory depression (from muscle weakness)
- Abdominal cramping
- Nausea
- Diarrhea

Diagnostic procedures for hyperkalemia include a history, physical examination, blood chemistry, 12-lead EKG, and ABGs. Management focuses on the identification and treatment of the cause (e.g., sodium bicarbonate to treat acidosis). If present, acidosis is treated prior to the hyperkalemia so that potassium can shift back into the cells and a true potassium level can be obtained. Calcium gluconate may be

administered to minimize dysrhythmias. Additionally, the following measures should be taken:

- Decrease dietary potassium intake
- Increase excretion, such as by the following methods:
  - Dialysis
  - Kayexalate (sodium polystyrene sulfonate, which increases gastrointestinal potassium excretion)
  - Intravenous fluids (dilute potassium levels and increase renal excretion)
  - Potassium-losing diuretics
- Facilitate cellular exchange by administering insulin (which may be given with intravenous dextrose to prevent blood glucose drops)

Hypokalemia

Hypokalemia occurs when potassium levels drop below 3.5 mEq/L. Hypokalemia typically results from excessive loss, inadequate intake, or increased potassium cellular uptake:

- Excessive loss as a result of one or more of the following:
  - Vomiting
  - Diarrhea
  - Nasogastric suctioning
  - Fistulas
  - Laxatives
  - Potassium-losing diuretics
  - Cushing's syndrome (decreases sodium excretion, which in turn increases potassium excretion)
  - Corticosteroids (decrease sodium excretion, which in turn increases potassium excretion)
- Deficient intake, such as occurs with the following:
  - Malnutrition
  - Extreme dieting
  - Alcoholism (can result in inadequate nutrition, nausea, and vomiting)
- Increased shift into the cell as occurs with the following:
  - Alkalosis (decreased serum hydrogen levels cause potassium to shift into the cells)
  - Insulin excess (increases potassium transportation into the cells)

Much like hyperkalemia, hypokalemia can affect several body systems because of potassium's functions, including the nervous, cardiac,

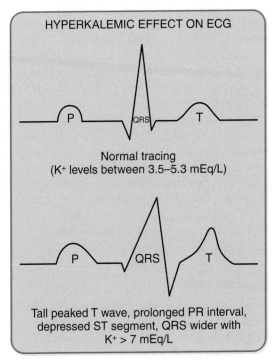

HYPERKALEMIC EFFECT ON ECG

P QRS T

Normal tracing
(K^+ levels between 3.5–5.3 mEq/L)

P QRS T

Tall peaked T wave, prolonged PR interval, depressed ST segment, QRS wider with $K^+ > 7$ mEq/L

FIGURE 6-5 Hyperkalemic effects on the electrocardiogram.

respiratory, and gastrointestinal systems. The severity of these effects reflects the extent of the hypokalemia. Clinical manifestations of hypokalemia are similar to those associated with hyperkalemia:

- Muscle weakness
- Paresthesia
- Hyporeflexia
- Leg cramps
- Weak, irregular pulse
- Hypotension
- Dysrhythmias (some of which are lethal)
- EKG changes (prolonged PR interval, depressed ST segment, flattened T wave, and a U wave [FIGURE 6-6; see the *Cardiovascular Function* chapter])
- Decreased bowel sounds
- Abdominal distension
- Constipation or ileus
- Cardiac arrest

Diagnostic procedures for hypokalemia include a history, physical examination, blood chemistry, 12-lead EKG, and ABGs. Management focuses on the identification and treatment of the cause (e.g., correcting any alkalosis). Additionally, strategies are directed at increasing the amount of potassium available to the body. Oral potassium is administered for mild cases, while diluted intravenous potassium is administered for more severe deficits.

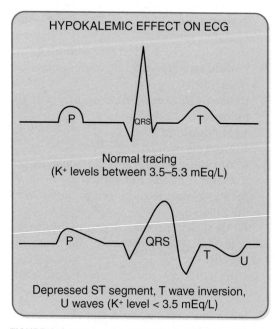

FIGURE 6-6 Hypokalemic effects on the electrocardiogram.

Calcium

Most of the body's **calcium** is found in the bones and teeth (99%). Most of the remaining stores (1%) are found in an ionized (unbound) form in the blood that can be used for physiological processes—for example, blood clotting, hormone secretion, receptor functions, nerve transmission, and muscular contraction. Calcium has an inverse relationship with phosphorus and a synergistic relationship with magnesium. When calcium levels go up, phosphorus goes down, and vice versa. Calcium needs magnesium to fully function as well as balance its effects.

Calcium is brought into the body through the absorption of dietary sources in the gastrointestinal tract, specifically the small intestines; therefore, conditions affecting intestinal absorption or surgical procedures that change the gastrointestinal tract (e.g., gastric bypass) can alter calcium absorption. Vitamin D aids in calcium absorption; it is primarily obtained through sun exposure and from fortified dairy products. Vitamin K also plays an important role in calcium regulation and bone formation (vitamin K binds to calcium in the bone); it is primarily found in green leafy vegetables. Calcium is found in large amounts in dairy products, salmon, sardines, green leafy vegetables, pinto beans, almonds, and figs, among other sources. The RDA of calcium is 800–1,200 mg/day; however, individuals' daily needs vary with certain conditions (e.g., pregnancy, childhood, and osteoporosis).

Calcium is excreted in the urine and stool. Levels of this electrolyte are regulated by the parathyroid hormones and calcitonin (a thyroid hormone). When serum calcium levels are low, parathyroid hormone mobilizes the bone calcium and pulls it into the bloodstream. To compensate for this shift, parathyroid hormone replaces this calcium by decreasing renal excretion and promoting intestinal absorption. Calcitonin, in contrast, regulates elevated calcium levels by pushing the excess calcium into the bone, decreasing intestinal absorption and increasing renal excretion.

Hypercalcemia

Hypercalcemia occurs when ionized calcium levels climb above 5 mEq/L. This imbalance may result from excessive calcium intake or calcium release from the bone as well as from inadequate excretion. Its causes include the following:

- Increased intake or release, including that caused by the following:
  - Calcium antacids (e.g., Tums)
  - Calcium supplements
  - Cancer (especially bone, but also lung, breast, ovarian, prostate, leukemia, and gastrointestinal cancers)
  - Immobilization
  - Corticosteroids
  - Vitamin D deficiency
  - Hypophosphatemia
- Deficit excretion, including that caused by the following:
  - Renal failure
  - Thiazide diuretics
  - Hyperparathyroidism

Clinical manifestations of hypercalcemia reflect decreased cell membrane excitability and are often nonspecific. The cardiac, nervous, musculoskeletal, gastrointestinal, and renal systems can all be affected by these high calcium levels. Clinical manifestations of hypercalcemia include the following signs and symptoms:

- Dysrhythmias (some of which can be fatal)
- EKG changes (short QT interval)
- Personality changes
- Confusion
- Decreased memory
- Headache
- Lethargy
- Stupor
- Coma
- Muscle weakness
- Decreased deep tendon reflexes
- Anorexia
- Nausea and vomiting
- Constipation
- Abdominal pain
- Pancreatitis
- Renal calculi (stones)
- Polyuria (high calcium levels interfere with ADH, resulting in increased water excretion)
- Dehydration

Diagnostic procedures include a history, physical examination, blood chemistry, and 12-lead EKG. Management of hypercalcemia focuses on identification and treatment of the underlying cause (e.g., dialysis for renal failure).

Additionally, strategies may be implemented to treat clinical manifestations (e.g., antidysrhythmic agents). Giving oral phosphate preparations, increasing mobility, and administering calcitonin can facilitate the movement of the excessive calcium out of the bloodstream and into the bone. Increasing intravenous fluid administration can increase renal excretion of calcium. Diuretics may be necessary to enhance this excretion further.

Hypocalcemia

Hypocalcemia occurs when ionized calcium levels fall below 4 mEq/L. This condition occurs as a result of increased losses or decreased intake of calcium:

- Excessive losses, including those associated with the following:
  - Hypoparathyroidism
  - Renal failure
  - Hyperphosphatemia
  - Alkalosis (as serum hydrogen levels decrease, calcium levels decrease)
  - Pancreatitis (decreases intestinal absorption of fat; calcium binds to the fat and is excreted)
  - Laxatives (decrease absorption)
  - Diarrhea
  - Other medications (e.g., diuretics, calcitonin, and gentamicin)
- Deficient intake, including that caused by the following:
  - Decreased dietary intake
  - Alcoholism (decreased diet and poor absorption)
  - Absorption disorders (e.g., Crohn's disease)
  - Hypoalbuminemia (much of calcium is bound to protein)

As opposed to hypercalcemia, hypocalcemia increases cell membrane excitability. The low calcium levels affect the cardiac, neurologic, musculoskeletal, respiratory, and gastrointestinal systems. Clinical manifestations of hypocalcemia include the following signs and symptoms:

- Dysrhythmias (some of which can be lethal)
- EKG changes (prolonged QT interval)
- Increased bleeding tendencies (e.g., bruising and petechia)
- Anxiety
- Confusion
- Depression

- Irritability
- Fatigue
- Lethargy
- Paresthesia
- Increased deep tendon reflexes
- Tremors
- Muscle spasms
- Seizures
- Laryngeal spasms
- Increased bowel sounds
- Abdominal cramping

In addition to these clinical manifestations, two signs specific to hypocalcemia may be present—Trousseau's and Chvostek's signs. To test for **Trousseau's sign**, arterial blood flow is occluded by using an inflated blood pressure cuff. The cuff is placed on the upper arm and inflated above the individual's usual systolic pressure measurement. The inflated cuff is left in place for approximately 3 minutes. The test is considered positive for increased neuromuscular irritability if it elicits a carpal spasm (flexed wrist and metacarpophalangeal joints, extended interphalangeal joints, and adducted thumb) (FIGURE 6-7). To test for **Chvostek's sign**, the healthcare practitioner taps the patient's facial nerve in front of the ear. A spasm or brief contraction of the corner of the mouth, nose, eye, and muscles in the cheek is considered a positive sign and indicates increased neuromuscular irritability (FIGURE 6-8).

Diagnostic procedures for hypocalcemia are similar to those for hypercalcemia. Management focuses on identification and treatment of the underlying cause. Calcium levels can be increased with oral supplements (in mild

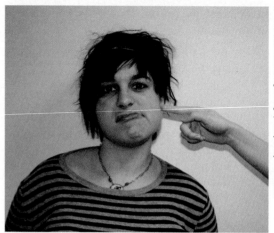

FIGURE 6-8 Chvostek's sign.

deficiencies) and intravenous calcium gluconate (in moderate to severe deficiencies). Vitamin D supplements can increase intestinal calcium absorption. Additionally, phosphorus intake may be decreased to bring calcium levels up.

Phosphorus

Most of the body's **phosphorus**, or phosphate, is found in the bones, with smaller quantities circulating in the bloodstream. As previously mentioned, phosphorus has an inverse relationship with calcium. Phosphorus plays a key role in bone and tooth mineralization, cellular metabolism, acid–base balance, and cell membrane formation, among other functions.

Phosphorus primarily enters the body through dietary sources, and its elimination mainly occurs in the urine. Foods with high phosphorus concentrations include dairy products, protein sources (e.g., chicken, beef, fish, and nuts), grains, and carbonated sodas. The RDA of phosphorus is approximately 1,000 mg/day. Absorption of phosphorus is decreased when it is ingested with foods containing calcium, magnesium, and aluminum—all of which bind with phosphorus.

Hyperphosphatemia

Hyperphosphatemia occurs when phosphorus levels climb above 4.5 mg/dL. It usually results from decreased excretion or increased intake of phosphorus:

- Deficient excretion, such as that caused by the following:
  - Renal failure
  - Hypoparathyroidism (decreases renal excretion)
  - Adrenal insufficiency

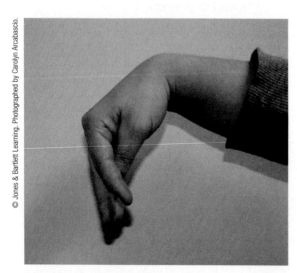

FIGURE 6-7 Trousseau's sign.

- Hypothyroidism
- Laxatives, especially those containing phosphorus (decrease calcium levels, which increases phosphorus levels)
- Excessive intake or cellular exchange, such as that caused by the following:
  - Cellular damage (e.g., burn, trauma, and chemotherapy)
  - Hypocalcemia
  - Acidosis (increased phosphorus shifts from the intracellular compartment to the intravascular compartment)

Clinical manifestations are similar to those observed with hypocalcemia and are rarely seen alone. Diagnostic procedures for hyperphosphatemia consist of a history, physical examination, and blood chemistry. Management includes identification and treatment of the underlying cause (e.g., dialysis for renal failure). Aluminum hydroxide and aluminum carbonate can bind to phosphorus and increase intestinal excretion. Additionally, treatment of hypocalcemia may be necessary.

Hypophosphatemia

Hypophosphatemia occurs when phosphorus levels drop below 2.5 mg/dL. This imbalance is usually caused by increased excretion or decreased intake of phosphorus:

- Excessive excretion or cellular exchange, such as that caused by the following:
  - Renal failure
  - Hyperparathyroidism (increases renal excretion)
  - Alkalosis (increased amounts of phosphorus shift from the intravascular compartment to the intracellular compartment)
- Deficient intake, such as that caused by the following:
  - Malabsorption
  - Vitamin D deficiency
  - Magnesium and aluminum antacids
  - Alcoholism
  - Decreased dietary intake (rare)

Clinical manifestations are similar to those associated with hypercalcemia. Diagnostic procedures include a history, physical examination, and blood chemistry. Management of hypophosphatemia focuses on the identification and treatment of the underlying cause (e.g., dialysis for renal failure). Phosphorus levels can be increased with administration of oral supplements (in mild deficiencies) and intravenous potassium phosphate (in moderate to severe deficiencies).

Magnesium

Magnesium is an intracellular cation that is mostly stored in the bone and muscle. This electrolyte helps maintain normal muscle and nerve function, regular cardiac rhythm, a healthy immune system, bone strength, blood glucose levels, and normal blood pressure; it is also involved in energy metabolism and protein synthesis. Magnesium has a direct relationship with calcium and an inverse relationship with phosphorus. It is obtained through dietary intake and excreted through the kidneys. Foods with a high magnesium content include green vegetables, legumes, nuts, seeds, and whole grains. The RDA for magnesium is approximately 400 mg per day.

Hypermagnesemia

Hypermagnesemia occurs when magnesium levels increase above 2.5 mEq/L. This imbalance is rare and usually results from renal failure or from excessive use of laxatives or antacids. Clinical manifestations of hypermagnesemia are similar to those of hypercalcemia. Diagnostic procedures include a history, physical examination, and blood chemistry. Treatment strategies consist of diuretics and dialysis to promote renal function. Additionally, administering intravenous calcium may be necessary to minimize the effects of magnesium (calcium is a direct antagonist of magnesium).

Hypomagnesemia

Hypomagnesemia results when magnesium levels drop below 1.8 mEq/L. Hypomagnesemia can result from inadequate intake, chronic alcoholism, malnutrition, pregnancy (e.g., preeclampsia), diarrhea, diuretics, and stress. Clinical manifestations of this condition are similar to those of hypocalcemia. Diagnostic procedures are the same as those used with hypermagnesemia. Treatment strategies include magnesium oral supplements for mild deficits and intravenous magnesium for more severe cases.

Acid–Base Balance

Acid–base stability is crucial to sustain life and maintain health. Acid–base balance is achieved through a variety of buffer systems and compensatory mechanisms. Body fluids, the kidneys, and the lungs all play pivotal roles in maintaining this balance. Acid–base balance is measured by examining pH, which is the concentration of hydrogen, and has a narrow safety margin (serum pH of 7.35–7.45). Acid–base imbalances can vary in severity based on the degree of pH change. Death can occur if serum pH levels fall below 6.8 or rise above 7.8. Changes in pH may be caused by a variety of conditions, including infection, organ failure, or trauma. In many cases, the acid–base fluctuations can cause more negative effects than the causative condition; therefore, the resulting acid–base imbalance is often corrected before treating the underlying condition.

Learning Points

Understanding ions' relationships with other ions can help you understand what is happening in the body.
- Sodium and potassium have an inverse relationship; thus, when one goes up, the other goes down.
- Calcium and phosphorus have an inverse relationship.
- Calcium and magnesium have a synergistic relationship, so one enhances the other.

pH Regulation

One way to measure serum hydrogen is by **pH**, which reflects acid–base status. The pH measure is a negative logarithm that reflects the hydrogen concentration; the higher the hydrogen concentration, the lower the pH number (**FIGURE 6-9**). Hydrogen is necessary for maintaining the cellular membranes and for enzyme activities. Acids are produced as a by-product of protein, carbohydrate, and fat metabolism. The acidic by-products are found

in body fluids as **volatile acids**, such as carbonic acid. Carbonic acid breaks down into hydrogen and bicarbonate. Additionally, an acidic **volatile gas** is produced as a by-product of cellular respiration, such as carbon dioxide (CO_2). Carbon dioxide is expelled through breathing, and the remaining volatile acid is converted to **nonvolatile acids** (e.g., hydrochloric acid, phosphoric acid, and sulfates) that are then excreted in the urine. Three systems work together to maintain acid–base balance—the buffers, respiratory system, and renal system.

Learning Points

The blood's pH must remain between 7.35 and 7.45 (**FIGURE 6-10**). The body's goal is to maintain a constant balance between incoming/produced acids and bases (similar to a faucet that is on) and eliminated acids and bases (such as an open drain). Imbalances lead to acidosis (the acid sink overflows) or alkalosis (the base sink overflows). Balance can be restored by increasing elimination (by draining the sink faster) and/or by decreasing flow (by slowing down the dripping faucet).

Buffers

Buffers are the chemicals that combine with an acid or a base to change pH. Buffering is an immediate reaction to counteract pH variations until compensation is initiated. The body has four major buffer mechanisms: the bicarbonate–carbonic acid system, the phosphate system, the hemoglobin system, and the protein system.

The **bicarbonate–carbonic acid system** is the most significant buffering mechanism in the extracellular fluid. Carbonic acid and

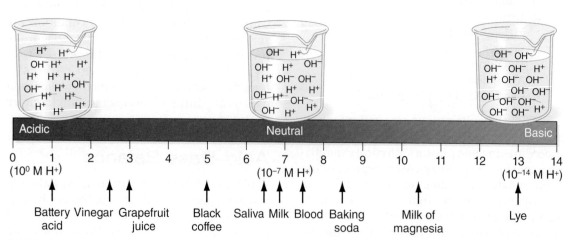

FIGURE 6-9 The pH scale.

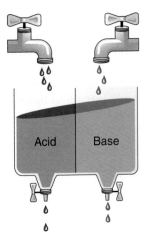

FIGURE 6-10 Acid–base balance.

bicarbonate (base) are the key players in this system. Carbon dioxide is a by-product of cellular metabolism. Once produced, it diffuses into the interstitial fluid and blood, where it reacts with water to form carbonic acid. The carbonic acid decomposes immediately, owing to the presence of the enzyme carbonic anhydrase, to form hydrogen ions and bicarbonate. Carbonic anhydrase is present at many sites in the body, including the lungs and kidneys. In the lungs, this reaction is reversed so that carbon dioxide can be expired along with water—a process that decreases the amount of carbonic acid. In the kidneys, the reaction forms hydrogen ions that are then excreted in the urine, and the bicarbonate is returned to the blood.

The **phosphate system** acts much like the bicarbonate–carbonic acid system. Phosphates are found in high concentrations in the intracellular fluid. Some of these phosphates act as weak acids, whereas others act as weak bases. Buffering in this system primarily takes place in the kidneys by accepting or donating hydrogen.

The **hemoglobin system** is a buffer found in the erythrocytes that works by binding to or releasing hydrogen and carbon dioxide. When combined with oxygen, hemoglobin tends to release hydrogen. Exposing hemoglobin to acid and lower oxygen concentrations in the capillaries causes it to release the oxygen that is bound to it (see the *Hematopoietic Function* chapter). Hemoglobin then becomes a weaker acid, taking up extra hydrogen. This change maintains the pH in the capillaries. The opposite change occurs when hemoglobin is exposed to the higher oxygen concentrations found in the lungs. As hemoglobin binds with oxygen, it becomes more acidic (more prone to release hydrogen). Hydrogen reacts with bicarbonate to

form carbonic acid, which is then converted to carbon dioxide and released into the alveoli.

The **protein system** is the most abundant buffering system. Proteins can act as either an acid or a base by binding to or releasing hydrogen, respectively. Proteins exist in the intracellular and extracellular fluids but are most abundant inside the cells. Hydrogen and carbon dioxide diffuse across the cell membrane to bind with proteins inside the cells, while albumin and plasma are the primary buffers in the intravascular space.

In addition to these systems, two positively charged ions—potassium and hydrogen—move in opposite directions in and out of the cell to balance pH there. When there is an extracellular excess of hydrogen, hydrogen moves inside the cell for buffering purposes; in exchange, potassium moves out of the cell. When there is an extracellular deficit of hydrogen, these ions move in the opposite directions. As mentioned in a previous section, potassium imbalances can lead to acid–base imbalances, and acid–base imbalances can lead to potassium imbalances.

Respiratory Regulation

The respiratory system manages pH deviations by changing carbon dioxide (acid) excretion. Speeding up respirations will lead to excretion of more carbon dioxide, thereby decreasing acidity. Slowing down respirations will lead to excretion of less carbon dioxide, thereby increasing acidity. Chemoreceptors that sense pH changes trigger this change in breathing pattern. The only way the lungs can remove acids is through the elimination of carbon dioxide from carbonic acid—the lungs cannot remove other acids. The respiratory system is also a mechanism that can respond quickly to pH imbalances, but its quick action is generally short lived. The respiratory system reaches its maximum response in 12–24 hours, but can maintain the changes in breathing pattern for only a limited time before becoming fatigued.

Renal Regulation

The renal system is the slowest mechanism to react to pH changes, taking hours to days to achieve its buffering effect, but it is the longest lasting. The kidneys respond to alterations in pH by changing the excretion or retention of hydrogen (acid) or bicarbonate (base). The renal system acts to balance pH levels by permanently removing hydrogen from the body. Additionally, the kidneys can reabsorb acids or bases as well as produce bicarbonate to correct pH imbalances.

Compensation

To maintain homeostasis, the body will take actions to compensate for the pH changes. The body never overcompensates; rather, the pH is adjusted so that it remains just within the normal range. The cause of the imbalance often determines the compensatory change. For instance, if pH is becoming more acidic because of lung disease that limits gas exchange (e.g., emphysema), then the renal system will kick in to compensate for this problem by releasing more bicarbonate and excreting more hydrogen. If a lung disease is increasing carbon dioxide excretion (e.g., hyperventilation), which will increase pH, then the kidneys will compensate by decreasing bicarbonate production and hydrogen excretion. In contrast, the lungs can compensate for problems that originate outside the lungs. For example, the lungs will decrease the rate and depth of respirations to retain more carbon dioxide when a condition increases the loss of acids (e.g., vomiting). If a condition increases the loss of bases (e.g., diarrhea), then the lungs will increase the rate and depth of respirations to excrete more carbon dioxide. If the kidneys and lungs cannot compensate to restore the pH levels to normal range, cellular activities are affected, leading to disease states.

Metabolic Acidosis

Metabolic acidosis results from a deficiency of bicarbonate (base) or an excess of hydrogen (acid) (**TABLE 6-2**). These conditions drop the pH below 7.35. Causes of metabolic acidosis include the following:

- Bicarbonate deficit, including that caused by the following:
  - Intestinal losses (e.g., diarrhea and fistulas)
  - Renal losses (e.g., renal failure)

TABLE 6-2	**Acid–Base Imbalances**	
	Acidosis	**Alkalosis**
Respiratory System		
Causes	Slow, shallow respirations Respiratory congestion	Hyperventilation
Effect	Increased $PaCO_2$	Decreased $PaCO_2$
Compensatory mechanism	Kidneys excrete more hydrogen and reabsorb more bicarbonate	Kidneys excrete less hydrogen and reabsorb less bicarbonate
Diagnostic findings	High $PaCO_2$ High bicarbonate Compensated: pH = 7.35–7.4 Decompensated: pH < 7.33	Low $PaCO_2$ Low bicarbonate Compensated: pH = 7.4–7.45 Decompensated: pH > 7.47
Metabolic System		
Causes	Diarrhea Renal failure Diabetic ketoacidosis Tissue hypoxia	Vomiting Excessive antacid use
Effect	Decreased bicarbonate	Increased bicarbonate
Compensatory mechanism	Rapid, deep respirations Kidneys excrete more hydrogen and increase bicarbonate absorption (when not involved)	Slow, shallow respirations Kidneys excrete less hydrogen and decrease bicarbonate absorption (when not involved)
Diagnostic findings	Low bicarbonate Low $PaCO_2$ Compensated: pH = 7.35–7.4 Decompensated: pH < 7.33	High bicarbonate High $PaCO_2$ Compensated: pH = 7.4–7.45 Decompensated: pH > 7.47

$PaCO_2$ = partial pressure of carbon dioxide; PO_2 = partial pressure of oxygen.

- Acid excess, including that caused by the following:
  - Tissue hypoxia resulting in lactic acid accumulation (e.g., shock and cardiac arrest)
  - Ketoacidosis (e.g., uncontrolled diabetes, excessive alcohol consumption, starvation, and extreme dieting)
  - Drugs and toxins (e.g., antifreeze, aspirin, and hyperalimentation)
  - Renal retention (e.g., renal failure)

Metabolic acidosis exists when the bicarbonate and pH levels are lower than normal (**TABLE 6-3**). Metabolic acidosis results from an existing problem; therefore, the characteristics of that condition are manifested along with the acidosis. Clinical manifestations of metabolic acidosis are often neurologic in nature but the gastrointestinal, cardiac, and respiratory systems can also be affected. These manifestations include the following signs and symptoms:

- Headache
- Malaise
- Weakness
- Fatigue
- Lethargy
- Coma
- Warm, flushed skin
- Nausea and vomiting
- Anorexia
- Hypotension
- Dysrhythmias
- Shock
- Kussmaul's respirations (deep, rapid respirations that develop in an attempt to eliminate excess acid by exhaling more carbon dioxide)

TABLE 6-3	Normal Serum Arterial Blood Gas Values*	
Blood Gas	**Normal Range**
pH	7.35–7.45
PaO_2	95–100 mm Hg
$PaCO_2$	35–45 mm Hg
Bicarbonate (HCO_3)	22–26 mEq/L
Base excess	–2.4 to +2.5 mEq/L
Arterial O_2 saturation	96–98%

*Values may vary slightly. PaO_2 = partial pressure of oxygen; $PaCO_2$ = partial pressure of carbon dioxide.

- Hyperkalemia (increased serum hydrogen levels cause potassium to shift out of the cells; lack of insulin in diabetic ketoacidosis impairs the transportation of potassium in the cell)

Learning Points

Compensation can be a challenge to understand. First, make sure you understand what the acids and bases are. Carbon dioxide and hydrogen are acids; bicarbonate is a base. The body will increase or decrease the excretion of these substances in an attempt to restore pH balance. If the body excretes more acid or produces more base, then the pH will become more alkaline. If the body retains more acid or produces less base, then the pH will become more acidic.

Two body systems can compensate for pH imbalances—the renal and respiratory systems. If the cause of the imbalance originates within one of those systems, then the other system will have to perform the role of the primary compensatory mechanism. The system that is the source of the pH imbalance will not be able to resolve its own problem. Thus, if the problem originates in the lungs, the kidneys will manage it. If the problem originates outside the lungs, the lungs will manage it.

Diagnostic procedures for metabolic acidosis include a history, physical examination, ABGs, blood chemistry, and CBC. Evaluation of the **anion gap** from the arterial blood gas results can be helpful in determining the cause of metabolic acidosis (**FIGURE 6-11**). The anion gap is used to identify the anions that are not measured. Conditions that cause metabolic acidosis because of excess acid will increase the anion gap; otherwise, the anion gap will remain normal. Under normal conditions, the sum of cations is approximately equal to the sum of anions in the extracellular fluid. Sodium is the most plentiful cation in the extracellular fluid, while bicarbonate and chloride are the most abundant anions. To determine the anion gap, the bicarbonate and chloride results are added together and subtracted from the sodium (sodium – [bicarbonate + chloride]). A normal anion gap is 6–9 mEq/L.

Identifying and treating the causative condition (e.g., antidiarrheal agents or dialysis) is vital to achieve successful patient outcomes. Treatment to correct the acidosis merely stabilizes the patient until the causative condition can be managed. Strategies to correct the acidosis include the following measures:

- Administering intravenous bicarbonate
- Correcting electrolyte disturbances such as hyperkalemia

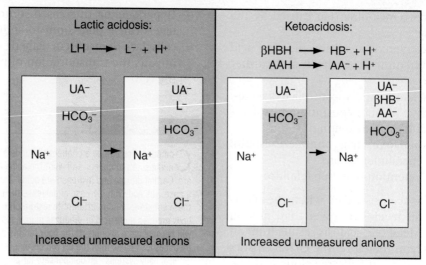

FIGURE 6-11 Anion gap with metabolic acidosis.

- Improving oxygenation (e.g., oxygen therapy and mechanical ventilation)
- Administering insulin (probably intravenous) to treat diabetic ketoacidosis

Metabolic Alkalosis

Metabolic alkalosis results from excess bicarbonate or deficient acid, or both (Table 6-2). These conditions cause the pH to rise above 7.45. Causes of metabolic alkalosis include the following:

- Excess bicarbonate, such as that caused by the following:
  - Excessive antacid use
  - Use of bicarbonate-containing fluids (e.g., lactated Ringer's solution)
  - Hypochloremia (increases bicarbonate reabsorption)
- Deficient acid, such as that caused by the following:
  - Gastrointestinal loss (e.g., vomiting or nasogastric suction)
  - Hypokalemia (low potassium levels cause hydrogen to shift inside the cells)
  - Renal loss (e.g., renal failure or diuretics)
  - Hypovolemia (decreases renal perfusion)
  - Hyperaldosteronism (excessive aldosterone increases renal excretion of hydrogen)

Metabolic alkalosis exists when the bicarbonate and the pH levels rise to greater than normal (Table 6-3). Much like metabolic acidosis, metabolic alkalosis manifestations generally occur in combination with the manifestations of the causative conditions (e.g., hypovolemia).

Clinical manifestations of metabolic alkalosis are mostly neurologic in nature but may also involve the respiratory and cardiac systems:

- Mental confusion
- Hyperactive reflexes
- Paresthesia
- Tetany
- Seizures
- Respiratory depression (respirations will decrease in an attempt to hold in more carbon dioxide)
- Dysrhythmias
- Coma

Diagnostic procedures for metabolic alkalosis include a history, physical examination, ABGs, blood chemistry, and CBC. Identifying and treating the causative condition (e.g., antiemetics or cessation of antacid use) is vital to achieve successful patient outcomes. Treatment to correct the alkalosis merely stabilizes the patient until the causative condition can be managed. Strategies to correct the alkalosis include the following measures:

- Adequate hydration, likely including intravenous fluids
- Correcting electrolyte disturbances such as hypokalemia and hypochloremia
- Cautious administration of Diamox (acetazolamide) (which increases bicarbonate excretion, but may increase potassium excretion as well)
- Administering arginine hydrochloride (which increases chloride levels)
- Administering a weak hydrochloric acid solution

Respiratory Acidosis

Respiratory acidosis results from carbon dioxide retention, which increases the amount of carbonic acid present and, in turn, decreases the pH level (Table 6-2). This increase in carbon dioxide usually follows a state of hypoventilation or decreased gas exchange in the lungs. Many conditions can cause hypoventilation and/or impair gas exchange:

- Acute asthma exacerbations
- Chronic obstructive pulmonary disease (emphysema and chronic bronchitis)
- Airway obstructions
- Pulmonary edema
- Pneumonia
- Drug overdose
- Respiratory failure
- Central nervous system depression

Respiratory acidosis exists when the carbon dioxide levels rise and the pH levels fall below normal (Table 6-3). Manifestations generally occur in combination with the manifestations of the causative condition (e.g., asthma). Carbon dioxide easily diffuses across the blood–brain barrier, causing the neurologic manifestations. Additionally, respiratory acidosis can affect the cardiac system. Clinical manifestations of respiratory acidosis include the following signs and symptoms:

- Headache
- Blurred vision
- Tremors
- Muscle twitching
- Vertigo (an illusion of motion)
- Irritability
- Disorientation
- Lethargy
- Coma
- Tachycardia leading to bradycardia
- Blood pressure fluctuations
- Diaphoresis

Diagnostic procedures for respiratory acidosis include a history, physical examination, ABGs, blood chemistry, CBC, and chest X-ray. Treatment centers on improving respiratory status by relieving hypoxia and hypercapnia. Strategies may include the following measures:

- Oxygen therapy
- Mechanical ventilation
- Positioning the patient for optimal ventilation (high Fowler's position)
- Bronchial hygiene measures (e.g., coughing, deep breathing, and chest physiotherapy)
- Bronchodilators
- Treatment of causative conditions (e.g., antibiotics for pneumonia)

Respiratory Alkalosis

Respiratory alkalosis results from excess exhalation of carbon dioxide, which in turn leads to carbonic acid deficits and increased pH (Table 6-2). Respiratory alkalosis generally occurs because of conditions that cause hyperventilation:

- Acute anxiety
- Pain
- Fever (which causes excessive oxygen utilization, increasing respirations)
- Hypoxia (e.g., oxygen deprivation and high altitudes)
- Gram-negative septicemia (which triggers the respiratory centers in the brain to increase respirations)
- Aspirin overdose (also triggers the medulla to increase respirations)
- Excessive mechanical ventilation
- Hypermetabolic states such as hyperthyroidism (which causes excessive oxygen utilization, increasing respirations)

Respiratory alkalosis exists when the carbon dioxide levels fall and the pH levels rise above normal (Table 6-3). Clinical manifestations reflect central nervous system irritability. Manifestations of hypercalcemia may be present secondary to calcium binding to protein. Clinical manifestations of respiratory alkalosis include the following signs and symptoms:

- Paresthesia
- Dizziness
- Vertigo (an illusion of motion)
- Syncope
- Muscle irritability and twitching
- Tetany
- Inability to concentrate
- Seizures
- Tachycardia
- Dysrhythmias
- Dry mouth
- Anxiety
- Excessive diaphoresis
- Coma

Diagnostic procedures for respiratory alkalosis include a history, physical examination, ABGs, blood chemistry, CBC, and chest X-ray. Treatment of the underlying cause and increasing carbon dioxide levels is crucial to improve patient outcomes. Often the solution is as simple

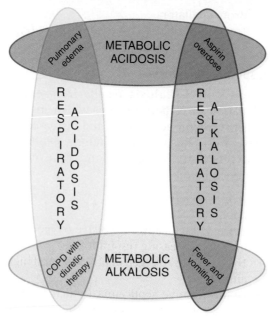

FIGURE 6-12 Mixed acid–base disorders.

as breathing into a paper bag—an intervention that allows carbon dioxide to be recirculated back to the lungs. Strategies that are more aggressive may be needed if the patient is unable to follow directions or is unconscious. They may include controlled mechanical ventilation and anxiety reduction interventions (e.g., sedatives and therapeutic communication).

Mixed Disorders

Mixed disorders occur when respiratory and metabolic disorders result in an acidotic or alkalotic state. Such an outcome occurs when both the respiratory and renal systems demonstrate an imbalance of acid or base. The severity of the pH imbalance depends on the degree of acid and base disturbances. Many conditions can create this synergistic effect (**FIGURE 6-12**). Such mixed disorders can make the patient critically ill, and can be complex to manage.

Arterial Blood Gas Interpretation

Arterial blood gases (ABGs) have traditionally been, and remain today, the principal diagnostic tool for evaluating acid–base balance (Table 6-2). ABG interpretation has mystified many nursing students and nurses since the invention of this measurement. Through simple steps, the ABG riddle can be solved, and the patient can receive appropriate care. First, descriptions of the results found on an ABG are in order, some of which have already been discussed:

- The pH measures the hydrogen concentration in the plasma.
- $PaCO_2$ (the partial pressure of carbon dioxide) indicates the adequacy of pulmonary ventilation.
- HCO_3 (bicarbonate) indicates the activity in the kidneys to retain or excrete bicarbonate.
- PaO_2 (the partial pressure of oxygen) indicates the concentration of oxygen in the blood.
- Base excess/deficit indicates the concentration of buffer—in particular, bicarbonate. Positive values indicate an excess of base or a deficit of acid. Negative values indicate a deficit of base or an excess of acid.

When interpreting an ABG result, focus on the pH, $PaCO_2$, and HCO_3. Interpreting ABGs involves looking for patterns and understanding what those patterns indicate, keeping in mind the patient's total clinical picture. Recall that $PaCO_2$ is an acid and HCO_3 is a base. More acid will lower the pH, whereas less acid will raise the pH. More base will raise the pH, whereas less base will lower the pH.

Now turning to the ABG results, use a systematic approach when examining it (**TABLE 6-4**). Make note of the patient's pH, $PaCO_2$, and HCO_3 on a piece of paper. Start by examining the pH. Is it high, low, or normal? This is half of the

TABLE 6-4	Arterial Blood Gas Interpretation			
Acid–Base Disorder	pH	$PaCO_2$	HCO_3	Compensation
Respiratory acidosis	< 7.4 (A)	> 45 mm Hg (A)	Normal	HCO_3 > 26 mEq/L (B)
Respiratory alkalosis	> 7.4 (B)	< 35 mm Hg (B)	Normal	HCO_3 < 22 mEq/L (A)
Metabolic acidosis	< 7.4 (A)	Normal	< 22 mEq/L (A)	$PaCO_2$ < 35 mm Hg (B)
Metabolic alkalosis	> 7.4 (B)	Normal	> 26 mEq/L (B)	$PaCO_2$ > 45 mm Hg (A)

puzzle. The pH will identify whether the condition is acidosis or alkalosis. If it is high, write a *B* for "basic" beside it. If the pH is low, write an *A* for "acidic." If it is normal, which side of normal is it? For results less than 7.4, write an *A*; for results greater than 7.4, write a *B*.

Next, check the $PaCO_2$. Is it high, low, or normal? In respiratory disturbances, pH and CO_2 move in opposite directions. If the CO_2 goes up, the pH goes down, and vice versa. Because CO_2 is an acidic influence, write an *A* if it is high and a *B* if it is low. If it is within normal range, write an *N* beside it.

Next, examine the HCO_3. Is it high, low, or normal? With metabolic disturbances, the pH and HCO_3 move in the same direction. Because HCO_3 is a base influence, write a *B* if it is high and an *A* if it is low. If it is within normal range, write an *N* beside it.

At this point, you should have three letters written down beside your patient ABG results. Now you just match up the *A*s and *B*s you have written down. Finally, determine if the body has been able to compensate. The results with the paired *A* or *B* is the primary change. The third unpaired result indicates the compensation. If the unpaired result is still normal, then it is **uncompensated**. If the unpaired result has changed to the opposite letter of the pairs and the pH is still abnormal, then it is **partially compensated**; if the pH has returned to normal, then it is **fully compensated**.

To review, these are the steps in ABGs interpretation:

1. Is the pH high, low, or normal?
   a. If pH > 7.4, write a *B* beside it for basic.
   b. If pH < 7.4, write an *A* beside it for acidic.
   c. Make note if pH is within normal limits (7.35–7.45).
2. Is the $PaCO_2$ high, low, or normal?
   a. If $PaCO_2$ is between 35 and 45 mm Hg, write an *N* beside it for normal.
   b. If $PaCO_2$ > 45 mm Hg, write an *A* beside it for acidic.
   c. If $PaCO_2$ < 35 mm Hg, write a *B* beside it for basic.
3. Is the HCO_3 high, low, or normal?
   a. If HCO_3 is between 22 and 26, write an *N* beside it for normal.
   b. If HCO_3 > 26 mEq/L, write a *B* beside it for basic.
   c. If HCO_3 < 22 mEq/L, write an *A* beside it for acidic.

4. Look for patterns:
   a. Two *A*s indicate acidosis. If one of the *A*s is CO_2, then the disorder is respiratory. If one of the *A*s is HCO_3, then the disorder is metabolic. In both cases, the other *A* is the pH.
   b. Two *B*s indicate alkalosis. If one of the *B*s is CO_2, then the disorder is respiratory. If one of the *B*s is HCO_3, then the disorder is metabolic. In both cases, the other *B* is the pH.
   c. Three *A*s or *B*s indicate a mixed disorder. All *A*s indicate mixed respiratory and metabolic acidosis. All *B*s indicate mixed respiratory and metabolic alkalosis.
5. Determine compensation:
   a. If the unpaired result is within normal range, then the disturbance is uncompensated.
   b. If the unpaired result is the opposite letter of the pairs but the pH is still abnormal, then the disturbance is partially compensated.
   c. If the unpaired result is the opposite letter and the pH has returned to normal range, then the disturbance is fully compensated.

Practice Arterial Blood Gas Interpretation

Practice 1

pH:	7.32	**A**
$PaCO_2$:	37 mm Hg	**N**ormal
HCO_3:	14 mEq/L	**A**

Practice 2

pH:	7.50	**B**
$PaCO_2$:	30 mm Hg	**B**
HCO_3:	24 mEq/L	**N**ormal

Practice 3

pH:	7.33	**A**
$PaCO_2$:	55 mm Hg	**A**
HCO_3:	28 mEq/L	**B**

Practice 4

pH:	7.47	**B**
$PaCO_2$:	48 mm Hg	**A**
HCO_3:	29 mEq/L	**B**

Practice 5

pH:	7.38	**A** (but within normal limits)
PaCo$_2$:	48 mm Hg	**A**
HCO$_3$:	29 mEq/L	**B**

Practice 6

pH:	7.44	**B** (but within normal limits)
PaCo$_2$:	49 mm Hg	**A**
HCO$_3$:	29 mEq/L	**B**

Practice 7

pH:	7.30	**A**
PaCo$_2$:	50 mm Hg	**A**
HCO$_3$:	19 mEq/L	**A**

Practice 8

pH:	7.49	**B**
PaCo$_2$:	32 mm Hg	**B**
HCO$_3$:	30 mEq/L	**B**

application to practice

Now that we have learned about fluid, electrolyte, and acid–base imbalances, let's put this knowledge into practice. After receiving reports on the following patients, which patient should you go see first?

- A 76-year-old female admitted 3 days ago with pneumonia; her most recent blood gases are pH 7.35, PaO$_2$ 90, HCO$_3$ 35, and PaCO$_2$ 29
- A 48-year-old male admitted yesterday with kidney stones, who complains of pain that is a 5 on a 0–10 scale
- A 52-year-old female admitted yesterday with acute renal failure; her most recent lab results are pH 7.3, PaO$_2$ 94, HCO$_3$ 15, PaCO$_2$ 44, K 6.1, Na 148, and osmo 369

- A 59-year-old male admitted 2 days ago with Stage III bronchiogenic carcinoma, who complains of nausea and pain that is a 6 on a 0–10 scale

Once again, you go through the usual thought process—who would die first, acute versus chronic conditions, Maslow's hierarchy of needs, and patient safety. Let's start with the 76-year-old female. If you analyze the arterial blood gases, you will find that these results are normal. This patient is relatively stable and probably can wait. Moving on to the 48-year-old male, he is in moderate pain and may need pain medicine, but nothing indicates anything life threatening is going on. Now consider the 52-year-old female

admitted with renal failure. When you analyze her arterial blood gases, you find that she is experiencing uncompensated metabolic acidosis. Also note that this patient's potassium is elevated. Given that both of these conditions can be life threatening, keep this patient on your short list. Finally, the 59-year-old male is experiencing a life-threatening cancer and is in pain, so this patient warrants being on the short list.

After considering all these patients, the two patients on your short list are experiencing life-threatening conditions. You should see the 52-year-old female with uncompensated metabolic acidosis first, because she is more acute than the 59-year-old male with lung cancer.

CHAPTER SUMMARY

Fluid, electrolytes, bases, and acids are constantly moving among body compartments. This movement is influenced by intake, output, cellular metabolism, and pathologic states. The body is equipped with numerous mechanisms to maintain fluid, electrolyte, and pH homeostasis among these compartments. When these mechanisms fail, conditions that threaten the individual's well-being arise. Early identification and action are crucial to improve the prognosis of the person encountering these conditions, and nurses play a pivotal role in managing this patient's plan of care.

REFERENCES

Baumberger-Henry, M. (2008). *Fluid and electrolytes* (2nd ed.). Sudbury, MA: Jones and Bartlett.

Chiras, D. (2011). *Human biology* (7th ed.). Burlington, MA: Jones & Bartlett Learning.

Chiras, R. K. (2008). *Anatomy and physiology: Understanding the human body*. Sudbury, MA: Jones and Bartlett.

Elling, B., Elling, K., & Rothenberg, M. (2004). *Anatomy and physiology*. Sudbury, MA: Jones and Bartlett.

Gould, B. (2015). *Pathophysiology for the health professions* (5th ed.). Philadelphia, PA: Elsevier.

Madara, B., & Pomarico-Denino, V. (2008). *Pathophysiology* (2nd ed.). Sudbury, MA: Jones and Bartlett.

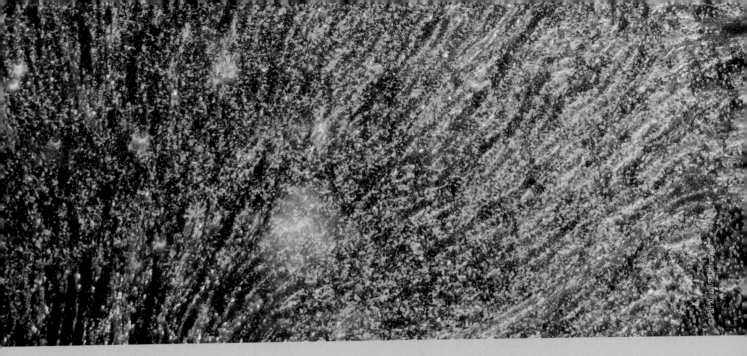

CHAPTER 7
Urinary Function

LEARNING OBJECTIVES

- Discuss normal urinary anatomy and physiology.
- Describe and compare renal alterations that alter urinary elimination.
- Describe and compare renal alterations that result in impaired renal function.

KEY TERMS

acute renal failure (ARF)
afferent arteriole
ammonia
anasarca
azotemia
benign prostatic hyperplasia (BPH)
bladder
bladder cancer
Bowman's capsule
calyx
chronic kidney disease (CKD)
chronic overdistension
cystitis
deamination
detrusor hyperreflexia

efferent arteriole
enuresis
erythropoietin
functional incontinence
glomerular filtration rate (GFR)
glomerulonephritis
glomerulus
gross total incontinence
hydronephrosis
intrarenal condition
micturition
mixed incontinence
nephritic syndrome
nephrolithiasis
nephron

nephrotic syndrome
neurogenic bladder
nocturnal enuresis
overactive bladder
overflow incontinence
polycystic kidney disease (PKD)
postrenal condition
prerenal condition
pyelonephritis
reflex incontinence
renal artery
renal capsule
renal cell carcinoma
renal cortex
renal hilum

renal pelvis
renal sinus
renin–angiotensin–aldosterone
retention
stress incontinence
transient incontinence
urea
uremia
ureter
urethra
urge incontinence
uric acid
urinary incontinence
urinary tract infection (UTI)
urination
Wilms' tumor

The urinary system plays a pivotal role in homeostasis. Structures of the urinary system include the kidneys, ureters, bladder, and urethra (FIGURE 7-1). This system regulates fluid volume, blood pressure, metabolic waste and drug excretion, vitamin D conversion, pH regulation, and hormone synthesis. This chapter focuses on normal and abnormal states of the urinary system. Disorders of this system can create imbalances in homeostasis quickly. Hence, these disorders require a prompt response to restore the body's delicate balance.

Anatomy and Physiology

The urinary system regulates fluid volume (see the *Fluid, Electrolyte, and Acid–Base Homeostasis* chapter), blood pressure (see the *Cardiovascular Function* chapter), metabolic waste and drug excretion, vitamin D conversion, pH balance (see the *Fluid, Electrolyte, and Acid–Base*

Homeostasis chapter), and hormone synthesis. It includes the kidneys, ureters, bladder, and urethra (**TABLE 7-1**).

The kidneys are bean-shaped organs about the size of a person's fists; they are positioned on either side of the vertebrae in retroperitoneal space. Connective tissue called the **renal capsule** surrounds the kidney. The area immediately beneath the capsule is known as the **renal cortex**; it contains the functional units of the kidney, the nephrons. The **renal artery** supplies each kidney with blood. The **renal hilum** is the opening in the kidney through which the renal artery and nerves enter and the renal vein and ureter exit. The hilum opens medially into a cavity called the **renal sinus**. The central portions of the renal sinuses enlarge to form the **renal pelvis**. Urine drains in a manner similarly to a funnel into the renal pelvis through tubes called **calyces**. The calyces drain urine into the **ureters**, which transport the urine using peristaltic actions to the **bladder**

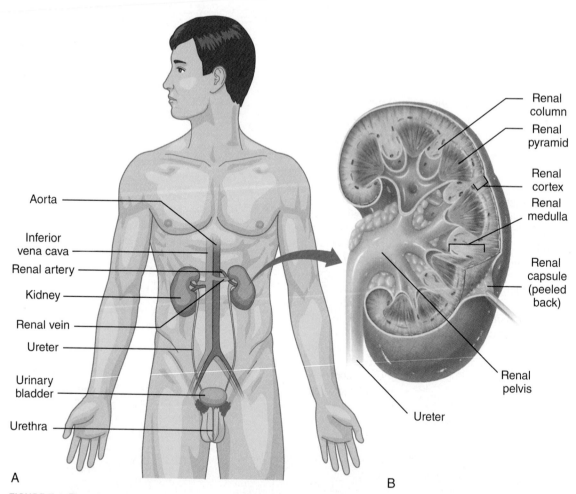

Aorta

Inferior vena cava

Renal artery

Kidney

Renal vein

Ureter

Urinary bladder

Urethra

A

Renal column

Renal pyramid

Renal cortex

Renal medulla

Renal capsule (peeled back)

Renal pelvis

Ureter

B

FIGURE 7-1 The urinary system. (a) Anterior view showing the relationship of the kidneys, ureters, urinary bladder, and urethra. (b) A cross section of the human kidney showing the cortex, medulla, and renal pelvis.

TABLE 7-1	Components of the Urinary System and Their Functions

Component	Function
Kidneys	Eliminate wastes from the blood; help regulate body water concentration; help regulate blood pressure; help maintain a constant blood pH
Ureters	Transport urine to the urinary bladder
Urinary bladder	Stores urine; contracts to eliminate stored urine
Urethra	Transports urine to the outside of the body

for storage. The muscular bladder serves as a reservoir for urine until it can be excreted. As the volume of urine in the bladder increases, the urine exerts pressure on the two bladder sphincters (internal and external) and stretch receptors in the bladder. A pressure of 200 to 300 mL on the sphincters and receptors sends nerve impulses to the brain, triggering the urge to urinate (FIGURE 7-2). **Urination**, or **micturition**, is a voluntary act; when urination is initiated, the bladder contracts and the external sphincter relaxes, forcing urine out through the **urethra**. The urethra is approximately 1.5 inches long in women and 6–8 inches long in men. The shorter urethra in women, in combination with use of a sitting position for urination, increases women's risk for developing urinary tract infections.

The kidneys are the primary site for carrying out the urinary system's functions. One kidney contains 1–2 million microscopic filtering units, or **nephrons**, to accomplish its functions (FIGURE 7-3). Each nephron is similar to a funnel with a long stem. It contains multiple sections (e.g., loop of Henle, proximal convoluted tubule, and distal convoluted tubule), and each of these sections is responsible for excreting or reabsorbing specific substances (**TABLE 7-2**). The proximal convoluted tubule of the kidney enlarges into a double-membrane chamber called **Bowman's capsule**. Bowman's capsule surrounds a cluster of capillaries referred to as the **glomerulus**. Blood enters the glomerulus

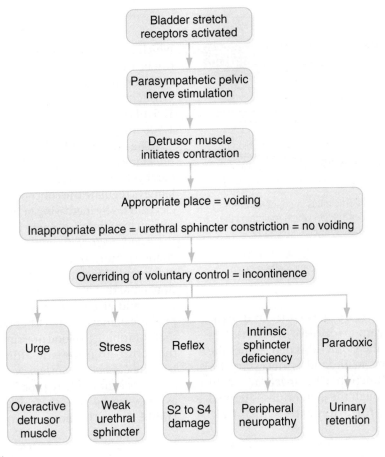

FIGURE 7-2 Urination.

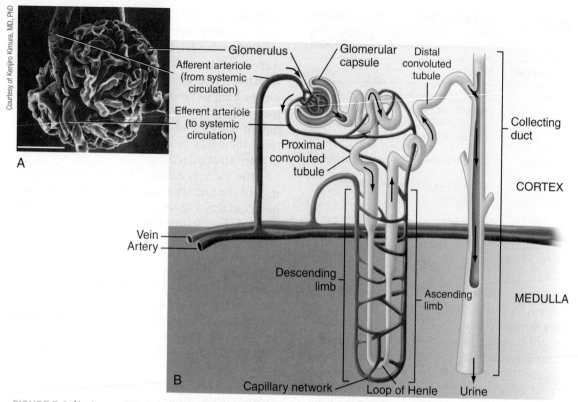

Courtesy of Kenjiro Kimura, MD, PhD

FIGURE 7-3 Nephrons of the kidney. Part of the nephron is located in the cortex, and part is located in the medulla. The electron micrograph to the left of the illustration is of a glomerulus from a human nephron.

TABLE 7-2	Components of the Nephron and Their Functions

Component	Function
Glomerulus	Mechanically filters the blood
Bowman's capsule	Mechanically filters the blood
Proximal convoluted tubule	Reabsorbs 75% of the water, salts, glucose, and amino acids
Loop of Henle	Participates in countercurrent exchange, which maintains the concentration gradient
Distal convoluted tubule	Site of tubular secretion of H^+, potassium, and certain drugs

through an **afferent arteriole** and exits through an **efferent arteriole** (**FIGURE 7-4**). This blood supply to the glomerulus determines the amount of urine made and is necessary for healthy renal function. The speed at which blood moves through the glomerulus is termed the **glomerular filtration rate (GFR)**. GFR,

which is the best measure of renal functioning, can be calculated using a formula that incorporates serum creatinine levels, age, gender, and ethnicity. Usually, GFR is approximately 125 mL/min, and urine output is approximately 1,500 mL/day.

The human body can excrete waste through the kidneys, skin, liver, and intestines, with the kidneys being the primary site for excretion. The kidneys regulate the concentration of water and electrolytes by increasing or decreasing their excretion to maintain stability within the body (see the *Fluid, Electrolyte, and Acid–Base Homeostasis* chapter). Hormones, such as antidiuretic hormone and aldosterone, alter this rate of excretion (**FIGURE 7-5**). In part, this mechanism of water and electrolyte regulation aids in blood pressure management. Other renal mechanisms that contribute to blood pressure control include the **renin–angiotensin–aldosterone** system (see the *Cardiovascular Function* chapter).

Cells continuously produce waste products as they carry out their internal processes (**TABLE 7-3**). The body removes these waste

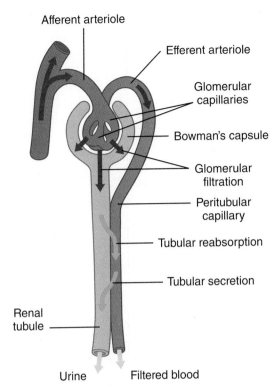

Afferent arteriole

Efferent arteriole

Glomerular capillaries

Bowman's capsule

Glomerular filtration

Peritubular capillary

Tubular reabsorption

Tubular secretion

Renal tubule

Urine   Filtered blood

FIGURE 7-4 The glomerulus of the kidneys. The nephron carries out three processes: glomerular filtration, tubular reabsorption, and tubular secretion. All three processes contribute to the filtering of the blood.

products to maintain homeostasis through urine formation. The three most significant metabolic wastes that the kidneys manage are ammonia, urea, and uric acid.

- **Ammonia**, a highly toxic chemical, results from the breakdown of amino acids in the liver. Amino acid breakdown generally occurs in the presence of an excess of protein or a deficit of carbohydrates in the diet; however, carbohydrate deficits are rare in industrialized countries except in persons on high-protein diets.
- When amino acids are broken down, the amino groups are stripped from the molecules in a process called **deamination**. These amino groups are converted to ammonia following deamination. Most of this ammonia is then converted to **urea** in the liver. Liver disease can impair this process, leading to extremely high levels of ammonia (see the *Gastrointestinal Function* chapter).
- **Uric acid** is another metabolism by-product produced by the liver. Uric acid results from the breakdown of nucleotides, the building

blocks of deoxyribonucleic acid (DNA). Excess uric acid levels can lead to gout, which results in uric acid crystal deposits in the joints (see the *Musculoskeletal Function* chapter).

Along with these waste products, other substances normally found in urine include sodium, potassium, and small amounts of protein and bacteria. Urine should be pale yellow and clear. Additional substances and changes in color or clarity can indicate renal pathology (**TABLE 7-4**). Multiple diagnostic tests can be performed to determine whether the kidneys are functioning properly.

The kidneys are also responsible for converting vitamin D into its active form. The inactive form of vitamin D is produced by the action of ultraviolet rays on cholesterol in the skin or is ingested. The active form created by conversion of vitamin D aids in calcium and phosphorus absorption. People with renal disease will have issues converting vitamin D into its active form.

Additionally, the kidneys regulate pH by secreting bicarbonate and excreting hydrogen (see the *Fluid, Electrolyte, and Acid–Base Homeostasis* chapter). They synthesize several hormones, including atrial natriuretic peptide (see the *Fluid, Electrolyte, and Acid–Base Homeostasis* chapter), erythropoietin, and renin (see the *Cardiovascular Function* chapter). The kidneys release **erythropoietin** in a response to hypoxia (e.g., anemia or cardiac or pulmonary disease); erythropoietin stimulates the bone marrow to produce more red blood cells. If iron stores are adequate, an increase in red blood cells increases the body's overall oxygen-carrying capacity, thus decreasing hypoxia.

With aging, the kidneys begin functioning less efficiently. This decreased functioning can be further exacerbated by the presence of chronic conditions (e.g., diabetes mellitus, hypertension, and arteriosclerosis). As a consequence, the aging individual may experience less filtration capability, leading to waste accumulation and loss of homeostatic regulation (e.g., fluid, electrolyte, and pH balance). Additionally, renal-related complications are common with these aging changes (e.g., anemia, hypertension, and osteoporosis). Aging persons may require alternative medication dosing (usually a smaller dose or doses spaced further apart) to prevent drug toxicity because of this impaired filtration.

ADH LEVEL	EFFECT ON KIDNEY
Increased ADH levels	Collecting ducts and the distal convoluted tubules become permeable to water; water moves out of ducts and into blood 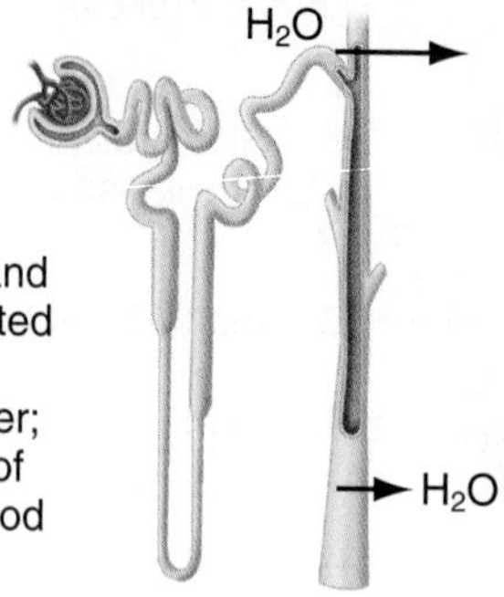 H_2O H_2O
Decreased ADH levels	Collecting ducts become impermeable to water; water is not reabsorbed from the filtrate and is excreted 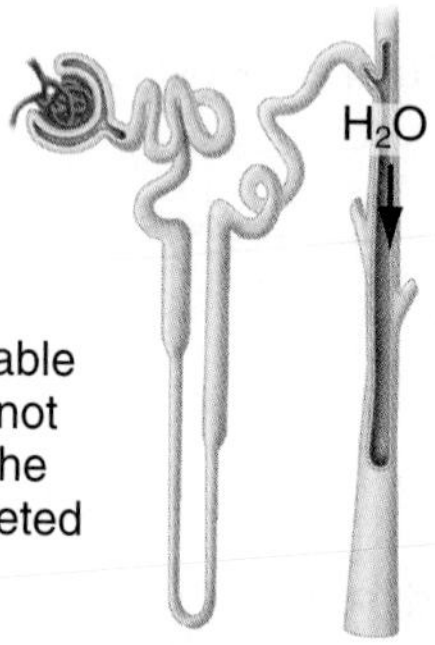 H_2O

ALDOSTERONE LEVEL	EFFECT ON KIDNEY
Increased aldosterone levels	Tubules increase reabsorption of sodium from the filtrate and decrease reabsorption of potassium; water and sodium thus move from filtrate into the blood, and excess potassium is excreted 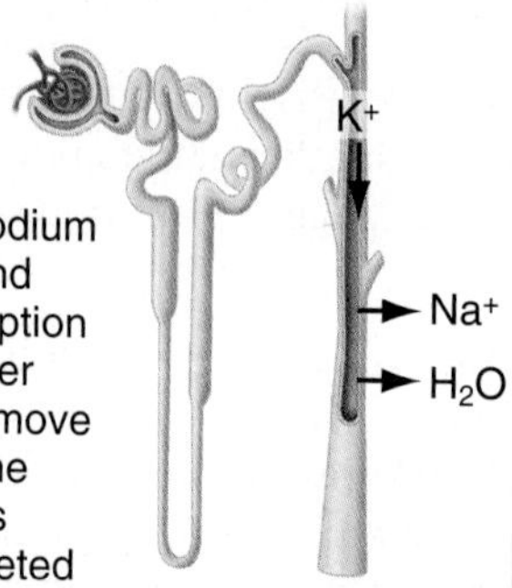 K^+ Na^+ H_2O
Decreased aldosterone levels	Tubular absorption of sodium and potassium is normal; water is not reabsorbed from the filtrate and is excreted 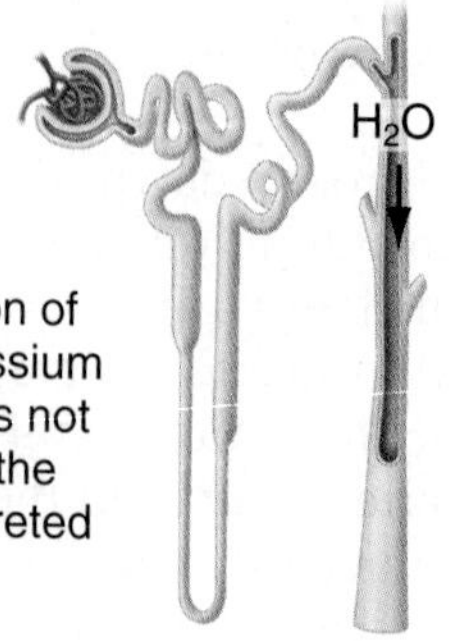 H_2O

FIGURE 7-5 Effects of antidiuretic hormone and aldosterone on the kidneys.

TABLE 7-3	Important Metabolic Wastes and Substances Excreted from the Body	

Chemical	Source	Organ of Excretion
Ammonia	Deamination (removal of amine group) of amino acids in liver	Kidneys
Urea	Derived from ammonia	Kidneys and skin
Uric acid	Nucleotide breakdown in liver	Kidneys
Bile pigments	Hemoglobin breakdown in liver	Liver (into small intestine)
Urochrome	Hemoglobin breakdown in liver	Kidneys
Carbon dioxide	Breakdown of glucose in cells	Lungs
Water	Food and water; breakdown of glucose	Kidneys, skin, and lungs
Inorganic ions*	Food and water	Kidneys and sweat glands

* Ions are not a metabolic waste product like the other substances shown in this table. Nonetheless, ions are excreted to maintain constant levels in the body.

TABLE 7-4	Renal Function Tests

Test	Related Physiology
BUN (blood urea nitrogen)	The end product of protein metabolism is urea, which is excreted entirely by the kidneys; therefore, BUN is an indication of liver and kidney function.
Serum creatinine	Creatinine forms when creatinine phosphate is used in skeletal muscle contractions. Because it is entirely excreted by the kidneys, the serum creatinine level is an indication of renal function. The creatinine level is not affected by hepatic function, so it is a more precise indication of renal function than is BUN. A 50% reduction in glomerular filtration rate (GFR) doubles the creatinine level.
24-hour urine collection for creatinine clearance	Measures GFR and is dependent upon renal artery perfusion and glomerular filtration (GF).
Urinalysis	Cloudy, foul-smelling, white blood cells (WBCs) = urinary tract infection (UTI). Dark yellow = dehydration. Acetone odor = diabetic ketoacidosis. Presence of protein = injured glomerular membrane. Glucose = diabetes mellitus. Ketones = fatty acid metabolism. Crystals = possible renal stone formation. Many hyaline casts = proteinuria. Cellular casts = nephrotic syndrome.
Intravenous pyelogram (IVP)	IV-administered, radiopaque dye allows the visualization of the kidneys, renal pelvis, ureters, and bladder.
PSA (prostatic-specific antigen)	PSA is a glycoprotein found in all prostatic epithelial cells. An increase may be indicative of prostatic enlargement; thus this test is used to screen for prostatic cancer and as an indicator of treatment success/failure.

UNDERSTANDING CONDITIONS THAT AFFECT THE URINARY SYSTEM

When considering alterations in the urinary system, organize them based on their basic underlying pathophysiology to increase understanding. Those pathophysiological concepts include those conditions that alter urinary elimination and impair renal function. Conditions that alter urination may include structural barriers (e.g., nephrolithiasis, congenital disorders, and tumors) or problems with the act of urination (e.g., incontinence). These conditions require interventions to promote urination (e.g., catheterization, bladder training, or surgery). Conditions that impair renal function include those disorders that prevent the kidneys from regulating fluid and electrolytes as well as excreting waste products and other substances. These conditions require interventions to maintain homeostasis (e.g., dialysis).

Conditions Resulting in Altered Urinary Elimination

The act of urination requires (1) a functioning bladder with stretch receptors that can sense the filling of the bladder with urine, (2) an intact parasympathetic pelvic nerve to transmit the signal, and (3) working detrusor muscles to initiate bladder contractions to expel the urine (Figure 7-2). The sympathetic nerve innervations to the detrusor muscle and internal sphincter prevent inappropriate stimulation of urination. Upper motor impulses can delay voiding by tightening the urethral sphincter. Although urination is mostly a voluntary act, voiding can be delayed only to a certain point. If the urge to void is ignored too long, bladder contractions take over the neural delaying mechanism and involuntary urination occurs.

Incontinence

Urination is a reflex in very young children, but it is controlled consciously in older children and adults. In children up to 3 years of age, urination is completely reflexive: Once the bladder expands, it empties. As children grow older, they learn to control urination. In older children and adults, the external sphincter is under conscious control—it will not relax until deliberately allowed to do so.

Older children and adults sometimes lose control over urination, resulting in a condition referred to as **urinary incontinence** (Figure 7-2). Urinary incontinence is a common and often embarrassing problem that has many causes. The types of incontinence and their causes are profiled here (**FIGURE 7-6**):

- **Enuresis** is the involuntary urination by a child after 4–5 years of age, when bladder control is expected. Most children have **nocturnal enuresis**, or bed-wetting, only. Enuresis can have psychological (e.g., anxiety) and structural (e.g., smaller than normal bladder) origins. Multiple strategies and treatments are available (e.g., motivation, support, alarm systems, and medications to concentrate urine at night), but usually the condition resolves in time with or without treatment.
- **Transient incontinence** refers to urinary incontinence resulting from a temporary condition. Such conditions include delirium, infection, atrophic vaginitis, use of certain medications (e.g., diuretics and sedatives), psychological factors (e.g., depression and anxiety), high urine output (e.g., overhydration), restricted mobility, fecal impaction, alcohol, and caffeine.

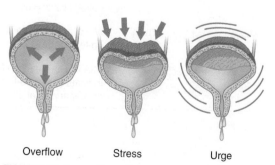

Overflow   Stress   Urge

FIGURE 7-6 Types of incontinence.

- **Stress incontinence** describes loss of urine from pressure (stress) exerted on the bladder by coughing, sneezing, laughing, exercising, or lifting something heavy. Stress incontinence occurs when the sphincter muscle of the bladder is weakened. In women, physical changes resulting from pregnancy, childbirth, and menopause can weaken the sphincter muscle. Additionally, women may develop a cystocele (bulging of the bladder through the vaginal wall; see the *Reproductive Function* chapter) because of these physical changes, which can also increase their risk for stress incontinence. In men, prostate removal can lead to this type of incontinence. Additional factors contributing to stress incontinence in both genders include obesity and chronic coughing. Obesity increases pressure on the bladder and surrounding muscles, weakening them. Chronic coughing (e.g., that caused by smoking and lung disease) can also increase stress on the urinary sphincter.

- **Urge incontinence** is a sudden, intense urge to urinate, followed by an involuntary loss of urine. The bladder muscle contracts and may give the individual only a few seconds' to a minute's warning before voiding. With urge incontinence, the need to urinate is felt often, including throughout the night. Urinary tract infections, bladder irritants, bowel conditions, smoking, Parkinson's disease, Alzheimer's disease, stroke, injury, and nervous system damage (e.g., that associated with multiple sclerosis) may all cause urge incontinence. **Overactive bladder** describes urge incontinence with no known cause.

- **Reflex incontinence** refers to urinary incontinence caused by trauma or damage to the nervous system (e.g., that caused by spinal cord injury above the second to fourth sacral vertebra, multiple sclerosis, and diabetes mellitus). **Detrusor hyperreflexia** is increased detrusor muscle contractility that occurs even though there is no sensation to void. With reflex incontinence, urgency is generally absent.

- **Overflow incontinence** is the result of an inability to empty the bladder, or **retention**. Other indications of overflow incontinence include dribbling urine and a weak urine stream. This type of incontinence may occur due to bladder damage, urethral blockage, nerve damage (e.g., that caused by diabetes mellitus), and prostate conditions. **Chronic overdistension**, also called nurse's bladder and teacher's bladder, occurs because of a perceived inability to interrupt work to void. This chronic avoidance of emptying the bladder results in detrusor muscle areflexia and overflow incontinence.

- **Mixed incontinence** occurs when symptoms of more than one type of urinary incontinence are experienced.

- **Functional incontinence** occurs in many older adults, especially people in nursing homes. In such a case, a physical or mental impairment prevents toileting in time. For example, a person with severe arthritis may not be able to undress quickly enough to prevent incontinence.

- **Gross total incontinence** refers to a continuous leaking of urine, day and night, or the periodic uncontrollable leaking of large volumes of urine. In these cases, the bladder has no storage capacity. This type of incontinence can occur because of anatomic defects, spinal cord or urinary system injuries, or a fistula (abnormal opening) between the bladder and an adjacent structure, such as the vagina.

Generally, risk factors for developing urinary incontinence include the following conditions:

- *Being female.* Women are more likely than men are to have stress incontinence. Pregnancy, childbirth, menopause, and normal female anatomy account for this difference. However, men with prostate conditions are at increased risk for urge and overflow incontinence.

- *Advancing age.* The muscles of the bladder and urethra lose some of their strength with age. Changes with age may also reduce bladder capacity and increase the risk of involuntary urination. However, incontinence is not inevitable with age, and incontinence is not normal at any age, except during infancy.

- *Being overweight.* Being obese or overweight increases the pressure on the bladder and surrounding muscles, weakening them and allowing urine to leak out under stress (e.g., stress caused by coughing or sneezing).

- *Smoking.* Chronic coughing associated with smoking can cause episodes of incontinence or aggravate incontinence that has other causes. Constant coughing puts stress on the urinary sphincter, leading to stress incontinence. Smokers are also at risk of developing overactive bladder.

- *Other diseases.* Renal disease or diabetes mellitus may increase the risk for incontinence because of changes in renal function and nerve innervations.

Urinary incontinence can lead to complications ranging from minor to severe in nature. Skin problems (e.g., rashes, skin infections, and ulcers) can result from the presence of constant moisture. Recurrent urinary tract infections can develop from incomplete emptying of the bladder. Additionally, urinary incontinence can negatively affect psychological health (e.g., it can cause poor self-image, embarrassment, sexual dysfunction, anxiety, and depression), and changes can occur in the individual's usual activities (e.g., work and exercise).

Diagnostic procedures for urinary incontinence include a history, physical examination, bladder diary, urinalysis, urine cultures, cystourethrogram (X-ray of the bladder and urethra), cystoscopy (visualization of the bladder with a small, lighted instrument), pelvic ultrasound, postvoid residual measurement, and urodynamic testing (which measures pressures in the bladder). Treatment for urinary incontinence depends on the type, underlying cause, and severity. Treatment and management strategies range from conservative to aggressive:

- Bladder training
- Scheduled toileting
- Fluid and diet management (e.g., avoiding alcohol, caffeine, or acidic foods; reducing liquid consumption; losing weight; or increasing physical activity)
- Pelvic floor muscle exercises (e.g., Kegel exercises)
- Electric stimulation (electrodes are temporarily inserted into the rectum or vagina to strengthen pelvic floor muscles through gentle electric stimulation)
- Medications (e.g., anticholinergics or estrogen replacement)
- Urethral inserts (small, tamponlike disposable devices or plugs inserted into the urethra)
- Pessary (a stiff ring inserted into the vagina to hold up the bladder)
- Radiofrequency therapy (a nonsurgical procedure that uses radiofrequency energy to heat tissue in the lower urinary tract, causing it to become firmer)
- Botulinum toxin type A (Botox) injections into the bladder muscle
- Bulking material injections (e.g., collagen, carbon-coated zirconium beads, Coaptite) into tissue surrounding the urethra
- Sacral nerve stimulator (an implanted device that emits painless electrical impulses that stimulate the sacral nerve)
- Artificial urinary sphincter (a fluid-filled ring implanted around the neck of the bladder that is controlled by a manual subcutaneous valve)
- Sling procedures (a surgically constructed pelvic sling or hammock around the bladder neck and urethra created by using strips of tissue, synthetic material, or mesh)
- Bladder neck suspension (a surgical procedure to raise and support the bladder in a more normal anatomic position)
- Absorbent pads and protective garments
- Urinary catheter (usually as an intermittent self-catheterization)
- Increased perineal hygiene
- Skin barrier creams
- Safety measures (e.g., move any rugs or furniture out of path to the restroom, adequate lighting, widening the bathroom doorway, and installing an elevated toilet seat)
- Acupuncture
- Hypnotherapy
- Herbal remedies (e.g., *Crataeva nurvala*, horsetail [*Equisetum*], aloe vera extract)
- Coping strategies and support

Neurogenic Bladder

Neurogenic bladder refers to all bladder dysfunction caused by an interruption of normal

---

Learning Points

Here is an easy acronym to remember the causes of acute urinary incontinence.

DRIPS

D = Delirium, dehydration, diapers

R = Retention, restricted mobility

I = Impaction, infection, inflammation

P = Pharmaceuticals (opiates and calcium antagonists cause urinary retention and constipation; anticholinergics cause retention; alpha-adrenergic antagonists cause reduced urethral resistance in women; diuretics increases urine production), psychologic problems (e.g., depression, neurosis, or anxiety)

S = Stool impaction (constipation) (Newman, 2010; Resnick & Yalla, 1998, p. 1045)

bladder nerve innervation. Many factors can disrupt bladder nerve innervations, including the following conditions:

- Brain or spinal cord injury
- Nervous system tumors
- Brain or spinal cord infections
- Dementia
- Parkinson's disease
- Spina bifida
- Diabetes mellitus
- Stroke
- Medications (e.g., antidepressants, antihistamines, analgesics, antihypertensives, and antiemetics)
- Vaginal childbirth
- Multiple sclerosis
- Chronic alcoholism
- Systemic lupus erythematosus
- Heavy metal poisoning
- Herpes zoster

Clinical manifestations of neurogenic bladder include symptoms of an overactive bladder (e.g., frequency and urgency) and an underactive bladder (e.g., hesitancy and retention). Diagnostic procedures for neurogenic bladder consist of a history, physical examination, bladder diary, urinalysis, urine cultures, cystourethrogram, cystoscopy, pelvic ultrasound, postvoid residual measurement, and urodynamic testing. Additionally, other procedures may be performed to determine the underlying cause (e.g., computed tomography [CT], magnetic resonance imaging [MRI]). Treatment strategies depend on the etiology and include those therapies previously discussed for incontinence.

Congenital Disorders

Abnormalities of the urinary and reproductive systems are the most common congenital defects (also see the *Reproductive Function* chapter). Because of these systems' close relationship, an abnormality in one system will often lead to an abnormality in the other. Numerous congenital disorders of the urinary system are possible, most of which are structural problems. Some defects cause no symptoms (e.g., both ureters draining one kidney and abnormal kidney positioning), whereas others are life threatening (e.g., renal agenesis [failure of an organ to develop in utero]). Problems with kidney development can be the most severe. The kidneys begin to develop in approximately the fifth week of gestation. Urine formation begins at 9 to 12 weeks' gestation. Urine is the main component of amniotic fluid, which is vital for normal fetal development.

Urinary Tract Infections

Urinary tract infections (UTIs) are extremely common and include any infections that begin in the urinary tract. According to the National Institutes of Health (NIH, 2012), UTIs are the second most frequently occurring infection. The lower urinary tract (bladder and urethra) is the most frequent site for the infection.

UTIs are caused by a direct invasion of the urinary tract by bacteria. Urine is an excellent medium for microorganism growth because of its protein content. Most bacteria that enter the urinary tract are quickly removed by the body before they cause symptoms. Notably, the urinary system includes several mechanisms to prevent infection: one-way valves where the ureters attach to the bladder; urination, which washes microbes out of the body; prostate secretions that slow bacterial growth in men; and the immune system. Occasionally, however, the bacteria resist the body's defenses and cause infection. Due to the high concentration of bacteria, most infections invade the urethra from the meatus in the perineal area. The microorganism can then ascend through the urethra to the bladder and then move along the ureters to the kidneys. Occasionally, microorganisms may invade the kidneys from the blood.

UTIs are most often caused by *Escherichia coli*, which is part of the normal intestinal flora. Virulent forms of *E. coli* can avoid being washed away during urination by attaching to the mucosa along the urinary tract. *E. coli* can gain access to the urinary tract due to the anus's close proximity to the urinary meatus, especially in women. In addition to this close proximity, women are more vulnerable to developing UTIs for the following reasons:

- Women have shorter urethras (so the microorganisms have a shorter distance to travel).
- Women usually urinate in a sitting position (which prevents full emptying of the bladder).
- Women may experience increased perineal tissue irritation from sexual activity, tampons, bubble baths, bathing suits, tight-fitting pants, and deodorants, as well as nylon, lace, and thong underwear.

Although men are less likely than women to experience a UTI, they are likely to have a recurrent UTI because the bacteria can hide deep inside prostate tissue. Other risk factors for developing UTIs include the following:

- Benign prostatic hypertrophy (causes urinary retention)
- Congenital urinary tract abnormalities (can alter urinary flow)
- Immobility (prevents complete bladder emptying, leading to urinary stasis)
- Urinary or bowel incontinence (can increase the potential for contamination of the urinary meatus)
- Renal calculi (obstruct urine output, leading to urinary stasis)
- Decreased cognition (increases the risk for incontinence and toileting issues)
- Pregnancy (the growing uterus puts pressure on the bladder, impairing urinary flow)
- Impaired immune response (e.g., diabetes mellitus)
- Impaired nerve innervations (e.g., spinal cord injuries)
- Urinary catheterization (provides a direct pathway to the urinary system; the most common source of nosocomial infections)
- Improper personal hygiene (increases the number of microorganisms)
- Using a diaphragm or spermicide for birth control (increases bacterial growth)
- Using unlubricated condoms (increases irritation)

Some UTIs may be asymptomatic, but general clinical manifestations, when present, include the following signs and symptoms:

- Urgency
- Dysuria
- Frequency
- Hematuria
- Bacteriuria
- Cloudy, foul-smelling urine
- Symptoms of infection (e.g., fever, chills, and fatigue)

Diagnostic procedures for UTIs include a history, physical examination, urinalysis, urine culture, cystoscopy, cystourethrogram (X-ray of the bladder and urethra while the bladder is full and during urination), complete blood count (CBC), and ultrasound, X-ray, CT, and MRI of the kidneys, ureters, and bladder. Treatment for UTI focuses on eradicating the microorganism with antibiotics. Additional strategies concentrate on prevention of UTIs:

- Increasing hydration, especially consumption of water and juices (increases flushing of the urinary tract)
- Avoiding irritants (e.g., bubble bath and deodorants)
- Performing proper perineal hygiene (women should clean from front to back, and uncircumcised men should retract the foreskin to clean the penis)
- Wearing cotton underwear
- Wearing loose-fitting clothing
- Not delaying urination
- Adequately emptying the bladder (especially after intercourse)
- Providing appropriate catheter care (when present)
- Probiotics (reestablish normal flora)

Cystitis

Cystitis refers to inflammation of the bladder. The inflammatory response is triggered, causing the bladder and urethra walls to become red and swollen. Infection most commonly initiates this response, but irritants (e.g., radiation and catheters) occasionally can activate it. In addition to the usual UTI symptoms, clinical manifestations of cystitis include abdominal pain and pelvic pressure. Diagnostic procedures and treatment regimens follow those usually seen for UTIs.

Pyelonephritis

Pyelonephritis refers to an infection that has reached one or both kidneys. The invading microorganisms usually ascend from the lower urinary tract but can also gain access from the bloodstream. *E. coli* is the most common culprit. In addition to having the same risk factors as UTIs, pyelonephritis is more common in those persons who require frequent medical attention, experience recurrent UTIs, or have contracted an antibiotic-resistant bacterial strain. With this condition, the kidneys become grossly edematous and structures fill with exudate, compressing the renal artery. Abscesses and necrosis can develop, impairing renal function and causing permanent damage. Pyelonephritis can be acute or chronic.

In addition to the usual UTI symptoms, clinical manifestations of pyelonephritis are more severe and include flank pain and increased blood pressure. Diagnostic procedures for pyelonephritis consist of a history, physical examination, urinalysis, urine and blood cultures, CBC, cystoscopy, intravenous pyelogram, CT, renal ultrasound, biopsy, and cystourethrogram.

With treatment, most cases of pyelonephritis will improve without any complications. Strategies include the usual UTI treatments, but long-term antibiotics (4–6 weeks) are typically required. Complications, if they occur, can involve chronic kidney disease, recurrent UTIs, and sepsis. Surveillance for development of complications and treatment of those complications that occur are also necessary.

Urinary Tract Obstructions

The urinary system is similar to the basic plumbing in any house. Blockages in any part of the plumbing system prevent the flow of the liquid, causing the system to back up. Many opportunities for blockages to occur exist throughout the urinary system, making urinary obstructions common. These blockages may be as simple as particulates collecting and forming stones to as complex as the growth of tumors.

Nephrolithiasis

Nephrolithiasis refers to the presence of renal calculi (kidney stones). Calculi are hard masses of crystals composed of minerals that the kidneys normally excrete (FIGURE 7-7). These stones, which can vary in size from as small as a grain of sand to as large as a golf ball, are the most common cause of urinary obstruction. Nephrolithiasis is more common in men and Caucasians. Generally, the calculi form in the renal pelvis, ureters, and bladder.

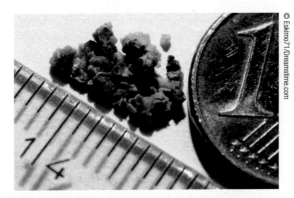

FIGURE 7-7 Renal calculi.

Calculi may contain various combinations of chemicals (**TABLE 7-5**). The most frequently encountered type of calculi contains calcium in combination with either oxalate or phosphate. Other types of calculi include struvite or infection stones, uric acid stones, and cystine stones. The calculi may be smooth or jagged, and they are usually yellow or brown.

In a healthy individual, urine contains chemicals that prevent these crystals from forming. Once the minerals begin to precipitate, they grow like a snowball being rolled in the snow. Conditions

TABLE 7-5	Types of Renal Calculi	
Type	**Causes**	**Treatment**
Calcium	Causes of calcium calculi include the following: • Increased absorption of calcium from the small bowel • Hyperparathyroidism • Inability of renal tubules to reabsorb calcium • Dietary excess of calcium • Chronic bowel disease that results in steatorrhea; fat then combines with calcium and renders the calcium unable to bind to oxalate, causing stone formation	Treatment depends on the cause and includes the following: • Cellulose phosphate or thiazide diuretics to decrease dietary absorption of calcium • Surgical resection of the parathyroid gland to reduce hyperparathyroidism • Thiazide diuretic therapy to correct renal tubular defects, resulting in the inability to reabsorb calcium • Purine dietary restrictions to reduce uric acid production • Increased fluid intake and treatment of chronic diarrhea
Struvite (magnesium–ammonium–phosphate)	Caused by urase-producing bacteria Urinary pH around 7.2 Usually large in size Texture is relatively soft Associated with frequent UTI More common in women	Prevention of UTI Percutaneous nephrolithotomy
Uric acid	Urine pH lower than 5.5 encourages insoluble urate salt formation Common causes include rapid and dramatic weight loss, and some malignancies	Large calculi can be dissolved by increasing the urine pH above 6.5 with potassium citrate (the solubility of urate salt is then increased)
Cystine	Abnormal excretion of cystine (amino acid), ornithine lysine, and arginine	Prevention: increase fluid intake and increase urine pH above 7.5

that increase the likelihood of the crystals forming include pH changes (e.g., a UTI), excessive concentration of insoluble salts in the urine (e.g., dehydration, bone disease, gout, renal disease, and dietary increases), and urinary stasis (e.g., immobility). Additional risk factors for developing nephrolithiasis include family history, obesity, hypertension, and diet (high-protein, high-sodium, or low-calcium diet).

Calculi usually cause symptoms only when they obstruct urine flow. This obstruction can lead to hydronephrosis (urine accumulation in the kidney). The movement of calculi through the urinary system can be quite painful and cause irritation of the urinary mucosa, increasing the risk for a UTI. Clinical manifestations of nephrolithiasis include the following signs and symptoms:

- Colicky pain (pain that fluctuates in intensity, with periods of pain lasting 20–60 minutes; often severe, this pain is due to the calculi scraping the ureter wall, and it is colicky due to ureter spasms that occur in an attempt to move the calculi along) in the flank area that radiates to the lower abdomen and groin
- Bloody, cloudy, or foul-smelling urine
- Dysuria
- Frequency
- Genital discharge
- Nausea and vomiting
- Fever and chills (if an infection is present)

Diagnostic procedures for nephrolithiasis consist of a history, physical examination, urine examination (urinalysis, culture, 24-hour urine collection), kidney–ureter–bladder X-ray, CT, ultrasound, intravenous pyelogram, calculi analysis, and serum studies (e.g., calcium, uric acid, and phosphate).

Treatment of nephrolithiasis is specific to the type of calculi present (Table 7-5); therefore, determining the type of calculi is crucial to resolve the current calculi and prevent future calculus development. To determine the type of calculi, all urine is strained to capture any passed calculi. Small stones can pass through the urinary system. Strategies to assist the passing of these calculi include increasing fluid intake to 2.5–3.5 L throughout the day and engaging in physical activity (if possible). The increased presence of fluid in the urinary system will expand the diameter of the ureters and urethra, easing the passing of the calculi. Larger calculi can be broken up to allow for passing of the smaller pieces. Procedures to disintegrate these calculi include extracorporeal shock wave lithotripsy (high-frequency sound waves are directed at the calculi to pulverize them), percutaneous nephrolithotomy (a laser is directed at a calculus with a fiber-optic scope), and ureteroscopy (a forceps is used to grab a calculus and remove it through a fiber-optic scope). Surgical removal of the calculi may be indicated in the following situations:

- The calculi do not pass after a reasonable period of time and cause constant pain.
- A calculus is too large to pass on its own or is lodged in a difficult location.
- The calculi obstruct urinary flow.
- The calculi cause ongoing UTIs, renal damage, or constant bleeding.
- The calculi have enlarged.

Treating the underlying cause (e.g., with antibiotics, antigout agents, or urine pH–modifying agents) of the calculi and pain management will also be necessary.

Recurrence is common with nephrolithiasis; therefore, prevention strategies are essential. Dietary changes are the mainstay of prevention, with the changes implemented being specific to the type of calculi (Table 7-5). Additional prevention strategies include adequate fluid intake (2–2.5 L per day) and physical activity.

Hydronephrosis

Hydronephrosis is an abnormal dilation of the renal pelvis and the calyces of one or both kidneys that occurs secondary to a disease (FIGURE 7-8). Diseases that obstruct urine flow are commonly associated with this condition, including nephrolithiasis, tumors, benign prostatic hyperplasia, strictures, and stenosis. Congenital urologic defects can also cause hydronephrosis, including reflux nephropathy, a congenital condition that causes backflow of urine into the kidneys. Unilateral renal involvement indicates an obstruction in one of the ureters, and bilateral renal involvement indicates an obstruction in the urethra.

Because urine is continuously forming, the presence and severity of clinical manifestations depend on the degree of urinary obstruction. Partial obstructions with mild hydronephrosis may not produce any initial symptoms. Complete obstruction with severe hydronephrosis, by comparison, applies direct pressure and compresses tissue and blood vessels, leading to atrophy, necrosis, and glomerular filtration cessation. When present, clinical manifestations include the following signs and symptoms:

- Colicky flank pain or pressure
- Bloody, cloudy, or foul-smelling urine

Myth Busters

Several common myths surround renal calculi and should be addressed.

Myth 1: Only men get renal calculi.

Although calculi formation is more common in men, rates among women are increasing.

Myth 2: Eating certain foods will cause calculi to form.

In general, eating certain foods will not cause calculi to form in persons who are not already susceptible to their formation.

Myth 3: Most renal calculi form from calcium, so dietary intake of calcium should be reduced.

For years, the medical community thought a low-calcium diet was the best way to prevent renal calculi, especially in those persons who already had stones, but recent research has changed that thinking. Studies have shown that low-calcium diets are not effective, and may actually be harmful, because they tend to increase the likelihood of low bone density and osteoporosis. Researchers now believe that more—rather than less—calcium is better, with normal amounts being best. So, drinking that glass of milk and cutting back on the hamburgers and chips may help reduce your risk of renal calculi!

Myth 4: If a person has renal calculi, then he or she is more likely to develop cholelithiasis (gallstones).

Not even close! Cholelithiasis and nephrolithiasis are not related at all—the "stones" form in different areas of the body. Typically, those individuals who are at greater risk for developing cholelithiasis are a different group from those who have renal calculi. Women, Native Americans, and Mexican Americans, people older than 60 years of age, and those on frequent diets are more likely to have gallstones.

Data from National Institutes of Health. (2002, November). Kidney stones. *The NIH Word on Health.*

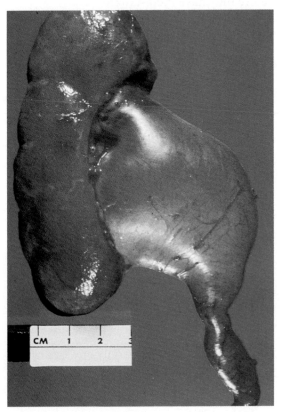

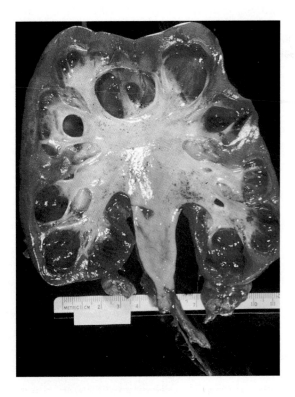

FIGURE 7-8 Hydronephrosis.

Courtesy of Leonard V. Crowley, MD, Century College

- Dysuria
- Decreased urine output
- Frequency
- Urgency
- Nausea and vomiting
- Abdominal distension
- UTIs

Diagnostic procedures for hydronephrosis include a history, physical examination, urinalysis, renal ultrasound, CT, intravenous pyelogram, and MRI. Prognosis depends on the severity of the hydronephrosis and early treatment. Treatment focuses on resolving the underlying cause, and facilitating urine flow will be necessary if UTIs develop. If the hydronephrosis is prolonged, permanent renal damage can occur to one or both kidneys.

Tumors

Benign tumors are rare in the urinary system; most urinary tumors are malignant. These tumors can occur at any point along the urinary system. Regardless of their location, tumors can obstruct urine flow and impair renal function in addition to leading to the consequences of cancer (e.g., metastasis, pain, and weight loss).

Wilms' Tumor

Wilms' tumor, or nephroblastoma, is a rare kidney cancer that primarily affects children. According to the National Cancer Institute (2016c), 500 new cases of Wilms' tumor are diagnosed each year. Wilms' tumor is the most common malignant tumor in children, with its peak incidence occurring around age 3–4 years. This tumor usually occurs in one kidney, but it can affect both (in 4–5% of cases). A second tumor may appear later in the remaining kidney. Wilms' tumor usually grows as a solitary mass that can become quite large (FIGURE 7-9).

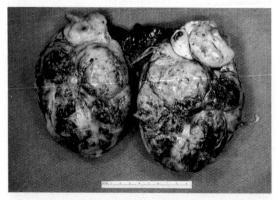

FIGURE 7-9 Wilms' tumor.
© University of Alabama at Birmingham Department of Pathology PEIR Digital Library (http://peir.net)

The exact cause of Wilms' tumor is unknown, but it is thought to arise in utero when the cells that normally form the kidneys fail to develop properly. This development issue can occur spontaneously or as a result of genetic changes. Notably, Wilms' tumor has been associated with genetic mutations on chromosome 11 as well as on the X chromosome. This type of cancer often occurs in conjunction with several congenital defects, including aniridia (absence of the iris of the eye), hemihypertrophy (enlargement of one side of the body), and urinary tract abnormalities (e.g., cryptorchidism and hypospadias). Even though it is rare, Wilms' tumor tends to run in families, intensifying its genetic connection. The risk of developing this tumor also seems to be higher in females and African Americans. In contrast, Asian Americans have a lower risk of developing Wilms' tumor than other ethnic groups.

Because of improved diagnostic procedures, Wilms' tumor can now be detected early, leading to an improved prognosis for children affected by this disease. The long-term survival rate is excellent with early detection and treatment. Unfortunately, Wilms' tumor may sometimes go undetected early because the tumor can grow quite large without causing pain; nevertheless, most of these tumors are diagnosed before they have metastasized.

Clinical manifestations of Wilms' tumor are similar to those of other cancers:

- Asymptomatic abdominal mass
- High blood pressure
- Hemihypertrophy
- Hematuria
- UTIs
- Abdominal pain (late)
- Nausea and vomiting
- Anorexia
- Bowel pattern changes (often constipation)
- Weight loss
- Fatigue

Diagnostic procedures for Wilms' tumor include a history, physical examination, renal ultrasound, BUN, creatinine, creatinine clearance, CBC, abdominal computerized tomography (CT), urinalysis, and biopsy. Once diagnosed, the following staging system guides treatment:

- *Stage I*: The cancer is in only one kidney and generally can be completely removed with surgery.
- *Stage II*: The cancer has metastasized to the tissues and structures near the kidney, but

it can still be completely removed by surgery.

- *Stage III*: The cancer has metastasized beyond the kidney area to nearby lymph nodes or other structures within the abdomen and may not be completely removed by surgery.
- *Stage IV*: The cancer has metastasized to distant structures, such as the lungs, liver, or brain.
- *Stage V*: Cancer cells are found in both kidneys.

The standard treatment for Wilms' tumor is surgery (e.g., simple, partial, or radical nephrectomy) and chemotherapy, but radiation therapy may be used if warranted by tumor histology. Coping strategies and support interventions (e.g., allowing play time and local support groups) will be beneficial for the family and child. Additionally, palpation of the abdomen should be avoided.

Renal Cell Carcinoma

Renal cell carcinoma is the most frequently occurring kidney cancer in adults (most common in those 50–70 years of age). The National Cancer Institute (2016b) estimates that nearly 63,000 new cases of renal cancer will be diagnosed in 2016, with more than 14,000 deaths attributed to this cancer. Renal cell carcinoma is a primary tumor arising from the renal tubule (**FIGURE 7-10**). Its exact cause is unknown. Risk factors for developing this type of cancer include being male, dialysis treatment, family history, hypertension, other kidney disease (e.g., horseshoe kidney and polycystic kidney disease), and smoking. Metastasis to the liver, lungs, bone, or nervous system is common at the time of diagnosis.

Renal cell carcinoma is typically asymptomatic in its early stages. When present, clinical manifestations include the following signs and symptoms:

- Painless hematuria (gross or microscopic)
- Abnormal urine color (dark, rusty, or brown)
- Dull, achy flank pain
- Urinary retention
- Palpable mass over the affected kidney
- Unexplained weight loss
- Anemia (if the tumor suppresses hormone secretion)
- Polycythemia (if the tumor secretes erythropoietin or an erythropoietin-like substance)
- Hypertension
- Paraneoplastic syndromes such as hypercalcemia (due to ectopic parathyroid hormone production by the tumor or bone metastasis) or Cushing's syndrome (increased adrenocorticotropic hormone)
- Fever

Diagnostic procedures for renal cell carcinoma are used to identify the presence of a tumor and determine whether metastasis has occurred. These procedures include a history, physical examination, urinalysis, CT, MRI, positron emission tomography (PET) scan, bone scan, chest X-ray, intravenous pyelogram, cystoscopy, renal arteriogram, biopsy, liver function panel, CBC, and blood chemistry.

Interestingly, renal cell carcinoma is one of the few tumors in which well-documented cases of spontaneous tumor regression in the absence of therapy exist, but such outcomes occur very rarely and may not lead to long-term survival (National Cancer Institute, 2016b). Partial or complete surgical removal of the kidney (nephrectomy) is recommended because the cancer is generally unresponsive to radiation or chemotherapy, although some newer chemotherapy agents (e.g., multikinase inhibitors) have shown promise in this indication. Hormone therapy and immunotherapy may have modest effects in shrinking the tumor. Prognosis is better when the condition is diagnosed prior to metastasis of the cancer.

Bladder Cancer

Bladder cancer refers to any cancer that forms in the tissue of the bladder. Most bladder cancers are transitional cell carcinomas (cancer beginning in the cells that make up the inner bladder lining). Other types include squamous cell carcinoma (cancer beginning in thin, flat cells) and

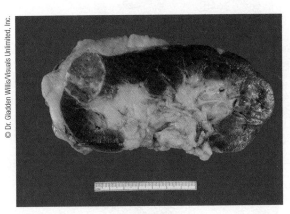

© Dr. Gladden Willis/Visuals Unlimited, Inc.

FIGURE 7-10 Renal cell carcinoma.

adenocarcinoma (cancer beginning in the cells that make and release mucus and other fluids). The cells that form squamous cell carcinoma and adenocarcinoma develop in the inner lining of the bladder because of chronic irritation and inflammation. This type of cancer usually evolves as multiple invasive tumors that extend through the bladder wall and surrounding structures. Metastasis to the pelvic lymph nodes, liver, and bone is common.

The National Cancer Institute (2016a) estimates that nearly 77,000 new cases of bladder cancer will be diagnosed in 2016, with more than 16,000 deaths being attributed to this cancer. Although bladder cancer most frequently occurs in older adults, it can occur at any age, and it is more common in men and Caucasians. Other persons at increased risk include those who work with chemicals (e.g., dye, rubber, hairdressing chemicals, and aluminum), smoke, have excessive use of analgesics, experience recurrent UTIs, have long-term catheter placement, and received chemotherapy or radiation.

Clinical manifestations of bladder cancer include the following:

- Painless hematuria (gross or microscopic)
- Abnormal urine color (dark, rusty, or brown)
- Frequency
- Dysuria
- Urge incontinence

- UTIs
- Back or abdominal pain

Diagnostic procedures are used to identify the presence of a tumor and determine whether metastasis has occurred. These procedures consist of a history, physical examination, urinalysis, CT, MRI, PET scan, bone scan, chest X-ray, intravenous pyelogram, cystoscopy, biopsy, and liver function panel. Even with early diagnosis and treatment, bladder cancer often reoccurs. Treatment strategies are based on staging and include surgical removal of the tumor, radiation, chemotherapy, and immunologic agents.

Benign Prostatic Hyperplasia

Although the prostate is a structure of the male reproductive system, diseases of the prostate can cause significant issues in the urinary system because of its close proximity to those structures (FIGURE 7-11). **Benign prostatic hyperplasia (BPH)**, also called benign prostatic hypertrophy, is a common, nonmalignant enlargement of the prostate gland that occurs as men age, usually appearing by age 50. Its exact cause is unknown, but declining testosterone and increasing estrogen levels are thought to cause prostatic stromal cell proliferation. This increase in proliferation enlarges the prostate gland. A second theory postulates that stem cells in the prostate do not mature and die as they are programmed to do (apoptosis) (see the *Cellular Function* chapter).

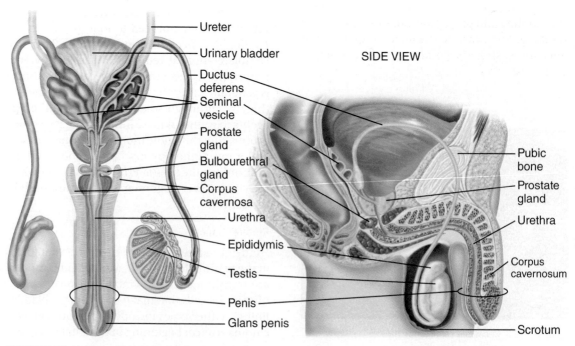

FRONT VIEW

- Ureter
- Urinary bladder
- Ductus deferens
- Seminal vesicle
- Prostate gland
- Bulbourethral gland
- Corpus cavernosa
- Urethra
- Epididymis
- Testis
- Penis
- Glans penis

SIDE VIEW

- Pubic bone
- Prostate gland
- Urethra
- Corpus cavernosum
- Scrotum

FIGURE 7-11 Urethra and prostate gland.

The resulting imbalance between dying cells and reproducing cells enlarges the prostate over time. As the prostate expands, it presses against the urethra like a clamp on a hose. Clamping the urethra obstructs urine flow, leading to urinary stasis and UTIs. The bladder wall becomes thick and irritated as urine overfills this organ. The bladder begins to contract with even small amounts of urine, and, over time, it loses its ability to empty completely.

Clinical manifestations of BPH are primarily urinary in nature, with the severity of these symptoms depending on the size of the prostate:

- Frequency
- Urgency
- Urinary retention
- Difficulty initiating urination
- Weak urinary stream
- Dribbling urine
- Nocturia
- Bladder distension
- Overflow incontinence
- Erectile dysfunction

BPH does not increase prostate cancer risk, but the clinical presentation is very similar to that of prostate cancer. Diagnostic procedures can determine whether the prostate enlargement is due to BPH or prostate cancer (see the *Reproductive Function* chapter). These procedures consist of a history, physical examination (including digital rectal examination), urine flow measures, urinalysis, prostate-specific antigen (PSA), rectal ultrasound, biopsy, cystoscopy, BUN, and creatinine.

Treatment centers on relieving the urinary obstruction and reestablishing sexual function (if possible). Strategies to improve urine flow include pharmacologic agents (e.g., alpha blockers and alpha$_5$-reductase inhibitors) to shrink or limit growth of the prostate. Herbal remedies (e.g., saw palmetto) have also been used, although only limited evidence supports their effectiveness. Other strategies to improve BPH symptoms include minimally invasive procedures such as laser therapy, transurethral needle ablation (TUNA), transurethral electrovaporization of the prostate (TURP), hyperthermia, high-density forced ultrasound (HIFU), intraurethral stents, and transurethral balloon dilation. Partial or complete surgical removal of the prostate gland may be necessary. Additionally, use of alcohol should be avoided because it can make symptoms worse.

Conditions Resulting in Impaired Renal Function

Polycystic Kidney Disease

Polycystic kidney disease (PKD) is an inherited disorder characterized by numerous, grapelike clusters of fluid-filled cysts in both kidneys (FIGURE 7-12). These cysts enlarge the kidneys while compressing and eventually replacing the functional kidney tissue. The exact trigger for the formation of the cysts is unknown.

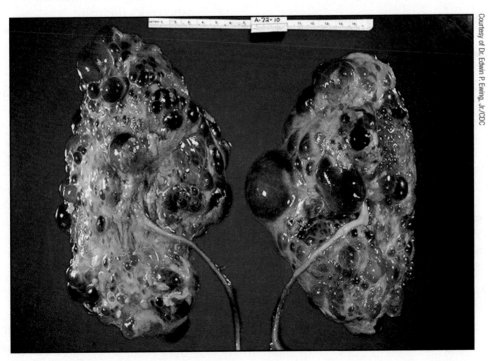

Courtesy of Dr. Edwin P. Ewing, Jr./CDC

FIGURE 7-12 Polycystic kidney disease.

Prognosis and progression of the disease vary widely, depending on the type of PKD. Autosomal dominant (see the *Cellular Function* chapter) PKD is the most common type; it has been mapped to mutations on the short arm of chromosomes 4 and 16. This form of PKD occurs in both children and adults, but it is much more common in adults, with symptoms often not emerging until middle age. Like most recessive conditions (see the *Cellular Function* chapter), autosomal recessive PKD is far less common. This type appears in infancy or childhood, tends to be extremely serious, and progresses rapidly, resulting in renal failure and generally causing death in infancy or childhood. PKD affects men and women equally.

Learning Points

The urinary system is a basic household septic system. The kidneys remove waste and unneeded substances from the blood to have them excreted. The kidneys collect these products in the form of urine much like a toilet, and flushing the toilet is much like what the kidneys do in sending the urine to the bladder. The bladder acts like a septic tank, holding the waste until the tank is full. When full, the bladder (and the septic tank) must be emptied.

When obstructions occur at any point in the urinary system, urine backs up, much like the septic system would do if obstructed. This backflow can cause severe damage in both cases: In the urinary system, the kidneys become damaged by the irritation and pressure of the excess urine; in the septic system, the house becomes damaged from the corrosive septic contents.

Clinical manifestations depend on the individual's age and the type of PKD. These manifestations reflect the structural changes associated with the disease and the resulting renal impairment. In neonates, manifestations include the following signs and symptoms:

- Potter facies: pronounced epicanthic folds (skin folds at the corner of the eyes on either side of the nose), pointed nose, small chin, and floppy, low-set ears
- Large, bilateral, symmetrical masses on the flanks
- Respiratory distress (caused by fluid accumulation from renal impairment)
- **Uremia** (waste accumulation due to renal impairment)

In adults, manifestations include the following signs and symptoms:

- Hypertension (due to activation of the renin–angiotensin–aldosterone system)
- Lumbar pain

- Increased abdominal girth
- Swollen, tender abdomen
- Grossly enlarged, palpable kidneys

Some other symptoms may affect both groups:

- Hematuria (due to impaired glomerular filtration)
- Nocturia (related to an inability to concentrate urine)
- Drowsiness (because of waste accumulation)

Other conditions that may occur in conjunction with PKD include brain aneurysms, cysts in other organs (especially the liver), and colon diverticula. Because of the renal impairment associated with this condition, PKD can lead to critical complications such as pyelonephritis, cyst rupture, retroperitoneal bleeding, and chronic kidney disease. Other, less serious complications include anemia, hypertension, and renal calculi (kidney stones).

Diagnostic procedures for PKD consist of a history, physical examination, urinalysis, blood chemistry, urography (kidney X-ray), abdominal ultrasound, CT, MRI, and intravenous pyelogram (X-ray of the kidneys, ureters, and bladder with the use of radioactive contrast media). PKD often progresses slowly, leading to end-stage renal disease. Treatment strategies focus on controlling symptoms and preventing complications:

- Pharmacology, including the following agents:
  - Antibiotics (when infections are present)
  - Analgesics (for pain)
  - Antihypertensive agents
  - Diuretics
- Adequate hydration
- Low-salt diet
- Surgically draining cystic abscesses or retroperitoneal bleeding
- Dialysis
- Kidney transplant

Inflammatory Disorders

The inflammatory process (see the *Immunity* chapter) can cause havoc in the urinary system, especially in the kidneys. The structures can become edematous and damaged due to the inflammatory mediators and their effects. These changes impair the kidneys' ability to function properly, leading to serious consequences.

Glomerulonephritis

Glomerulonephritis is a bilateral inflammatory disorder of the glomeruli that typically follows a streptococcal infection. Other risk factors include immunodeficiency and the presence of chronic inflammatory conditions (e.g., systemic lupus erythematosus). Affecting men more than women, glomerulonephritis is a leading cause of chronic kidney disease in the United States; the inflammatory changes (e.g., congestion and cell proliferation) impair the kidneys' ability to excrete waste and excess fluid. Glomerulonephritis can be acute or chronic. Many forms of glomerulonephritis have been identified, with nephrotic and nephritic syndromes being the most prevalent (FIGURE 7-13).

Nephrotic Syndrome

Nephrotic syndrome occurs when antibody–antigen complexes lodge in the glomerular membrane, triggering activation of the complement system. This condition is caused by systemic diseases that damage the kidneys (e.g., systemic lupus erythematosus, hepatitis B, and diabetes mellitus), by infections (e.g., streptococcal infections and mononucleosis), as a reaction to medications (e.g., gold therapy and nonsteroidal anti-inflammatory drugs), and idiopathically. The inflammatory changes result in increased glomerular capillary permeability, leading to marked proteinuria, lipiduria, hypoalbuminemia, and massive generalized edema (**anasarca**). The high level of protein in the urine indicates impaired glomerular filtration. The loss of protein in the urine contributes to low serum levels (hypoalbuminemia) and gives the urine a dark and cloudy (smoky or coffee-colored) appearance. Additionally, immunoglobulins are excreted in the urine; this loss of immune cells, in turn, increases the individual's risk for

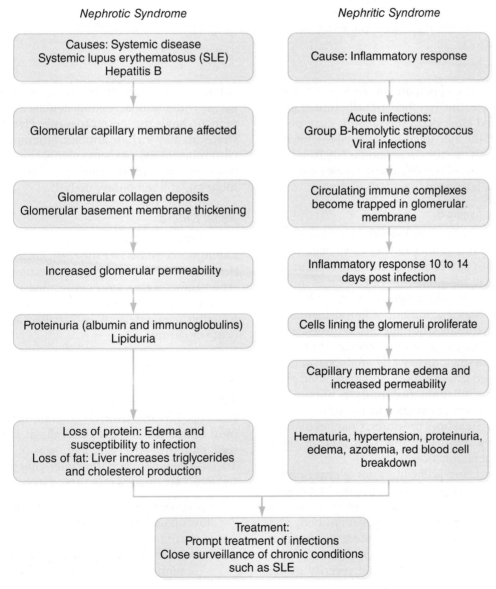

FIGURE 7-13 Nephrotic and nephritic syndrome.

A 13-year-old boy presented to the clinic complaining of a sore throat that persisted for 2 days. After those 2 days, he developed fever, nausea, and malaise. A throat culture revealed the presence of Group A beta hemolytic streptococci, and the child was started on antibiotic therapy. The child's symptoms gradually improved, but approximately 2 weeks later, he returned to the clinic because the fever, nausea, and malaise returned. He became tachypneic and short of breath. The mother noted that his eyes were puffy, his ankles were swollen, and his urine was dark and cloudy.

On examination, the child's blood pressure was 148/100 mm Hg,

his pulse was 122 beats/min, and his respirations were 35/min. Orbital and ankle edema were present. Rales (abnormal breath sounds) were auscultated bilaterally in the chest, but no heart murmurs were found. Slight tenderness to percussion over the flank areas was noted.

A chest X-ray showed evidence of congestion and edema in the lungs. The patient's hematocrit was 37% and his WBC was 11,200/mm^3. Blood urea nitrogen was 48 mg/dL (normal is less than 20 mg/dL). Urinalysis results showed that the patient's protein was 2+ (24-hour excretion was 0.8 g), specific gravity was 1.012, and there were moderate amounts of RBCs and

WBCs in the urine. Serum albumin was 4.1 g/dL (normal is 3.5–4.5).

1. Which evidence supports the conclusion that this patient has a kidney disease?
2. Which clinical pattern of kidney disease does this patient have? Can you explain the symptoms?
3. Which morphologic changes would you expect in the kidney?
4. What is the prognosis? What are the possible short- and long-term complications of this disease? Is it necessary to hospitalize the patient?

infection. To compensate for the loss of protein in the urine, the liver increases albumin, triglyceride, and cholesterol production—a response that puts the individual at increased risk for atherosclerosis (see the *Cardiovascular Function* chapter). The loss of protein also decreases colloidal pressure, leading to the massive edema.

Nephritic Syndrome

Nephritic syndrome refers to inflammatory injury to the glomeruli that can occur when antibodies interact with normally occurring antigens in the glomeruli. Diseases that initiate the inflammatory response (e.g., infection) cause nephritic syndrome. Clinical manifestations of nephritic syndrome include gross hematuria, urinary casts and leukocytes, low GFR, **azotemia** (buildup of waste products), oliguria (decreased urine output), and high blood pressure. The inflammatory injury results in red blood cells being excreted in the urine, which changes circulatory pressures. Changes in these pressures result in a low GFR and, in turn, impair renal function.

Diagnostic procedures for glomerulonephritis consist of a history, physical examination, urinalysis, blood chemistry, serum antibody levels (e.g., antinuclear antibody and rheumatoid factor), erythrocyte sedimentation rate (ESR), CT, and renal biopsy. Treatment depends on the type, cause, and severity of the

glomerulonephritis. In many cases, recovery occurs with minimal residual damage. Children tend to have the best prognosis. Treatment strategies may include antibiotic therapy, corticosteroids, blood pressure management (e.g., diuretics, angiotensin-converting enzyme inhibitors), and temporary dialysis.

Renal Failure

The pivotal role that the kidneys play in maintaining homeostasis (see the *Fluid, Electrolyte, and Acid–Base Homeostasis* chapter) becomes clear when these organs stop performing that role. *Renal failure* refers to the kidneys' inability to function adequately; it is classified as either acute or chronic.

Acute Renal Failure

Acute renal failure (ARF), also termed acute kidney injury, refers to a sudden loss of renal function. This loss, which is generally reversible, most commonly occurs in critically ill, hospitalized patients. ARF has a mortality rate of 10–60% depending on the underlying etiology. Its causes are divided into three categories:

1. **Prerenal conditions**, which disrupt blood flow on its way to the kidneys:
   - Extremely low blood pressure or blood volume (e.g., hemorrhage, sepsis, dehydration, shock, and traumatic injury)

- Heart dysfunction (e.g., myocardial infarction and heart failure)

2. **Intrarenal conditions**, which directly damage the structures of the kidneys:
   - Reduced blood supply within the kidneys (e.g., atherosclerosis)
   - Hemolytic uremic syndrome (associated with infection with certain strains of *E. coli*, in which bacterium toxins damage small blood vessels; it is the leading cause of acute kidney failure in children)
   - Renal inflammation (e.g., glomerulonephritis and acute interstitial nephritis [usually associated with an allergic reaction to certain nephrotoxic medications])
   - Toxic injury (usually from alcohol, cocaine, heavy metals, solvents, fuels, chemotherapy drugs, and contrast dyes)

3. **Postrenal conditions**, which interfere with the urine excretion:
   - Ureter obstruction (e.g., nephrolithiasis and tumors)
   - Bladder obstruction and dysfunction (e.g., BPH, tumors, and nerve innervation disruption)

In addition to these causes, other factors that can increase the risk of developing ARF include advanced age, autoimmune disorders, and liver disease.

ARF has an abrupt onset (usually over a period of 48 hours) and progresses through four phases. The individual is usually asymptomatic in the initial phase. Although renal damage is occurring, the nephrons that are still functioning compensate for those that are not. During the second (oliguric) phase, impaired glomerular filtration leads to solute and water reabsorption. This reabsorption decreases daily urine output to approximately 400 mL or less, such that waste products begin to accumulate (uremia). The second phase can last a few days to a few weeks. In the third (diuretic) phase, renal function gradually returns as healing and cellular regeneration occur. Diuresis occurs due to tubular damage that impairs the kidneys' ability to concentrate the urine. Daily urine output in this phase can be as much as 5 L. The excessive urine output can lead to dehydration and electrolyte imbalances. The third phase can last days to weeks. In the recovery stage, glomerular function gradually returns to normal. This final stage can persist for 3–12 months. Depending on the age and overall health of the individual, full renal function may be regained.

As previously mentioned, the initial phase of ARF is asymptomatic. As renal function is lost, however, symptoms appear. Clinical manifestations vary depending on the ARF phase. In the oliguric phase, manifestations are as follows:

- Decreased urine output
- Electrolyte disturbances (usually increased levels)
- Fluid volume excess
- Azotemia
- Metabolic acidosis

In the diuretic phase, manifestations include:

- Increased urine output
- Electrolyte disturbances (usually decreased levels)
- Dehydration
- Hypotension

In the recovery phase, symptoms begin resolving.

Diagnostic procedures for ARF include those to identify both the renal injury and its underlying cause. These procedures consist of a history, physical examination, BUN, creatinine, blood chemistry, arterial blood gases, urinalysis, CBC, renal ultrasound, and biopsy. Treatment strategies for ARF vary depending on the phase. For instance, different fluid and electrolyte disturbances occur in the second and third phases, requiring different strategies for these phases. Some patients with ARF may require temporary dialysis until renal recovery occurs. Other supportive strategies include the following measures:

- A diet that is high in calories and carbohydrates but restricted in protein, sodium, potassium, and phosphates
- Hypertension management
- Anemia treatment with synthetic erythropoietin
- Infection prevention strategies (e.g., hand washing, limiting visitors, and aseptic technique)

Chronic Kidney Disease

Chronic kidney disease (CKD) tends to consist of a gradual loss of renal function that is irreversible. During the disease process, nonoperational scar tissue replaces injured nephrons. An estimated 23 million adults are living with CKD in the United States (NIH, 2013). Several conditions, including those in the following list, can initiate the slow, progressive destruction of the nephrons:

- Diabetes mellitus (type 1 and type 2) is the leading cause of CKD in the United States because of the vascular damage it produces (see the *Endocrine Function* chapter).
- Hypertension is another common cause of CKD in the United States; it can damage the glomeruli and ultimately cause the damaged nephrons to lose their ability to filter waste from the blood.
- Urine obstructions (e.g., nephrolithiasis and BPH) can block urine flow, increasing pressure in the kidneys and reducing their function.
- Renal diseases (e.g., polycystic kidney disease, pyelonephritis, and glomerulonephritis) damage nephrons in a variety of ways.
- Renal artery stenosis (narrowing or blockage of the artery that supplies the kidneys) impairs blood flow and leads to kidney damage.
- Ongoing exposure to toxins (e.g., fuel, solvents, and lead) and nephrotoxic medications (e.g., many antibiotics, chemotherapy, and nonsteroidal anti-inflammatory drugs) can cause direct damage as these agents circulate through the kidneys.
- Sickle cell disease can damage the kidneys by impairing renal blood flow as the sickled blood cells clump together in the renal arteries.
- Systemic lupus erythematosus causes direct damage to the renal tissue as the autoantibodies destroy the body's own cells.
- Smoking hardens the blood vessel walls throughout the body, especially in the tiny vessels of the kidney, and triggers vasoconstriction; both of these changes cause chronic ischemia and necrosis.
- With aging, the kidneys generally become less efficient and are exposed to more conditions that can cause damage.

CKD generally evolves through five stages that are identified based on GFR. In the first stage, kidney damage is present but the GFR is normal or high (greater than 90). The GFR begins falling as the patient progresses through stage II (GFR 60–89), stage III (GFR 30–59), and stage IV (GFR 15–29). Eventually, the patient reaches kidney failure in stage V, as the GFR drops to less than 15 or the patient begins dialysis. Clinical manifestations begin to appear slowly as the renal function declines by 50%. Even with the declining GFR, the kidneys can maintain relatively normal function to a point because the surviving nephrons hypertrophy and increase their rates of filtration, reabsorption, and secretion. Over time, however, waste products begin to accumulate as renal function declines. Additionally, the kidneys lose the ability to concentrate the urine, maintain blood pressure control, and secrete erythropoietin. Multiple systems are affected as these changes develop (**TABLE 7-6**). These complications worsen as the renal function declines.

Clinical manifestations are complex and dependent on the degree of renal function lost. These manifestations also reflect the complications associated with CKD (Table 7-6). As mentioned, CKD is often asymptomatic initially because the remaining nephrons compensate for those lost to the disease. Clinical manifestations develop insidiously as 50% of the nephrons are destroyed. These manifestations include the following signs and symptoms:

- Hypertension (see the *Cardiovascular Function* chapter)
- Polyuria with pale urine (early)
- Oliguria or anuria (absent urine output) with dark-colored urine (late)
- Anemia
- Bruising and bleeding tendencies
- Electrolyte imbalances, specifically hyperkalemia, hypocalcemia, hypomagnesemia, and hyperphosphatemia
- Muscle twitches and cramps (related to hypocalcemia and hyperphosphatemia; see the *Fluid, Electrolyte, and Acid–Base Homeostasis* chapter)
- Pericarditis, pericardial effusion, pleuritis, and pleural effusion (secondary to uremia)
- Heart failure (see the *Cardiovascular Function* chapter)
- Respiratory distress and abnormal breath sounds (due to pulmonary edema associated with heart failure; see the *Cardiovascular Function* chapter)
- Sudden weight change (usually increased because of fluid retention)
- Edema of the feet and ankles (due to fluid retention)
- Azotemia
- Peripheral neuropathy, restless leg syndrome, and seizures
- Nausea and vomiting
- Anorexia
- Malaise
- Fatigue and weakness
- Headaches that seem unrelated to any other cause

TABLE 7-6   Complications of Chronic Kidney Disease

System	Etiology	Treatment
General appearance	Tired, weak, sallow skin color due to anemia and toxins	Dialysis and Epogen
Integumentary	Itching (uremic frost) occurs in an attempt to remove toxins from the body	Dialysis and palliative care
Sensory	Metallic taste in mouth and fishy breath odor (uremic fetor) due to toxins	Dialysis
Cardiopulmonary	Hypertension	
	Related to salt and water retention, erythropoietin (20% of patients on this therapy develop CKD), or increased renin production Accelerated renal damage if not controlled Heart failure develops	Limiting salt and fluids Angiotensin-converting enzyme (ACE) inhibitors, angiotensin II receptor blockers, calcium-channel blockers, and beta blockers Blood pressure goal is 120/80 mm Hg
	Pericarditis	
	Result of metabolic toxins	Hemodialysis
	Chest pain, fever, friction rub, and decreased cardiac output	
	Heart failure (in 75% of patients needing dialysis)	
	Result of increased workload of the heart (left ventricular hypertrophy) secondary to anemia, dialysis (shunting of blood), fluid overload, hypertension, and atherosclerosis	Salt and fluid restriction Diuretics (loop) ACE inhibitors and angiotensin II receptor blockers
Hematologic	Coagulopathy	
	Platelet dysfunction due to abnormal aggregation and adhesion Bleeding time increases Platelet count slightly decreased May have petechiae or purpura	Desmopressin (causes release of factor VIII from endothelial cells)—used before surgery
	Anemia	
	Related to decreased erythropoietin production (occurs when glomerular filtration rate falls below 20–25 mL/min) and iron deficiency Hemodialysis causes some red blood cell destruction	Epogen if hematocrit is below 33% (hemoglobin levels should increase no more than 1 g/dL every 3–4 weeks so hypertension does not develop) Intravenous iron for patients on dialysis (oral absorption of iron is poor)
Gastrointestinal	Anorexia, nausea, vomiting, and hiccups—related to metabolic toxins	Dialysis
Endocrine	Decreased libido, impotence, and infertility	
	Decreased estrogen levels in women—they do not ovulate Decreased testosterone levels in men	Dialysis and a healthy diet may restore fertility
	Glucose intolerance	
	Peripheral insulin resistance	
	Serum insulin high	
	Kidneys cannot clear insulin from bloodstream	Patients with diabetes may require lower doses of hypoglycemic agents

(continues)

TABLE 7-6 Complications of Chronic Kidney Disease (*continued*)

System	Etiology	Treatment
Mineral metabolism	Renal osteodystrophy (disorder of calcium, phosphorus, and bone) leading to bone pain, fractures, muscle weakness, and calcium deposits in the blood vessels, soft tissue, heart, and lungs	
	Low glomerular filtration rate leads to slower phosphorus excretion, so calcium excretion increases	Restrict dietary phosphorus
	Parathyroid hormone secretion rises and causes a high bone turnover rate	Administer phosphorus-binding drugs such as calcium carbonate
	In stage V, excess hydrogen ions are buffered by leaching of large stores of calcium phosphate and calcium carbonate from the bones = bone demineralization	Vitamin D (suppresses parathyroid hormone)
Neurologic	Uremic encephalopathy	
	Appears when glomerular filtration rate falls below 10–15 mL/min or because of hyperparathyroidism	Dialysis
	Symptoms: poor concentration (first sign) that progresses to confusion, asterixis, weakness, nystagmus, and hyperreflexia	
	Peripheral neuropathy (restless leg syndrome, distal pain, and loss of deep tendon reflexes)	
	Impotence and autonomic dysfunction	
Metabolic	Hyperkalemia	
	Glomerular filtration rate below 10–20 mL/min	Monitor cardiac status
	Hemolysis, trauma, and acidosis	Administer calcium chlorides, insulin, glucose (insulin moves potassium into cells), bicarbonate, or an exchange resin
	Diet high in citrus fruits/juices	
	Medications such as ACE inhibitors and nonsteroidal anti-inflammatory drugs	Dietary potassium restriction
Acid–base disorders	Damaged kidneys	
	Cannot produce enough ammonia or buffer hydrogen ions	Maintain serum bicarbonate above 21 mEq/L by giving alkali supplements such as sodium bicarbonate, calcium bicarbonate, or sodium citrate
	Arterial pH generally between 7.33 and 7.37	
	Excess hydrogen ions are buffered by large stores of calcium phosphate and calcium carbonate from the bones	

- Sleep disturbances
- Decreased mental alertness
- Flank pain
- Jaundice
- Persistent pruritus
- Recurrent infections (due to an impaired immune response because of uremia)

Diagnosis of CKD is often difficult because the initial symptoms are vague and nonspecific. Diagnostic procedures focus on identifying the disease and any complications that have developed as a result of its development. These procedures include a history, physical examination, urinalysis, blood chemistry (especially creatinine and BUN), CT, MRI, renal ultrasound, biopsy, CBC, and arterial blood gases.

The main goal of CKD treatment is to stop or slow disease progression, usually by controlling the underlying cause. Additionally, strategies to treat and prevent complications will be necessary (Table 7-6). Doses of any medications will likely need adjustments; with limited excretion capability, medication toxicity is probable when the usual doses are given. Without treatment, CKD has a mortality rate of 100%. Conservative management strategies are employed early, but evolve into more aggressive measures as renal function declines.

application to practice

Now that we have discussed conditions of the urinary system, let's put this knowledge into practice. After receiving reports on the following patients, which patient should you assess first?

- A 32-year-old female admitted yesterday with recurrent UTI who is not responding to therapy and complains of dysuria and hesitancy
- A 48-year-old male admitted yesterday with nephrolithiasis who complains of pain rated as a 5 on a 0–10 scale
- A 38-year-old female admitted 2 hours ago who was involved in a motor vehicle accident and has hematuria

- A 62-year-old male 2 days post transurethral electrovaporization of the prostate (TURP)

Once again, you go through the usual thought process—who would die first, acute versus chronic conditions, Maslow's hierarchy of needs, and patient safety. Let's start with the 32-year-old patient. UTI is acute but not generally life threatening. Keep her on the short list, though. Moving on to the 48-year-old patient, nephrolithiasis is not life threatening, but it is acute. Additionally, this patient is experiencing some moderate pain. We should keep him on the short list, too. For the 38-year-old patient,

hematuria can be concerning because she was in a motor vehicle accident. The kidneys likely experienced trauma that could lead to acute renal failure, which can be life threatening. This patient would likely take priority over the first two, but take a look at the last patient before you make your final decision. The 62-year-old patient is 2 days postoperative. The critical time period is likely passed, and the TURP procedure is generally minimally invasive. Prostate issues would not likely be life threatening in the short term. After considering all the patients to be assessed, you should see the 38-year-old female first.

CHAPTER SUMMARY

The urinary system maintains homeostasis through a complex filter (kidney) that can regulate pH, fluid, electrolytes, and blood glucose. Additionally, the urinary system is the main site for excreting waste products and other harmful substances obtained from the food and water ingested orally. A functioning urinary system is crucial to maintaining health, and disease in this system

can have detrimental effects on other systems and the body as a whole. Prevention and early treatment of these diseases are paramount to avoiding these consequences. Maintaining a healthy lifestyle (e.g., drinking plenty of fluids, avoiding harmful chemicals, preventing sexually transmitted infection, exercising, and smoking cessation) can help preserve urinary health.

REFERENCES

AAOS. (2004). *Paramedic: Anatomy and physiology*. Sudbury, MA: Jones and Bartlett.

Baumberger-Henry, M. (2008). *Fluid and electrolytes* (2nd ed.). Sudbury, MA: Jones and Bartlett.

Chiras, D. (2011). *Human biology* (7th ed.). Burlington, MA: Jones & Bartlett Learning.

Crowley, L. V. (2012). *An introduction to human disease* (9th ed.). Burlington, MA: Jones & Bartlett Learning.

Elling, B., Elling, K., & Rothenberg, M. (2004). *Anatomy and physiology*. Sudbury, MA: Jones and Bartlett.

Gould, B. (2015). *Pathophysiology for the health professions* (5th ed.). Philadelphia, PA: Elsevier.

Madara, B., & Pomarico-Denino, V. (2008). *Quick look nursing: Pathophysiology* (2nd ed.). Sudbury, MA: Jones and Bartlett.

National Cancer Institute. (2016a). Bladder cancer treatment (PDQ). Retrieved from http://www.ncbi.nlm.nih.gov /pubmedhealth/PMH0032608/

National Cancer Institute. (2016b). Renal cell cancer treatment (PDQ): Health professional version. Retrieved from http://www.cancer.gov/types/kidney/hp/kidney -treatment-pdq#link/_228_toc

National Cancer Institute. (2016c). Wilms tumor and other childhood kidney tumors treatment (PDQ): Health professional version. Retrieved from http://www.cancer.gov /types/kidney/hp/wilms-treatment-pdq#section/all

National Institutes of Health (NIH). (2002, November). Renal calculi. *Word on Health*.

National Institutes of Health (NIH). (2012). Urinary tract infection in adults. Retrieved from https://www.niddk.nih .gov/health-information/health-topics/urologic-disease /urinary-tract-infections-in-adults/Pages/facts.aspx

National Institutes of Health (NIH). (2013). Chronic kidney disease and kidney failure. Retrieved from http://report.nih .gov/NIHfactsheets/ViewFactSheet.aspx?csid=34&key=C

National Institutes of Health (NIH). (2015). Polycystic kidney disease. Retrieved from https://www.niddk.nih.gov /health-information/health-topics/kidney-disease/polycystic- kidney-disease-pkd/Pages/facts.aspx

Newman, D. K. (2010). Causes of acute incontinence. Retrieved from http://www.seekwellness.com/m /incontinence/incontinence-causes.htm

Professional guide to pathophysiology (3rd ed.). (2010). Philadelphia, PA: Lippincott Williams & Wilkins.

Resnick, N., & Yalla, S. (1998). Geriatric incontinence and voiding dysfunction. In P. C. Walsh, A. B. Retik, E. D. Vaughan, & A. J. Wein (Eds.), *Campbell's urology* (7th ed., p. 1045) Philadelphia, PA: W.B. Saunders.

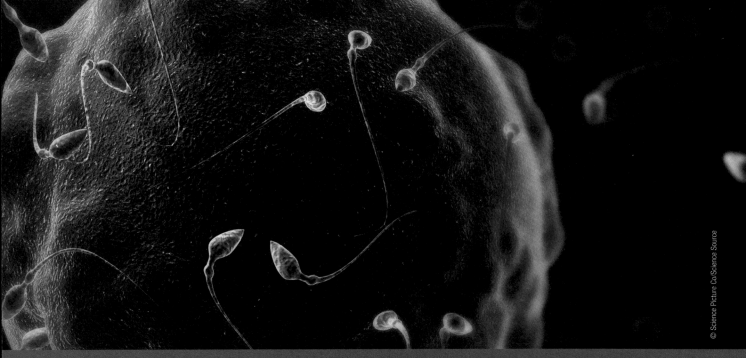

CHAPTER 8
Reproductive Function

LEARNING OBJECTIVES

- Discuss normal reproductive anatomy and physiology.
- Describe congenital reproductive disorders.
- Describe issues with fertility.
- Describe and compare common menstrual disorders.

- Discuss various disorders of the reproductive structures.
- Describe and compare infectious disorders of the reproductive system.
- Describe and compare cancers of the reproductive system.

KEY TERMS

amenorrhea	dysmenorrhea	human papillomavirus (HPV)	metrorrhagia
ampulla	ectopic pregnancy	hydrocele	mons pubis
anteflexed	ectopic testes	hymen	myometrium
areola	ejaculation	hypospadias	nipple
areolar gland	ejaculatory duct	impregnation	oligomenorrhea
ascending testicle	endometrial cancer	infertility	oogenesis
Bartholin's glands	endometriosis	labia majora	orgasm
breast cancer	endometrium	labia minora	ovarian cancer
candidiasis	epididymis	lactation	ovarian cyst
cervical cancer	epididymitis	latent herpes genitalis	ovaries
cervix	epispadias	latent syphilis	ovulation
chancre	erectile dysfunction (ED)	leiomyoma	paraphimosis
chlamydia	fallopian tubes	mammary glands	parturition
chordee	fibrocystic breast disease	mastitis	pelvic inflammatory
clitoris	foreskin	meatus	disease (PID)
condylomata acuminatum	genital herpes	menopause	penile cancer
Cowper's glands	gestation	menorrhagia	penis
cryptorchidism	gonorrhea	menstrual cycle	perimetrium
cystocele	herpes simplex virus (HSV)	menstruation	phimosis

placenta
polycystic ovary syndrome
polymenorrhea
premenstrual dysphoric
    syndrome (PMDD)
premenstrual syndrome
    (PMS)
priapism
primary herpes genitalis
primary syphilis
prodrome
prolactin

prostate cancer
prostate gland
prostatitis
recurrent herpes genitalis
rectocele
retractile testicle
retroflexed
scrotum
secondary syphilis
semen
seminal vesicles

sexually transmitted
    infection (STI)
shedding herpes genitalis
Skene's gland
smegma
spermatic cord
spermatocele
spermatogenesis
syphilis
tertiary syphilis
testes
testicular cancer

testicular torsion
testosterone
trichomoniasis
uterine prolapse
uterus
vagina
varicocele
vas deferens
vestibule
vulva
zygote

The reproductive system is composed of the structures responsible for procreation; therefore, a healthy reproduction system is necessary for the survival of the species. This system is responsible for transmitting genetic material to offspring (see the *Cellular Function* chapter). The male reproductive system generates sperm and transports it to the female reproductive system. The female reproductive system produces ova. When a sperm fertilizes an ovum, the female reproductive system nurtures and safeguards the embryo as it develops into a fetus, with this process lasting until birth. The primary difference between the two systems is the varying hormone levels, which cause the reproduction system to develop differently—the male reproductive system is generally external, whereas the female reproductive system is internal.

Anatomy and Physiology

Normal Male Reproductive System

The male reproductive system includes organs involved in the generation (**spermatogenesis**) and transportation of sperm. These organs include the penis, scrotum, testes, duct system, and accessory glands (**FIGURE 8-1**; **TABLE 8-1**). In addition to producing sperm, the male reproduction system produces sex hormones (mostly testosterone) that give males their distinct characteristics (e.g., facial hair, increased muscle mass, and low voice pitch). Parts of the male reproductive system work with the urinary system to aid in urinary elimination (e.g., the urethra). Because the male reproductive and urinary systems are integrated, disorders in one system generally affect the other system (see the

Urinary Function chapter for more discussion of the urinary system).

Penis

The **penis** is part of the male external genitalia; it contains erectile tissue that fills with blood during sexual arousal. The penis deposits sperm in the female reproductive system during sexual intercourse. The penis consists of three cylinders—the corpus spongiosum (which contains the urethra) and two copora cavernosa (**FIGURE 8-2**). The penis structure includes the root, shaft, and glans (enlarged tip). Penis length can vary considerably, but the average length is 2–5 inches when flaccid and 4–7 inches when erect. Penis appearance can also vary from person to person (**FIGURE 8-3**).

TABLE 8-1	The Male Reproductive System
Component	**Function**
Testes	Produce sperm and male sex steroids
Epididymides	Store sperm
Vas deferens	Conduct sperm to urethra
Sex accessory glands	Produce seminal fluid that nourishes sperm
Urethra	Conducts sperm to outside of the male body
Penis	Organ of copulation
Scrotum	Provides proper temperature for testes

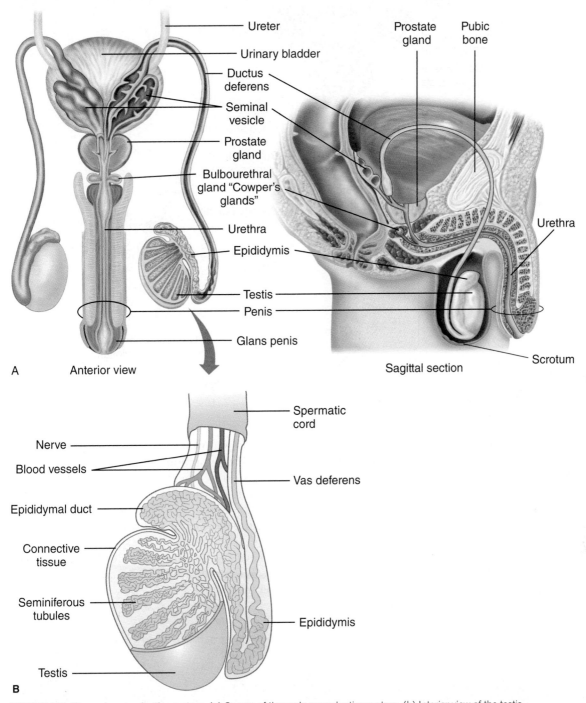

FIGURE 8-1 The male reproductive system. (a) Organs of the male reproductive system. (b) Interior view of the testis.

A sheath of loose skin, called the **foreskin**, covers the glans penis at birth. The foreskin is often surgically removed (circumcision) shortly after birth for hygienic, cultural, or religious reasons. The glans produces an oily secretion that can combine with dead skin to form a cheesy substance called **smegma**. If the smegma is not regularly removed from under the foreskin, the penis can become irritated and infected. The glans also has an opening, or **meatus**, that allows for **ejaculation** (propulsion of sperm-containing fluid) and urination.

Scrotum

The **scrotum** is a sac of skin just below the penis that contains the testes, epididymides, and lower spermatic cords. The scrotum maintains the proper testicular temperature for

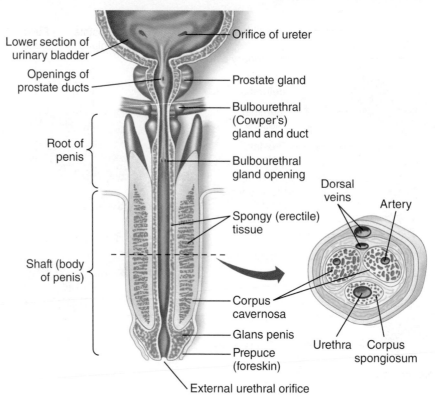

FIGURE 8-2 Anatomy of the penis.

spermatogenesis by contracting to draw the testes closer to the body to warm them, and relaxing to drop the testes farther from the body to cool them.

Testes

The **testes**, or gonads, produce sperm and the sex hormones. Spermatogenesis develops in most males by 16 years of age. The testes form in the abdominal cavity in utero and descend into the scrotum in approximately the seventh month of gestation when stimulated by rising testosterone levels. Occasionally, they will descend shortly after birth (usually by 3 months of age). Seminiferous tubules produce sperm, and the **epididymis** stores sperm until ejaculation (up to 6 weeks). The sperm mature during storage, making them capable of swimming. The testes can produce approximately 50,000 sperm per minute.

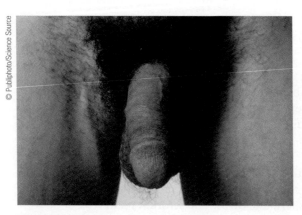
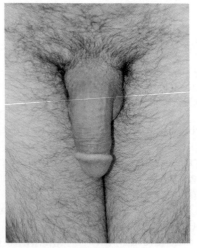
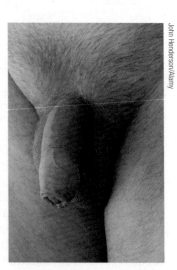

FIGURE 8-3 Variations of the male genitalia.

The testes produce hormones (especially testosterone) in their Leydig cells. Exposure to increased **testosterone** levels gives males their classic secondary sex characteristics (e.g., facial hair and deep voice) and sex drive. Testosterone also regulates metabolism and protein anabolism (encourages skeletal growth and muscle development), inhibits pituitary secretion of the gonadotropins (follicle-stimulating hormone and interstitial cell-stimulating hormone), and promotes potassium excretion and renal sodium reabsorption. Additionally, testosterone contributes to male pattern baldness and acne in some men.

Duct System

The male reproductive system contains a complex tube structure to deliver sperm from the testes to the female reproductive system. This duct system includes the epididymis, vas deferens, spermatic cord, ejaculatory duct, and urethra. Once they are mature, sperm leave the epididymis and travel to the **vas deferens**. The testicular artery and venous plexus, lymph vessels, nerves, connective tissue, and cremaster muscle (which contracts or relaxes the scrotum) surround the vas deferens; together, these structures make up the **spermatic cord**. The vas deferens widens at the prostate, forming a pouch called the **ampulla**. The ampulla joins the **seminal vesicles** (a pair of pouches that secrete an alkaline ejaculatory fluid containing sugar, protein, and prostaglandins to nurture and protect the sperm) to form the **ejaculatory duct**. The sperm and the ejaculatory fluid join in the vesicles to form **semen**. The semen flows from the ejaculatory duct to the urethra, where it is propelled from the penis during sexual intercourse.

Accessory Glands

The primary function of the accessory reproductive glands is to facilitate ejaculation. Sexual stimulation initiates the ejaculatory process. When a male is sexually stimulated, his sperm travel from the epididymis to the vas deferens and then to the seminal vesicles. Fluid from the **prostate gland** (a chestnut-shaped gland located at the base of the urethra) mixes with the sperm and secretions of the seminal vesicles. This prostate fluid further decreases the ejaculatory fluid's acidity, increases sperm motility, and prolongs sperm life. The alkaline medium counteracts the acidity of vaginal secretions that would otherwise kill the sperm. The **Cowper's glands** (two pea-sized glands found adjacent to the urethra) secrete another alkaline fluid into the urethra to neutralize acidity caused by urine transportation. The Cowper's gland secretions can sometimes be seen at the meatus before ejaculation. This secretion aids in lubrication of the penis during sexual intercourse and may contain some sperm left over from a previous ejaculation; therefore, these secretions can cause pregnancy even if the penis is withdrawn prior to ejaculation.

The actual expulsion of semen from the penis is the result of motor neurons stimulating muscular contractions of the glands and ducts of the reproductive system—particularly the ampulla, seminal vesicles, and bulbocavernosus muscle (the muscle surrounding the corpus spongiosum). During ejaculation, a valve at the bladder closes to prevent urine from entering the urethra and killing the sperm. An **orgasm**, the climax of pleasurable sensations, usually accompanies the ejaculation. Ejaculated semen contains sperm (about the volume of a pinhead) and secretions (about a tablespoon) from the seminal vesicles, prostate, and Cowper's glands. One ejaculation contains approximately 300 million sperm.

Normal Female Reproductive System

The female reproductive tract is a complex system that includes organs to manage the generation of eggs (**oogenesis**), transportation of eggs (**ovulation**) for fertilization (**impregnation**), support of fetal development (**gestation**), birth of the fetus (**parturition**), and feeding of the offspring (through **lactation**). To accomplish all these functions, the female reproductive system requires a delicate hormone balance and operational organs. These organs include the ovaries, fallopian tubes, uterus, vagina, external genitalia, and mammary glands (**FIGURE 8-4**; **FIGURE 8-5**; **FIGURE 8-6**; **FIGURE 8-7**). In addition to facilitating the system's function, the hormones (specifically estrogen and progesterone) produced by the female reproductive system give females their distinct characteristics (e.g., enlarged breasts, wide hips, and high-pitched voice).

The female reproductive system is located in a hub of activity in the body. This system is intimately intertwined with the physiologic functions of nearby structures in the female pelvis. The female pelvis contains organs of the urinary and gastrointestinal system along with organs for reproduction; thus, the female pelvis is the site for urination, defecation, menstruation, ovulation, copulation (sexual intercourse), impregnation, pregnancy, and

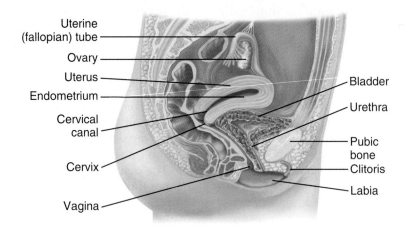

FIGURE 8-4 Side view of the female reproductive system.

parturition. Because of the close proximity of these three systems, problems in one system can lead to problems in the others.

Ovaries

The **ovaries** are paired, almond-shaped organs located on each side of the uterus (Figure 8-5; **FIGURE 8-8**). Two ligaments (suspensory and ovarian ligaments) and the mesovarium (fold in the peritoneum) hold the ovaries in place. The

ovaries produce hormones (primarily estrogen and progesterone) that regulate reproductive function and secondary sex characteristics (e.g., enlarged breasts, wide hips, and high-pitched voice).

The ovaries also contain the precursors to mature eggs (oocytes). During oogenesis, the oocytes mature into ova (mature eggs). By the 30th week of gestation, the female fetus has approximately 7 million follicles (biological

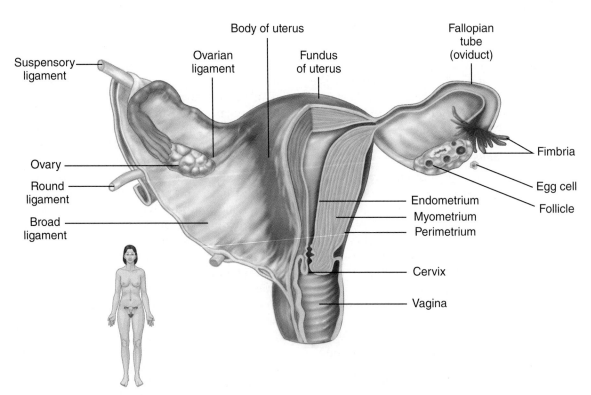

FIGURE 8-5 Front view of the female reproductive system.

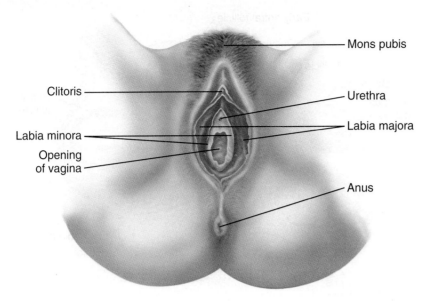

FIGURE 8-6 The female external genitalia.

units, each containing a single oocyte). These 7 million follicles degenerate to approximately 2 million follicles by birth. By puberty, only approximately 400,000 follicles remain. During the reproductive years, the follicles mature as they are exposed to pituitary hormones—specifically, follicle-stimulating hormone (FSH) and luteinizing hormone (LH). During the ovulation phase of the menstrual cycle, the mature follicle ruptures, releasing the

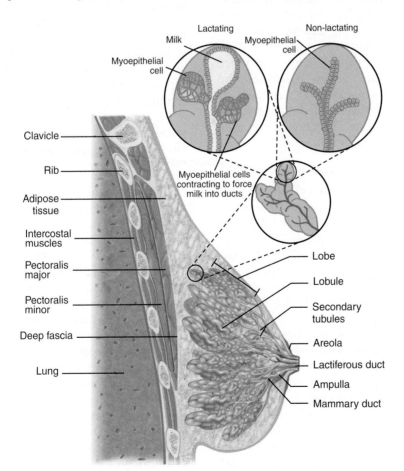

FIGURE 8-7 The female mammary glands.

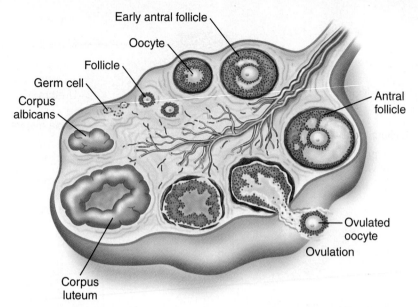

Early antral follicle

Oocyte

Follicle

Germ cell

Corpus albicans

Antral follicle

Ovulated oocyte

Ovulation

Corpus luteum

FIGURE 8-8 Structure of the ovary.

mature ovum into the fallopian tubes (**FIGURE 8-9**). The ovum travels to the uterus for fertilization by the sperm. Fewer than 500 of each woman's ova mature and become potentially fertile. Although approximately a dozen follicles begin developing during each cycle, usually only one makes it to ovulation. Multiple births (e.g., twins or triplets) may occur when more than one ovum is produced, released, and fertilized. Once the mature follicle releases the ovum, the empty follicle (called the corpus luteum) secretes progesterone to signal the endometrium to prepare for fertilization.

Fallopian Tubes

The **fallopian tubes** are two cylindrical structures that extend from the fundus of the uterus to near the ovaries. The ends of the tubes near the ovaries are fimbriated (fringe-like) to capture the ovum after ovulation. The tubes use a ciliary and muscular action to move the ovum toward the uterus as well as to assist sperm in moving from the uterus toward the ovum that is likely still in one of the tubes. If fertilization occurs, the same ciliary and muscular action moves the fertilized egg (**zygote**) from the tube to the uterus for implantation (**FIGURE 8-10**). Occasionally, the zygote does not reach the uterus but rather becomes implanted outside the uterus (called an **ectopic pregnancy**). The most common site for ectopic pregnancies is the fallopian tubes. Ectopic pregnancies cannot develop normally and can be life threatening.

Uterus

The **uterus** is a hollow, pear-shaped organ held in place by the broad, round, and uterosacral ligaments. Usually, the uterus is tilted forward (**anteflexed**) over the bladder, but it is tilted backward (**retroflexed**) in approximately 20% of women. Women with retroflexed uteruses are more likely to experience menstrual discomfort, but should not experience any unusual fertility issues.

During pregnancy, the fetus grows and develops inside the uterus. The thick uterine wall consists of three layers that serve to carry, nurture, and deliver the fetus.

- The **endometrium** is the inner mucosal lining of the uterus, which undergoes hormonal changes to facilitate and maintain pregnancy. During pregnancy, a vascular organ (called the **placenta**) develops to nourish the fetus through the umbilical cord (which contains two arteries and one vein). The placenta attaches to the endometrium on one side and surrounds the fetus on the other (**FIGURE 8-11**). The uterus expels the placenta within a few minutes after birth.
- The **myometrium** is the middle layer of the uterus; it consists of smooth muscle and a vascular system. During pregnancy, the vascular system radically increases to support the fetus. During childbirth, the myometrium contracts to push the fetus out through the vaginal canal. After childbirth or abortion (spontaneous or induced

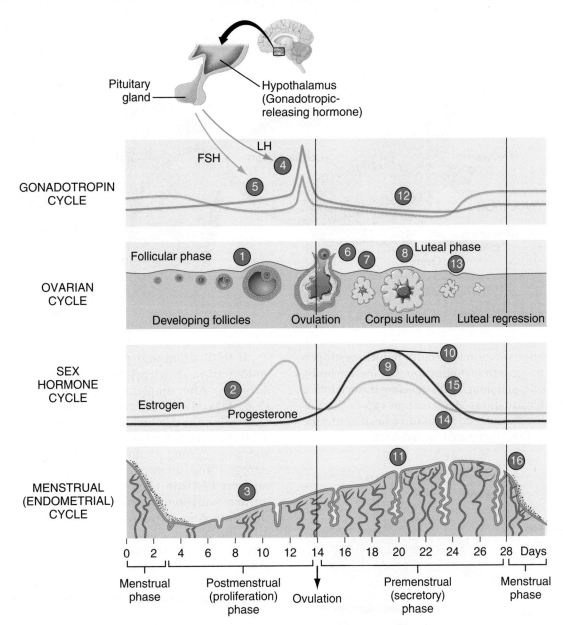

Pituitary gland

Hypothalamus (Gonadotropic-releasing hormone)

LH

FSH

4

5

GONADOTROPIN CYCLE

12

Follicular phase

1

Luteal phase

6 7

8

13

OVARIAN CYCLE

Developing follicles   Ovulation   Corpus luteum   Luteal regression

SEX HORMONE CYCLE

10

9

15

2

14

Estrogen

Progesterone

MENSTRUAL (ENDOMETRIAL) CYCLE

11

16

3

0   2   4   6   8   10   12   14   16   18   20   22   24   26   28   Days

Menstrual phase

Postmenstrual (proliferation) phase

Ovulation

Premenstrual (secretory) phase

Menstrual phase

FIGURE 8-9 The menstrual cycle.

pregnancy termination), this layer contracts to constrict blood vessels and control bleeding.

- The **perimetrium** is the outer, serous layer that covers all of the fundus and part of the corpus, but none of the **cervix** (the narrow opening from the uterus to the vagina). The incomplete coverage of this layer allows for surgical access into the uterus without requiring an incision into the peritoneum (the membrane that lines the abdominal cavity).

The **menstrual cycle** is a series of monthly changes that begin at puberty and continue through the reproductive years. The average age

of onset of menstruation (menarche) is approximately 13 years. Hypothalamus maturation and subsequent hormone increases trigger the menstrual cycle. Initiation of this cycle is marked by the onset of **menstruation** (shedding of the endometrium). The menstrual cycle is usually a 28-day cycle that consists of three phases—the menstrual, proliferative (estrogen dominated), and secretory (progesterone dominated) phases.

At the end of the secretory phase, the uterus is ready to receive and nourish a zygote. If fertilization does not occur, estrogen and progesterone levels increase, while FSH and LH levels decrease. Lower FSH and LH levels cause

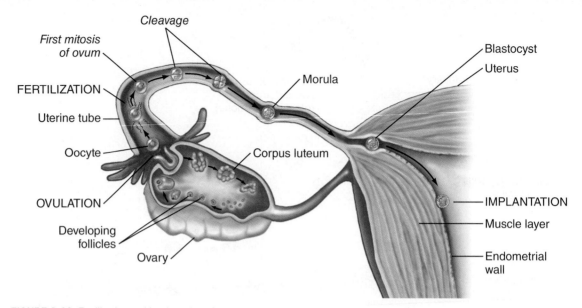

FIGURE 8-10 Fertilization and implantation of the embryo.

the corpus luteum to atrophy, reducing estrogen and progesterone production. The uterine lining thickens and sloughs off, signaling the beginning of menstruation. Menstruation expels the unfertilized ovum and maintains a healthy uterine lining that is prepared for fertilization.

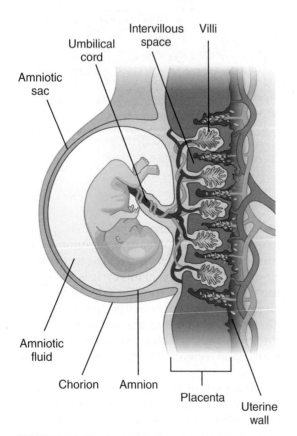

FIGURE 8-11 The developing placenta and embryo.

If fertilization and pregnancy occur, the endometrium thickens and vascularization develops. After implantation of the zygote (5–6 days after fertilization), the placenta secretes human chorionic gonadotropin to stimulate the corpus luteum to continue estrogen and progesterone production. The continued estrogen and progesterone production will suppress FSH and LH production, preventing further ovulation and menstruation. Human chorionic gonadotropin secretion continues until the placenta fully develops and begins making its own estrogen and progesterone, a phase that usually begins by the end of the first trimester.

The menstrual cycle continues to be repeated throughout a woman's reproductive years until estrogen levels begin to decline with age. As a result of the decreased estrogen levels, ovulation and menstruation become less frequent and more erratic. This change in the menstrual cycle usually begins between 45 and 55 years of age. **Menopause** refers to the complete cessation of the menstrual cycle. In addition to changes in the menstrual cycle, the declining estrogen levels associated with menopause can cause the following manifestations:

- Atrophy of the breasts and internal reproductive organs
- Decreased vaginal secretions (which can make sexual intercourse painful)
- Behavioral changes (e.g., irritability and depression)
- Headaches

- Insomnia
- Hot flashes
- Night sweats
- Decreased bone density

These manifestations can vary in severity, but in most cases they are mild and improve with time. Hormone replacement therapy can decrease severity of the symptoms, but careful consideration should be given prior to initiating such therapy because it is associated with an increased risk of breast cancer, thrombus (blood clot), and stroke.

Vagina

The **vagina** is a hollow, tunnel-like structure located between the bladder and the rectum and extends from the cervix to the external genitalia. This muscular canal is usually 2–4 inches in length, and it has the ability to expand in width (e.g., during parturition). The vagina serves as a passageway for sperm to travel to the fallopian tubes, for the body to discharge menstrual fluid, and to birth the fetus. Sperm enter the vagina when the male partner inserts his penis during sexual intercourse. Ejaculation propels the semen into this canal, where the sperm begin their journey to the fallopian tubes. In the mucosal lining of the vagina, **Skene's glands** secrete a protective, lubricating fluid during sexual intercourse. Tactile stimulation of the vagina is generally thought to produce the female orgasm.

The vagina may contain a thin connective tissue that covers the external vaginal opening to some degree, called the **hymen** (**FIGURE 8-12**). All hymens have openings large enough to permit menstrual flow passage or tampon insertion, but the openings are generally too small to permit an erect penis to enter without tearing. Tearing of the hymen does not usually cause significant discomfort, but it may cause a few drops of blood to be noticed. In addition to sexual intercourse, physical activity can partially or completely tear the hymen; therefore, the absence or presence of the hymen is not a reliable indicator of virginity.

External Genitalia

The external female genitalia contain several structures that are collectively referred to as the **vulva**. These structures include the mons pubis, labia majora, labia minora, clitoris, and vestibule. The size, color, and shape of these structures as well as hair distribution and skin texture can vary significantly from person to person (**FIGURE 8-13**). The **mons pubis** is the pad of fat over the pubic bone (symphysis pubis) that becomes covered with hair after puberty. The **labia majora** are the two large, fatty skin folds that protect the perineum and aid in lubrication; they become prominent and darkened after puberty. The **labia minora** are two small, firm skin folds just inside the labia majora; they have a rich blood and nerve supply. The two labia minora connect at their upper portion to form the **clitoris**. The clitoris is very sensitive to stimulation and becomes filled with blood during sexual arousal. It contains two corpora cavernosa, similar to the penis. **Bartholin's glands** lie just within the labia minor and provide lubrication during sexual intercourse. The **vestibule** refers to the area that contains the urethral and vaginal opening.

Mammary Glands

The **mammary glands** are located in the breast. Although both males and females have mammary glands, they are functioning structures only in females. The mammary glands are not a reproductive organ per se, but they can have a

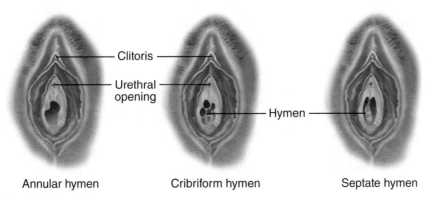

FIGURE 8-12 The various types of hymens.

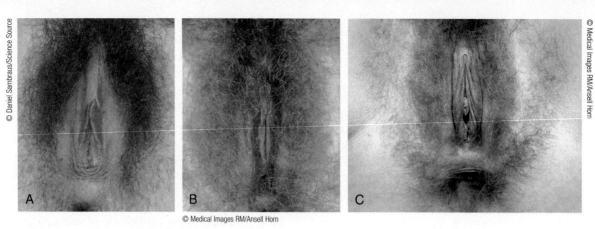

© Daniel Sambraus/Science Source

© Medical Images RM/Ansell Horn

© Medical Images RM/Ansell Horn

FIGURE 8-13 Variations of the female genitalia.

role in sexual arousal and provide nourishment to the newborn. Each breast contains 15–20 clusters of milk-secreting mammary glands that open into the nipple. The mammary glands do not make milk unless stimulated to do so. **Prolactin**, a hormone released by the anterior pituitary gland, prompts milk production. During pregnancy, increased estrogen levels trigger prolactin secretion, which matures the mammary glands and prepares them for milk production. After childbirth, prolactin secretion initially decreases as the estrogen levels return to nonpregnancy levels, but the newborn's suckling then stimulates increased prolactin production.

Each breast in both sexes contains a **nipple** surrounded by an **areola** (area of pigmentation). The **areolar glands** produce secretions that protect and lubricate the nipple and areola during breastfeeding.

Congenital Disorders

Abnormalities of the urinary and reproductive system are the most common congenital defects. Because of these systems' close relationship, an abnormality in one system will often lead to an abnormality in the other. Additionally, fetal development of both systems is intertwined. The reproductive system continues its development until birth; however, even though the system is formed at birth, it is incapable of reproduction until it matures during puberty. Numerous congenital disorders of the reproductive system are possible, most of which are structural problems. Some disorders cause mild symptoms (e.g., epispadias and hypospadias), whereas others may cause infertility and gender ambiguity (e.g., testicular or ovarian agenesis).

Epispadias

Epispadias refers to the condition in which the urethral meatus occurs on the dorsal (upper) surface of the penis instead of the end (**FIGURE 8-14**). The urethral opening may extend the entire length of the penis. Additionally, the penis may be shorter, be wider, or have an abnormal curve. Epispadias is rare (1 in 117,000 newborn boys) and usually develops during the first month of gestation (Jayachandran, Bythell, Platt, & Rankin, 2011). This malformation can also affect females (1 in 484,000 newborn girls), with the meatus often being placed in the clitoris. Epispadias is more likely to cause urination problems in men and sexual dissatisfaction in women. Men with epispadias are not necessarily infertile, but they may have trouble propelling the semen adequately during ejaculation. Both males and females with epispadias are at increased risk for urinary tract infections.

Urinary defects, such as bladder exstrophy (in which part or all of the bladder is present outside the body) (**FIGURE 8-15**), often occur with this type of congenital condition. Classic bladder exstrophy occurs in 3.3 per 100,000 births. Exstrophy–epispadias complex (EEC) refers to a spectrum of congenital abnormalities that includes epispadias, classic bladder exstrophy, cloaca exstrophy (the bladder and intestines are exposed at birth), and several variations. EEC occurs due to a rupture of fetal tissue (the cloacal membrane) during the first trimester. The prevalence of this condition ranges from 1 per 10,000 births (EEC involving classic exstrophy) to 1 per 200,000 births (EEC involving cloaca exstrophy).

The exact cause of epispadias and EEC is unknown, but these defects are thought to result from an event occurring early in pregnancy. Risk

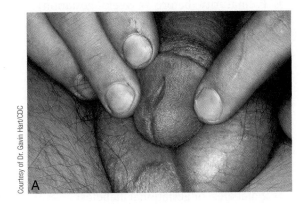

A

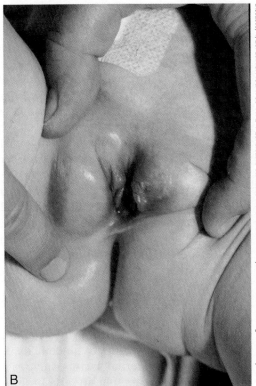

Reproduced from Ebert, A., Reutter, H., Ludwig, M., & Rösch, W.H. (2009). The exstrophy-epispadias complex. *Orphanet Journal of Rare Diseases*, 4, 23. doi:10.1186/1750-1172-4-23. Creative Commons license available at http://creativecommons.org/licenses/by/2.0

B

FIGURE 8-14 Epispadias. (a) Male. (b) Female.

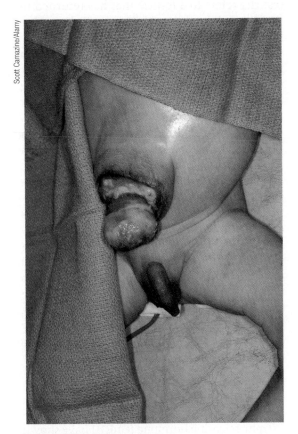

FIGURE 8-15 Bladder exstrophy.

factors include parental history of epispadias or exstrophy (500 times greater risk than the general population) and maternal factors including young age, high parity, and smoking.

Diagnosis of epispadias is typically made through a physical examination. Other procedures may be used to identify associated conditions and determine the severity of this congenital defect, including intravenous pyelogram (IVP) (X-ray of the kidneys, bladder, and ureters using radioactive isotopes), pelvic X-ray, computed tomography (CT), magnetic resonance imaging (MRI), and ultrasound of the urinary system and genital structures. In males, surgical procedures may be performed that use the foreskin to repair the defect, but urinary incontinence is common in postoperative patients. In patients with EEC, the goal is to protect the external structures (e.g., prevent injury, cover with plastic wrap, and mist tents) until repair can be done. Surgical repair of EEC may also include closure of the abdominal wall and urinary or intestinal diversions. Multiple procedures may be required to achieve the desired cosmetic outcome, urine flow control, and sexual function.

Hypospadias

Hypospadias refers to the condition in which the urethral meatus is on the ventral (under) surface of the penis instead of the end (**FIGURE 8-16**). According to the Centers for Disease Control and Prevention (CDC, 2016a), hypospadias is a commonly occurring congenital defect (5 out of 1,000 newborn boys). Like epispadias, hypospadias can vary in severity, and the opening can extend along the length of the penis. Males with this condition may also have a downward curvature of the penis, called **chordee**, that becomes apparent with an erection. Hypospadias does not usually affect females, but it can be the cause of gender ambiguity. This ambiguity may lead to inappropriate surgical gender assignment. Genetic studies prior to any gender assignment procedures can minimize this risk.

The exact cause of hypospadias is unknown, but it is thought to result from a combination of environmental exposure (e.g., medication exposure in utero) and genetic vulnerability. Risk increases with maternal factors such as age greater than 35 years, obesity, use of fertility treatments, and hormone therapy just before or during pregnancy.

Diagnosis of hypospadias is made through a physical examination. Imaging tests (e.g., MRI, CT, X-rays, and ultrasound) may be performed to identify other congenital defects. Surgical repair (often in stages) can improve the penis's appearance as well as urinary and sexual function. Surgery can be done as early as 4 months of age but should be undertaken before 18 months of age.

Cryptorchidism

Cryptorchidism is a congenital condition in which one or both testes do not descend from the abdomen to the scrotum prior to birth (**FIGURE 8-17**). Usually the undescended testes remain along the path of descent, but they can also deviate from that path (**ectopic testes**). Approximately 2–5% of full-term males are born with one or two undescended testicles. Rarely, both testes are undescended. Risk factors for cryptorchidism include:

- Prematurity (before 37 weeks' gestation)
- Low birth weight
- Small size for gestational age
- Multiple fetuses (e.g., twins)
- Family history of cryptorchidism or other problems of genital development
- Maternal estrogen exposure during first trimester
- Maternal alcohol use during pregnancy
- Maternal cigarette smoking or secondhand smoke exposure during pregnancy
- Maternal diabetes (type 1 diabetes, type 2 diabetes, or gestational diabetes)
- Parental exposure to some pesticides

Occasionally, a testicle that descended normally by birth may disappear later in childhood, often due to muscular reflexes that develop in puberty. A **retractile testicle** moves back and forth between the scrotum and the lower abdomen. In this case, the testicle is easily returned to the scrotum through gentle manipulation. An **ascending testicle**, or acquired undescended testicle, refers to a testicle that has returned to the lower abdomen and cannot easily be guided back into the scrotum.

Diagnostic procedures for cryptorchidism include a history, physical examination, self-testicular examinations (the condition places the individual at increased risk for testicular cancer later in life), abdominal ultrasound, MRI, laparoscopy (visualization using a small camera through a small abdominal incision), and open abdominal exploratory surgery. Additionally, hormone levels and genetic studies can distinguish potential causes and complications.

In most cases, the testes descend by 9 months of age without treatment. Cryptorchidism treatment should be done by 6 months of age to prevent permanent damage to the testicles and improve fertility during later life. Testes that do not naturally descend into the scrotum before birth are considered abnormal, and the individual is at increased risk for cancer and infertility even with repair. Treatment strategies include the following measures:

- Manual manipulation
- Hormonal therapy (specifically human chorionic gonadotropin [hCG] and gonadotropin-releasing hormone [GnRH] have shown promise in eliciting testicle descent)

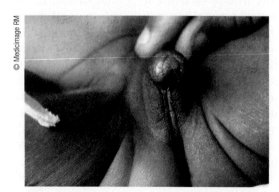

© Medicinage RM

FIGURE 8-16 Hypospadias.

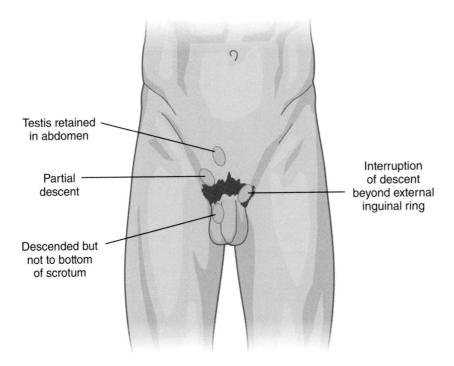

Testis retained
in abdomen

Partial
descent

Descended but
not to bottom
of scrotum

Interruption
of descent
beyond external
inguinal ring

FIGURE 8-17 Potential sites for cryptorchidism.

- Surgical repair (either laparoscopic or open)
- Orchiectomy (testicle removal)
- Testicle implants
- Hormone replacement (specifically testosterone if the testicle is removed or damaged)

Infertility Issues

Infertility describes a biological inability to contribute to reproduction. The ability to conceive and support a fetus requires functioning male and female reproductive systems. If a couple has been unsuccessful in conceiving after 1 year of actively trying, they should consult a fertility expert.

Male problems that can lead to infertility include decreased sperm or sperm abnormalities, hormone deviations, and physical impediments. Diagnostic procedures for infertility in males include a history, physical examination, sperm analysis, complete blood count (CBC), cultures of penal drainage (if infection is suspected), hormone analysis (e.g., FSH, LH, thyroid-stimulating hormone [TSH], testosterone, and prolactin), and imaging studies (e.g., ultrasound and vasography).

Female infertility problems include ovulation dysfunction, hormone deviations, physical obstructions (e.g., stenosis or tumors of the fallopian tubes or cervix), uterine defects (e.g., positioning or placenta development), and severe reproductive tract infections. Diagnostic procedures for infertility in females include a history, physical examination, ovulation testing, hyterosalpingography (X-ray of the uterus with radioactive isotopes), ovarian reserve testing (determines the quality and quantity of eggs available), hormone analysis (e.g., FSH, LH, TSH, prolactin, estrogen, and progesterone), imaging studies (e.g., ultrasound and hysterosonography), and genetic testing.

Treatment for infertility includes the following measures:

- Lifestyle modifications (e.g., weight loss, stress reduction, smoking cessation)
- Endocrinopathies
  - hCG, GnRH, testosterone, and estrogen supplements
  - Estrogen receptor blockers (increase GnRH secretion)
  - Dopamine antagonists (inhibit prolactin release)
  - Gonadotropins (stimulate gonadal steroid hormones)
- Immunotherapy for males with antisperm antibodies
- Alpha-sympathomimetics for males with retrograde ejaculation (closes bladder neck)

- Collagen injections to the bladder neck
- Sperm treatment to wash and concentrate sperm
- Antimicrobial therapy (if infection is present)
- Coenzyme Q (may increase sperm quantity and quality)
- Metformin (decreases insulin resistance, making ovulation more likely to occur)
- Intrauterine insemination
- In vitro fertilization

Erectile Dysfunction

Erectile dysfunction (ED), or impotence, refers to the inability to attain or maintain a penile erection sufficient to complete sexual intercourse. Although ED can occur at any age, this problem is most common in older men. ED can be transient or permanent, depending on the etiology. An erection results from psychological, neurologic, and vascular processes; ED can result from dysfunctions in any of these areas. Psychological causes include the following:

- Anxiety
- Depression
- Guilt
- Stress
- Feelings of inadequacy
- Relationship issues

Physiologic causes include the following:

- Circulatory impairment (e.g., arteriosclerosis)
- Diabetes mellitus
- Multiple sclerosis
- Prostate disease (e.g., benign prostatic hypertrophy or prostate cancer)
- Hypertension
- Neurologic dysfunction (e.g., spinal cord injury, Parkinson's disease, or cerebral trauma)
- Certain medications (e.g., antihypertensive and antipsychotic agents)
- Low testosterone levels
- Alcohol and tobacco use
- Liver cirrhosis

Diagnostic procedures for ED consist of a history, physical examination, hormone analysis (e.g., testosterone, LH, TSH, and prolactin), ultrasound (e.g., penis, testicles, transrectal), dynamic infusion cavernosometry and cavernosography (X-ray of the penis after injecting contrast dye into penile blood vessels), and specific tests for chronic diseases (e.g., diabetes mellitus, hypertension, and arteriosclerosis).

A variety of treatment options are available, some of which are costly and are not covered by most insurance plans. When ED has a physiologic origin, identifying and resolving the cause is the priority. Treatment strategies include the following measures:

- Psychological counseling
- Testosterone replacement
- Phosphodiesterase inhibitors (e.g., sildenafil [Viagra], tadalafil [Cialis], and vardenafil [Levitra])
- Other medications (e.g., adrenergic antagonists)
- Herbal remedies (e.g., ginkgo, ginseng, saw palmetto)
- Prostaglandin E injections directly into the corpus cavernosum
- Penis pumps (or vacuum devices)
- Surgical penile implants
- Vascular surgery

Disorders of the Testes and Scrotum

Disorders of the testes and scrotum are usually structural in origin, and some can cause infertility (e.g., cryptorchidism). These disorders can be acquired or congenital, and most can be resolved with minimal residual effects.

Phimosis

Phimosis occurs when the foreskin cannot be retracted from the glans penis. Not being able to retract the foreskin is common during the first 3 years of age, but the foreskin should become retractable as the child grows. Scarring resulting from poor hygiene, infections, and inflammation can all cause phimosis. Elderly men are at risk of this condition due to loss of skin elasticity and infrequent erections. Phimosis can lead to urinary obstruction and pain.

Paraphimosis refers to a condition in which the foreskin is retracted and cannot be returned over the glans penis. Paraphimosis may occur when the foreskin is forcibly retracted or when the patient or caregiver forgets to replace the foreskin during hygiene. In paraphimosis, the penis becomes constricted and the glans becomes edematous. If paraphimosis is not resolved, the lack of blood flow can lead to gangrene, making it a medical emergency.

Treatment strategies for both phimosis and paraphimosis include circumcision, topical steroid cream, and foreskin stretching.

Priapism

Priapism is a prolonged, painful erection. The unwanted, unrelenting erection is not a result of sexual stimulation. Priapism usually results from either too much blood shunting within the corpus cavernosum (referred to as nonischemic or high-flow priapism) or blood becoming trapped in the penis (referred to as ischemic or low-flow priapism). Priapism is most common in boys between 5 and 10 years old and in men 20 to 50 years of age. Priapism occurs in conjunction with a variety of blood, circulatory, and nervous dysfunctions:

- Sickle cell anemia (most common cause in pediatric cases)
- Leukemia
- Trauma
- Tumors (e.g., prostate, bladder, and renal carcinomas; melanoma)
- Diabetes mellitus
- Spinal cord injuries
- Neurologic diseases (e.g., multiple sclerosis and stroke)
- Medications (e.g., phosphodiesterase inhibitors, anticoagulants, and antianxiety agents)
- Alcohol and illicit drugs (e.g., cocaine, ecstasy, and marijuana)
- Poisonous venom (e.g., from a scorpion or black widow)

Diagnostic procedures can identify the type of priapism. They include a history, physical examination, abdominal and penile ultrasound, penile arterial blood gases (ABGs), CBC, toxicology tests, and CT. An erection lasting more than 4 hours is considered a urologic emergency, warranting immediate medical attention. Without medical attention, priapism can lead to ischemia, necrosis, ED, and infertility.

Treatment focuses on managing the underlying cause and varies depending on the type of priapism. Strategies for ischemic (low-flow) priapism include the following:

- Needle aspiration of blood
- Injection of medications directly into the penis (e.g., alpha-adrenergic sympathomimetic agents)
- Surgical placement of a shunt

Strategies for nonischemic (high-flow) priapism include the following:

- Cold application
- Lower abdominal pressure
- Surgical repair of trauma

Additional interventions regardless of type include the following:

- Analgesics
- Sedation
- Hydration
- Urinary catheterization

Hydrocele

A **hydrocele** is an accumulation of fluid between the layers of the tunica vaginalis (the membrane covering the testes) or along the spermatic cord (**FIGURE 8-18**). This condition can affect one or both testes. A hydrocele often occurs as a congenital defect, affecting approximately 10% of newborn males. In this case, the vas deferens does not close properly as the testes descend into the scrotum and fluid drains from the abdomen. A congenital hydrocele usually disappears without treatment by 1 year of age. An inguinal hernia—a condition in which a section of the intestine passes through the abdominal wall—commonly occurs in infants with hydroceles. Adult men can acquire a hydrocele because of inflammation, infection, trauma, and tumors.

Hydroceles are usually painless, but the scrotum feels heavy. The swelling generally worsens over the course of the day. This scrotum enlargement can be differentiated from other testicular disorders (e.g., testicular cancer) through transillumination (transmission of light through tissue). Hydroceles will transilluminate light, whereas solid tumors will not (**FIGURE 8-19**).

Diagnostic procedures for hydroceles consist of a history, physical examination (including transillumination), and ultrasound. In most cases, the hydrocele resolves without any action other than treating the underlying cause. Strategies to encourage reabsorption of the fluid include scrotal elevation (on a rolled towel), sitz baths (warm-water treatments for the perineum), and heat/cold application. Large amounts of fluid can compromise testicular blood flow, requiring aspiration or surgical removal (hydrocelectomy) of the fluid.

Spermatocele

A **spermatocele** is a benign, sperm-containing cyst that develops between the testis and the epididymis (**FIGURE 8-20**). Usually the cyst is painless and small, but it can grow quite large, leading to increased discomfort. Additionally, the cyst is moveable and may transilluminate light. The exact cause of this common condition is

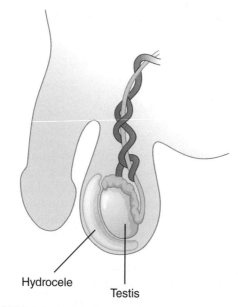

FIGURE 8-18 Hydrocele.

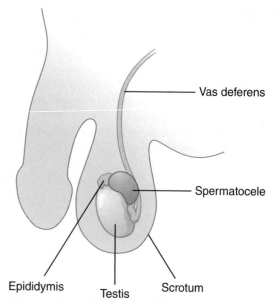

FIGURE 8-20 Spermatocele.

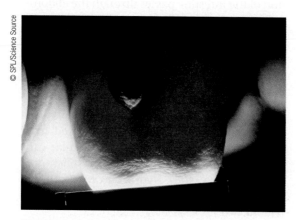

FIGURE 8-19 Transillumination of hydrocele.

unknown, but it is thought to be caused by a blockage of the duct system, infection, inflammation, or trauma. Diagnostic procedures are similar to those for hydroceles. The cyst usually does not cause problems but may require surgical removal (spermatocelectomy) if the cyst is large.

Varicocele

A **varicocele** is a dilated vein in the spermatic cord (**FIGURE 8-21**). Much like varicose veins in the leg (see the *Cardiovascular Function* chapter), this condition results from valve issues that allow blood to pool in the veins. These valve issues can be caused by congenital defects (e.g., incompetent or absent valves) or obstructions (e.g., tumors and thrombi). Varicoceles are more common in men ages 15–25 and are typically seen on the left side of the scrotum. For unknown

reasons, they occur more frequently in infertile men (approximately 40% greater risk). Additionally, varicoceles are the most common cause of low sperm counts and decreased sperm quality because of testicular ischemia. Varicoceles that appear suddenly in an older man may be caused by a renal tumor that has blocked blood flow. Varicoceles are much more common (approximately 80–90%) in the left testicle than in the right testicle because of several anatomic factors (e.g., the angle at which the left testicular vein enters the left renal vein, a lack of effective antireflux valves at the left testicular and renal vein juncture, and increased renal vein pressure). Some varicoceles may be mild and asymptomatic, whereas extensive varicoceles can be tender and painful. The dilated veins give the scrotum a "bag of worms" feeling upon palpation, and the blood pooling may give a sense of heaviness in the scrotum. Additionally, men with varicoceles may experience fertility issues.

Diagnostic procedures for varicoceles are similar to those for hydroceles. Treatment is often unnecessary unless the varicocele causes discomfort. Treatment strategies include scrotal support (e.g., wearing briefs or a jock strap), surgical repair (open or laparoscopic), embolectomy, and sclerotherapy (injection of an irritant into the vein that causes the vessel to harden and fade).

Testicular Torsion

Testicular torsion refers to an abnormal rotation of the testes on the spermatic cord

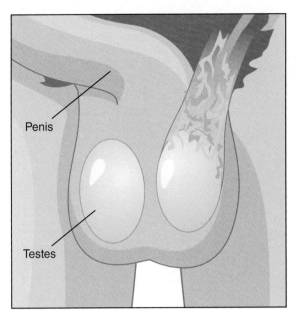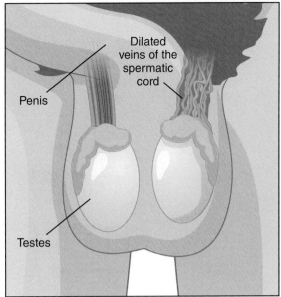

Dilated
veins of the
spermatic
cord

Penis

Penis

Testes

Testes

FIGURE 8-21 Varicocele.

(FIGURE 8-22). Sudden scrotal edema and pain develop as the twisting compresses the blood vessels, leading to ischemia and necrosis. Immediate treatment is required to restore blood flow and minimize testicular damage.

Testicular torsion is more common during the first year of life and at the beginning of puberty. It is most frequently caused by trauma, but can also occur after strenuous exercise or spontaneously, especially in males whose testicles are not secured in the scrotum due to congenital differences. The primary manifestation is sudden, severe testicular pain (usually unilateral) with or without a predisposing event. Other manifestations may include scrotal swelling, nausea, vomiting, dizziness, hematospermia (bloody semen), and a testicular mass.

Diagnostic procedures include a history, physical examination, testicular Doppler ultrasound (to determine blood flow), and scrotal ultrasound. Surgery will be required to treat testicular torsion and should be performed within 6 hours to prevent testicular necrosis. Manual manipulation may be used to untwist the testes, but surgery will be required to secure the testicle and prevent reoccurrence.

Menstrual Disorders

The female menstrual cycle can vary from person to person. The duration and the amount of menstrual bleeding fluctuate to some degree, but a standard pattern can be expected. The usual duration of menstruation is 4–6 days, and the usual amount of bleeding for the entire menstruation is approximately 30 mL. Irregular or abnormal bleeding may be harmless, merely uncomfortable, or an indication of serious problems. These conditions may or may not require treatment.

Amenorrhea refers to the absence of menstruation. With this condition, menstruation may have never occurred (primary) or may have ceased (secondary). The amenorrhea is considered primary if menstruation has not occurred by 16 years of age. Genetic disorders (e.g., Turner's syndrome) and congenital defects (e.g., uterine agenesis and hypothalamic conditions) can result in failure of menstruation to start when expected. Hypothalamic tumors, stress, sudden weight loss, extreme reduction in body fat (such as caused by eating disorders or incurred by athletes), anemia, and chemotherapy can halt menstruation by changing hormone levels. Normal causes of amenorrhea include pregnancy, lactation, and menopause. Management of amenorrhea focuses on identification and treatment of the underlying cause.

Dysmenorrhea is painful menstruation. Most women experience some discomfort during menstruation, but with dysmenorrhea, the cramping pain impairs usual daily activities. The pain begins at the conclusion of ovulation and continues through menstruation. Primary dysmenorrhea may appear at the first menstrual cycle and often has no known etiology. Dysmenorrhea may also appear later in life secondary to

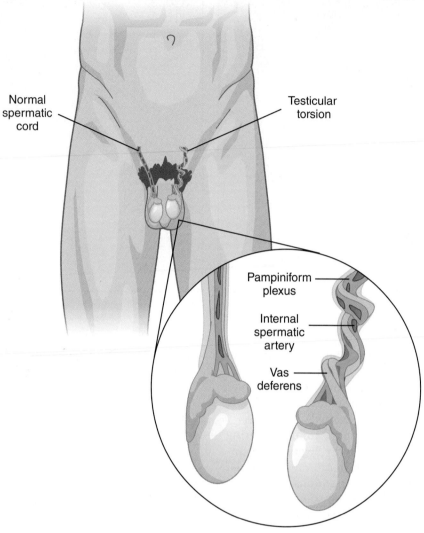

FIGURE 8-22 Testicular torsion.

a number of conditions (e.g., endometriosis or reproductive cancers). In many cases of dysmenorrhea (especially the primary type), the condition resolves following childbirth. Excessive prostaglandin secretion produces strong uterine muscle contractions and blood vessel constriction, intensifying the normal uterine ischemia associated with menstruation. These contractions and ischemia generate strong, intermittent abdominal pain that can radiate to the back, legs, and perineum. Excessive prostaglandins can also cause nausea, vomiting, diarrhea, headaches, and dizziness. Diagnostic procedures may be performed to identify the dysmenorrhea and underlying cause—specifically, a history, physical examination, pelvic ultrasound, laparoscopy, and hysteroscopy. Treatment strategies focus on relieving the discomfort and resolving the underlying etiology. These strategies include analgesics

(especially nonsteroidal anti-inflammatory drugs [NSAIDs] because they inhibit prostaglandin secretion), oral contraceptives (which prohibit ovulation), and heat application.

Several abnormal bleeding patterns are possible, most of which usually result from a lack of ovulation. However, these conditions can be related to hormone imbalances and pathologic conditions (e.g., reproductive cancers). Any changes in menstrual bleeding pattern warrant investigation. **Menorrhagia** describes an increased menstrual blood flow amount (approximately 80 mL per menstruation) and duration (usually 8–10 days). **Metrorrhagia** refers to vaginal bleeding between menstrual periods in premenopausal women. A short (less than 21 days) menstrual cycle, known as **polymenorrhea**, results in frequent menstruation; a long (more than 42 days) menstrual cycle, known as **oligomenorrhea**, results in infrequent menstruation.

Premenstrual syndrome (PMS) refers to a group of physical and emotional symptoms that affect many women for reasons not fully understood. According to the NIH (2013), approximately 15 out of 20 girls and women who menstruate suffer from some degree of PMS. PMS occurs more often in women between their late 20s and late 40s who have at least one child, a personal or family history of major depression, and a history of postpartum depression or affective mood disorder. Clinical manifestations of PMS include irritability, depression, mood swings, fatigue, headache, abdominal bloating, changes in bowel pattern, joint pain, breast tenderness, weight gain, and sleep disturbances; these symptoms usually begin 5–11 days before menstruation. Premenstrual dysphoric syndrome (PMDD) is a severe form of PMS that is characterized by severe depression, tension, and irritability. Diagnostic procedures for PMS center on a thorough history (focusing on gynecologic complaints) and physical examination. Treatment strategies are individualized and often include hormone therapy, diuretics, antidepressants (especially selective serotonin reuptake inhibitors), analgesics (specifically NSAIDs), and comfort measures (e.g., heat application, warm baths, rest, and light exercise). Additional measures include the following:

- Decreasing consumption of caffeine, soda, chocolate, fat, processed sugars, and alcohol
- Increasing consumption of fluids, specifically water and juice
- Eating small, frequent meals that are high in whole grains, vegetables, and fruit but low in sodium and sugar
- Supplementing vitamin B_6, calcium, and magnesium

Disorders of Pelvic Support

Muscles, ligaments, and fascia normally support the bladder, uterus, and rectum in the female pelvis. These supportive structures weaken with age, excessive stretching (e.g., childbirth), and trauma. Decreasing hormone levels at the onset of menopause can further atrophy these structures. With weakened support, the organs can shift out of normal position. In many women, more than one organ is affected.

Myth Busters

Menstruation has long been a source of myths, misconceptions, and old wives' tales. Because of their history, these misconceptions are often difficult to change.

Myth 1: You should not wash your hair or take a bath during menstruation.

There is absolutely no reason why you should not wash your hair or take a bath during menstruation! In fact, a warm bath may actually decrease discomfort by relaxing uterine muscles.

Myth 2: You cannot get pregnant if you have sex during menstruation.

Do not bet on it! While the odds of becoming pregnant are the highest near ovulation, pregnancy can occur anytime during the menstrual cycle.

Myth 3: Sex is unhealthy during menstruation.

Some women may feel uncomfortable having sexual intercourse during menstruation, but there is no medical reason not to have sex during menstruation. In fact, sexual intercourse may relieve discomfort.

Myth 4: You should not get your feet wet during menstruation.

There is no medical basis for this old wives' tale. This myth was made popular by some historical educational materials.

Myth 5: Women who are menstruating can catch colds easily and should avoid cold water or iced drinks.

Being cold may make abdominal cramping worse, but there is no increased incidence of colds during menstruation.

There are numerous other myths surrounding menstruation; these are just the more popular ones.

Cystocele

A **cystocele** occurs when the bladder protrudes into the anterior wall of the vagina. For this reason, a cystocele may be identified as a prolapsed bladder. The weakened pelvic support that results in this condition often results from excessive straining (e.g., childbirth, chronic constipation, and heavy lifting). The abnormal positioning prevents the bladder from completely emptying; therefore, recurrent cystitis (bladder infection) is common. Cystoceles vary in severity, and mild cases can be asymptomatic. Clinical manifestations of a cystocele include the following:

* Visualization of the bladder from the vaginal opening (**FIGURE 8-23**)
* Feeling of fullness in the pelvis or vagina
* Stress incontinence
* Urinary retention, frequency, and urgency
* Pain or urine leakage during sexual intercourse

Diagnostic procedures for cystoceles consist of a history, physical examination, and voiding cystourethrogram (X-ray of the bladder during urination). Treatment strategies include pessary devices (vaginally inserted rings that support the bladder), surgical repair, estrogen therapy (if the woman is postmenopausal), incontinence interventions (e.g., bladder training and protective garments), Kegel exercises (isometric exercises to strengthen the pelvic muscles), and avoidance of straining.

Rectocele

A **rectocele** occurs when the rectum protrudes through the posterior wall of the vagina. The rectocele may be large enough to bulge through the vaginal opening. Although any condition that strains the fascia can contribute to rectoceles, most occur after menopause because of decreasing levels of estrogen. Rectoceles may be

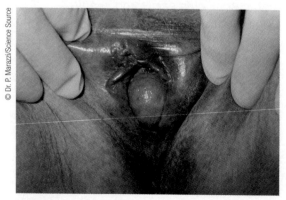

FIGURE 8-23 Cystocele.

© Dr. P. Marazzi/Science Source

uncomfortable, but they are rarely painful. Mild cases are usually asymptomatic, but when present, clinical manifestations include the following:

* Visualization of the rectum from the vaginal opening
* Feeling of fullness in the pelvis or vagina
* Difficulty defecating
* Rectal pressure
* Bowel incontinence

Diagnostic procedures for rectoceles are similar to those used for cystoceles. Treatment strategies include surgical repair, estrogen therapy (if postmenopausal), bowel training, and avoidance of straining.

Uterine Prolapse

Uterine prolapse refers to the descent of the uterus or cervix into the vagina. Uterine prolapse results from conditions that stretch or weaken the pelvic support (e.g., childbirth, aging, obesity, chronic cough, and chronic constipation). Uterine prolapse varies in severity and is classified using the following system:

* First degree—the cervix has dropped into the vagina
* Second degree—the cervix is apparent at the vaginal opening
* Third degree—the cervix and uterus bulge through the vaginal opening

Uterine prolapse is usually asymptomatic in its early stages, but as the uterus descends, clinical manifestations appear:

* Visualization of the cervix or uterus from the vaginal opening
* Feeling of fullness in the pelvis or vagina
* Difficult or painful sexual intercourse
* Vaginal bleeding
* Difficulty with urination and defecation

Diagnostic and treatment strategies for uterine prolapse are similar to those used for cystoceles and rectoceles.

Disorders of the Uterus

The uterus is a crucial organ for reproduction in females. Conditions that affect the uterus include benign or malignant tumors (e.g., leiomyomas and cervical cancer), congenital disorders (e.g., abnormal uterine positioning), infection (e.g., pelvic inflammatory disease), and hormonal imbalances that may affect menstruation and fertility.

Endometriosis

With **endometriosis**, the endometrium begins growing in areas outside the uterus. Although such ectopic endometrial tissue most commonly occurs in the fallopian tubes, ovaries, and peritoneum, it can be found anywhere in the body. The abnormal endometrial tissue continues to act as it normally would during menstruation (e.g., thickening, breaking down, and bleeding) even though it is outside the uterus. Without an outlet, the blood becomes trapped and irritates the surrounding tissue. Pain, cysts, scarring, and adhesions (fibrotic tissue that binds organs together) develop because of the inflammation, with the scarring and adhesions often resulting in infertility.

The exact cause of endometriosis is unclear, but numerous theories have been proposed. One theory holds that menstrual blood containing endometrial cells flows back through the fallopian tubes (retrograde menstruation), takes root, and grows. Another theory proposes that the bloodstream carries endometrial cells to other sites in the body. Other theories speculate that a predisposition toward endometriosis may be carried in the genes of certain families, or an inappropriate immune response may contribute to endometriosis development. Other theories suggest that certain cells (responsible for embryonic reproductive development) are present within the abdomen of some women and retain their ability to become endometrial cells with genetic or environmental influences later in life.

Risk factors for endometriosis include early onset of menstruation, late onset of menopause, nulliparity (never having had children), metrorrhagia, low body mass index, and having a closed hymen. Clinical manifestations depend on the severity of the endometriosis, but often worsen as the endometriosis progresses (**FIGURE 8-24**). Endometriosis begins developing at the onset of menstruation and advances over time. Most cases are diagnosed in patients between 25 and 35 years of age. Clinical manifestations of endometriosis include the following symptoms:

- Dysmenorrhea
- Menorrhagia
- Pelvic pain
- Dyschezia (pain with bowel movements)
- Pain during or after sexual intercourse
- Infertility

Mild

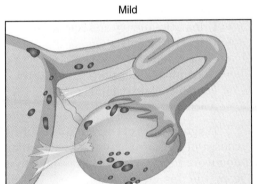

Moderate

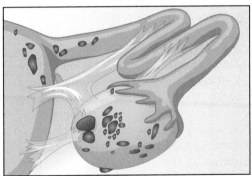

Severe

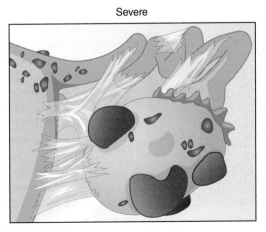

FIGURE 8-24 Stages of endometriosis.

Diagnostic procedures for endometriosis consist of a history, physical examination, laparoscopy, and pelvic ultrasound. Treatment strategies focus on minimizing discomfort and maximizing childbearing potential (if desired):

- Analgesics (particularly NSAIDs)
- Hormone therapy (e.g., contraceptive agents, gonadotropin-releasing hormone agonists and antagonists, and androgens)
- Surgical repair (laparoscopy or hysterectomy)

Leiomyomas

A **leiomyoma**, or uterine fibroid, is a firm, rubbery growth of the myometrium (**FIGURE 8-25**). Leiomyomas are the most common benign tumors in women, and they are classified according to their location (**FIGURE 8-26**). According to the NIH (2011), at least 25% of women have symptomatic leiomyomas, but as many as 50% of all women have "fibroids" (either symptomatic or asymptomatic) by the age of 50. Leiomyomas are more frequent in African Americans. Other risk factors include obesity, advancing age, hypertension, and nulliparity. The cause of leiomyomas is unknown, but most seem to grow during the menstruation years in the presence of estrogen and shrink after menopause. Tumor growth was thought to increase during pregnancy, but recent research suggests that growth actually levels off during pregnancy. Leiomyomas usually occur as multiple well-defined, unencapsulated masses. Although they do not usually interfere with fertility, they do increase the risk of spontaneous abortion and preterm labor slightly. The risk for fertility and pregnancy problems increases as the tumor size increases.

Most leiomyomas are asymptomatic and go undetected. Clinical manifestations depend on the leiomyoma size, which can range from

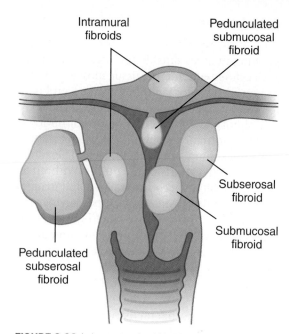

FIGURE 8-26 Leiomyoma classification.

microscopic to weighing several pounds. When present, clinical manifestations include the following symptoms:

- Menorrhagia
- Metrorrhagia
- Pain in the pelvis, back, or legs
- Urinary frequency and retention
- Urinary tract infections
- Constipation
- Abdominal distension
- Pain during sexual intercourse
- Anemia

Diagnostic procedures for leiomyomas consist of a history, physical examination, abdominal and transvaginal ultrasound, hysteroscopy (uterine endoscopy), biopsy (to rule out malignancy), laparoscopy, CT, MRI, and CBC. Generally, most leiomyomas are harmless and do not require treatment. Symptom severity and childbearing intentions should be considered when choosing treatment options. Treatment strategies include simple monitoring, hormone therapy (e.g., gonadotropin-releasing hormone agonists, progesterone, and androgen), analgesics (e.g., NSAIDs), surgery (e.g., myomectomy [removal of the fibroid] or hysterectomy), myolysis (laparoscopic laser treatment), endometrial ablation (using heat to destroy the uterine lining), and uterine artery embolization (which obstructs uterine blood supply). Additionally, anemia treatment (e.g., iron supplements and blood transfusions) may be necessary.

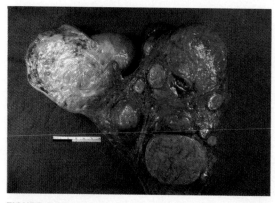

FIGURE 8-25 Leiomyomas.
© University of Alabama at Birmingham Department of Pathology PEIR Digital Library (http://peir.net)

Disorders of the Ovaries

A variety of benign and malignant conditions can affect the ovaries. Ovarian disorders can be congenital (e.g., hypogonadism and Turner's syndrome) or acquired (e.g., ovarian cancer), but many have a genetic basis. These disorders can affect the women's hormonal balance and fertility status.

Ovarian Cysts

Ovarian cysts are benign, fluid-filled sacs on the ovary. Often the cyst forms during the ovulation process. Instead of the follicle releasing the egg, the fluid stays in the follicle, creating a cyst (referred to as a functional cyst). In most cases, these cysts are harmless and disappear without treatment. On occasion, however, they rupture, causing discomfort. This common condition most frequently occurs during the childbearing years. Complications are rare, but ovarian cysts can lead to hemorrhage, peritonitis, infertility, and amenorrhea.

When present, abdominal pain or discomfort is the most prevalent clinical manifestation. Pain occurs when the cyst bleeds, ruptures, twists, or exerts pressure on nearby structures. Pain may also be associated with bowel movements and sexual intercourse. Other clinical manifestations include abnormal menstrual bleeding and abdominal distension.

Polycystic ovary syndrome is a condition in which the ovary enlarges and contains numerous cysts. Although the exact cause is unknown, this condition has been linked to hormone (e.g., androgen, estrogen, and LH increases; FSH decreases) and endocrine (e.g., hypothalamus and pituitary) abnormalities. Clinical manifestations include infertility (anovulation), amenorrhea, hirsutism (abnormal facial and body hair), acne, and male-pattern baldness. Polycystic ovary syndrome increases the risk for developing obesity, diabetes mellitus, cardiovascular disease, and cancer (especially endometrial and breast cancers).

Diagnostic procedures for ovarian cysts consist of a history, physical examination, abdominal ultrasound, CT, MRI, laparoscopy, CA-125 levels (to screen for ovarian cancer), biopsy (to rule out ovarian cancer), and hormone levels (including LH, FSH, estradiol, and testosterone). Most cysts will resolve in 8–12 weeks. When warranted, treatment strategies include the following measures:

- Hormone therapy (e.g., oral contraceptives)
- Analgesics (e.g., NSAIDs)
- Management of metabolic (e.g., diabetes mellitus) and other disorders
- Surgery (e.g., laparoscopy)

Disorders of the Breasts

Breast disorders can be benign (e.g., fibrocystic breast disease) or malignant (e.g., breast cancer), but most are not life threatening; however, malignancies should always be ruled out when breast symptoms are noted. These conditions can affect lactation, breastfeeding, and self-image.

Fibrocystic Breast Disease

Fibrocystic breast disease refers to the presence of numerous benign nodules in the breast. These firm, moveable masses become more prominent and painful during menstruation because of hormone fluctuations. This change in breast tissue is so common (affecting more than 60% of women) that many healthcare professionals consider it a normal variation. Although the exact cause is unknown, the condition is thought to be a result of hormones. Fibrocystic breast disease is more frequent during the childbearing years and is rare after menopause. Some contributing factors may be family history, a high-fat diet, consumption of chocolate, and excessive caffeine intake, but no scientific evidence has been obtained to confirm these links.

Clinical manifestations of fibrocystic breast disease usually worsen just before menstruation and ease just after menstruation onset. These manifestations vary in severity and include the following:

- Dense, irregular and bumpy breast tissue (usually more noticeable in the outer upper part of the breast)
- Dull, heavy breast pain and tenderness (usually bilateral; may be constant or intermittent)
- Feeling of breast fullness
- Occasional nonbloody nipple discharge

Diagnostic procedures for fibrocystic breast disease consist of a history, physical examination, mammogram, breast ultrasound, and biopsy (to rule out breast cancer). Usually no treatment is required. When necessary, treatment strategies are largely symptomatic and include needle aspiration of fluid, surgical removal of cysts, analgesics (e.g., NSAIDs or acetaminophen), a supportive bra, heat/cold application, limitation of dietary fat, and avoidance of caffeine and chocolate (although research is inconclusive about this strategy). Vitamin E, vitamin B_6, magnesium, and evening primrose oil may improve symptoms, but the use of these supplements remains controversial. Additionally, oral contraceptives can minimize symptoms.

Mastitis

Mastitis refers to an inflammation of the breast tissue that can be associated with infection and lactation. This condition usually develops within 6 weeks of childbirth. In most cases, a staphylococcal or streptococcal bacterium is introduced to the nipple through the breastfeeding process, but mastitis can also occur in the absence of lactation or breastfeeding. Impaired nipple or skin integrity increases the likelihood of mastitis developing. The infection usually invades the breast's fatty tissue, triggering an inflammatory response (e.g., edema, redness, warmth). The edema puts pressure on the milk ducts, causing pain and palpable lumps. Despite popular belief to the contrary, breastfeeding can occur in the presence of mastitis, but it may be uncomfortable. In some cases, however, flow of milk may become blocked and abscesses can develop.

Clinical manifestations usually appear suddenly and include the following signs and symptoms:

- Breast tenderness, swelling, redness, and warmth (FIGURE 8-27)
- Breast lumps
- Pain or a burning sensation continuously or while breastfeeding
- Flu-like symptoms (e.g., fever, malaise, chills, nausea, and vomiting)
- Nipple discharge (usually purulent)
- Enlarged nearby axillary lymph nodes

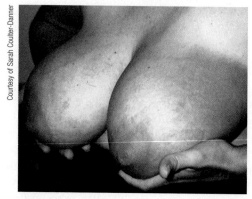

Courtesy of Sarah Coulter-Danner

FIGURE 8-27 Mastitis.

Diagnostic procedures for mastitis include a history, physical examination, and cultures (drainage and/or breastmilk). Treatment strategies consist of antibiotic therapy, adequate hydration, rest, analgesics (e.g., acetaminophen and NSAIDs), supportive bra, heat/cold application, adequate milk expression, and needle aspiration. During treatment, breastfeeding is safe and should be encouraged (except if the mother is HIV positive).

Miscellaneous Infections

Infections can occur at any point along the reproductive tract. Such infections often originate in the urinary tract, but reproductive tract infections can also migrate to the urinary system. Many of these infections are easily resolved, but if untreated, some can have detrimental effects (e.g., infertility).

Prostatitis

Prostatitis refers to inflammation of the prostate, which can be either acute or chronic. Prostatitis may be caused by a variety of conditions (e.g., bacteria, sperm, trauma, stress, and urinary catheter) that trigger the inflammatory process. The prostate has protective mechanisms to prevent ascending infection such as the flushing action of urination and ejaculation. Additionally, it contains secretions that have an antimicrobial action (possibly attributable to their zinc content). Owing to its close proximity to the urinary system, the prostate is often invaded by a pathogen from this system. Prostatitis is more common in young and middle-aged men, and immune-compromised states and a history of sexually transmitted infections (especially chlamydia and gonorrhea) increase the risk of this condition.

Prostatitis is classified into four categories:

- Category 1: Acute bacterial prostatitis
  - Usually seen in younger men
  - Usually results from a urinary tract infection (often *Escherichia coli*)
  - Least common
  - Easiest to diagnose and treat, but can be life threatening
- Category 2: Chronic bacterial prostatitis
  - Usually results from recurrent urinary tract infection
  - Relatively uncommon
  - Persists longer than 3 months
  - Indolent (causes little to no pain)

- Category 3: Chronic prostatitis/chronic pelvic pain
  - No clear etiology and may be noninflammatory
  - No bacteria are present, but immune cells can be found
  - Most common and least understood
  - Manifestations last longer than 3 months; can disappear and reappear without warning
- Category 4: Asymptomatic inflammatory prostatitis
  - No clear etiology
  - No bacteria are present, but immune cells can be found
  - May be associated with infertility

Clinical manifestations of prostatitis vary depending on the type. These manifestations include the following signs and symptoms:

- Dysuria
- Difficulty urinating, such as dribbling or hesitancy
- Urinary frequency and urgency
- Nocturia
- Pain in the abdomen, groin, lower back, perineum, or genitals
- Painful ejaculation
- Indications of infection such as fever, chills, and myalgia (with acute bacterial prostatitis)
- Recurrent urinary tract infections (with chronic bacterial prostatitis)

Diagnostic procedures for prostatitis consist of a history, physical examination (including a digital rectal examination), urinalysis, sperm analysis, cultures (urine and prostate discharge), cystoscopy, and transrectal ultrasound. Treatment varies depending on the type. These strategies include long-term organism-specific antibiotic therapy, analgesics (e.g., NSAIDs and acetaminophen), antipyretics, adequate hydration, sitz bath, and prostatic massage.

Epididymitis

Epididymitis describes an inflammation of the epididymis, the duct connecting the testes to the vas deferens. Ascending bacterial infections or sexually transmitted infections usually initiate this inflammatory process. Bacteria, most commonly *Escherichia coli*, frequently spread to the epididymis from the urinary system. Gonorrhea and chlamydia are the typical sexually transmitted culprits. Urinary tract infections are the most frequent etiology in older men, whereas sexually transmitted infections are more frequent in younger men. Rare triggers of this type of inflammation include tuberculosis and the antidysrhythmic medication amiodarone (Cordarone). Risk factors for developing epididymitis include the following conditions:

- Being uncircumcised
- Recent surgery or a history of structural problems in the urinary tract
- Urinary catheterization
- Sexual intercourse with more than one partner and failure to use condoms

The inflammatory and infectious process can lead to abscesses, fistulas (the cutaneous scrotal type), infertility, testicular necrosis, and chronic epididymitis. Clinical manifestations of epididymitis reflect the inflammatory and infectious processes:

- Indicators of infection (e.g., fever, chills, and myalgia)
- Scrotal tenderness, erythema, and edema (which can become severe)
- Prehn's sign (elevating the scrotum relieves pain)
- Penile discharge
- Bloody semen
- Painful ejaculation
- Dysuria
- Groin pain

Diagnostic procedures for epididymitis focus on identifying the causative agent and consist of a history, physical examination, CBC, ultrasound, urinalysis, cultures (urine and penile discharge), sexually transmitted infection testing (e.g., gonorrhea and chlamydia), and inflammatory markers (e.g., C-reactive protein and erythrocyte sedimentation rate). Treatment strategies center on eliminating the infection and decreasing discomfort. These interventions include the following measures:

- Antibiotic therapy
- Analgesics (especially NSAIDs)
- Bed rest
- Scrotal support (wearing briefs instead of boxer underwear) and elevation (on a rolled towel)
- Cold application
- Screening and treatment of sexual partners

Candidiasis

Candidiasis is a yeast infection caused by the common fungus *Candida albicans*. This condition usually occurs as an opportunistic infection (see the *Immunity* chapter) that can arise anywhere in the body (especially the skin and the gastrointestinal tract), but the focus of the discussion here is the infection's effects on the reproductive system.

In the reproductive system, candidiasis most frequently occurs in the vagina and is a common cause of vaginitis (inflammation of the vagina). *Candida* and many other microorganisms are part of the normal flora present in the vagina, which usually exist in a balanced state. Imbalance may occur in the presence of vaginal pH changes; normally, the vagina is slightly acidic. Antibiotic therapy can increase vaginal pH (making it more alkaline), leading to yeast overgrowth. Bubble baths and feminine products can also alter the delicate pH balance. Other factors contributing to such imbalance include decreased immune response (e.g., corticosteroid medications) and increased glucose in the vaginal secretions (e.g., pregnancy, oral contraceptives, diabetes mellitus, and obesity). Candidiasis is not sexually transmitted, but men may develop mild symptoms after having sexual intercourse with an infected partner. These symptoms in males will usually resolve without treatment.

Clinical manifestations of candidiasis include the following signs and symptoms:

- A thick, white vaginal discharge that resembles cottage cheese
- Vulvular erythema and edema
- Vaginal and labial itching (can be intense) and burning
- White patches on the vaginal wall
- Dysuria
- Painful sexual intercourse

Candidiasis can mimic other vaginal infections; therefore, diagnostic procedures are used as part of the differential diagnosis. Diagnostic procedures include a history, physical examination (including a pelvic examination), and discharge culture.

Treatment focuses on reestablishing normal flora balance, minimizing tissue irritation, and increasing comfort. Most cases of candidiasis can be treated at home and without medical supervision. Self-management is not recommended in the following situations:

- Symptoms are moderate or severe
- Fever or pelvic pain is present
- Negative history for candidiasis
- Pregnancy
- The presence or possible presence of other vaginal infections

If self-management strategies are not successful, a healthcare provider should be consulted. Treatment strategies can also be used for prevention of candidiasis:

- Antifungal agents (available in oral, parenteral, and vaginal cream or suppository forms; some are available without a prescription)
- Perineum care (including cleaning from front to back, keeping the perineum area clean and dry, avoiding soap and rinsing with water only, and taking warm—not hot—baths)
- Avoid douching
- Resist the urge to scratch
- Eat yogurt with live cultures or take *Lactobacillus acidophilus* tablets (these can also be taken with antibiotics to prevent candidiasis)
- Practice safe sex (tissue irritation increases the risk for contracting a sexually transmitted infection)
- Avoid use of feminine hygiene sprays, fragrances, or powders in the genital area
- Avoid wearing extremely tight-fitting clothing (which may cause irritation)
- Wear cotton underwear or cotton-crotch panty hose and avoid underwear made of silk or nylon (these materials are not very absorbent and restrict airflow, increasing sweating in the genital area and irritation)
- Use feminine pads instead of tampons during menstruation
- Control blood glucose (if diabetic)

Pelvic Inflammatory Disease

Pelvic inflammatory disease (PID) is a general term that refers to an infection of the female reproductive system. According to the CDC (2016b), PID diagnoses have declined in recent years, but an average of 5% of all U.S. women will have PID in their lifetime.

In this infection, bacteria usually ascend through the reproductive tract from the vagina. PID can be either acute or chronic, and most commonly results from a sexually transmitted infection (usually gonorrhea or chlamydia). Bacteria may also breach the reproductive tract during childbirth, endometrial procedures (e.g., surgery or intrauterine implants), and abortions (spontaneous or induced). Douching also increases the risk of developing PID. Acute bacterial invasions are more likely to occur immediately following menstruation, when the endometrium is more vulnerable. Less frequently, bacteria can invade from the circulatory system or surrounding structures.

Whatever its source, the infection triggers the inflammatory response, resulting in mucosal irritation, edema, and purulent exudate. The edema and exudate can obstruct the reproductive structures, and the exudate can migrate to the peritoneal cavity, increasing the risk of peritonitis (see the *Gastrointestinal Function* chapter). Abscesses and septicemia (bacterial blood infection) can develop and become life threatening. Adhesions and strictures frequently result from PID, leading to chronic pelvic pain, ectopic pregnancies, infertility, and problems with surrounding structures.

Clinical manifestations of PID vary slightly depending on whether the infection is acute or chronic. These manifestations include the following signs and symptoms:

- Indications of infection such as fever, chills, myalgia, and leukocytosis (with acute forms)
- Pain or tenderness in the pelvis, lower abdomen, or lower back (sudden and severe with acute forms)
- Abnormal vaginal and cervical discharge (usually purulent)
- Bleeding after sexual intercourse
- Painful sexual intercourse
- Urinary frequency
- Dysuria
- Dysmenorrhea
- Amenorrhea
- Metrorrhagia
- Anorexia
- Nausea and vomiting

Diagnostic procedures for PID consist of a history, physical examination, discharge culture, Papanicolaou (Pap) smear, CBC, pelvic ultrasound, CT, and laparoscopy. Aggressive treatment is necessary to prevent complications. Treatment strategies include the following measures:

- Antibiotic therapy
- Screen and treat sexual partners (to prevent spreading and reinfection)
- Practice safe sex (to prevent spreading and reinfection)
- Avoid douching (which spreads the infection to the upper reproductive tract)
- Treat abscesses (needle aspiration or surgical removal)
- Follow-up reexamination (to ensure that infection is completely resolved)
- Infertility evaluation

Sexually Transmitted Infections

Sexually transmitted infections (STIs), sometimes referred to as sexually transmitted diseases (STDs), encompass a broad range of infections that can be contracted through sexual contact (including oral–genital contact, anal contact, and vaginal intercourse). More than 30 different sexually transmissible bacteria, viruses, and parasites have been identified; some of these pathogens can also be transmitted from mother to child during pregnancy and childbirth as well as through blood contact (e.g., human immunodeficiency virus [HIV; see the *Immunity* chapter] and syphilis). Some STIs are easily eradicated with appropriate treatment (e.g., chlamydia and gonorrhea), whereas others persist for a lifetime (e.g., genital herpes and condylomata acuminata).

The CDC (2014) estimates that approximately 20 million new STIs are diagnosed each year in the United States—almost half of them among people 15–24 years of age. More than 110 million men and women are estimated to be living with an STI across the nation. Laws mandate that three STIs be reported to the CDC: chlamydia, gonorrhea, and syphilis. In 2014, increases were seen in the prevalence of all three of these nationally reported STIs. Other STIs are not required to be reported (e.g., genital herpes and condylomata acuminata); therefore, their actual prevalence may be much higher than the CDC's estimates.

STI prevalence rates vary depending on the geographic region within and outside the United States. STI rates have been increasing in the United States despite education efforts directed toward their prevention. Some of this increase may be attributed to changes in societal attitudes toward sex and pregnancy (e.g., less fear and more media inundation) as well as changes in screening practices.

Bacterial STIs

Bacterial STIs are common and are usually treated with minimal residual effects. Screening generally focuses on identifying the causative organism through cultures of exudate, rapid assay tests, and fluorescent antibody tests. Treatment of bacterial STIs usually requires a simple course of antibiotics. If taken properly, the antibiotics will resolve the infection. Reinfection is common, but it can be minimized by refraining from sexual activity until bacteria are eradicated, by practicing safe sex (e.g., using condoms and dental dams), and by sexual partners receiving treatment.

Chlamydia

Chlamydia is caused by *Chlamydia trachomatis*, an intracellular parasite that requires a host cell to reproduce. Chlamydia is the most commonly reported STI in the United States; more than 1.4 million cases were reported to the CDC in 2014. Chlamydia prevalence rates have been steadily increasing in the United States for the past 20 years (**FIGURE 8-28**). According to the CDC (2015), chlamydia rates are high across all groups and regions in the United States, but the burden of chlamydia is the highest in women, African Americans, and persons living in District of Columbia.

Chlamydia can be transmitted through sexual contact and from mother to child during childbirth. Many times, it is transmitted to the child in the form of neonatal conjunctivitis (an eye infection that can lead to blindness) and pneumonia. Complications of chlamydia include PID, epididymitis, prostatitis, infertility, neonatal conjunctivitis, and ectopic pregnancy. Additionally, the bacterium invades the epithelial lining of the reproductive tract, causing inflammation that can increase the patient's risk for contracting other STIs.

Often called the silent STI, chlamydia is usually asymptomatic in both males and females. When present, clinical manifestations include the following signs and symptoms:

- Dysuria
- Penile, vaginal, or rectal discharge (usually purulent)
- Testicular tenderness or pain
- Rectal pain
- Painful sexual intercourse

Because of this STI's high prevalence and potential to cause neonatal complications, it is recommended that all pregnant women be screened for chlamydia and receive treatment if they are found to be infected. Diagnostic procedures include a history, physical examination, and cultures. Treatment usually consists of antibiotics such as azithromycin (Zithromax), doxycycline, or erythromycin. Sexual partners should also be screened and treated. Additionally, avoiding vaginal childbirth by electing to have a cesarean section delivery may decrease mother-to-child transmission rates.

Gonorrhea

Gonorrhea (referred to colloquially as the clap) is caused by *Neisseria gonorrhoeae*, an aerobic bacterium that has developed many drug-resistant strains. Although rates of gonorrhea had been declining for 20 years (**FIGURE 8-29**), incidence of this STI seems to have started increasing again; gonorrhea remains a very commonly reported disease to the CDC. According to the CDC (2014), gonorrhea rates are highest in men, American Indians/Alaska Natives, and persons living in District of Columbia.

The *N. gonorrhoeae* bacterium attaches to the epithelial mucosa of the vagina, mouth, or anus, causing irritation and inflammation. Gonorrhea is transmissible through sexual contact and from mother to infant during childbirth. Mother-to-child transmission usually results in neonatal conjunctivitis. Outside the body, the bacterium dies within a few seconds.

Complications of gonorrhea include PID, epididymitis, prostatitis, infertility, neonatal conjunctivitis, and ectopic pregnancy. Additionally, gonorrhea can spread to other locations in the body; in such a case, complications may include arthritis (usually of the hands, wrists, ankles, knees, and elbows), dermatitis

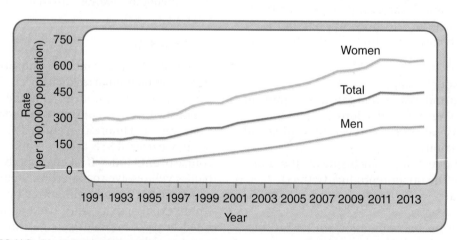

FIGURE 8-28 U.S. chlamydia prevalence rates.

Reproduced from Centers for Disease Control and Prevention. (2015). Sexually transmitted disease surveillance. Retrieved from https://www.cdc.gov/std/stats14/figures/1.htm

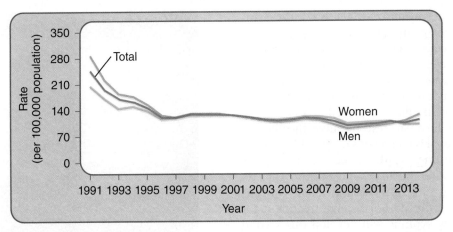

FIGURE 8-29 U.S. gonorrhea prevalence rates.

Reproduced from Centers for Disease Control and Prevention. (2015). Sexually transmitted disease surveillance. Retrieved from http://www.cdc.gov/std/stats14/figures/13.htm

(usually of the hands and lower extremities), and endocarditis.

Gonorrhea is often asymptomatic. Clinical manifestations, if they occur, usually do not appear until 2–10 days after the infection has taken hold. Men are more likely than women to experience symptoms. When present, clinical manifestations include the following signs and symptoms:

- Dysuria
- Urinary frequency or urgency
- Penile, vaginal, or rectal discharge (white, yellow, or green) (colloquially referred to as the drip) (**FIGURE 8-30**)
- Redness or edema at the urinary meatus (in men)
- Testicular tenderness or pain
- Rectal pain
- Painful sexual intercourse
- Pharyngitis
- White blisters that darken and disappear (Figure 8-30)

Diagnostic procedures include a history, physical examination, and cultures. Treatment for gonorrhea usually consists of antibiotics such as azithromycin (Zithromax), doxycycline, or erythromycin.

Syphilis

Syphilis is an ulcerative infection caused by *Treponema pallidum*, a spiral-shaped (spirochete) bacterium that requires a warm, moist environment to survive (**FIGURE 8-31**). Syphilis is transmitted through skin or mucous membrane contact with infected, ulcerative lesions (**chancres**). Additionally, the bacterium can cross from the mother through the placental barrier to the fetus after the fourth month of gestation (congenital syphilis). Syphilitic lesions also provide an opportunity for other STIs to invade.

Syphilis occurs in several stages, each with its own clinical manifestations:

- **Primary syphilis** is the first stage. Painless chancres (usually one) form at the site of infection about 2–3 weeks after the initial

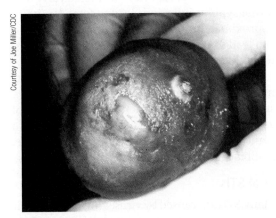

FIGURE 8-30 Characteristic lesions and discharge associated with gonorrhea.

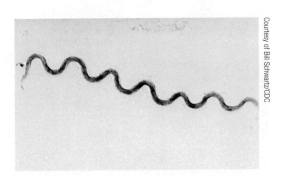

FIGURE 8-31 *Treponema pallidum*, the spirochete that causes syphilis.

infection is acquired (**FIGURE 8-32**). The chancres often go unnoticed and disappear about 4–6 weeks later, even without treatment. The bacteria become dormant, and no other symptoms are present. Because the individual may not test positive during this stage, the test should be repeated at a later date. Even if he or she tests negative, the infected individual is contagious during this stage.

- **Secondary syphilis** occurs about 2–8 weeks after the first chancres form. Approximately 33% of those individuals with infection who do not receive treatment for primary syphilis will develop this second stage, which is characterized by a generalized, nonpruritic, brown-red rash (**FIGURE 8-33**). Other symptoms include malaise, fever, and patchy hair loss. These symptoms will often go away without treatment, and again, the bacteria become dormant. The individual will test positive (if untreated) and is contagious during this stage, especially with direct contact with the rash.

- **Latent or tertiary syphilis** is the final stage of syphilis. The early latency stage begins when the secondary symptoms disappear and lasts 1–4 years. The late latency stage can last for years as the infection spreads to the brain, nervous system, heart, skin, and bones. The infection can cause blindness, paralysis, dementia, cardiovascular disease, pathological fractures, and death. The individual will test positive (if untreated) and is contagious only during the early part of this stage.

Syphilis prevalence rates in the United States have remained constant for the last 50 years for all three stages (**FIGURE 8-34**). According to the CDC (2014), syphilis rates are highest in men, American Indians/Alaska Natives, men

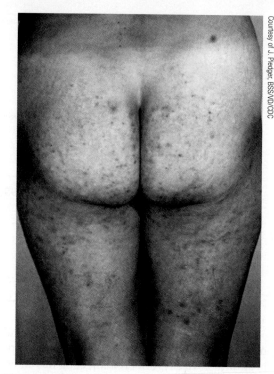

FIGURE 8-33 Skin rash characteristic of secondary syphilis.

who have sex with men (MSM), and persons living in the District of Columbia.

In utero, the fetus is protected from syphilis by a membrane known as Langhans layer for the first 4 months of the pregnancy. Consequently, screening and treating the mother prior to the fourth month of gestation can significantly decrease the likelihood that the fetus will contract the infection. Diagnostic procedures include a history, physical examination, and serum antibodies (e.g., Venereal Disease Research Laboratory [VDRL] test or rapid plasma reagin [RPR]). Positive (if treated) and high-risk women should be retested for syphilis in the last trimester of the pregnancy. Untreated early maternal syphilis infections lead to fetal demise in approximately 40% of cases. Congenital syphilis can lead to multiple defects affecting the bones, teeth, liver, lungs, and nervous system.

For nonpregnant women and men, treatment should begin early—at the first sign of a suspicious lesion. Treatment usually consists of antibiotics such as penicillin (preferred), a penicillin derivative, doxycycline, or tetracycline. Antibiotics are useless for latent-phase syphilis.

Viral STIs

Many STIs are caused by viruses. In terms of their severity, these infections can range from minor (e.g., condylomata acuminata) to life threatening

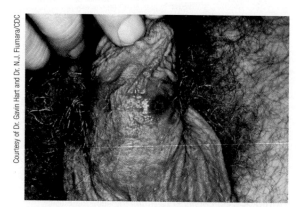

FIGURE 8-32 Chancre characteristic of primary syphilis.

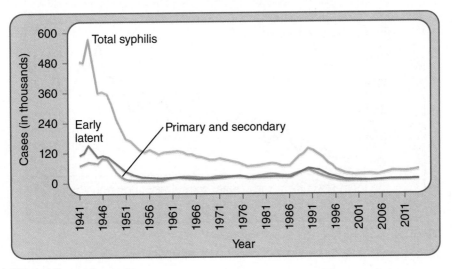

FIGURE 8-34 U.S. syphilis prevalence rates.

Reproduced from Centers for Disease Control and Prevention. (2015). Sexually transmitted disease surveillance. Retrieved from http://www.cdc.gov/std/stats14/figures/31.htm

(e.g., HIV). Viral STIs can also lead to several reproductive cancers (e.g., human papillomavirus). These types of infections are the most difficult STIs to treat because viruses are highly adaptive and elusive. Treatment options for the various infections depend on the causative virus.

Genital Herpes

Genital herpes is an infection that causes blisters (vesicles) on the genitals and in the reproductive tract. Genital herpes is caused by the **herpes simplex virus (HSV)**, which belongs to a family containing more than 70 herpes viruses. Some more common viruses in this family include cytomegalovirus (which can cause mental retardation and fetal demise with maternal infections), varicella-zoster virus (which causes chickenpox and shingles), and Epstein-Barr virus (which can cause lymphoma).

HSV occurs in two forms—HSV type 1 and HSV type 2. Generally, HSV type 1 infections occur above the waist, whereas HSV type 2 infections occur below the waist. HSV type 1 infection most frequently manifests as a cold sore (a small blister on the mouth or nose). Most cases of genital herpes (70%) are caused by HSV type 2. HSV type 2 infections can also spread above the waist, and HSV type 1 infections can spread below the waist through oral–genital sexual contact. HSV type 2 is also transmissible through direct skin-to-skin contact. Although the risk of transmission is greatest when lesions are present, HSV can be spread when lesions are not apparent. HSV type 2 is also transmissible from mother to child.

Contracting genital herpes during pregnancy creates the greatest risk to the fetus (e.g., spontaneous abortion). HSV can also be transmitted to the infant during childbirth if an active genital herpes infection is present at the time of delivery. Transmission of this infection during childbirth can result in encephalitis and brain damage. If lesions are present at the time of birth, a cesarean section should be performed to minimize these risks. Rarely, HSV can be transmitted to the fetus through the placenta, causing an infection prior to birth. Pregnant women should be monitored for genital herpes throughout their pregnancy.

Genital herpes is not a reportable disease to the CDC; however, data from healthcare clinics indicate that the prevalence of genital herpes has been increasing for the last 50 years, albeit with declining numbers of cases (incidence) occurring in the most recent years (**FIGURE 8-35**). According to the CDC (2014), rates of genital herpes are highest in women and African Americans.

Both types of HSV infections are characterized by recurrent episodes of the lesions. Most people with HSV type 2 will experience reoccurrence of the lesions; however, recurrence is much less frequent with HSV type 1. The virus causes an initial infection at the entry site, but then travels along the dermatome to the nerve root, where it remains protected and dormant until the next outbreak (reoccurrence), which will occur at the same site. In either case, the lesions appear and progress similarly. Recurrent episodes begin with a tingling or burning sensation at the site just before the lesion appears (**prodrome**). The lesions first appear as vesicles surrounded by erythema. These vesicles rupture,

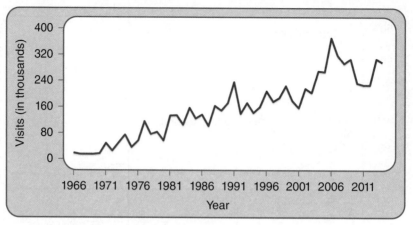

FIGURE 8-35 Genital herpes–related clinic visits in the United States.

leaving behind a painful ulcerative lesion with watery exudate (**FIGURE 8-36**). Ultimately, a crust forms over the ulcer, and it heals spontaneously in 3–4 weeks. Because genital herpes creates an opening in the skin, the individual is at risk for contracting other STIs.

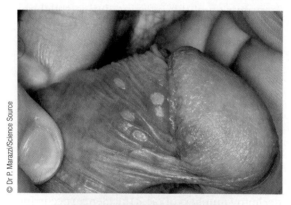

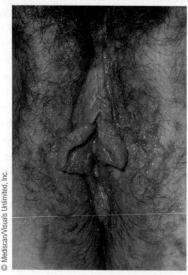

FIGURE 8-36 Genital herpes blisters on the external genitalia.

Genital herpes progresses through four stages:

1. **Primary herpes genitalis** is the first stage. This stage begins at the actual time of infection and antibody development. The time from exposure to this primary infection can range from 2 to 20 days. This first occurrence of the infection can be either very painful or completely asymptomatic (75% of cases). When present, clinical manifestations associated with this stage include a painful lesion, malaise, low-grade fever, and groin lymph node enlargement.
2. **Latent herpes genitalis** begins once the antibodies are formed. Antibodies do not protect an individual against reinfection, but they do tend to make the recurrent episodes less severe. During this phase, the virus travels up the nerve root and becomes dormant (**FIGURE 8-37**). The individual is asymptomatic while the virus is dormant.
3. **Shedding herpes genitalis** is the third stage. During this stage, the virus is reactivated but produces no symptoms. It is being excreted from the body, however, and can be transmitted to another person through sexual contact. This stage occurs infrequently—in fewer than 1% of cases.
4. **Recurrent herpes genitalis** is characterized by the reactivation of the virus and clinical manifestations. During this stage, the virus travels back down the nerve root to the skin and causes a blister at the same site as with the first stage. The number of reoccurrences varies from none to many in a lifetime. Factors that can trigger a reoccurrence include stress, menstruation, and illness.

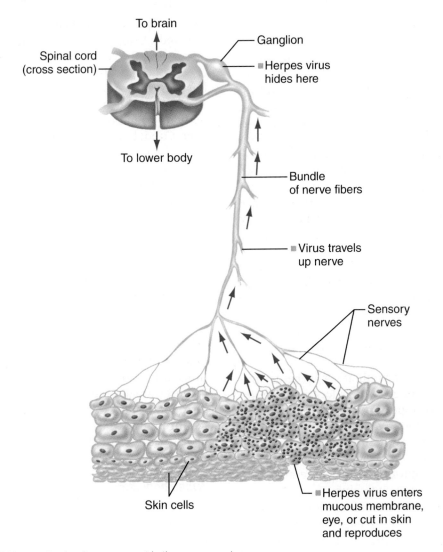

To brain

Spinal cord
(cross section)

Ganglion

■ Herpes virus
hides here

To lower body

Bundle
of nerve fibers

■ Virus travels
up nerve

Sensory
nerves

Skin cells

■ Herpes virus enters
mucous membrane,
eye, or cut in skin
and reproduces

FIGURE 8-37 Herpes simplex virus movement in the nervous system.

Diagnostic procedures for genital herpes include a history, physical examination, tissue and secretion cultures, Pap smears, and polymerase chain reaction test (which detects the presence of HSV and determines type). Genital herpes is a significant public concern because the lesions and symptoms are not always apparent, transmission can occur with or without symptoms, and no cure exists. Genital herpes can cause a great deal of psychological stress for patients because of the ongoing fear of outbreaks and the need to disclose the information about their infection status to partners.

Treatment options (e.g., antiviral medications) that can suppress the number of outbreaks as well as minimize the severity and duration of reoccurrences are available. Avoiding reoccurrence triggers, especially stress, can also prevent outbreaks. Implementing stress reduction strategies (e.g., yoga, meditation, journaling, and distraction) is advised. Secondary bacterial infections can develop from the lesions, so proper hygiene (e.g., washing the area with soap and water several times a day, keeping the area dry, and wearing loose-fitting clothing and cotton underwear) is advised during outbreaks. Additionally, genital herpes increases the risk for reproductive cancers in women (especially cervical cancer), so Pap smears should be performed every 6–12 months. Because the risk of transmission is highest when lesions are present, sexual activity should be avoided during outbreaks. Due to the lifelong implications of genital herpes, prevention is the best treatment strategy. Prevention strategies center on safe sex practices (e.g., using condoms, limiting sexual partners).

Condylomata Acuminata

Condylomata acuminata, or genital warts, are benign growths caused by **human papillomavirus (HPV)**. More than 70 different types of HPV exist, several of which can cause condylomata acuminata. Condylomata acuminata can occur on the external genitals, vaginal wall, cervix, anus, thighs, lips, mouth, and throat. In addition to condylomata acuminata, HPV infection can lead to the development of reproductive (e.g., cervical and penile) and anal cancers. HPV can have an incubation period that lasts up to 6 months. The immune system clears most HPV within 2 years (about 90%), though some infections persist.

Most sexually active men and women will contract HPV at some point in their lives. Condylomata acuminata are not reportable to the CDC; however, data from healthcare clinics indicate that condylomata acuminata prevalence has been increasing for nearly 50 years (**FIGURE 8-38**).

Condylomata acuminata may be asymptomatic, depending on their location. The lesions vary in appearance, texture, and size (**FIGURE 8-39**; **FIGURE 8-40**). Growths can be raised, flat, rough, smooth, flesh-colored, white, gray, pink, cauliflower-like, large, or barely visible. Additional symptoms may include abnormal bleeding, discharge, or itching.

Diagnostic procedures for condylomata acuminata include a history, physical examination, Pap smear, tissue biopsy, and polymerase chain reaction test. While there are no treatments for HPV itself, treatments exist for the serious conditions that HPV can cause. A vaccine is available to prevent HPV infections. Because of the cancer risk, this vaccine is recommended for both males and females (ideally to be administered around 11 or 12 years of age, before sexual activity is initiated). Using condoms and dental dams can also reduce the risk of HPV transmission.

Most condylomata acuminata are harmless, but they can be removed for aesthetic purposes. Removal of the growths will not cure the underlying condition, so the growths may reappear. Condylomata acuminata can be removed using chemicals (e.g., podophyllin), cryosurgery (freezing the tissue with liquid nitrogen), electrocauterization (heating the tissue with electricity), laser therapy (burning the tissue with a light), or surgical excision.

As with other STIs, sexual partners of individuals with HPV infection should also be screened and treated. Condylomata acuminata can be fatal if transmitted to infants at birth, so cesarean section deliveries are advised for pregnant women with this STI.

Protozoan STIs

Like candidiasis infections, protozoan infections often arise when the body's natural defenses are altered; unlike candidiasis, however, some of these infections can be transmitted through sexual contact. Protozoan STIs are usually easily treated and resolve with minimal issues.

Trichomoniasis

Trichomoniasis (colloquially referred to as the trich) is caused by *Trichomonas vaginalis*, a one-celled anaerobic organism. This extracellular parasite can burrow under the mucosal lining. In men, the organism primarily resides in the urethra and causes no symptoms. In women, the organism resides in the vagina and the infection becomes symptomatic when vaginal microbial imbalance occurs. The *T. vaginalis*

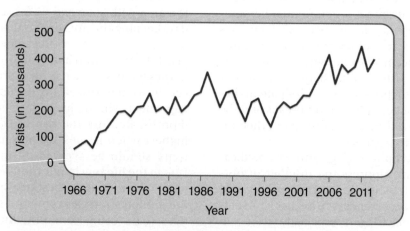

FIGURE 8-38 Genital warts–related clinic visits in the United States.

Reproduced from Centers for Disease Control and Prevention. (2015). Sexually transmitted disease surveillance. Retrieved from http://www.cdc.gov/std/stats14/figures/50.htm

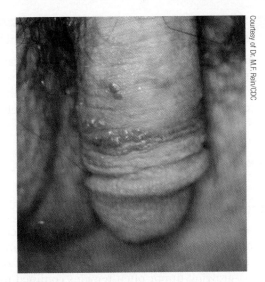

FIGURE 8-39 Genital warts on the penis.

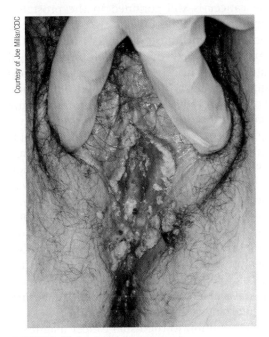

FIGURE 8-40 Genital warts on the vagina.

organism cannot survive in the mouth or the rectum.

In addition to sexual contact, trichomoniasis can be contracted through prolonged moisture exposure (e.g., bathing suits and protective garments). Trichomoniasis is not reportable to the CDC, but data from healthcare clinics indicate that trichomoniasis rates in women have been controlled for the last 40 years (**FIGURE 8-41**).

In men, trichomoniasis does not usually generate symptoms and resolves in a few weeks without treatment. In women, the primary clinical manifestation is copious amounts of odorous, frothy, white or yellow-green vaginal discharge. This discharge can irritate the vagina and vulva. Additional symptoms may include itching, painful intercourse, and dysuria.

Diagnostic procedures for trichomoniasis include a history, physical examination, and Pap smear. Trichomoniasis is easily treated with metronidazole (Flagyl), an antibiotic that treats bacteria and parasite infections. Sexual partners should also be treated to prevent reinfection. Untreated or prolonged infections can increase the risk of cervical cancer.

Cancers

Malignancies of the reproductive system may either originate in the reproductive tract or spread there from other sites. Some of these cancers have high rates of successful treatment (e.g., testicular cancer), whereas others have high mortality rates (e.g., ovarian cancer). Typical cancer diagnosis, staging, and treatments are generally utilized with these tumors (see the *Cellular Function* chapter).

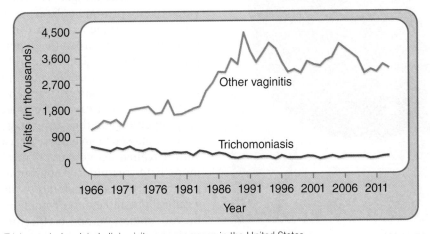

FIGURE 8-41 Trichomoniasis-related clinic visits among women in the United States.

Myth Busters

A common misconception is that condoms protect users against all STIs. While condoms are highly effective against most STIs, some of these infections have been known to spread despite condom use. STIs that can spread through skin-to-skin contact even with a condom in place include HPV, HSV, and syphilis. Additional strategies, such as obtaining the HPV vaccine, receiving genital herpes suppression therapy, and treating syphilis early, can decrease the likelihood of contracting and spreading these infections.

Penile Cancer

Penile cancer is a rare malignancy. Its exact cause is unknown, but risk is thought to be increased by the presence of smegma, being uncircumcised, poor hygiene, phimosis, and HPV infections. Penile cancer appears as a thick, gray-white lesion (Bowen's lesion) or a red, shiny lesion (erythroplasia of Queyrat) (**FIGURE 8-42**). Prognosis is good with early diagnosis and treatment, but a penectomy (removal of the penis) may be required if the cancer is extensive or does not respond to the usual cancer treatments (e.g., chemotherapy, radiation, and surgical excision).

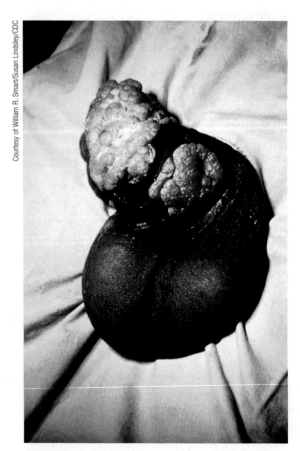

Courtesy of William R. Smart/Susan Lindsley/CDC

FIGURE 8-42 Penile cancer.

Prostate Cancer

Prostate cancer is the most common cancer among men, particularly African Americans (American Cancer Society, 2016). This kind of slow-growing tumor often remains confined to the prostate (80% of cases are diagnosed while the cancer is still confined to the prostate), improving the prognosis. Prostate cancer is the second leading cause of cancer deaths in the United States, but the 5- and 10-year survival rates for this disease are improving. Prognosis improves with early diagnosis and treatment and worsens with advancing age. Increased screening may contribute to these newly improved survival rates. The exact cause of prostate cancer remains unknown, but men's risk is thought to increase with a history of STIs, family history, consumption of high-fat diet, and androgen hormone replacement (some tumors are androgen dependent).

As the tumor grows, the prostate enlarges and impedes the urethra; therefore, prostate cancer presents with similar clinical manifestations as benign prostatic hyperplasia (e.g., urinary difficulties and erectile dysfunctions) (see the *Urinary Function* chapter). Additional manifestations may include bloody semen and hematuria.

In addition to the usual cancer diagnostic procedures (e.g., biopsy), measurements of prostate-specific antigen (whose level is elevated in any prostate enlargement), free prostate-specific antigen (which can differentiate between benign prostatic hypertrophy and prostate cancer), and prostatic acid phosphatase (which is high in prostate cancer) may be performed. Prostate cancer treatment follows the path of the usual cancer treatments and can vary depending on the cancer stage. If the cancer is diagnosed in an early stage, careful observation (called active surveillance) instead of immediate treatment is appropriate for many patients. Treatment includes a combination of a radical prostatectomy (complete prostate removal), radiation, and orchiectomy (removal of the testes) or antitestosterone drug therapy.

These treatments often impact the patient's quality of life due to their side effects or complications (e.g., urinary and erectile dysfunctions), which may be short or long term in duration. Researchers are exploring new biologic markers in an effort to improve the differential diagnosis between indolent and aggressive prostate cancer so as to minimize unnecessary treatment of the indolent variant (American Cancer Society, 2016).

Testicular Cancer

Testicular cancer is an uncommon cancer. Young (15–35 years old) and Caucasian men are at higher risk of developing this type of cancer than other groups. Most cases of testicular cancer occur as a slow-growing (seminoma) tumor, but some cases occur as a fast-growing (nonseminoma) tumor. Risk for developing testicular cancer is thought to be increased by family history, infection, trauma, tobacco use, testicular abnormalities (e.g., atrophy or dysgenesis), and cryptorchidism. Testicular cancer usually affects one testicle, but can affect both. Metastasis, when it happens, usually occurs to the nearby lymph nodes, lungs, liver, bone, and brain.

Testicular cancer is often asymptomatic. When present, clinical manifestations usually include a hard, painless, palpable mass that does not transilluminate; testicular discomfort or pain; testicle enlargement; and gynecomastia (female-like breast).

Testicular cancer is highly curable even when it has metastasized to other sites. Early diagnosis and treatment enhance prognosis. Monthly self-testicular examinations are the cornerstone of early detection. Other diagnostic procedures include measurement of tumor markers such as alpha fetoprotein, beta human chorionic gonadotropin, and lactate dehydrogenase. In most cases, an orchiectomy is advised, but chemotherapy and radiation may also be used to treat this disease. Testicular cancer can reoccur in the remaining testicle, so self-testicular examinations and follow-up are crucial.

Breast Cancer

Breast cancer is the most common malignancy in women and the second leading cause of cancer death in women (American Cancer Society, 2016). While breast cancer can occur in men, its rates are highest in Caucasian women, although African American women are most likely to die from it. Other factors that increase the risk of this type of cancer include advancing age, early onset of menstruation, family history (although not always present), genetic predisposition (defects on the *BRCA1* and *BRCA2* genes), obesity, chest-wall radiation, and excessive alcohol consumption (more than one to two drinks per day). Exogenous estrogen exposure (e.g., oral contraceptives, hormone replacement therapy) may increase the risk for breast cancer, although current formulations have minimized this risk.

Most breast cancers originate in the duct system, but such a malignancy may also arise in the lobules (structures that produce milk). The tumor can infiltrate the surrounding tissue and adhere to the skin, causing dimpling. In its early stages, the tumor moves freely, but it becomes fixed as the cancer progresses. Most tumors are estrogen dependent, and metastasis usually occurs to nearby axillary lymph nodes. Because metastasis can occur early, in most cases several nodes are affected at the time of diagnosis. Widespread metastasis quickly follows to the lungs, brain, bone, and liver.

In its early stages, breast cancer is often asymptomatic. Symptoms arise as the tumor grows. In men, symptoms usually include a breast mass and breast tenderness or pain. Clinical manifestations of breast cancer in women include the following signs and symptoms:

- Mass in the breast or axillary that is hard, has uneven edges, and is usually painless
- Change in the size, shape, or feel of the breast or nipple (e.g., redness, dimpling, or puckering that looks like the peel of an orange) (**FIGURE 8-43**)
- Nipple drainage that may be bloody, clear to yellow, green, or purulent

Indications that the cancer has metastasized include bone pain, skin ulcers, edema in the arm next to the affected breast, and weight loss.

Early diagnosis and treatment are crucial to positive outcomes. Monthly self-breast examinations are the cornerstone of early detection—in fact, women discover most tumors during this examination. Another diagnostic procedure specific to breast cancer is the mammogram, but like other screening tools, it is not perfect. Most (95%) of the 10% of women who have abnormal mammograms do not have cancer (American Cancer Society, 2016). Currently, the American Cancer Society's (2016) recommendations are that women at average risk who are 40–44 years of age should be given the choice for an annual mammogram; those 45–54 years of age should have annual mammograms; and those 55 years of age and older should have biennial or annual mammograms. Women in high-risk groups

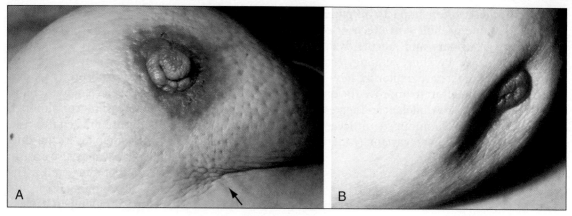

FIGURE 8-43 Changes in the breast caused by advanced breast cancer.
Courtesy of Leonard V. Crowley, MD, Century College

should start annual mammograms sooner (typically age 30) in addition to receiving annual MRI.

Recent advances in breast cancer treatments (especially in chemotherapies) have significantly increased survival rates for this disease. Treatment strategies vary depending on the stage, but usually breast cancer requires an aggressive, multimethod treatment (e.g., chemotherapy, radiation, surgery, and hormone therapy) to improve outcomes. The life-threatening nature of breast cancer, along with the changes in body image that result from treatment, can increase the need for coping and support interventions (e.g., support groups and counseling).

Cervical Cancer

Cervical cancer rates have been declining in recent years with advancements in screening. The Pap smear—the long-standing cervical screening method—can now detect precancerous changes (dysplasia). Procedures can be performed to remove these precancerous cells, limiting the likelihood of these changes progressing to permanent malignant changes (**FIGURE 8-44**). The precancerous cells are 100% treatable; however, malignant changes can return if carcinogen exposure continues. Almost all cervical cancers are caused by HPV infection; therefore, most risk factors for cervical cancer are the same as those that increase the risk of contracting HPV (e.g., having multiple sex partners and not practicing safe sex). According to the National Cancer Institute (2016), Hispanic women have the highest incidence of cervical cancer, while African American women have the highest mortality rates from this disease.

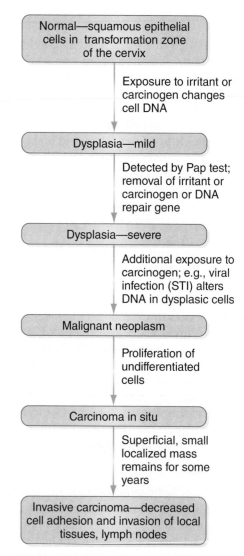

FIGURE 8-44 Development of cervical cancer.
Modified from Gould, B. (2014). *Pathophysiology for the health professions* (5th ed.). Philadelphia, PA: Elsevier. Copyright Elsevier 2015.

Early-stage cervical cancer is usually asymptomatic. When present, clinical manifestations include the following signs and symptoms:

- Continuous vaginal discharge, which may be pale, watery, pink, brown, bloody, or foul smelling
- Abnormal vaginal bleeding between menstruation, after intercourse, or after menopause
- Menorrhagia

Indications of advanced cervical cancer include the following conditions:

- Anorexia
- Weight loss
- Fatigue
- Pelvic, back, or leg pain
- Unilateral lower-extremity edema
- Heavy vaginal bleeding
- Leaking of urine or feces from the vagina
- Bone fractures

The Pap smear remains the cornerstone of early cervical cancer detection. Administration of the HPV vaccine, however, may prevent the cancer. Precancerous and early malignant changes can be treated using a loop electrosurgical excision procedure, cryotherapy, and laser therapy.

Advanced cancer will require chemotherapy, radiation, and surgery (usually a hysterectomy). The survival rate is usually 100% when cervical cancer is treated early, but the rate decreases as the disease advances.

Endometrial Cancer

Endometrial cancer, or cancer of the uterus, is a common malignancy in women. According to the American Cancer Society (2016), endometrial cancer is the fourth most frequent cancer in women, and the sixth leading cause of cancer death in women, with a 5-year survival rate of approximately 82% in most cases. Caucasian women have the highest prevalence rates, but African American women have the highest mortality rates. The exact cause of this disease is unknown, but excessive estrogen exposure may be a major factor in its development. Additional risk factors for developing endometrial cancer include obesity, diabetes mellitus, and hypertension.

The most significant finding indicating the possible presence of endometrial cancer is abnormal painless vaginal bleeding (the cancer erodes the endometrium), especially after menopause. Additional clinical manifestations include nonbloody vaginal discharge, pelvic

Myth Busters

Several misconceptions around breast cancer warrant discussion.

Myth 1: Breast implants, use of antiperspirant, and wearing underwire bras increase breast cancer risk.

There is *no* evidence that links these factors to breast cancer. Breast implants can make it more difficult to detect tumors with a self-breast examination depending on the surgical technique used to insert the implants. Placing the implants behind the muscle wall can improve the ability to detect any tumors. Nevertheless, breast implants, antiperspirant, and underwire bras do *not* increase breast cancer risk.

Myth 2: Only older women need to worry about breast cancer.

Breast cancer risk does increase with age, but women of *all* ages can develop breast cancer.

Myth 3: Breast cancer always runs in families.

Family history does increase the likelihood of developing breast cancer, but *most* women who develop breast cancer *do not* have a family history of breast cancer.

Myth 4: There is no need to worry about breast cancer if no *BRCA1* and *BRCA2* mutation is present.

BRCA1 and *BRCA2* mutations do increase breast cancer risk, but 90–95% of women who are diagnosed with breast cancer *do not* have either a family history or this genetic mutation.

Data from American Cancer Society. (2016). What are the risk factors for breast cancer? Retrieved from http://www.cancer.org/cancer/breastcancer /detailedguide/breast-cancer-risk-factors

Now that we have discussed conditions of the reproductive system, let's put that knowledge into practice. While working in the emergency department, the following patients need to be triaged. Which patient would have the highest priority?

- A 55-year-old man with a chancre on his genitals
- A 20-year-old man with a swollen, painful scrotum who has a history of a recent mumps infection
- A 65-year-old man with a history of prostate cancer and palpable bladder distension
- A 19-year-old man who has had an erection for "10 or 11 hours" and is complaining of severe pain

Once again, you go through the usual thought process—who would die first, acute versus chronic conditions, Maslow's hierarchy of needs, and patient safety. Most of the conditions affecting the reproductive are not immediately life threatening; however, many conditions can be medical emergencies because they threaten body function.

Let's start with the 55-year-old man with a chancre on the penis. Chancres may indicate the presence of any of several STIs, none of which are life threatening. STIs are acute, however, so keep this patient on your short list. Now consider the 20-year-old man with the swollen scrotum. Mumps often causes inflammation of the testes (orchitis). Neither condition is life threatening, but they are acute. Keep this patient on the short list, too. Next, consider the 65-year-old man with prostate cancer and bladder distension. Cancer is chronic, but the bladder distension is an acute change. Urinary retention is common with prostate problems, but it is not life threatening. Even so, this person should remain on the short list. Finally, consider the 19-year-old man with the prolonged erection. Priaprism is a medical emergency because the penis may develop necrosis. Although all of these patients are experiencing acute problems, the 19-year-old is experiencing the most severe issue and should be seen first to have a chance to save bodily functioning.

pain, weight loss, palpable abdominal mass, and pain during sexual intercourse.

The Pap smear does not detect cancers above the cervix, and a simple screening test is not available for endometrial cancer. Instead, biopsy is the diagnostic procedure of choice when this malignancy is suspected. If diagnosed early, endometrial cancer can be successfully treated with chemotherapy, radiation, surgery (hysterectomy), and hormone therapy.

Ovarian Cancer

Ovarian cancer is a relatively common cancer in women. According to the American Cancer Society (2016), ovarian cancer incidence rates have declined, but this disease remains the fifth leading cause of cancer death in women. Prevalence and mortality rates are the highest in Caucasian women. Ovarian cancer causes concern because there is no reliable screening test for this disease, it is difficult to treat, and it has often metastasized at the time of diagnosis. However, advances in treatment are improving the survival rates (5-year survival rates are approximately 46%). Risk factors for developing ovarian cancer include genetic predisposition (defects on the BRCA1 and BRCA2 genes), advancing age, infertility, excessive estrogen exposure, obesity, and androgen hormone therapy.

Early clinical manifestations of ovarian cancer are vague and include abdominal distension, pelvic pain, and eating disturbances. Additional symptoms consist of bowel pattern changes, gastrointestinal discomfort (e.g., gas, indigestion, and nausea), pain during sexual intercourse, malaise, urinary frequency, and menstruation changes.

CA-125, a protein that is produced in response to several conditions, including ovarian cancer, is often examined as a part of the diagnostic and treatment process. Because it is not specific to ovarian cancer, a biopsy is still required for definitive diagnosis. During treatment, a declining CA-125 level is considered a favorable response to interventions. Surgery and chemotherapy are the preferred treatment strategies. Surgery may include a bilateral salpingo-oophorectomy (removal of both ovaries and fallopian tubes) and a hysterectomy.

CHAPTER SUMMARY

The reproductive systems in males and females are responsible for procreation and hormone balance. Disorders of the reproductive system range from harmless to life threatening. These disorders are most often infections or tumors (benign and malignant). Reproductive function is closely connected with the endocrine, cardiovascular, and nervous systems and, therefore, can affect those systems. Maintaining reproductive health can decrease the likelihood of issues within this system. Strategies to promote reproductive health include practicing safe sex; abstaining from alcohol, smoking, and illicit drug use; maintaining a healthy weight; and limiting exposure to radiation and chemicals.

REFERENCES

AAOS. (2004). *Paramedic: Anatomy and physiology*. Sudbury, MA: Jones and Bartlett.

American Cancer Society. (2016). Cancer facts and figures 2016. Retrieved from http://www.cancer.org/acs/groups /content/@research/documents/document/acspc-047079.pdf

Centers for Disease Control and Prevention (CDC). (2014). Sexually transmitted disease surveillance. Retrieved from https://www.cdc.gov/std/stats14/std-trends-508.pdf

Centers for Disease Control and Prevention (CDC). (2015). Chlamydia statistics. Retrieved from https://www.cdc.gov /std/chlamydia/stats.htm

Centers for Disease Control and Prevention (CDC). (2016a). Facts about hypospadias. Retrieved from http://www.cdc .gov/ncbddd/birthdefects/Hypospadias.html#ref

Centers for Disease Control and Prevention (CDC). (2016b). Pelvic inflammatory disease. Retrieved from https://www.cdc .gov/std/pid/stdfact-pid-detailed.htm

Chiras, D. (2011). *Human biology* (7th ed.). Burlington, MA: Jones & Bartlett Learning.

Elling, B., Elling, K., & Rothenberg, M. (2004). *Anatomy and physiology*. Sudbury, MA: Jones and Bartlett.

Gould, B. (2015). *Pathophysiology for the health professions* (5th ed.). Philadelphia, PA: Elsevier.

Greenger, J., Bruess, C., & Conklin, S. (2014). *Exploring the dimensions of human sexuality* (5th ed.). Sudbury, MA: Jones and Bartlett.

Jayachandran, D., Bythell, M., Platt, M., & Rankin, J. (2011). Register based study of bladder exstrophy-epispadias complex: Prevalence, associated anomalies, prenatal diagnosis and survival. *Journal of Urology, 186*(5), 2056–2000.

Moini, J. (2016). *Anatomy and physiology for health professionals* (2nd ed.). Burlington, MA: Jones & Bartlett Learning.

National Cancer Institute. (2016). Cervical cancer. Retrieved from http://seer.cancer.gov/statfacts/html/cervix.html

National Institutes of Health (NIH). (2011). Uterine fibroids. Retrieved from http://www.ncbi.nlm.nih.gov/pubmedhealth /PMH0001912/

National Institutes of Health (NIH). (2013). Premenstrual syndrome. Retrieved from http://www.ncbi.nlm.nih.gov /pubmedhealth/PMH0072449/

Professional guide to pathophysiology (3rd ed.). (2010). Philadelphia, PA: Lippincott Williams & Wilkins.

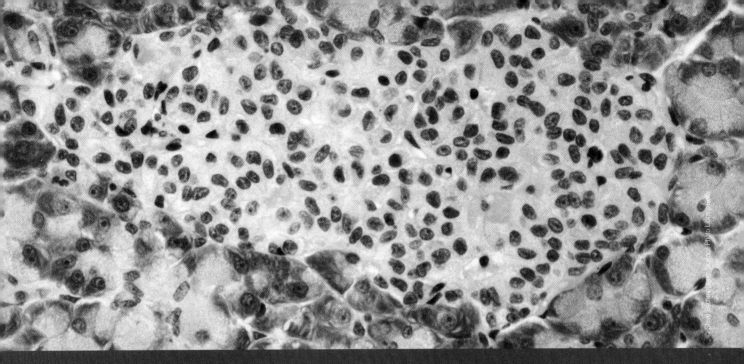

CHAPTER 9
Gastrointestinal Function

LEARNING OBJECTIVES

- Discuss normal gastrointestinal anatomy and physiology.
- Describe and compare congenital defects of the gastrointestinal system.
- Compare and contrast disorders of the upper gastrointestinal system.

- Describe and compare disorders of the gallbladder, liver, and pancreas.
- Compare and contrast disorders of the lower gastrointestinal system.
- Describe and compare cancers of the gastrointestinal system.

KEY TERMS

achlorhydria
acute gastritis
appendicitis
appendix
ascites
aspiration
atrophic gastritis
bile
cecum
celiac disease
cholecystitis
cholelithiasis
chronic gastritis
chyme
cirrhosis
cleft lip
cleft palate
colon
colorectal cancer

constipation
Crohn's disease
Curling's ulcer
Cushing's ulcer
defecation
diarrhea
diverticula
diverticular disease
diverticulitis
diverticulosis
duodenal ulcer
dysphagia
emesis
esophageal cancer
esophagus
feces
frank blood
gallbladder
gastric cancer

gastric ulcer
gastritis
gastroenteritis
gastroesophageal reflux disease (GERD)
hematemesis
hepatic artery
hepatitis
hepatobiliary system
hiatal hernia
infantile hypertrophic pyloric stenosis (IHPS)
inflammatory bowel disease (IBD)
intestinal obstruction
irritable bowel syndrome (IBS)
jaundice
large intestine

liver
liver cancer
lower esophageal sphincter (LES)
mastication
melena
mesentery
mucosa
mucus
muscle layer
nausea
occult blood
oral cancer
pancreas
pancreatic cancer
pancreatitis
paralytic ileus
parietal peritoneum layer
peptic ulcer disease (PUD)

peristalsis
peritoneal cavity
peritoneum
peritonitis
portal hypertension

portal vein
pyloric sphincter
pyloric stenosis
rectum
retching

rugae
serosa
small intestine
stomach
stress ulcer

submucosa layer
ulcerative colitis
visceral peritoneum layer
vomiting
vomitus

T[he GI system, gastroint]estinal system, or diges-
[tive] system, consists of structures
and el[...] [digestion,
cesses [...] [...] [water, and
electro[...] [required in the body's p]hysiologic
activit[...] [structures of the GI system in]clude an
alime[ntary canal through which] [food] is passed
and [accessory organs that aid] [in] [digestion
(FIGUR[E 9-2). The alimentary canal in]cludes the
oral ca[vity, pharynx, esophagus, stoma]ch, small
intestine, large intestine, and anus. The accessory organs include the salivary glands, liver,
gallbladder, bile ducts, and pancreas.

Disorders of the GI system can result in nutritional deficits and metabolic imbalances.
These conditions vary from mild (e.g., constipation) to [life-threatening (e.g. pancreatitis)] in severity, a[...] [...] specific
manifes[...] [...] [discussion] in the
system'[...] [sections].

Anatomy and Physiology

The GI [tract is divided into upper and] lower
divisio[ns, which will be further disc]ussed in
upcomi[ng sections. Additionally, the] liver,
gallbla[dder, and pancreas are coll]ectively
referre[d to as the hepatobiliary s]ystem
because of their close proximity to each other
and their complementary functions. The walls

of the GI tract have four layers (**FIGURE 9-3**). The
mucosa is the innermost layer that produces
mucus. **Mucus** facilitates movement of the GI
contents and protects the GI tissue from the
extreme pH conditions of the GI tract (the stomach's pH is in the range of 1–2) necessary for
digestion. The epithelial mucosa cells have a
high turnover rate because of erosion associated
with food passage and the highly acidic environment. The **submucosa layer** consists of connective tissue that includes blood vessels, nerves,
lymphatics, and secretory glands. The **muscle
layer** includes circular and longitudinal smooth
muscle layers. This layer contracts in a wavelike
motion to propel food through the GI tract, an
action called **peristalsis**. The **serosa** is the outer
layer of the wall.

The **peritoneum** is the large serous membrane that lines the abdominal cavity. The outer
parietal peritoneum layer covers the abdominal wall as well as the top of the bladder and
uterus. The inner **visceral peritoneum layer**
encases the abdominal organs. This double-
walled membrane is similar to the pericardial
sac (see the *Cardiovascular Function* chapter) and
the pleural membrane (see the *Respiratory Function* chapter). The **peritoneal cavity** is the
space between these two layers; it contains serous fluid to decrease friction and facilitate
movement. The **mesentery** is a double-layer
peritoneum containing blood vessels and nerves

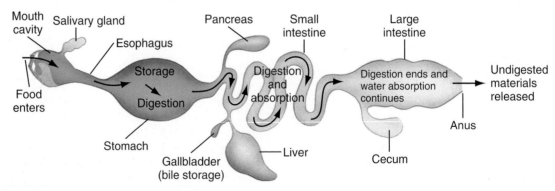

FIGURE 9-1 Functions of the gastrointestinal system.

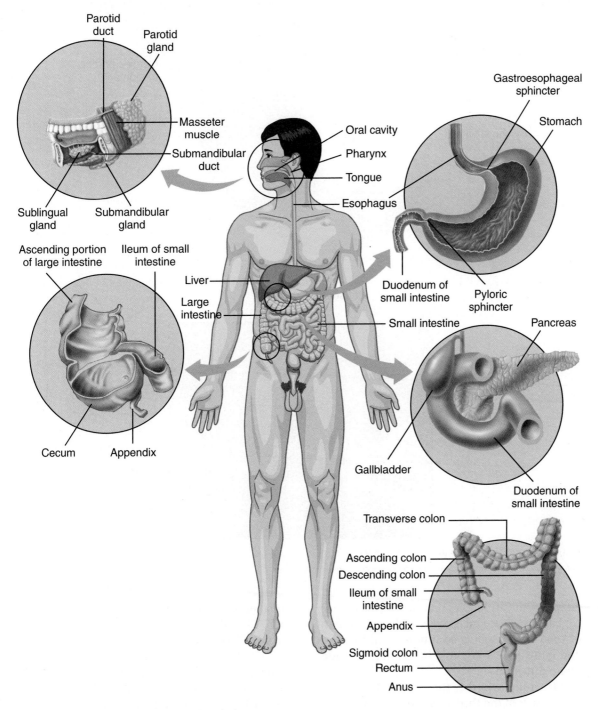

FIGURE 9-2 The structures of the gastrointestinal system.

that supplies the intestinal wall. It supports the intestines while allowing flexibility to accommodate peristalsis and varying content volumes.

Upper Gastrointestinal Tract

The upper GI tract includes the oral cavity, pharynx, esophagus, and stomach (Figure 9-2). Food usually enters the GI tract through the mouth (consumption), where chemical and mechanical digestion begins. Issues with the mouth or swallowing can create a need to bypass the mouth and esophagus and introduce the food or a food supplement directly into the stomach or small intestine. Chewing, or **mastication**, pulverizes the food into small pieces, and saliva from the salivary glands moistens and further breaks down the food (**TABLE 9-1**). Saliva contains

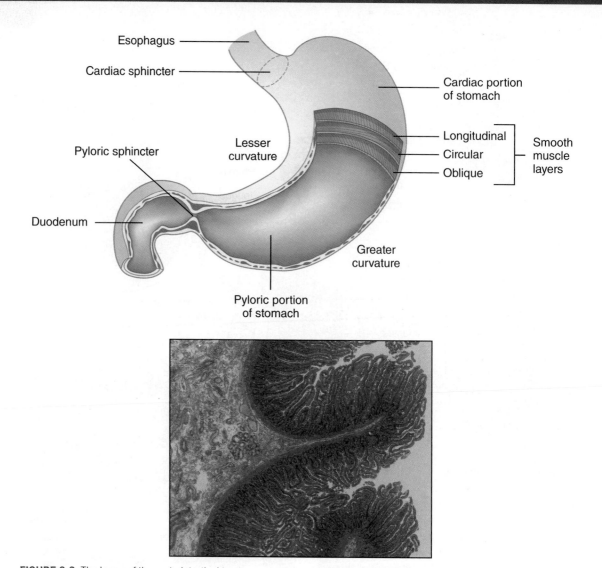

Esophagus

Cardiac sphincter

Cardiac portion of stomach

Pyloric sphincter

Lesser curvature

Longitudinal

Circular

Oblique

Smooth muscle layers

Duodenum

Greater curvature

Pyloric portion of stomach

FIGURE 9-3 The layers of the gastrointestinal tract.

Photo: © Donna Beer Stolz, PhD, Center for Biologic Imaging, University of Pittsburgh Medical School

enzymes and antibodies that can kill or neutralize bacteria. The smell, taste, feel, and thought of food trigger saliva secretion. Healthy teeth and gums play a key role in maintaining adequate nutrition.

The tongue pushes the semisolid food mass to the back of the throat, where it is swallowed (**FIGURE 9-4**). Food passing the trigeminal and glossopharyngeal nerves initiates the swallowing reflex. These nerves relay information to the swallowing center in the medulla; the swallowing center then coordinates the movement of the food from the mouth through the esophagus to the stomach with cranial nerves V, IX, X, and XII. This orchestrated movement prevents food from entering the nearby trachea and lungs (a phenomenon called **aspiration**). The **esophagus** has muscular rings to move the food toward the stomach (**FIGURE 9-5**). As the food nears the stomach, the **lower esophageal sphincter (LES)**

relaxes to allow the food to enter the stomach. The LES also prevents the stomach contents from refluxing into the esophagus.

The **stomach** is an expandable food and liquid reservoir. When it is empty, the stomach wall shrinks, forming wrinkles called **rugae** (**FIGURE 9-6**). As the stomach fills, the rugae unfold and the wall stretches to accommodate a volume up to 2 to 4 liters. Inside the stomach, hydrochloric acid and enzymes (Table 9-1) further chemically digest the food, and peristaltic churning further mechanically digests the food. This new food mixture is referred to as **chyme**. The highly acidic nature of chyme aids in digestion and destroys bacteria. The epithelial cells of the stomach's inner lining are densely packed together to prevent damage to the tissues through contact with the acidic stomach contents. For additional protection, numerous glands are located in the stomach that coat the inner lining with a

TABLE 9-1	Digestive Juices and Actions	
Source	**Type**	**Action**
Salivary glands	Bicarbonate	Moistens food
	Salivary lipase	Digests fat
Stomach	Hydrochloric acid	Digests protein
		Kills bacteria
	Pepsin	Digests protein
	Gastric lipase	Digests fat
	Intrinsic factor	Aids in absorption of vitamin B_{12} in the small intestine
	Mucus	Protects stomach lining
Liver	Bile acids	Dissolves fats
	Cholesterol	Excreted in bile
	Phospholipids	Aids in absorption of fats
	Immunoglobulins	Acts as antibodies
Pancreas	Bicarbonate	Protects digestive enzymes
		Neutralizes acid
	Water	Carries enzymes
	Amylase	Digests starch and glycogen
	Lipases	Digests fats
	Proteases	Digests protein

thick layer of mucus. Nutrients are not absorbed in the stomach; instead, the food is simply prepared for absorption. However, alcohol is absorbed in the stomach. Chyme leaves the stomach through the **pyloric sphincter** in small (1–3 mL), intermittent amounts. As it passes through the pyloric sphincter into the duodenum, liver and pancreatic secretions (Table 9-1) are added to continue the digestion process. Much like the LES, the pyloric sphincter prevents reflux of bile from the small intestines into the stomach.

Liver

The **liver** is an organ that is a hub of activity. This large organ performs as many as 500 different functions. Some of the liver's primary roles are vital for homeostasis and include the following:

- Metabolize carbohydrates, protein, and fats
- Synthesize glucose, protein (albumin), cholesterol, triglycerides, and clotting factors
- Store glucose (glycogen), fats (lipids), and micronutrients (e.g., iron, copper, and vitamin B_{12}) and release them when needed
- Detoxify the blood of potentially harmful chemicals (e.g., alcohol, nicotine, and medications)
- Maintain intravascular fluid volume through the production of circulating proteins (see the *Fluid, Electrolyte, and Acid–Base Homeostasis* chapter)
- Metabolize medications to prepare them for excretion
- Produce bile (necessary for emulsification of fat and fat-soluble vitamins)
- Inactivate and prepare hormones for excretion
- Remove damaged or old erythrocytes from blood to recycle iron and protein
- Serve as a blood reservoir (stores approximately 450 mL of blood that can be used when needed)
- Convert fatty acids to ketones

A tough membrane (Glisson's capsule) protects this crucial organ. The liver has a dual blood supply. The **hepatic artery** carries oxygenated blood from the general circulation to the liver at a rate of approximately 300 mL per minute to nourish the liver. The **portal vein** carries partially deoxygenated blood from the stomach, pancreas, and spleen, as well as from the small and large intestines, to the liver at a rate of approximately 1,000 mL per minute so that the liver can process nutrients and digestion by-products.

The liver is one of the body's few organs that can regenerate. As much as 75% of the liver tissue can be lost or removed, yet the remaining liver tissue can slowly regenerate into a whole liver again. This regeneration occurs primarily due to certain liver cells (hepatocytes) that act as stem cells. A single hepatocyte can divide into two daughter cells. During regeneration, steps

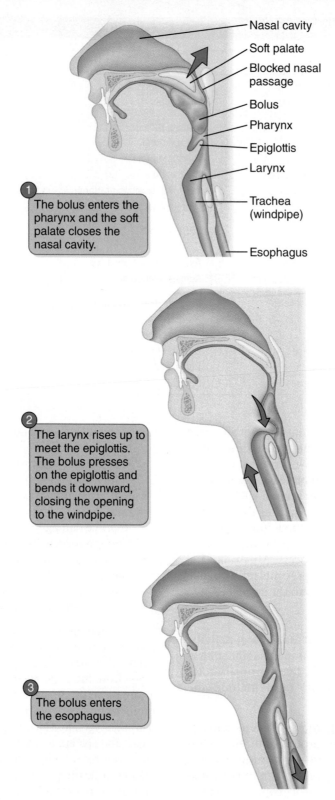

FIGURE 9-4 Swallowing.

should be taken to protect the liver from damage (e.g., avoiding hepatotoxic medications and substances).

In addition to providing regeneration capabilities, the hepatocytes produce bile and perform most of the liver's other activities. The hepatocytes constantly produce bile at a rate of approximately 600–1,200 mL per day. **Bile** is a green or yellowish liquid that contains water, bile salts (formed from cholesterol), conjugated

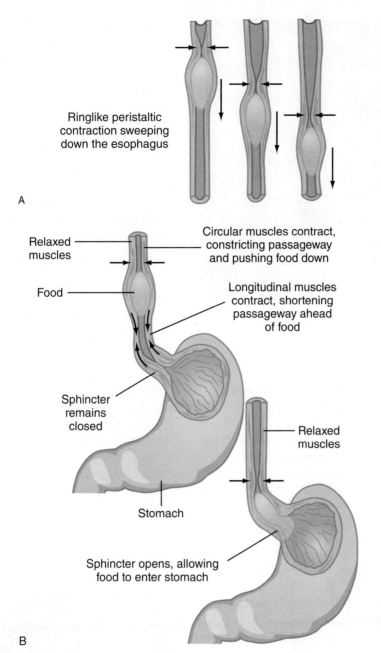

Ringlike peristaltic contraction sweeping down the esophagus

A

Relaxed muscles

Circular muscles contract, constricting passageway and pushing food down

Food

Longitudinal muscles contract, shortening passageway ahead of food

Sphincter remains closed

Relaxed muscles

Stomach

Sphincter opens, allowing food to enter stomach

B

FIGURE 9-5 Peristalsis. (a) Peristaltic contractions in the esophagus propel food into the stomach. (b) When food reaches the stomach, the gastroesophageal sphincter opens, allowing food to enter.

bilirubin, cholesterol, and electrolytes (including bicarbonate). Bile salts are necessary to emulsify fats and fat-soluble vitamins (A, D, E, and K) so that they can be absorbed in the small intestine. The distal ileum reabsorbs most of the bile and returns it to the liver through the portal vein for recycling. The bicarbonate ions in the bile neutralize the acidic gastric contents so that the intestinal and pancreatic enzymes can perform their functions. The bile flows from the liver through a duct system to either the **gallbladder** for storage or on to the duodenum.

The gallbladder is a small (usually no larger than a golf ball), saclike organ located on the under-surface of the liver that serves as a reservoir for bile. In addition to storing the bile, the gallbladder concentrates it by removing water. The presence of chyme in the small intestine triggers the gallbladder to contract, releasing bile into yet another duct system, where it travels to the small intestine. If the gallbladder requires surgical removal, the bile constantly flows directly from the liver to the small intestine.

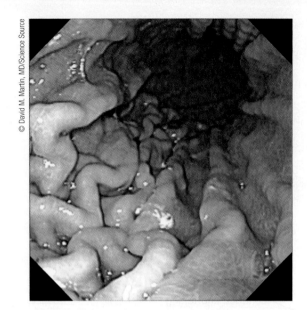

FIGURE 9-6 Rugae of the stomach.

Pancreas

The **pancreas** is an organ that is nestled underneath the stomach and liver. It has exocrine and endocrine functions. The exocrine functions include producing enzymes, electrolytes (e.g., bicarbonate ions), and water necessary for digestion (Table 9-1). A duct system carries

these substances to the duodenum to join the chyme. The endocrine functions (see the *Endocrine Function* chapter) include producing hormones (insulin and glycogen) to help regulate blood glucose, thereby maintaining homeostasis.

Lower Gastrointestinal Tract

The lower GI tract comprises the small intestine (duodenum, jejunum, and ileum), large intestine (cecum, colon, and rectum), and anus (Figure 9-2). The **small intestine** is the longest section of the GI tract (approximately 20 feet long in adults). This length allows for adequate nutrient absorption as the small intestine continues the digestion process. In the small intestine, the enzymes that have been secreted into the GI tract break the large food molecules into smaller molecules, which are then absorbed. These smaller molecules are transported to the circulatory and lymphatic system. Muscular rings slowly move the food mixture through the small intestine using a peristaltic wave motion. The wall of the small intestine contains numerous circular folds (plicae circulars) covered with villi and microvilli (**FIGURE 9-7**). These projections increase the surface area available for absorption of nutrients. Each villus contains capillaries, nerves,

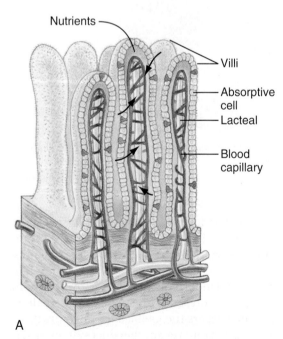

Nutrients

Villi

Absorptive cell

Lacteal

Blood capillary

A

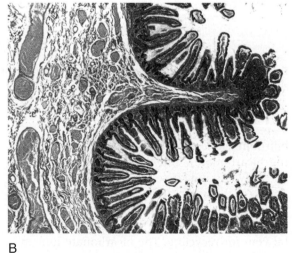

B

FIGURE 9-7 Villi of the small intestines.

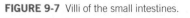
Photo: © Donna Beer Stolz, PhD, Center for Biologic Imaging, University of Pittsburgh Medical School

and lymphatic vessels that play key roles in this absorption. The small intestine also contains cells that secrete fluid to neutralize pH and enzymes to facilitate digestion. Much like the stomach, the small intestine produces a large amount of protective mucus.

After making its long journey through the small intestine, the chyme ultimately reaches the large intestine (in approximately 3–5 hours). The **large intestine** is approximately 5 feet long and does not contain villi. The small intestine ends in a pouch called the **cecum**. The **appendix** is also attached to the cecum. This small, wormlike structure seemingly has no function, but does have plenty of potential to cause harm. The **colon** makes up most of the large intestine. Unlike the coiled small intestine, the colon has three relatively straight sections—termed the ascending, transverse, and descending colon.

The mixture entering the colon from the small intestine includes water, unabsorbed food molecules, indigestible food remnants (e.g., cellulose), and electrolytes (sodium and potassium). The colon absorbs 90% of the water and electrolytes, and *Escherichia coli* feed off the undigested or unabsorbed food remnants. *E. coli* organisms constitute a large population of bacteria normally found in the GI tract. These bacteria synthesize several key vitamins (e.g., vitamins B_{12}, B_1, B_2, and K) that are later absorbed by the large intestine. As the chyme moves through the colon, it changes into **feces**. Feces contain the remaining undigested or unabsorbed remnants along with bacteria (one-third of the feces). Feces also introduce mucus (approximately 300 mL daily) to aid in bowel movements, even in times of decreased dietary intake. Because the feces are more dense than the contents in the small intestines, the colon's muscular rings must be thicker to propel the feces until they reach the **rectum** (this usually takes approximately 18 hours). The rectum serves as a reservoir to store the feces.

Much like the bladder (see the *Reproductive Function* chapter), the rectum expands when feces enter this area, stimulating the stretch receptors in the rectal wall. These receptors send an impulse through the spinal cord to elicit the **defecation** reflex. During defecation, the internal and external anal sphincters relax and the rectum contracts to expel the feces. Defecation is consciously controlled (except in infants) and may require assistance from abdominal muscles. Defecation control requires both appropriate muscular and nervous function. The urge to defecate can be delayed up to a point, but the longer the feces remain in the large intestine, the more water from them will be absorbed, making the feces more difficult to expel.

In addition to the nerves that control defecation, the sympathetic and parasympathetic nervous systems innervate the GI tract. Activation of the sympathetic nervous system slows digestive activity, whereas activation of the parasympathetic nervous system increases digestive activity.

Gastrointestinal Changes Associated with Aging

The GI system undergoes a few, usually minor, changes with aging. The stomach lining may shrink and become inflamed, leading to **atrophic gastritis**. Stomach acid production can decrease (**achlorhydria**), occasionally because of atrophic gastritis. Achlorhydria can cause vitamin B_{12} deficiency and slow digestion. Changes in the liver associated with age include reduced blood flow, delayed drug clearance, and a diminished capacity to regenerate damaged liver cells. Additionally, changes in the metabolism and absorption of lactose, calcium, and iron can occur. In particular, the small intestine absorbs less calcium with advancing age, so increased calcium intake is needed to prevent bone mineral loss and osteoporosis. The production of some enzymes, such as lactase (which aids in the digestion of lactose, a sugar found in dairy products), declines with age. Peristalsis also decreases with age, increasing the risk of constipation.

Learning Points

The GI tract is another system in the body that is much like basic household plumbing. Normally, food enters the tubular system and moves in one direction until the waste products are expelled. Peristaltic movement keeps the system flowing in the right direction, but conditions can sometimes slow, cease, or reverse this movement. Problems can occur when food moves too rapidly or too slowly through the system. Much like household plumbing, the whole system backs up and overall health can be significantly impacted if an occlusion occurs. If the system is backing up, intake should cease until functioning returns. Remember, *what goes in must come out!*

When considering alterations in the GI system, organizing them based on their basic underlying pathophysiology can increase understanding. These concepts are based on the two major underlying pathological issues—altered nutrition and impaired elimination. Conditions that alter nutritional status include issues with consuming (e.g., cleft lip), digesting (e.g., pancreatitis), and absorbing (e.g., celiac disease) food. Regardless of the cause of the altered nutrition, the end result is similar—inadequate nutritional states in which individuals may be underweight and vitamin deficient. Conditions impairing elimination generally focus on constipation and diarrhea. These issues may be either the primary condition or a symptom of another condition. Additionally, conditions that cause altered nutrition may cause issues with elimination.

Disorders of the Upper Gastrointestinal Tract

Disorders of the upper GI tract generally cause issues with nutrition and range in severity from mild to life threatening. These disorders can be congenital (e.g., cleft lip/palate or pyloric stenosis) or acquired (e.g., peptic ulcers). Depending on their severity, most of these disorders can be resolved or managed with minimal residual effects.

Congenital Defects

Congenital defects of the digestive system often affect the upper GI tract. These congenital disorders are common and not usually life threatening, but they may cause nutritional and self-image issues.

Cleft Lip and Palate

Cleft lip and cleft palate are relatively common congenital defects of the mouth and face that are apparent at birth. The Centers for Disease Control and Prevention (CDC, 2015a) estimates that cleft palate without cleft lip occurs 1 in every 2,650 births in the United States, and cleft lip with or without cleft palate occurs 1 in every 4,440 births. These conditions usually develop between the fourth and ninth weeks of gestation and are multifactorial in origin. Such defects have been associated with genetic mutations, maternal diabetes, drugs (e.g., anticonvulsants), toxins, viruses, vitamin deficiencies, and cigarette smoking. Clefts are most frequent in children of Native American, Hispanic, and Asian descent, whereas African American children are the least likely to have a cleft. Males are twice as likely as females to have a cleft lip. Females, however, are twice as likely as males to have a cleft palate. A cleft lip and palate can affect the appearance of an individual's face and may lead to feeding issues, speech problems, ear infections (otitis media), and hearing problems. The conditions may vary in severity from a small notch in the lip to a complete groove that runs into the roof of the mouth and nose (**FIGURE 9-8**). These defects may occur either separately or together.

Cleft lip may appear unilaterally or bilaterally (on either side of the midline of the upper lip). This defect results from failure of the maxillary processes and nasal elevations or upper lip to fuse during development. Cleft palate results from failure of the hard and soft palates to fuse in development, creating an opening between the oral and nasal cavities. In addition to lip and palate deformities, teeth and nose malformations may be present. Feeding problems result from

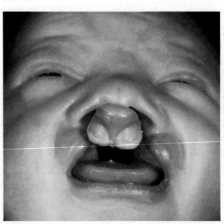

FIGURE 9-8 Cleft lip and palate.

these deficits due to an insufficient ability to suck. An infant with a cleft lip and/or palate is also at high risk for aspiration when the nasal cavity is open. The inability to make sounds using the lips and tongue impairs speech development.

Diagnostic procedures for cleft lip/palate consist of a history, physical examination, and prenatal ultrasound. Treatment strategies for cleft lip/palate include temporary measures (e.g., special nipples or dental appliances) until surgical procedures are recommended. Surgical repair of the defect is necessary to close the gap. Cleft lip repair is recommended before age 3 months, and cleft palate repair is recommended by 18 months of age. Follow-up procedures are often necessary from 2 years through the adolescent years. Cosmetic plastic surgery can improve the appearance of the defect. Surgical repair in utero is currently being explored. The major advantage of surgical repair before birth is little or no scarring. Speech therapy, including language and eating interventions, and orthodontist consultation can promote normal growth and development. Additionally, a multidisciplinary team (including an audiologist and a pediatrician) is frequently required to manage severe cases.

Pyloric Stenosis

Pyloric stenosis, also known as **infantile hypertrophic pyloric stenosis (IHPS)**, is a narrowing and obstruction of the pyloric sphincter. The pyloric sphincter muscle fibers become thick and stiff, making it difficult for the stomach to empty food into the small intestines. This condition can be present at birth, or it may develop later in life (rare in children older than 6 months). Most cases present at approximately 3 weeks of life. The exact cause of pyloric stenosis is unknown, but it is thought to be multifactorial—that is, a combination of environmental and hereditary factors. Recently, exposure to macrolides in early infancy has demonstrated a strong association with increased pyloric stenosis risk. Evidence also suggests that use of azithromycin and erythromycin in infants increases this risk. Although it is the most common cause of intestinal obstructions in infancy, pyloric stenosis is relatively uncommon (occurring in 2–4 infants per 1,000 births) (Singh & Sinert, 2015). Pyloric stenosis is most common in Caucasians and in males.

Clinical manifestations of pyloric stenosis usually appear within several weeks after birth. In the congenital form, the hypertrophied pyloric muscle can be palpated as a hard, olive-shaped mass in the abdomen (right upper quadrant), and vomiting (usually after every feeding, often projectile, and sometimes with hematemesis being noted) is usually the first symptom. Additional manifestations include the following signs and symptoms:

- Regurgitation
- Persistent hunger (often wants to eat soon after vomiting)
- Irritability (caused by persistent hunger)
- Belching
- Wavelike stomach contractions (result from the increased peristaltic effort to pass food through the narrowed areas)
- Small, infrequent stools
- Abdominal pain
- Failure to gain weight
- Dehydration, electrolyte imbalances, and pH disturbances (usually metabolic alkalosis)
- Jaundice (yellowing of the skin)

Diagnostic procedures for pyloric stenosis include a history, physical examination, abdominal ultrasound, barium X-ray, endoscopy, arterial blood gases (to identify and monitor pH disturbances), and blood chemistry (to identify and monitor fluid and electrolyte imbalances). Surgical repair called pyloromyotomy is recommended to open the sphincter, but balloon dilation may be used in high-surgical-risk infants. Additionally, fluid, electrolyte, and pH imbalances may need correction. Signs and symptoms usually resolve within 24 hours of surgical repair. In most cases, feedings are restarted within 8 hours of surgery.

Dysphagia

Dysphagia, or difficulty swallowing, usually develops secondary to a condition that causes mechanical obstruction of the esophagus or impaired esophageal motility (**FIGURE 9-9**). Numerous conditions can lead to dysphagia:

- Mechanical obstructions, including those caused by the following:
  - Congenital atresia (congenital separation of the upper and lower esophagus)
  - Esophageal stenosis or stricture (may be developmental or acquired)
  - Esophageal diverticula (outpouching of the esophageal wall)
  - Tumors (esophageal or of nearby structures)
- Neurologic disorders, including those caused by the following:
  - Stroke
  - Cerebral damage (e.g., traumatic brain injury)

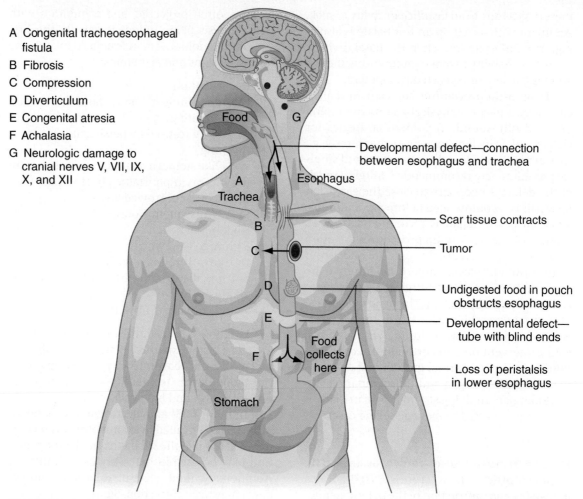

A Congenital tracheoesophageal fistula
B Fibrosis
C Compression
D Diverticulum
E Congenital atresia
F Achalasia
G Neurologic damage to cranial nerves V, VII, IX, X, and XII

Food
G
Developmental defect—connection between esophagus and trachea
Esophagus
A
Trachea
B
Scar tissue contracts
C
Tumor
D
Undigested food in pouch obstructs esophagus
E
Developmental defect—tube with blind ends
F
Food collects here
Loss of peristalsis in lower esophagus
Stomach

FIGURE 9-9 Causes of dysphagia.

- Achalasia (failure of the LES to relax because of loss of innervations)
- Parkinson's disease
- Alzheimer's disease
- Huntington's disease
- Cerebral palsy
- Multiple sclerosis
- Amyotrophic lateral sclerosis (ALS)
- Guillain-Barré syndrome
- Muscular disorders, including those caused by muscular dystrophy

Dysphagia can also have iatrogenic causes, resulting from many head and neck surgeries and procedures (e.g., laryngectomy, tracheostomy, endotracheal intubation, esophageal dilatation, radiation) as well as medications. Medications that relax the muscles, suppress the nervous system, or damage the mucosa may cause dysphagia (e.g., sedatives, narcotics, antipsychotics, nonsteroidal anti-inflammatory drugs, potassium chloride tablets). Dysphagia has likewise been associated with several psychiatric conditions, including anxiety,

depression, somatoform disorders, hypochondriasis, conversion disorders, and eating disorders.

Clinical manifestations include a sensation of food being stuck in the throat, choking, coughing, "pocketing" food in the cheeks, difficulty forming a food bolus, delayed swallowing, and painful swallowing (odynophagia). Dysphagia not only causes alterations in nutrition, but also poses an aspiration risk. Diagnostic procedures focus on identifying the underlying cause and consist of a history, physical examination, barium swallow, chest and neck X-rays, esophageal pH measurement, esophageal manometry (pressure measurement), flexible endoscopic evaluation of swallowing with sensory testing (FEESST; uses a small, lighted camera to view the mouth and throat while examining how the swallowing mechanism responds to such stimuli as a puff of air, food, or liquids), videofluoroscopic swallow study (VFSS; a videotaped X-ray of the entire swallowing process in which foods or liquids along with the mineral barium are consumed), and esophagogastroduodenoscopy (EGD; visualization of the esophagus, stomach, and duodenum using a small, lighted camera). Treatment strategies are specific for the causative condition but usually include speech therapy. Additionally, interventions are employed to maintain the patient's nutritional status and prevent aspiration (e.g., soft or pureed foods, thickened liquids, small bites, and no use of straws).

Vomiting

Vomiting, or **emesis**, is the involuntary or voluntary forceful ejection of chyme from the stomach up through the esophagus and out the mouth. Vomiting is a common event that results from a wide range of conditions. It may be protective (e.g., with drug overdose or infections) or result from reverse peristalsis (e.g., with intestinal obstructions). Increased intracranial pressure (see the *Neural Function* chapter) can cause sudden projectile vomiting. Additionally,

vomiting may be associated with other symptoms such as severe pain (e.g., migraines or renal calculi). The medulla coordinates vomiting, and drugs, toxins, and chemicals can stimulate this vomiting center.

Regardless of the cause, vomiting requires the collaboration of several structures (**FIGURE 9-10**). Involuntary vomiting occurs through the following sequence:

1. A deep breath is taken.
2. The glottis closes and the soft palate rises.
3. Respirations cease to minimize the risk of aspiration.
4. The gastroesophageal sphincter relaxes.
5. The abdominal muscles contract, squeezing the stomach against the diaphragm and forcing the chyme upward into the esophagus.
6. Reverse peristaltic waves eject chyme out of the mouth.

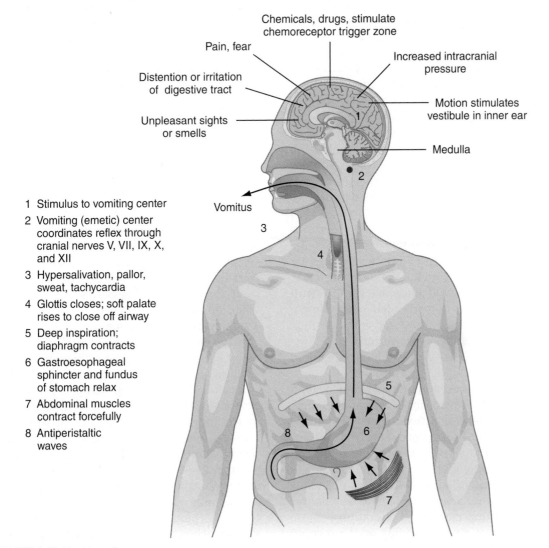

1 Stimulus to vomiting center
2 Vomiting (emetic) center coordinates reflex through cranial nerves V, VII, IX, X, and XII
3 Hypersalivation, pallor, sweat, tachycardia
4 Glottis closes; soft palate rises to close off airway
5 Deep inspiration; diaphragm contracts
6 Gastroesophageal sphincter and fundus of stomach relax
7 Abdominal muscles contract forcefully
8 Antiperistaltic waves

Chemicals, drugs, stimulate chemoreceptor trigger zone
Pain, fear
Distention or irritation of digestive tract
Unpleasant sights or smells
Increased intracranial pressure
Motion stimulates vestibule in inner ear
Medulla
Vomitus

FIGURE 9-10 Vomiting reflex.

Vomiting may be preceded by **nausea** (a subjective urge to vomit) or **retching** (a strong unproductive effort to vomit). Recurrent vomiting can be exhausting because of the strong muscular contractions. Additionally, recurrent vomiting can lead to fluid, electrolyte, and pH imbalances (see the *Fluid, Electrolyte, and Acid–Base Homeostasis* chapter). Aspiration of chyme into the lungs can cause serious damage and inflammation. This event can occur if the individual is supine or unconscious when vomiting occurs. Aspiration can also occur when the vomiting or cough reflex is suppressed from drugs (e.g., anesthesia or narcotics) or disease (e.g., stroke).

The characteristics of the contents vomited (called **vomitus**) are significant and can illuminate the underlying cause of the vomiting event. **Hematemesis** describes the condition in which blood is present in the vomitus. Blood in vomitus has a characteristic brown, granular appearance similar to coffee grounds. This appearance results from protein in the blood being partially digested in the stomach. Blood in the stomach is irritating to the gastric mucosa, so the stomach attempts to expel it. Hematemesis can occur from a number of conditions that are capable of causing upper GI bleeding (e.g., gastric ulcers and esophageal varices). Yellow- or green-colored vomitus usually indicates the presence of bile. This type of vomitus can occur as a result of a GI tract obstruction. A deep brown color of vomitus may indicate content from the lower intestine, possibly fecal. This type of vomitus frequently results from intestinal obstruction. Conditions that impair gastric emptying (e.g., pyloric stenosis) can cause recurrent vomiting of undigested food.

The force with which the vomiting occurs is important. Projectile vomiting occurs when the vomitus exits the mouth with such force that it is propelled over a short but significant distance. It is often sudden, with excessive vomitus with each attack, and not preceded with nausea. Projectile vomiting is associated with intestinal obstructions, delayed gastric emptying, increased intracranial pressure, poisoning, and overeating.

Diagnostic procedures for vomiting focus on identifying causative agents as well as fluid, electrolyte, and pH imbalances (usually metabolic alkalosis). These procedures vary and may include a history, physical examination, and blood chemistry, among others. Treatment strategies center on the cessation of vomiting, maintaining hydration, restoring acid–base balance, and correcting electrolyte alterations. These strategies may vary depending on the severity of the vomiting:

- Antiemetic medications (e.g., dimenhydrinate [Dramamine], ondansetron [Zofran], and promethazine [Phenergan])
- Oral or intravenous fluid replacement
- Correcting any electrolyte imbalances (see the *Fluid, Electrolyte, and Acid–Base Homeostasis* chapter)
- Restoring acid–base balance (see the *Fluid, Electrolyte, and Acid–Base Homeostasis* chapter)

Hiatal Hernia

A **hiatal hernia** occurs when a section of the stomach protrudes upward through an opening (hiatus) in the diaphragm toward the lung (**FIGURE 9-11**). The hiatus develops from weakening of the diaphragm muscle, frequently resulting from increased intrathoracic pressure (e.g., coughing, vomiting, or straining to defecate) or increased intra-abdominal pressure (e.g., pregnancy and obesity). Other causes of a hiatus include trauma and congenital defects. Risk factors associated with hiatal hernias include advancing age and smoking. Small hiatal hernias may go undetected and rarely cause problems. Large hiatal hernias can cause chyme to reflux into the esophagus, irritating the mucosa. When the stomach protrudes through the diaphragm, it creates a pouch. Chyme collects in this pouch, causing mucosa inflammation.

A hiatal hernia by itself rarely causes symptoms. Clinical manifestations reflect inflammation of the esophagus and stomach due to reflux of gastric acid, air, or bile. These manifestations include indigestion, heartburn (pyrosis), frequent belching, nausea, chest pain, strictures, and dysphagia. Manifestations worsen with recumbent positioning, eating (especially after large meals), bending over, and coughing. Conversely, these symptoms often improve when standing. Additionally, a soft upper abdominal mass (protruding stomach pouch) may be visualized especially when intra-abdominal pressure is increased (e.g., coughing, laughing, straining).

Diagnostic procedures for hiatal hernia consist of a history, physical examination, barium swallow, upper GI tract X-rays, manometry (measures the movement and pressure in the esophagus and stomach through a small nasogastric tube), and EGD. Treatment strategies focus on relieving inflammation by decreasing regurgitation of chyme and healing the mucosa. Such strategies include eating small frequent meals (six small meals per day), avoiding alcohol, assuming a high Fowler's position after meals, sleeping with the head of the bed elevated 6 inches, smoking cessation, losing weight (if overweight), reducing stress (stress increases

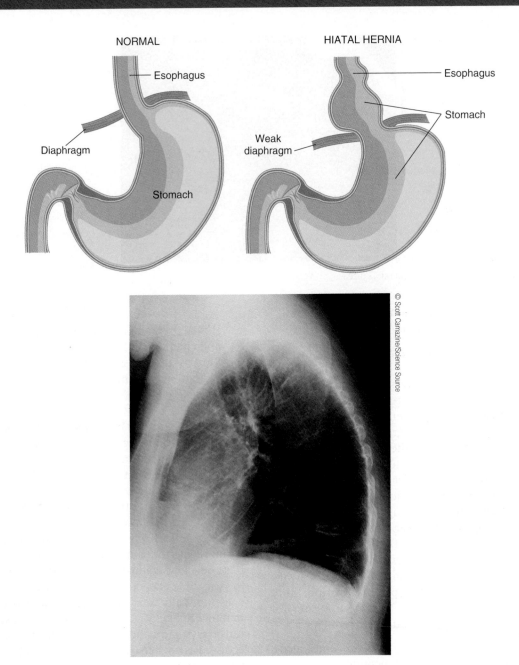

NORMAL

HIATAL HERNIA

FIGURE 9-11 Hiatal hernia.

gastrointestinal ischemia), as well as taking antacids, acid-reducing agents (e.g., histamine$_2$ blockers and proton pump inhibitors), and mucosal barrier agents. Surgical repair may be necessary for hiatal hernias not relieved by these strategies.

Gastroesophageal Reflux Disease

Gastroesophageal reflux disease (GERD) is a condition where chyme periodically backs up from the stomach into the esophagus. Occasionally, bile can back up into the esophagus. The presence of these gastric secretions irritates the esophageal mucosa (**FIGURE 9-12**). This gastric backflow occurs because the LES opens resulting in decreased LES pressure or increased stomach pressure. These pressure changes may originate from a number of sources:

- Certain foods (e.g., chocolate, caffeine, carbonated beverages, citrus fruit, tomatoes, spicy or fatty foods, and peppermint)
- Alcohol consumption
- Nicotine
- Hiatal hernia
- Obesity
- Pregnancy
- Certain medications (e.g., nitrates, sedatives, beta blockers, calcium-channel blockers, and anticholinergics)

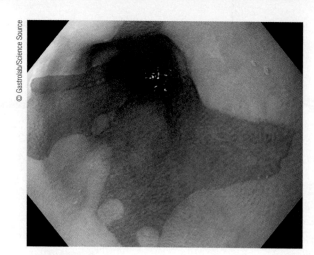

FIGURE 9-12 Gastroesophageal reflux disease.

- Nasogastric intubation
- Delayed gastric emptying

GERD varies in severity depending on the degree of LES weakness. Clinical manifestations include heartburn (early), epigastric pain (usually after a meal or when recombinant), dysphagia, nausea (usually after eating), dry cough, laryngitis, pharyngitis, regurgitation of food, and sensation of a lump in the throat. The pain associated with GERD is often confused with angina (see the *Cardiovascular Function* chapter) and may warrant steps to rule out cardiac disease. GERD can result in esophagitis, strictures, ulcerations, esophageal cancer, and chronic pulmonary disease (e.g., asthma).

Diagnostic procedures for GERD consist of a history, physical examination, barium swallow, EGD, esophageal pH monitoring, and esophagus manometry. Treatment strategies focus on balancing pressures and reducing acid:

- Avoiding triggers (e.g., trigger foods, alcohol, medications, and nicotine)
- Avoiding medications that cause gastric irritation (e.g., aspirin and nonsteroidal anti-inflammatory drugs [NSAIDs])
- Avoiding clothing that is restrictive around the waist
- Eating small, frequent meals and avoiding eating 2–3 hours before bedtime
- Assuming high Fowler's position for 2–3 hours after meals
- Losing weight
- Reducing stress
- Elevating the head of the bed approximately 6 inches
- Antacids (e.g., Maalox and Tums)
- Acid-reducing agents (e.g., proton pump inhibitors and histamine₂ blockers)
- Mucosal barrier agents

- Herbal therapies (e.g., licorice, slippery elm, and chamomile)
- Surgery (e.g., Nissen fundoplication or implantation of a Linx device)

Gastritis

Gastritis refers to an inflammation of the stomach's mucosal lining. The inflammation can involve the entire stomach or a region. This condition can be either acute or chronic; each type has its own presentation. **Acute gastritis** can be a mild, transient irritation, or it can be a severe ulceration with hemorrhage. It usually develops suddenly and is likely to be accompanied by nausea and epigastric pain. **Chronic gastritis**, in contrast, develops gradually and can last for months to years. It is likely to be accompanied by a dull epigastric pain and a sensation of fullness after minimal intake. In some cases, chronic gastritis can be asymptomatic. Gastritis can be further categorized as erosive (resulting from an imbalance between the aggressive and defensive factors that maintain the integrity of the gastric mucosa) or nonerosive (generally caused by *Helicobacter pylori* infections). **Gastroenteritis** refers to inflammation of the stomach and intestines usually resulting from an infection or allergic reaction.

Helicobacter pylori infection is the most common cause of chronic gastritis. This common bacterium spreads from person to person, but the majority of those individuals infected do not experience gastritis. In other cases, *H. pylori* embeds itself in the mucous layer, activating toxins and enzymes that causes inflammation. *H. pylori* is equipped with flagella that help it move, molecules that help it adhere, and enzymes that neutralize the gastric acid in its immediate vicinity. Why some people experience complications from *H. pylori* infections and others do not is not clear;

however, genetic vulnerability and lifestyle behaviors (e.g., smoking and stress) may increase susceptibility to the bacterium's effects. Other organisms that can be transmitted through food and water contamination and cause gastritis include *E. coli*, *Salmonella*, rotavirus, and amoebas.

Long-term use of NSAIDs (e.g., ibuprofen [Advil, Motrin], naproxen [Aleve]) can cause acute and chronic gastritis by reducing cyclooxygenase, a key substance that helps preserve the mucosal lining. Excessive alcohol consumption can also irritate and erode the mucosal lining. Severe stress due to major surgery, traumatic injury, burns, or severe infections can cause acute gastritis because of tissue ischemia and decreased gastric motility resulting from the stress response (see the *Immunity* chapter). Autoimmune conditions (e.g., Hashimoto's disease, Addison's disease, type 1 diabetes, and pernicious anemia) can create autoantibodies that attack the cells of the stomach lining. Other chronic diseases (e.g., HIV/AIDS, Crohn's disease, parasitic infections, scleroderma, and liver or renal failure) may be associated with chronic gastritis.

The clinical manifestations of gastritis reflect inflammation of the mucosal lining. These symptoms include indigestion, heartburn, epigastric pain, abdominal cramping, nausea, vomiting, anorexia, fever, and malaise. The presence of hematemesis and dark, tarry stools can indicate ulceration and bleeding. Chronic gastritis increases the risk for peptic ulcers, gastric cancer, anemia, and hemorrhage.

Diagnostic procedures for gastritis consist of a history, physical examination, upper GI tract X-ray, EGD, serum *H. pylori* antibodies levels, *H. pylori* breath test, complete blood count (CBC; to identify anemia), and stool analysis (*H. pylori* and occult blood). Acute gastritis is often self-limiting and resolves within 3 days. Treatment strategies vary depending on the underlying etiology. For instance, bacterial infections require antibiotic therapy. Chronic disease management is important to limit any complications associated with this inflammation. In addition to etiology-specific interventions, pharmacologic management may include antacids, acid-reducing agents, and mucosal barrier agents. Other strategies include those used to address GERD.

Peptic Ulcers

Peptic ulcer disease (PUD) refers to lesions affecting the lining of the stomach or duodenum (accounts for approximately 80% of cases) (**FIGURE 9-13**). The incidence of PUD has been declining in recent years, but it remains a common condition that affects approximately 4.5 million people in the United States each year (Anand, 2015). Risk factors for developing PUD include advancing age, NSAID use, *H. pylori* infections (most common cause), chronic disease (especially pulmonary and renal), and certain gastric tumors (e.g., those associated with Zollinger-Ellison syndrome). Other contributing factors include those associated with development of GERD (e.g., stress, smoking, and alcohol use).

Ulcers vary in severity from superficial erosions to complete penetration through the GI tract wall. Regardless of its etiology, PUD develops because of an imbalance between destructive forces (e.g., excess acid production) and protective mechanisms (e.g., decreased mucus production).

Duodenal ulcers are most commonly associated with excessive acid or *H. pylori* infections. Patients with duodenal ulcers typically present with epigastric pain that is relieved in the presence of food. **Gastric ulcers** (stomach ulcers), by comparison, are less frequent but more deadly. These ulcers are often associated with malignancy and NSAID use. In contrast to duodenal ulcers, the pain experienced with gastric ulcers typically worsens with eating. **Stress ulcers** is a term used to describe PUD that develops because of a major physiological stressor on the body (e.g., large burns, trauma, sepsis, surgery, or head injury). Stress ulcers associated with burns are generally called **Curling's ulcers**, whereas stress ulcers associated with head injuries are generally called **Cushing's ulcers**. Stress ulcers develop due to local tissue ischemia, tissue acidosis, entry of bile salts into the stomach, and decreased GI motility. Such ulcers most frequently develop in the stomach, and multiple ulcers can form within hours of the precipitating event. Often hemorrhage is the first indicator of a stress ulcer because the ulcer develops rapidly and tends to be masked by the primary problem.

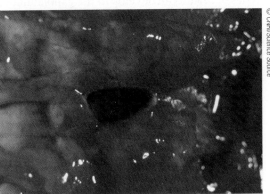

© CNRI/Science Source

FIGURE 9-13 Peptic ulcer.

Complications of PUD may involve GI hemorrhage, obstruction, perforation, and peritonitis. Clinical manifestations of PUD resemble those associated with other conditions of GI inflammation (e.g., gastritis and GERD):

- Epigastric or abdominal pain
- Abdominal cramping
- Heartburn
- Indigestion
- Chest pain
- Nausea and vomiting (may include hematemesis)
- Dark, tarry stools
- Fatigue
- Weight loss

Diagnostic procedures for PUD consist of a history, physical examination, upper GI tract X-ray, EGD, serum *H. pylori* antibody levels, *H. pylori* breath test, CBC (to identify anemia), and stool analysis (*H. pylori* and occult blood). Treatment strategies include those discussed for gastritis. Additionally, surgical repair may be necessary for perforated or bleeding ulcers.

Prevention is crucial with stress ulcers to improve patient outcomes. Prophylactic medications (e.g., acid-reducing agents) are administered to persons at risk for developing stress ulcers.

Cholelithiasis

Cholelithiasis, or gallstones, is a common condition (affecting 10% to 20% of all people in the United States) in which stones (calculi) of varying sizes and shapes form inside the gallbladder (Heuman, Allan, & Mihas, 2016) **(FIGURE 9-14)**. Cholelithiasis is more common in fair-skinned women. Other risk factors include advancing age, obesity, diet (high fat, high cholesterol, and low fiber), rapid weight loss (like that associated with bariatric surgery), pregnancy, hormone replacement, certain chronic diseases (e.g., diabetes mellitus, hyperlipidemia, and liver disease), and long-term parenteral nutrition. Three types of calculi can develop in the gallbladder or nearby ducts (**TABLE 9-2**; **FIGURE 9-15**), and the presence of calculi can cause inflammation or infection in the biliary system (**cholecystitis**).

Small calculi are often asymptomatic and excreted with the bile. Larger calculi are likely to obstruct bile flow and cause clinical manifestations. Prolonged obstruction of bile flow can lead to gallbladder rupture, fistula formation, gangrene, hepatitis, pancreatitis, and carcinoma. Gallstone disease is responsible for approximately 10,000 deaths annually in the United States—7,000 are attributed to acute complications and 3,000 are

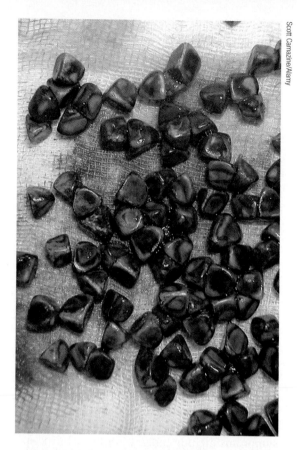

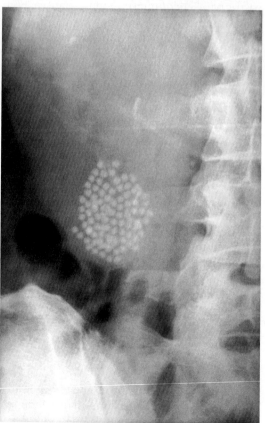

FIGURE 9-14 Cholelithiasis.

TABLE 9-2	Types of Cholelithiasis
Type	**Characteristics**
Cholesterol	Most common
	Can be small or large, single or multiple
	Can cause obstruction, pain (biliary colic), and jaundice
	Strong association with female hormones
	Increased incidence with obesity, extreme dieting, and hypercholesterolemia
Bilirubin (pigmented)	Usually multiple, small, black stones
	More common in Asians and in persons with chronic diseases that cause hemolysis (e.g., sickle cell anemia)
Mixed	Usually found in large numbers
	Bilirubin center surrounded by cholesterol and calcium

attributed to gallbladder cancer (Heuman et al., 2016). Manifestations of cholelithiasis include the following signs and symptoms:

- Biliary colic (abdominal cramping and pain that worsens after a fatty meal)
- Abdominal pain (especially in the right upper and middle upper quadrants; may radiate to the back or right shoulder)
- Abdominal distension
- Nausea and vomiting
- Jaundice (yellowing of the skin)
- Clay-colored stools (due to the lack of bile)

- Fever
- Leukocytosis

Diagnostic procedures for cholelithiasis consist of a history, physical examination, abdominal X-ray, gallbladder ultrasound, abdominal computed tomography (CT), endoscopic retrograde cholangiopancreatography (ERCP), magnetic resonance cholangiopancreatography (MRCP), percutaneous transhepatic cholangiogram (PTCA), bilirubin levels, liver function tests, pancreatic enzymes, and laparoscopy. Treatment strategies focus on removing the calculi, restoring bile flow, and preventing reoccurrence:

- Low-fat diet
- Medications to dissolve the calculi (e.g., bile acids)
- Antibiotic therapy (if infection is present)
- Nasogastric tube with intermittent suction (to facilitate abdominal decompression in the presence of an obstruction)
- Lithotripsy (e.g., extracorporeal shock wave)
- Surgically created opening for drainage (choledochostomy)
- Laparoscopic removal of calculi or gallbladder

Disorders of the Liver

Disorders of the liver are usually serious and often life threatening. The liver's involvement in so many of the body's activities results in a situation that can be complex to manage when this organ's functions become disrupted. Liver disorders are often acquired through ingestion of hepatotoxic substances (e.g., medications or alcohol) or infections.

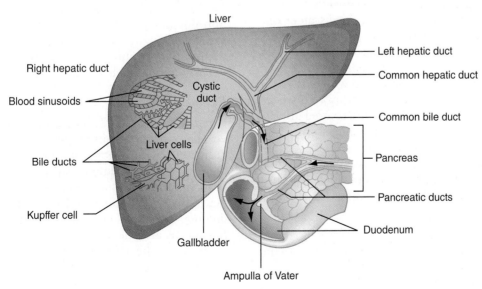

FIGURE 9-15 Location of cholelithiasis.

Hepatitis

Hepatitis is an inflammation of the liver that can be caused by infections (usually viral), alcohol, medications (e.g., acetaminophen [Tylenol], antiseizure agents, and antibiotics), or autoimmune disease (e.g., systemic lupus erythematosus, rheumatoid arthritis, and scleroderma). Hepatitis can be acute, chronic, or fulminant (such as in liver failure). Additionally, this disease can be active or nonactive. People with nonviral hepatitis usually recover, but some people develop liver failure, liver cancer, or cirrhosis. Nonviral hepatitis is not contagious, whereas viral hepatitis is contagious. Like individuals with nonviral hepatitis, people with viral hepatitis usually recover in time with no residual damage. However, advancing age and comorbidity increase the likelihood of liver failure, liver cancer, or cirrhosis in these patients. Both viral and nonviral hepatitis can result in hepatic cell destruction, necrosis, autolysis, hyperplasia, and scarring.

Viral hepatitis accounts for approximately 50% of all cases of acute hepatitis in the United States (Buggs & Dronen, 2014). There are five types of viral hepatitis, each with its own characteristics (**TABLE 9-3**). In the United States, viral hepatitis is most commonly caused by hepatitis A, hepatitis B, and hepatitis C. According to the CDC (2015b), rates of hepatitis A and B declined from 2000 to 2014, whereas hepatitis C cases have increased since 2000.

Acute hepatitis proceeds through four distinct phases—an asymptomatic incubation phase and three symptomatic phases. Clinical manifestations for each symptomatic phase include the following signs and symptoms:

- Prodromal phase: Starts 2 weeks after exposure to the virus; includes viral symptoms such as nausea, vomiting, malaise, anorexia, low-grade fever, and headache
- Icteric phase: Begins 1–2 weeks after the prodromal phase and lasts up to 6 weeks; includes jaundice, dark tea-colored urine or clay-colored stools, hepatomegaly, and right upper quadrant pain
- Recovery phase: Resolution of jaundice approximately 6–8 weeks after exposure; the liver may remain enlarged for as long as 3 months

Chronic hepatitis is characterized by continued hepatic disease lasting longer than 6 months. Its symptom severity and disease progression vary depending on the degree of liver damage.

An individual can live with chronic hepatitis for years but his or her health can quickly deteriorate with declining liver integrity. Fulminant hepatitis is an uncommon, rapidly progressing form that can quickly lead to liver failure, hepatic encephalopathy, or death within 3 weeks.

Diagnostic procedures for hepatitis include a history, physical examination, serum hepatitis profile, liver function tests, clotting studies, liver biopsy, and abdominal ultrasound. Treatment strategies concentrate on prevention, and vaccinations are the cornerstone of hepatitis prevention. Vaccinations are available for hepatitis A and B. Hepatitis A vaccination is recommended for all children starting at age 1 year, travelers to certain countries, men who have sex with men (MSM), intravenous drug users, persons with long-term liver disease, persons requiring repeated blood transfusions (e.g., those with hemophilia), and others at risk for exposure (e.g., living with someone who is hepatitis A positive). Hepatitis B vaccination is recommended for all infants beginning at birth, older children and adolescents who were not vaccinated previously, and adults at risk of developing this form of hepatitis (e.g., healthcare workers, MSM, and intravenous drug users). Prevention also includes limiting exposure to the virus (e.g., by limiting exposure to blood, body fluids, and feces).

Once viral hepatitis is contracted, there is no method of destroying the virus. Most cases of hepatitis A and E will resolve with no treatment. The other types of viral hepatitis can be treated with interferon injections to improve the immune response (see the *Immunity* chapter) and antiviral medications to decrease viral replication. Additional strategies include rest, adequate nutrition (a diet high in carbohydrates, protein, and vitamins), increased hydration, paracentesis (needle aspiration of fluid accumulation in the abdomen), and liver transplant.

Cirrhosis

Cirrhosis refers to chronic, progressive, irreversible, diffuse damage to the liver resulting in decreased liver function (**FIGURE 9-16**). This condition can be caused by hepatitis and all those factors that can lead to hepatitis (e.g., alcohol, hepatotoxic medications, and autoimmune conditions). Hepatitis C infection and chronic alcohol abuse are the most frequent causes of cirrhosis in the United States (Wolf, 2015). Eventually, the damage leads to fibrosis, nodule formation, impaired blood flow, and bile

chapter) commonly develop in the esophagus (**FIGURE 9-18**) and abdomen. Nearby organs utilizing the same circulation (e.g., the spleen, pancreas, and stomach) enlarge as pressures rise. Bleeding, either slow or severe, can occur along these overstretched vessels—particularly in the esophagus. Esophageal bleeding has a high mortality and reoccurrence rate. Fluid accumulates in the peritoneal cavity (a condition referred to as **ascites**) as the portal hypertension pushes fluid back into the abdominal cavity and the damaged liver can no longer produce sufficient amounts of albumin (a protein responsible for maintaining colloidal pressure and fluid balance in the vessels; see the *Fluid, Electrolyte, and Acid–Base Homeostasis* chapter). Changes in protein metabolism result in decreased protein clotting factors, muscle wasting, and hyperlipidemia. Changes in glucose metabolism can lead to hyperglycemia or hypoglycemia.

Bile accumulation in the liver causes inflammation and necrosis. Because it cannot flow through the duct system to the intestine, bile enters the bloodstream and causes **jaundice**. Fats cannot be digested and fat-soluble vitamins cannot be absorbed without the presence of bile. Additionally, the stools become clay colored without the presence of bile. The kidneys attempt to compensate for the excessive bile in the blood by increasing excretion, causing the urine to become dark. The excessive bile is also excreted in the sweat, causing bile salts to accumulate on the skin. These bile salts cause intense itching. Estrogen builds up in both sexes, as the liver can no longer inactivate the hormone. Excessive estrogen produces female characteristics in men and irregular menstruation in women. Numerous toxins and waste products also accumulate as the liver fails to detoxify the blood. In particular, the buildup of ammonia produces neurologic impairment that presents as confusion, disorientation, and hand tremors. Ulcers and GI bleeding occur as the excessive bile and inflammation impair the mucosa. GI bleeding, in combination with a high-protein diet, renal failure, and infection, can cause protein

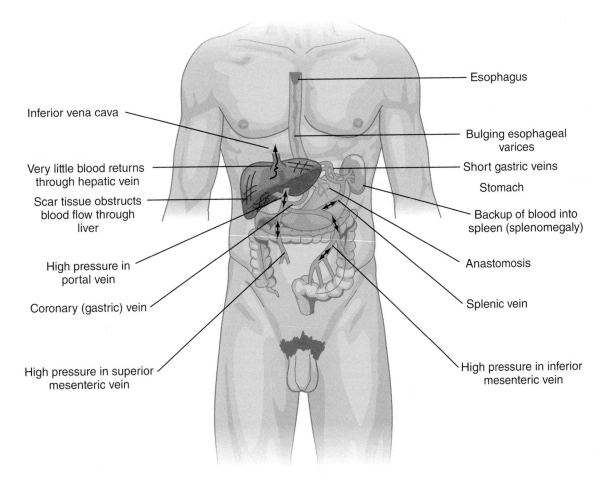

FIGURE 9-18 Development of esophageal varices.

levels to increase. Excessive protein levels lead to the rapid onset of encephalopathy. Spontaneous bacterial peritonitis may also occur because of compromised host defenses and bacterial overgrowth common in persons with cirrhosis.

Diagnostic procedures for cirrhosis include a history, physical examination, liver biopsy, abdominal X-ray, abdominal ultrasound, abdominal CT, abdominal magnetic resonance imaging (MRI), CBC, liver enzyme panel, EGD, clotting studies, stool examination (for occult blood), and endoscopy (to identify esophageal varices). Treatment strategies for cirrhosis are complex and vary depending on the underlying cause. Hepatitis-related cirrhosis is treated with antiviral agents and interferon. Alcohol, drugs, and hepatotoxic medications should be completely avoided. Nutritional imbalances (usually treated with total parenteral nutrition [TPN]) and metabolic dysfunction are corrected to manage complications and promote optimal health. Bile acid–binding agents can aid bile excretion. Portal hypertension is treated with a surgically implanted shunt. Fluid restriction, a low-sodium diet, diuretics, paracentesis, and shunts may be used to treat ascites. Esophageal varices are treated with endoscopic bands, shunts, or sclerotherapy. Antacids and acid-reducing agents can minimize GI inflammation. Strategies to treat encephalopathy are directed at eliminating the source of protein breakdown. Lactulose, a type of laxative, can promote ammonia excretion in the stools. Antibiotics can be given to suppress intestinal flora and decrease endogenous ammonia production.

A liver transplant usually offers the best outcome for individuals with cirrhosis, but not all patients are candidates for this therapy. Alcoholics must refrain from all alcohol consumption for a minimum of 6 months to be considered for transplant. Some hepatitis infections (hepatitis B more so than C) can return after transplant, so patients with such infections may not be considered as good candidates for this treatment. Additionally, patients with any evidence of cancer are not considered transplant candidates.

Disorders of the Pancreas

Disorders of the pancreas are frequently grave. The pancreas has a significant role in maintaining homeostasis by regulating electrolytes, water, and glucose. As a consequence, conditions affecting the pancreas can have a global impact on the individual's health. Most often, the gallbladder is affected by pancreatic disorders because of the intricate relationship between these two organs.

Pancreatitis

Pancreatitis is an inflammation of the pancreas that can be either acute or chronic. Causes of pancreatitis include cholelithiasis (the most common acute cause), alcohol abuse (the most common chronic cause), biliary dysfunction, hepatotoxic drugs, metabolic disorders (e.g., hypertriglyceridemia, hyperglycemia), trauma, renal failure, endocrine disorders (e.g., hyperthyroidism), pancreatic tumors, and penetrating peptic ulcer. When the pancreas is injured or its function is disrupted, pancreatic enzymes (phospholipase A, lipase, and elastase) leak into the pancreatic tissue and initiate autodigestion. Trypsin and elastase are activated proteolyses that, along with lipase, break down tissue and cell membranes, resulting in edema, vascular damage, hemorrhage, and necrosis. Pancreatic tissue is replaced by fibrosis, which causes exocrine and endocrine changes and dysfunction of the islets of Langerhans.

Acute pancreatitis is considered a medical emergency (**FIGURE 9-19**). The mortality rate from this condition is approximately 15%, but increases with advancing age and comorbidity. The following serious complications can also develop with acute or chronic pancreatitis:

- Acute respiratory distress syndrome (ARDS; see the *Respiratory Function* chapter)—acute pancreatitis can trigger the release of chemicals that lead to this life-threatening event.
- Diabetes mellitus (see the *Endocrine Function* chapter)—chronic pancreatitis can damage insulin-producing cells in the pancreas.
- Infection—acute pancreatitis can make the pancreas vulnerable to bacteria and infection; pancreatic infections are serious and require intensive treatment such as surgery to remove the infected tissue.
- Shock (see the *Cardiovascular Function* chapter)—infection and the release of miscellaneous immune mediators can trigger shock in patients with acute pancreatitis.
- Disseminated intravascular coagulation (DIC; see the *Hematopoietic Function* chapter)—DIC can be triggered by similar pathways as those that trigger ARDS and shock.
- Renal failure (see the *Urinary Function* chapter)—shock and activation of the renin–angiotensin system lead to decreased renal perfusion.
- Malnutrition—both acute and chronic pancreatitis can decrease pancreatic enzyme production, and these enzymes are necessary for

K.S. is a 35-year-old man who has been homeless for the past 5 years. He presents to the health department complaining of flulike symptoms and abdominal pain. K.S. has multiple tattoos and piercings. He admits to intravenous drug use and unprotected sexual behavior with multiple partners. Blood tests reveal that K.S.'s liver enzymes are elevated. The healthcare provider suspects some type of hepatitis.

1. Considering K.S.'s lifestyle, which type or types of hepatitis has he most likely contracted?

    A. Hepatitis A
    B. Hepatitis B
    C. Hepatitis C
    D. Hepatitis B or hepatitis C

2. How would you expect a differential diagnosis of hepatitis to be confirmed?

    A. Presence of viral particles in stool
    B. Presence of the specific hepatitis virus in the blood
    C. Presence of the specific hepatitis antibodies in the blood
    D. Development of jaundice

Tests confirm that K.S. has hepatitis B, and treatment is initiated. K.S. returns to the health department 2 weeks later with his girlfriend, who is exhibiting similar symptoms.

3. Which of the following factors likely explains the onset of the girlfriend's symptoms?

    A. They probably ate the same food.
    B. They likely obtained the virus from contaminated water.
    C. They probably infected each other through sexual contact or drug activity.
    D. They likely became infected because of poor living conditions.

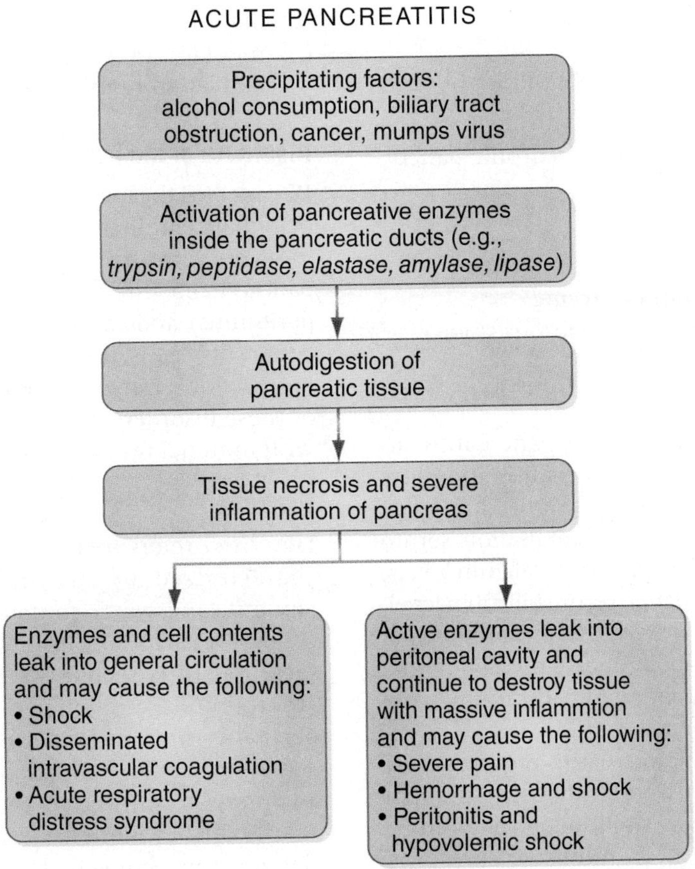

ACUTE PANCREATITIS

Precipitating factors: alcohol consumption, biliary tract obstruction, cancer, mumps virus

↓

Activation of pancreative enzymes inside the pancreatic ducts (e.g., *trypsin, peptidase, elastase, amylase, lipase*)

↓

Autodigestion of pancreatic tissue

↓

Tissue necrosis and severe inflammation of pancreas

Enzymes and cell contents leak into general circulation and may cause the following:
• Shock
• Disseminated intravascular coagulation
• Acute respiratory distress syndrome

Active enzymes leak into peritoneal cavity and continue to destroy tissue with massive inflammtion and may cause the following:
• Severe pain
• Hemorrhage and shock
• Peritonitis and hypovolemic shock

FIGURE 9-19 Effects of acute pancreatitis.

digestion and absorption; malnutrition and weight loss may occur, even when food intake remains stable.

- Pancreatic cancer—long-standing inflammation caused by chronic pancreatitis can initiate cellular mutations.
- Pseudocyst or abscess—acute pancreatitis can cause pancreatic fluids and necrotic debris to collect in cystlike pockets; a large pseudocyst or abscess that ruptures can cause complications such as internal bleeding and infection (e.g., peritonitis).

Clinical manifestations vary depending on whether the pancreatitis is acute or chronic. Manifestations of acute pancreatitis are usually sudden and severe; in contrast, manifestations of chronic pancreatitis tend to be insidious. Monitoring for the development of complications is crucial to achieve positive patient outcomes. Clinical manifestations of acute pancreatitis include the following symptoms:

- Upper abdominal pain that radiates to the back, worsens after eating, and is somewhat relieved by leaning forward or pulling the knees toward the chest
- Nausea and vomiting
- Mild jaundice
- Low-grade fever
- Blood pressure and pulse changes (may be increased or decreased)

Clinical manifestations of chronic pancreatitis include these symptoms:

- Upper abdominal pain
- Indigestion
- Losing weight without trying
- Steatorrhea (oily, fatty, odorous stools)
- Constipation
- Flatulence

Diagnostic procedures for pancreatitis include those to verify the pancreatitis and those to identify complications. These procedures may consist of a history, physical examination, serum amylase and lipase levels, serum calcium levels, CBC, liver enzymes panel, serum bilirubin level, arterial blood gases (ABGs), stool analysis (lipid and trypsin levels), abdominal X-ray, abdominal CT, abdominal MRI, abdominal ultrasound, and ERCP.

Management of pancreatitis requires early treatment and aggressive strategies to prevent complications. Patients will likely need to be closely monitored in an intensive care unit. This monitoring should include frequent measurement of vital signs (temperature, pulse, blood pressure, and respiration rate) and strict measurement of intake and output (usually hourly). Treatment strategies include the following measures:

- Resting the pancreas by fasting, administering intravenous nutrition (e.g., TPN), and gradually advancing the diet from clear liquids as tolerated to a low-fat diet
- Pancreatic enzyme supplements when the diet is resumed
- Maintaining hydration status with intravenous fluids
- Inserting a nasogastric tube with intermittent suction for persistent nausea and vomiting
- Antiemetic agents (if vomiting is present)
- Pain management (usually includes intravenous narcotic agents and analgesics)
- Antacids and acid-reducing agents
- Anticholinergic agents (which reduce vagal stimulation, decrease GI motility, and inhibit pancreatic enzyme secretion)
- Antibiotic therapy (if infection is present)
- Insulin (which treats hyperglycemia secondary to temporary or permanent pancreatic damage and TPN)
- Identifying and treating complications early (e.g., blood transfusions for hemorrhage, dialysis for renal failure, airway management for ARDS, surgical drain for abscesses, and laparotomy for biliary obstruction)

Disorders of the Lower Gastrointestinal Tract

Disorders of the lower GI tract can alter nutrition or impair elimination. These conditions range in severity from mild (e.g., diarrhea and constipation) to life threatening (e.g., appendicitis and peritonitis) and can be either congenital (e.g., celiac disease) or acquired (e.g., intestinal obstruction). Depending on their severity, most of these disorders can be resolved or managed with minimal residual effects.

Diarrhea

Diarrhea refers to a change in bowel pattern characterized by an increased frequency, amount, and water content of the stool. This condition can result from an increase in fluid secretion (it is secretory), a decrease in fluid absorption (it is osmotic), or an alteration in GI peristalsis (motility is affected). Diarrhea can be acute or chronic (lasting longer than 4 weeks), and may be attributed to many conditions. Acute diarrhea is often caused by viral or bacterial infections but can also be triggered by certain medications (e.g., antibiotics, antacids, and laxatives). Depending on the cause, acute diarrhea is usually self-limiting. Causes of chronic diarrhea include inflammatory bowel diseases (e.g., Crohn's disease and ulcerative colitis), malabsorption syndromes (e.g., celiac disease), endocrine disorders (e.g., thyroid disorders), chemotherapy, and radiation.

Clinical manifestations of diarrhea vary depending on the underlying etiology. When this condition originates in the small intestine, stools are large, loose, and provoked by eating. Diarrhea originating in the small intestine is usually accompanied by pain in the right lower quadrant of the abdomen. When diarrhea originates in the large intestine, stools are small and frequent. Diarrhea originating in the large intestine is frequently accompanied by pain and cramping in the left lower quadrant of the abdomen. Acute diarrhea is generally infectious in origin and accompanied by cramping, fever, chills, nausea, and vomiting. Blood, pus, or mucus may be present in the stool, which can aid in

diagnosis. Blood in the stool may present as **frank blood** (bright, red blood on the surface of the stool), **occult blood** (small amounts of blood hidden in the stool), or **melena** (dark, tarry stool from a significant amount of bleeding higher up in the GI tract). Additionally, bowel sounds may be hyperactive. Fluid, electrolyte, and pH (usually metabolic acidosis) imbalances frequently develop regardless of whether the diarrhea is acute or chronic (see the *Fluid, Electrolyte, and Acid–Base Homeostasis* chapter).

Diagnostic procedures for diarrhea focus on identifying the underlying cause and any complications. These procedures may include a history (including usual bowel pattern and completion of the Bristol Stool Chart [**FIGURE 9-20**]), physical examination, stool analysis (including cultures and occult blood), CBC, blood chemistry, ABGs, and abdominal ultrasound.

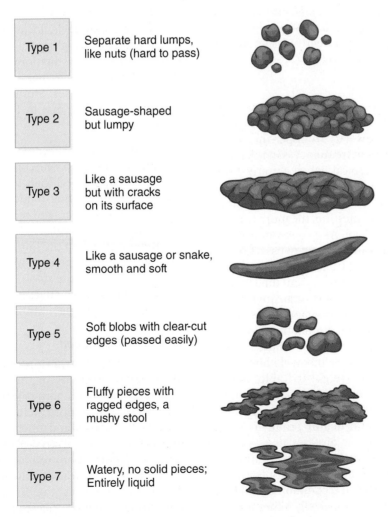

Type 1	Separate hard lumps, like nuts (hard to pass)
Type 2	Sausage-shaped but lumpy
Type 3	Like a sausage but with cracks on its surface
Type 4	Like a sausage or snake, smooth and soft
Type 5	Soft blobs with clear-cut edges (passed easily)
Type 6	Fluffy pieces with ragged edges, a mushy stool
Type 7	Watery, no solid pieces; Entirely liquid

FIGURE 9-20 Bristol Stool Chart.

Reference: Lewis, S., & Heaton, K. (1997). Stool form scale as a useful guide to intestinal transit time. *Scandinavian Journal of Gastroenterology, 32*(9), 920–924.

Treatment strategies vary depending on the underlying etiology. Acute diarrhea with infectious origins usually improves with fasting. Generally, food consumption slows GI motility, allowing bacterial and viral toxins to increase. As toxin levels rise, diarrhea can become more severe. In addition to avoiding food consumption, antidiarrheal agents may be withheld for the same reason. Antibiotics may be necessary depending on the infectious agent. In noninfectious diarrhea, antidiarrheal agents slow GI motility and increase fluid absorption. Some additional medications that may be administered include anticholinergic and antispasmodic agents. When oral intake is recommended, a clear liquid diet is usually ordered until the diarrhea subsides. At that time, the diet is advanced to a regular diet as tolerated. Dietary fiber can be used to manage chronic diarrhea; the fiber acts like a sponge to absorb the excess water and increase bulk in the stool. Maintaining hydration status and correcting electrolyte and pH imbalances is crucial to managing acute or chronic diarrhea (see the *Fluid, Electrolyte, and Acid–Base Homeostasis* chapter). Meticulous skin care can maintain skin integrity, especially in cases of bowel incontinence.

Constipation

Constipation refers to a change in bowel pattern characterized by infrequent passage of stool. Bowel patterns vary from person to person, so the decrease in frequency is in reference to the individual's typical bowel pattern. With constipation, the stool remains in the large intestine longer than usual. The longer the stool remains in the large intestine, the more water is removed from the stool. As a consequence, the stool becomes hard and difficult to pass. Constipation is often caused by a low-fiber diet, inadequate physical activity, insufficient fluid intake, delaying the urge to defecate, or laxative abuse (which smooths intestinal rugae). Stress (sympathetic nervous system stimulation slows GI motility) and travel can also contribute to constipation or other changes in bowel habits. Diseases of the bowel (e.g., irritable bowel syndrome), pregnancy, certain medications (e.g., narcotics, anticholinergic agents, and iron supplements), mental health problems (e.g., depression), neurologic diseases (e.g., stroke, Parkinson's disease, and spinal cord injuries), and colon cancer can cause constipation as well. In addition, constipation is common in children who are toilet training, especially if they are not ready for training or are scared of toileting.

Constipation may involve pain during the passage of a bowel movement, inability to pass stool after straining or pushing for more than 10 minutes, or no bowel movements for more than 3 days. Additionally, bowel sounds may be hypoactive. The passage of large, wide stools may tear the mucosal membrane of the anus, especially in children. This tearing can cause bleeding and an anal fissure to develop. Chronic constipation can lead to pH disturbances (usually metabolic alkalosis; see the *Fluid, Electrolyte, and Acid–Base Homeostasis* chapter), hemorrhoids (swollen, inflamed veins in the rectum or anus), diverticulitis, impaction, intestinal obstruction, and fistulas.

Diagnostic procedures for constipation focus on identifying the underlying cause. These procedures consist of a history (including usual bowel pattern and completion of the Bristol Stool Chart [Figure 9-20]), physical examination (may include a digital examination), abdominal X-ray, upper GI series, barium swallow, colonoscopy (for visualization of the large intestine), and proctosigmoidoscopy (for visualization of the lower bowel).

Treatment strategies focus on reestablishing the individual's usual bowel pattern and preventing future constipation episodes. These strategies may involve managing or removing any underlying causes. Strategies to treat and prevent constipation may include the following measures:

- Increasing dietary fiber (e.g., vegetables, fruit, and whole grains) with concomitant increase in hydration (specifically water and juices)
- Avoid constipating foods (e.g., processed sugar, white flour, and red meat)
- Increasing physical activity
- Defecating when the initial urge is sensed
- Taking stool softeners (incorporates lipids and water into the stool)
- Limited use of laxatives and enemas
- Digitally removing the impaction (if present)

Intestinal Obstruction

An **intestinal obstruction** refers to blockage of intestinal contents in the small intestine (where it is most common) or the large intestine. Intestinal obstructions have two types of causes—mechanical and functional. Mechanical obstructions consist of physical barriers, whereas functional obstructions result from GI tract dysfunction. Mechanical obstructions can occur due to foreign bodies, tumors, adhesions, hernias, intussusception (telescoping of a portion of the intestine into another portion), volvulus (twisting of the intestine), strictures, Crohn's disease, diverticulitis, Hirschsprung's disease (also known as congenital megacolon), and fecal impaction (**FIGURE 9-21**). Tumors, adhesions, and hernias account for approximately 90% of all mechanical small intestine obstructions. Tumors, diverticulitis, and volvulus are the most common causes of mechanical large intestine obstructions. Functional obstructions, also called **paralytic ileuses**, usually result from neurologic impairment (e.g., spinal cord injury); intra-abdominal surgery complications; chemical, electrolyte, and mineral disturbances; intra-abdominal infections (e.g., peritonitis and pancreatitis); abdominal blood supply impairment; renal and lung disease; and use of certain medications (e.g., narcotics).

Depending on the cause and location, intestinal obstructions can develop either suddenly or gradually. Additionally, the obstruction can be either partial or complete. Chyme and gas initially accumulate at the site of the blockage. Over time, saliva, gastric juices, bile, and pancreatic secretions begin to collect as the blockage lingers. This GI fluid buildup increases serum electrolytes and protein and causes abdominal distension and pain. Intestinal blood flow can become impaired, leading to strangulation and necrosis. Intestinal contents will begin to seep into the abdomen as the pressure at the blockage increases. These complications are more likely to develop with a complete obstruction. If a complete obstruction goes untreated, death can occur within hours due to shock and cardiovascular collapse. Additional complications include perforation, pH imbalances, and fluid disturbances.

The following manifestations are a result of the GI tract blockage (**FIGURE 9-22**):

- Abdominal distension
- Abdominal cramping and colicky pain
- Nausea and vomiting (usually gastric or bile contents)
- Constipation
- Diarrhea (some of the intestinal liquid passes around the obstruction)

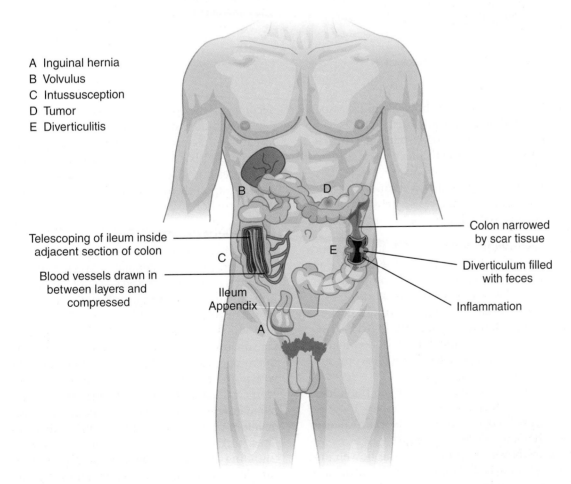

A Inguinal hernia
B Volvulus
C Intussusception
D Tumor
E Diverticulitis

Telescoping of ileum inside adjacent section of colon

Blood vessels drawn in between layers and compressed

Ileum
Appendix

Colon narrowed by scar tissue

Diverticulum filled with feces

Inflammation

FIGURE 9-21 Causes of intestinal obstruction.

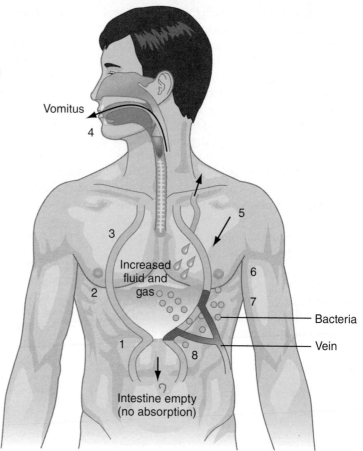

1 Site of obstruction
2 Increased fluid and
   gas lead to distention
3 Distention causes increased
   peristalsis to force contents
   past obstruction, leading to
   colicky pain
4 Severe vomiting from
   distention and pain leads
   to dehydration and
   electrolyte imbalance
5 Increased pressure on
   wall causes more fluid
   to enter intestine
6 Decreased blood pressure
   and hypovolemic shock
   as fluid shift into intestine
   continues (third spacing)
7 Continued pressure on
   intestinal wall causes
   edema and ischemia
   of wall and decreased
   peristalsis
8 Prolonged ischemia causes
   increased permeability and
   necrosis of wall; intestinal
   bacteria and toxins leak
   into blood and peritoneal
   cavity (peritonitis)

Vomitus

Increased
fluid and
gas

Bacteria

Vein

Intestine empty
(no absorption)

FIGURE 9-22 Effects of intestinal obstruction.

- Borborygmi (audible bowel sounds; associated with mechanical obstruction)
- Intestinal rushes (forcible intestinal contractions; associated with mechanical obstruction)
- Decreased or absent bowel sounds
- Restlessness, diaphoresis, tachycardia progressing to weakness, confusion, and shock

Diagnostic procedures for intestinal obstruction are directed at identifying the obstruction, the underlying etiology, and complications. These manifestations consist of a history (including the usual bowel pattern), physical examination, blood chemistry, ABGs, CBC, abdominal CT, abdominal X-ray, abdominal ultrasound, barium enema, sigmoidoscopy, and colonoscopy.

Treatment strategies depend on the underlying cause. Such strategies generally focus on correcting fluid, electrolyte, and pH imbalances (see the *Fluid, Electrolyte, and Acid–Base Homeostasis* chapter); decompressing the bowel; and reestablishing bowel movements. A nasogastric tube with intermittent suctioning is inserted to decompress the bowel and relieve vomiting. The patient should fast and receive TPN until bowel function is restored. Ambulation can help restore peristalsis. Laxatives should not be used in most cases until the obstruction is resolved. Surgery is frequently necessary to relieve mechanical obstruction.

Appendicitis

Appendicitis refers to an inflammation of the vermiform appendix (**FIGURE 9-23**). This inflammation is most often caused by an infection. The inflammation process triggers local tissue edema, which obstructs the small structure. Additional causes include inflammatory bowel disease and constipation. As fluid builds inside the appendix, microorganisms proliferate. The appendix fills with purulent exudate, and the stretched, edematous wall compresses area blood vessels. With blood flow compromised, ischemia and necrosis develop. The pressure inside the appendix escalates, forcing bacteria and toxins out to surrounding structures. Abscesses and peritonitis can develop as bacteria escape, and gangrene can result from the worsening necrosis. The

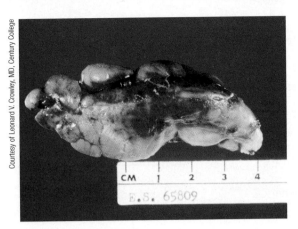

Courtesy of Leonard V. Crowley, MD, Century College

FIGURE 9-23 Appendicitis.

pressure inside the appendix will continue to intensify until the appendix ruptures or perforates, releasing its contents. This release can accelerate peritonitis, which can be life threatening.

Clinical manifestations reflect the pathogenesis characteristic of appendicitis. These manifestations vary significantly in severity, from asymptomatic to sudden and severe. The first symptom is often pain near the umbilicus. As swelling increases, the pain tends to move to the lower right quadrant of the abdomen (McBurney point). The pain gradually intensifies (over approximately 12–24 hours). It is often aggravated by movement, so patients tend to guard their abdomen. Due to normal anatomic variations, this pain may occur anywhere in the abdomen. The pain will temporarily subside if the appendix ruptures, but then will return and escalate as peritonitis develops. Nausea, vomiting, abdominal distension, and bowel pattern changes can also be associated with appendicitis. Other manifestations reflect the inflammation and infectious process (e.g., fever, chills, and leukocytosis). Additionally, the patient should be monitored for signs and symptoms of peritonitis (e.g., abdominal rigidity, tachycardia, and hypotension).

Urgent diagnosis and treatment are crucial for positive patient outcomes. Diagnostic procedures include a history, physical examination, CBC, abdominal ultrasound, abdominal X-ray, abdominal CT, and laparoscopy. Because of the life-threatening nature of appendicitis, surgery remains the cornerstone of treatment. In fact, appendicitis is one of the most common indications for emergency surgery in the United States. Performing the surgery prior to rupture of the appendix is paramount. Prior to rupture, the surgery can be performed through laparoscopy

with minimal risk. If the appendix ruptures, an open surgical procedure is necessary to ensure all of the appendix fragments and infectious materials are removed. Extensive irrigation of the abdominal cavity is performed to flush out any remaining bacteria. The wound may be left open to heal by secondary intention so as to decrease the risk of infection. Tubes may be inserted to drain any abscesses. Long-term antibiotic therapy may be necessary to prevent and resolve any infections. Analgesics will be necessary to manage pain before and after surgery. Additionally, the patient should avoid activities that increase intra-abdominal pressure (e.g., straining and coughing).

Peritonitis

Peritonitis is an inflammation of the peritoneum, the membrane that lines the abdominal wall and abdominal organs. Peritonitis usually presents as an acute condition, and treatment centers on resolving the underlying cause. The inflammation may result from chemical irritation (e.g., ruptured gallbladder or spleen) or direct organism invasion (e.g., appendicitis and peritoneal dialysis) (**FIGURE 9-24**). Chemical irritation will lead to a bacterial invasion if not quickly treated. The inflammatory response triggered by the chemical increases intestinal wall permeability. In turn, the increased permeability allows for passage of enteric bacteria. Necrosis or perforation of the intestinal wall also creates an opportunity for an enteric bacteria invasion.

Several protective mechanisms are activated along with the inflammatory response in an attempt to localize the problem. These mechanisms include producing a thick, sticky exudate that bonds nearby structures and temporarily seals them off. Abscesses may form as the body attempts to wall off the infections. Peristalsis may slow down as a response to the inflammation, decreasing the spread of toxins and bacteria. These mechanisms merely slow the progression, however. If the underlying cause is not treated, the condition can become critical as sepsis and shock develop.

Clinical manifestations reflect the inflammatory and infectious processes under way. These manifestations tend to be sudden and severe. The classic manifestation of peritonitis is abdominal rigidity. A rigid, boardlike abdomen develops because of a reflexive abdominal muscle spasm that occurs in response to the peritoneal inflammation. Inflamed tissue creates abdominal tenderness and pain. Large volumes

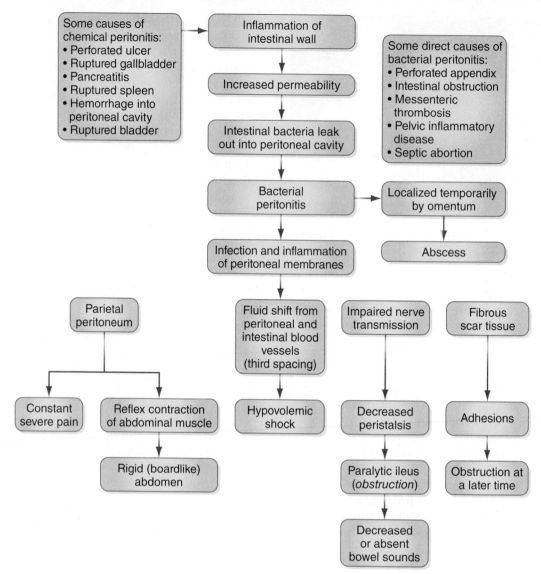

FIGURE 9-24 Development of peritonitis.

of fluid can leak into the peritoneal cavity (a phenomenon called third spacing), leading to hypovolemic shock (see the *Cardiovascular Function* chapter). This fluid contains protein and electrolytes, making it an optimal medium for bacterial growth. Nausea and vomiting are common responses to the intestinal irritation. Persistent inflammation impairs nerve conduction, which decreases peristalsis. This decreased peristalsis can, in turn, lead to intestinal obstruction. Sepsis develops as the bacteria and toxins migrate to the circulatory system through the inflamed membranes. Fever, malaise, and leukocytosis occur because of the infectious process. Additionally, the patient should be monitored for signs of sepsis and shock (e.g., tachycardia, hypotension, restlessness, and diaphoresis).

Diagnostic procedures for peritonitis consist of a history, physical examination, CBC, abdominal X-ray, abdominal ultrasound, abdominal CT, paracentesis with peritoneal fluid analysis, and laparotomy. Treatment strategies vary based on the underlying cause. The patient's prognosis depends on the underlying cause along with the implementation of early and aggressive treatment. Management often includes surgical repair of the chemical leak and draining of the infected fluid. Long-term antibiotic therapy specific to the causative organism will be required. In addition, correction of any fluid and electrolyte imbalance may be required. Insertion of a nasogastric tube with intermittent suction can relieve abdominal distension and treat intestinal obstructions. TPN will be necessary to maintain nutritional status until the peritonitis is resolved.

Celiac Disease

Celiac disease (also known as celiac sprue or gluten-sensitive enteropathy) is an inherited, autoimmune, malabsorption disorder. Although it is considered primarily a childhood disease, this condition can develop at any age. Celiac disease results from a combination of the immune response to an environmental factor (gliadin) and genetic predisposition. It is relatively uncommon in the United States, affecting about 1 in 3,000 people. Celiac disease is most common in Caucasians and in females.

Tropical sprue is a related disorder that occurs in tropical regions, especially India, Southeast Asia, Central America, South America, and the Caribbean. It is thought to be caused by a bacterial, viral, parasitic, or amoebic infection. Unlike celiac disease, which becomes a lifelong condition, tropical sprue can be resolved with antibiotic therapy.

Celiac disease results from a defect in the intestinal enzymes that prevent further digestion of gliadin—a product of gluten digestion. Gluten is an ingredient of grains (e.g., wheat, barley, rye, and oats). The combination of digestive dysfunction and immune activities creates a toxic environment for the intestinal villi. The villi atrophy and flatten, resulting in decreased enzyme production and making less surface area available for nutrient absorption (**FIGURE 9-25**). Eventually, the malnutrition associated with celiac disease can cause vitamin deficiencies that deprive the brain, peripheral nervous system, bones, liver, and other organs of vital nourishment. These nutritional deficits, in turn, can lead to other illnesses:

- Anemia
- Arthralgia (bone and joint pain)
- Myalgia (muscle pain)
- Bone disease (e.g., osteoporosis, kyphoscoliosis, and fractures)

- Dental enamel defects and discoloration
- Intestinal cancers
- Depression
- Growth and development delays in children
- Hair loss
- Hypoglycemia
- Mouth ulcers
- Increased bleeding tendencies (e.g., bruising and nose bleeds)
- Neurologic disorders (e.g., seizures and peripheral neuropathy)
- Skin disorders (e.g., dermatitis herpetiformis and eczema)
- Vitamin or mineral deficiency, single or multiple nutrient (e.g., iron, folate, vitamin B_{12}, and vitamin K)
- Endocrine disorders (e.g., menstrual dysfunction, thyroid disease, type 1 diabetes, and adrenal insufficiency)

Clinical manifestations of celiac disease vary significantly from person to person—a factor that often delays diagnosis. In infants, clinical manifestations generally appear as cereals are added to their diet (usually around 4–6 months of age). Most of the clinical manifestations are GI in nature, but occasionally there are no GI symptoms. The GI clinical manifestations may include the following symptoms:

- Abdominal pain
- Abdominal distension, bloating, gas, and indigestion
- Anorexia
- Constipation or diarrhea (may be chronic or occasional)
- Changes in appetite (usually decreased)
- Lactose intolerance (common upon diagnosis; usually goes away following treatment)
- Nausea and vomiting
- Steatorrhea
- Unexplained weight loss (although people can be overweight or of normal weight upon diagnosis)
- Signs of vitamin deficiencies (e.g., bruising, fatigue, hair loss, paresthesia, and mouth ulcers)

Manifestations that are not GI in nature may include irritability, lethargy, malaise, and behavioral changes. Additionally, the individual with celiac disease should be monitored for development of complications.

Diagnostic procedures for celiac disease consist of a history, physical examination, celiac blood panel, EGD, and duodenal biopsy. The celiac blood panel includes the immunoglobulin

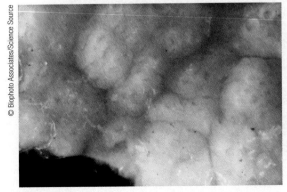

FIGURE 9-25 Effects of celiac disease on intestinal villi.

A antibody–endomysium antibodies, immuno-globulin A antigliadin antibodies, deaminated gliadin peptide antibody, immunoglobulin A antitissue transglutaminase, lactose tolerance test, and D-xylose test.

Dietary management is the cornerstone of treatment. Most people (approximately 90%) with celiac disease are effectively managed by eliminating gluten from their diet. Dietary changes may also be used as a part of diagnosis. The individual is given a gluten-free diet to assess whether the symptoms improve. A gluten-free diet involves avoiding wheat and wheat products—rice and corn can be substituted. Once gluten is removed from the diet, the intestinal mucosa will return to normal after a few weeks. Even when symptoms are controlled with diet, the individual with celiac disease remains at risk for intestinal cancers; consequently, he or she should be periodically monitored for cancer development. Additionally, long-term support may be necessary for children and parents of children with celiac disease.

Inflammatory Bowel Disease

Inflammatory bowel disease (IBD) describes chronic inflammation of the GI tract, usually the intestines. IBD is chiefly seen in women, Caucasians, persons of Jewish descent, and smokers. It encompasses two disorders—Crohn's disease and ulcerative colitis. Both conditions are characterized by periods of exacerbations and remissions that can vary in severity.

The exact cause of IBD is unknown, but this disease is thought to be caused by a genetically associated autoimmune state that has been activated by an infection. Immune cells located in the intestinal mucosa are stimulated to release inflammatory mediators (e.g., histamine, prostaglandins, leukotrienes, and cytokines). These mediators alter the function and neural activity of the secretory and smooth muscle cells in the GI tract. Fluid, electrolyte, and pH imbalances develop. IBD can be painful, debilitating, and life threatening.

Even though the two forms of IBD are similar, some differences between them warrant discussion.

Crohn's Disease

Crohn's disease is an insidious, slow-developing, progressive condition that often emerges in adolescence. Its exact cause is unknown, but T-cell activation leading to tissue damage has been implicated. This condition usually affects the intestines, but it may occur anywhere along the GI tract. Crohn's disease is characterized by patchy areas of inflammation involving the full thickness of the intestinal wall and ulcerations. These patchy areas and ulcerations, often called skip lesions, are separated by areas of normal tissue (**FIGURE 9-26**). The ulcers combine to form fissures divided by nodules (thickened elevations), giving the intestinal wall a cobblestone appearance. Eventually, the entire wall becomes thick and rigid,

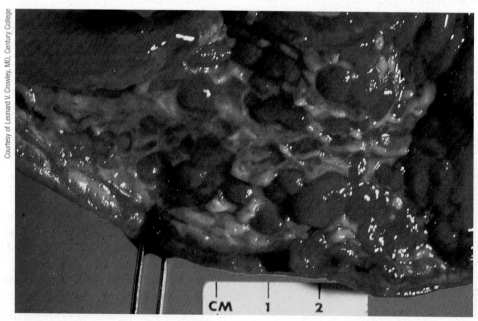

Courtesy of Leonard V. Crowley, MD, Century College

FIGURE 9-26 Crohn's disease.

and the intestinal lumen becomes narrowed and potentially obstructed. Granulomas—that is, nodules consisting of epithelial and immune cells—develop on the intestinal wall and nearby lymph nodes because of the chronic inflammation. Over time, the damaged intestinal wall loses the ability to process and absorb food. The inflammation also stimulates intestinal motility, decreasing digestion and absorption.

Complications of Crohn's disease include the following conditions:

- Malnutrition
- Anemia (especially iron-deficiency anemia because of the malnutrition)
- Fistulas
- Adhesions
- Abscesses
- Intestinal obstruction
- Perforation
- Anal fissure
- Fluid, electrolyte, and pH imbalances
- Delayed growth and development (in children)

Clinical manifestations of Crohn's disease reflect the inflammatory process and the digestive dysfunction. These manifestations, which intensify during exacerbations, include the following symptoms:

- Abdominal cramping and pain (typically in the right lower quadrant and may occur with defecation)
- Diarrhea (usually watery)
- Steatorrhea
- Constipation (as the intestinal lumen narrows)
- Palpable abdominal mass (thickened intestinal wall)
- Melena (if ulcers begin bleeding)
- Anorexia
- Mouth ulcers
- Weight loss
- Indications of inflammation (e.g., fever, fatigue, arthralgia, and malaise)

Diagnostic procedures for Crohn's disease consist of a history, physical examination, stool analysis (including cultures and occult blood), CBC, blood chemistry, C-reactive protein levels, erythrocyte sedimentation rate, abdominal X-ray, abdominal CT, abdominal MRI, barium studies (swallow and enema), sigmoidoscopy, colonoscopy, and biopsy. Treatment strategies focus on nutritional support, symptom relief, and complication minimization. Dietary management usually includes (1) a low-residue, high-calorie, high-protein diet; (2) oral nutritional supplements (e.g., Ensure and Sustacal); (3) multivitamin supplements; and (4) TPN as the disease progresses. Pharmacologic management usually includes (1) antidiarrheal agents; (2) aminosalicylates (5-ASAs; to treat mild to moderate inflammation); (3) glucocorticoids (to treat moderate to severe inflammation); (4) immune modulators (to suppress inflammatory response); (5) biologic agents (to treat severe unresponsive Crohn's disease); (6) analgesics; and (7) antibiotics (if infection is present). Surgical intestine resection may be necessary as the disease progresses and complications develop. Additional strategies involve stress management (e.g., exercise, meditation, deep breathing, biofeedback, and acupuncture) and support (e.g., group involvement and counseling).

Ulcerative Colitis

Ulcerative colitis is a progressive condition of the rectum and colon mucosa that usually develops in the second or third decade of life. Inflammation triggered by T-cell accumulation in the colon mucosa causes epithelium loss, surface erosion, and ulceration. The ulceration begins in the rectum and extends in a continuous segment to involve the entire colon. Ulcerative colitis rarely affects the small intestine. The mucosa becomes inflamed, edematous, and frail. Necrosis of the epithelial tissue (specifically at the base of the crypts of Lieberkühn) can result in abscesses, known as crypt abscesses. As the body attempts to heal, granulation tissue forms, but the tissue remains fragile and bleeds easily. The ulcers merge together, creating large areas of stripped mucosa. Nutritional, fluid, electrolyte, and pH imbalances develop due to the lack of an adequate surface area for absorption. Complications of ulcerative colitis include the following conditions:

- Malnutrition
- Anemia
- Hemorrhage
- Perforation
- Strictures
- Fistulas
- Pseudopolyps
- Toxic megacolon (life-threatening condition caused by rapid dilation of the large intestine)
- Colorectal carcinoma
- Liver disease (because of inflammation and scarring of the bile ducts)
- Fluid, electrolyte, and pH imbalances

Clinical manifestations of ulcerative colitis reflect the inflammatory process and digestive dysfunction. As is the case with Crohn's disease, these manifestations intensify during exacerbations. Manifestations usually include the following symptoms:

- Diarrhea (usually frequent [as many as 20 daily], watery stools containing blood and mucus)
- Tenesmus (persistent rectal spasms associated with the need to defecate)
- Proctitis (inflammation of the rectum)
- Abdominal cramping
- Nausea and vomiting
- Weight loss
- Indications of inflammation (e.g., fever, fatigue, arthralgia, and malaise)

Diagnostic procedures for ulcerative colitis consist of a history, physical examination, stool analysis (including cultures and occult blood), CBC, blood chemistry, C-reactive protein levels, erythrocyte sedimentation rate, abdominal X-ray, abdominal CT, abdominal MRI, barium enema, colonoscopy, and biopsy. Similar to Crohn's disease, treatment strategies focus on nutritional support, symptom relief, and complication minimization. Dietary management usually includes (1) a high-fiber, high-calorie, high-protein diet; (2) oral nutritional supplements (e.g., Ensure or Sustacal); (3) multivitamin supplements; and (4) TPN as the disease progresses. Pharmacologic management usually includes (1) antidiarrheal agents; (2) antispasmodics; (3) anticholinergics; (4) aminosalicylates (to treat mild to moderate inflammation); (5) glucocorticoids (to treat moderate to severe inflammation); (6) immune modulators (to suppress inflammatory response); (7) biologic agents; (8) analgesics; and (9) antibiotics (if infection is present). Surgical intervention (e.g., ileostomy or colostomy) may be necessary as the disease progresses and complications develop. Additional strategies involve stress management (e.g., exercise, meditation, deep breathing, biofeedback, and acupuncture) and support (e.g., group involvement and counseling).

Irritable Bowel Syndrome

Irritable bowel syndrome (IBS) refers to a chronic GI condition characterized by exacerbations associated with stress. IBS includes alterations in bowel pattern and abdominal pain not explained by structural or biochemical abnormalities. In contrast to IBD, IBS is less serious, is noninflammatory, and does not cause permanent intestinal damage (**TABLE 9-4**). IBS is more common in women than in men. Its exact cause is unknown, but three theories of its etiology include altered GI motility, visceral hyperalgesia, and psychopathology. IBS is thought to be an intensified response to stimuli that is characterized by increased intestinal motility and contractions. People with IBS may have a low tolerance for stretching and pain in the intestinal smooth muscle, causing them to respond to stimuli to which people without IBS do not respond. Complications of IBS include hemorrhoids, nutritional deficits, social issues, and sexual discomfort.

Clinical manifestations vary from person to person. Stress, mood disorders (e.g., anxiety and depression), food (e.g., chocolate, alcohol, dairy products, carbonated beverages, vegetables, and fruits), and hormone changes (e.g., menstruation) often worsen symptoms. These manifestations usually include the following symptoms:

- Abdominal distension, fullness, flatus, and bloating
- Intermittent abdominal pain exacerbated by eating and relieved by defecation
- Chronic and frequent constipation, usually accompanied by pain
- Chronic and frequent diarrhea, usually accompanied by pain
- Nonbloody stool that may contain mucus
- Bowel urgency
- Intolerance to certain foods (usually gas-forming foods and those containing sorbitol, lactose, and gluten)
- Emotional distress
- Anorexia

Diagnosis is based on clinical presentation (**TABLE 9-5**) and is often made by excluding other GI and psychological disorders. Diagnostic procedures consist of a history (including bowel pattern and Rome III criteria), stool analysis (including cultures and occult blood), celiac blood panel, abdominal X-ray, abdominal CT, abdominal MRI, barium studies (swallow and enema), sigmoidoscopy, colonoscopy, and biopsy.

Treatment focuses on management of symptoms and may vary depending on those symptoms. Pharmacologic strategies may include antidiarrheal agents, laxatives, antispasmodics, and antidepressants. Other strategies involve avoiding triggers, maintaining adequate fiber intake, stress management (through techniques such as exercise, meditation, deep breathing, biofeedback, and acupuncture), and support (e.g., group involvement, counseling, and psychotherapy).

TABLE 9-4	Comparison of Inflammatory Bowel Disease and Irritable Bowel Syndrome		
	Inflammatory Bowel Disease		**Irritable Bowel Syndrome**
	Ulcerative Colitis	**Crohn's Disease**	
Epidemiology	Abrupt onset	Insidious onset	Late teens/early adulthood
	Peak ages 15 to 30	15 to 40	
	Caucasian > African American	Female > male	Female > male
	Female > male		
Pathology	Possible autoimmune infection may precipitate familial tendency	Possible autoimmune infection may precipitate genetic predisposition	Cause unknown
	Continuous, irregular superficial inflammation of mucosal layer of colon and rectum	Skipping ulcerations involving mucosal and submucosal layers along the entire GI tract; 50% involve small intestine/colon	Bowel has increased response to stimuli and visceral hypersensitivity
		Strictures/fistulas common	Altered perception of central nervous system
Signs and Symptoms			
Abdominal pain	Intermittent, mild crampy tenderness	Crampy or steady	Sharp, burning; may be diffuse or left lower quadrant
		Periumbilical or right lower quadrant	
Mass present	No	Common	No
Bleeding	Common	Occasionally	No
Diarrhea	Frequent watery stools with blood and mucus	Chronic, recurrent, may have some blood	Intermittent, predominant
			Symptom varies with individual
Perianal lesions	No	One-third develop perianal abscesses or fistulas	No
Weight loss	With severe diarrhea	Common	No
Fever/malaise	During severe exacerbation	With exacerbation and abscess formation	No
Psychological	As a result of long-standing disease	As a result of long-standing disease	Exacerbation with stressful situations
Course/prognosis	75–80% relapse after first attack	Recurrent, progressive	Chronic, intermittent
	Most have mild to moderate disease	Typically need surgery after 7 years to treat/repair fistulas or abscesses	Rare functional limitations
	Routine colonoscopy with biopsy after having the disease for 7–8 years because of increased colon cancer risk	Shortened life span	

Diverticular Disease

Diverticular disease refers to conditions related to the development of diverticula. **Diverticula** (singular: *diverticulum*) are outwardly bulging pouches of the intestinal wall that develop when mucosa sections or large intestine submucosa layers herniate through a weakened muscular layer (**FIGURE 9-27**). Diverticula may be congenital or acquired. They are thought to be caused by a low-fiber diet that results in chronic constipation. The muscular wall can become weakened from the prolonged effort of moving hard stools. Pressure increases in the intestine in an attempt to propel the stool, forcing the mucosa through areas of weakness. Diverticular disease is rare in developing countries where high-fiber diets are typical, but is more common in developed countries where processed foods and low-fiber diets are widely consumed. In addition to diet, poor bowel habits (e.g., straining and delaying defecation) can contribute to developing diverticula.

TABLE 9-5	Rome III Criteria

Twelve weeks within 12 months (need not be consecutive) of abdominal pain or discomfort that has two of three features:

1. Relieved by defecation
2. Onset associated with changes in stool frequency
3. Onset associated with changes in stool form or appearance

Symptoms That Support Diagnosis of IBS

Abnormal stool frequency (> 3/day or < 3/week)

Abnormal stool form (lumpy and hard or watery and loose)

Abnormal stool passage (straining, urgency, feeling of incomplete evacuation)

Passage of mucus

Bloating or feeling of abdominal distension

Most cases of diverticular disease are asymptomatic and are discovered incidentally. **Diverticulosis** describes asymptomatic diverticular disease, usually with multiple diverticula present. **Diverticulitis** refers to a state in which diverticula have become inflamed, usually because of retained fecal matter. It can result in potentially fatal obstructions, infection, abscess, perforation, peritonitis, hemorrhage, and shock. Diverticulitis often remains asymptomatic until the condition becomes serious. When they appear, clinical manifestations usually include abdominal cramping, followed by passing a large quantity of frank blood. Bleeding may last hours or days before spontaneously ceasing. Most people with diverticulitis (approximately 80%) will experience only a single episode of bleeding and require no further treatment. Persistent or

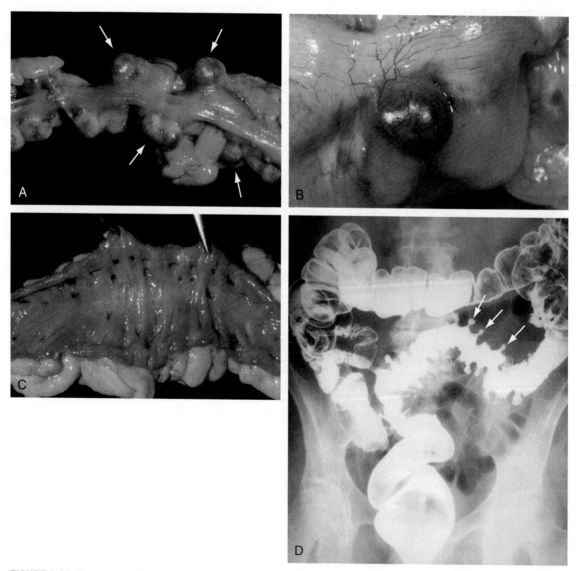

FIGURE 9-27 Diverticula. (a) Exterior of the colon illustrating several diverticula projecting through the wall of the colon. (b) A closer view of the diverticulum. (c) Interior of the colon, illustrating openings of multiple diverticula. (d) Diverticula of the colon demonstrated by injection of barium contrast material into the colon.

Courtesy of Leonard V. Crowley, MD, Century College

recurrent bleeding, however, requires further actions. In addition to bleeding, other clinical manifestations that may be present include a low-grade fever, abdominal tenderness (usually in the left lower quadrant), abdominal distension, constipation, obstipation (severe constipation usually caused by an intestinal obstruction), nausea, vomiting, a palpable abdominal mass, and leukocytosis.

Diagnostic procedures for diverticular disease consist of a history, physical examination, stool analysis (including that for occult blood), abdominal ultrasound, abdominal CT, abdominal MRI, colonoscopy, barium enema, and biopsy. Treatment strategies include consumption of a high-fiber diet, adequate hydration, proper bowel habits (e.g., defecating when urge is sensed and not straining), stool softeners, antibiotics (if infection is present), analgesics, and colon resection. A low-residue diet (i.e., avoiding foods with seeds, nuts, and corn) is thought to help, but no evidence supports this notion. Food intake is usually decreased when active bleeding is present, and blood transfusions may be necessary depending on the amount of blood loss.

Cancers

Malignancies of the GI system may originate in the GI tract or spread there from other sites. These cancers can lead to altered nutrition as well as impaired elimination depending on their location. Some GI cancers have moderate treatment success rates (e.g., colorectal cancer), whereas others have high mortality rates (e.g., oral and pancreatic cancer). Typical cancer diagnosis, staging, and treatments are usually employed with cancers involving the GI system (see the *Cellular Function* chapter).

Oral Cancer

Oral cancer can occur anywhere in the mouth, but most cases involve squamous cell carcinomas of the tongue and mouth floor (FIGURE 9-28). Approximately 75% of cases can be attributed to use of smoked and smokeless tobacco. Alcohol consumption also significantly increases the risk of developing oral cancer. Combined alcohol and tobacco use can increase this risk by as much as 100-fold. Additional risk factors include viral infections (especially with human papillomavirus), immunodeficiencies, inadequate nutrition, poor dental hygiene, chronic irritation (e.g., from dentures), and exposure to ultraviolet light (as in cancer of the lips).

Incidence rates of oral cancer have slightly decreased since 1980. Men are twice as likely as

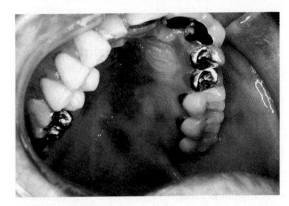

FIGURE 9-28 Oral cancer.

Courtesy of CDC/Sol Silverman, Jr., DDS, University of California, San Francisco

women to develop oral cancer. According to the American Cancer Society (2016), oral cancer is the eighth most frequent cancer in men. Prevalence and mortality rates are the highest in African American men; however, overall mortality rates have decreased since 1980.

In its early stages, oral cancer is very treatable. Unfortunately, most cases are advanced by the time the diagnosis is made because the cancer tends to be hidden. Oral cancer has a 5-year survival rate of 63%—a rate that has significantly improved since 1990.

Oral cancer usually appears initially as a painless, whitish thickening that develops into a nodule or an ulcerative lesion. Multiple lesions may be present. These lesions persist, do not heal, and bleed easily. Additional manifestations include a lump, thickening, or soreness in the mouth, throat, or tongue as well as difficulty chewing or swallowing food. Oral cancer often metastasizes to the neck lymph nodes and the esophagus.

Treatment primarily consists of surgery and radiation, but surgery may be difficult depending on the location. Chemotherapy may be added for patients with advanced disease. Speech therapy is often necessary after treatment to improve chewing, swallowing, and speech.

Esophageal Cancer

Much like oral cancer, esophageal cancer is usually a squamous cell carcinoma or adenocarcinoma, and it most often affects men. Incidence rates of esophageal cancer have remained steady, but the mortality rates have increased since 1980. According to the American Cancer Society (2016), esophageal cancer is the seventh leading cause of cancer death in men, even though it did not make the list of top 10 cancers in men. Rates are fairly equal across racial and ethnic groups.

The distal esophagus is the most common site at which this cancer develops. Esophageal cancer is associated with chronic irritation (e.g., GERD, achalasia, hiatal hernia, alcohol abuse, and use of smoked and smokeless tobacco) and obesity. These tumors can grow to match the circumference of the esophagus, creating a stricture, or they can grow out into the lumen of the esophagus, creating an obstruction. Complications include esophageal obstruction, respiratory compromise, and esophageal bleeding.

Esophageal cancer is usually asymptomatic in its early stages, delaying its diagnosis and treatment. Because of the usually late diagnosis, the prognosis is poor for patients with esophageal cancer. Clinical manifestations, when present, typically include dysphagia, odynaphagia, chest pain (not related to eating), weight loss, hematemesis, and halitosis. Surgery is the treatment of choice, but chemotherapy and radiation are also frequently included in management. Speech therapy will likely be necessary following treatment.

Gastric Cancer

Gastric cancer occurs in several forms, but adenocarcinoma (an ulcerative lesion) is the most frequently encountered type. Incidence and mortality rates of gastric cancer in the United States have declined since 1980. Nevertheless, gastric cancer remains extremely prevalent worldwide (it is the fifth most common type of cancer) and is the third most deadly cancer worldwide (World Health Organization [WHO], 2015). Japan has particularly high rates of gastric cancer. Gastric cancer is prevalent in men and Asians and Pacific Islanders, but mortality rates are highest among African American men. Gastric cancer has a 5-year survival rate of approximately 29%.

Gastric cancer is strongly associated with increased intake of salted, cured, pickled, preserved (containing nitrates and nitrites), and smoked foods. A low-fiber diet and constipation can increase the risk of developing this cancer because they prolong the time over which the intestinal wall is exposed to these substances. Additional risk factors include family history, *H. pylori* infections, smoking, pernicious anemia, chronic atrophic gastritis, and gastric polyps.

Gastric cancer is asymptomatic in its early stages, which often delays its diagnosis and treatment. When present, clinical manifestations include the following symptoms:

- Abdominal pain and fullness
- Epigastric discomfort
- Palpable abdominal mass
- Dark stools, possibly melena
- Dysphagia that worsens over time
- Excessive belching
- Anorexia
- Nausea and vomiting
- Hematemesis
- Premature abdominal fullness after meals
- Unintentional weight loss
- Weakness and fatigue

Surgical removal of the stomach (gastrectomy) is the only curative treatment. Chemotherapy and radiation are also used as curative and palliative measures. Nutritional support (e.g., TPN) and supplements (e.g., vitamin B_{12} and iron) will be needed before, during, and after treatment.

Liver Cancer

Liver cancer most commonly occurs as a secondary tumor that has metastasized from the breast, lung, or other GI structures (**FIGURE 9-29**). Incidence and mortality rates of liver cancer in the United States have tripled since 1980. According to the American Cancer Society (2016), liver cancer is the 10th most common cancer in men and the 5th deadliest cancer in men. Worldwide, liver cancer is the 2nd most common cancer (WHO, 2015). Most primary tumors are caused by chronic cirrhosis or hepatitis. Liver cancer is most prevalent among men as well as Asians and Pacific Islanders. It has a 5-year survival rate of approximately 17%.

Liver cancer may either be asymptomatic or produce mild symptoms initially. Clinical manifestations are similar to those of other liver diseases:

- Anorexia
- Fever
- Jaundice
- Nausea and vomiting

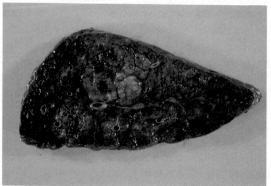

FIGURE 9-29 Liver cancer.

- Abdominal pain (usually in the upper right quadrant)
- Hepatomegaly
- Splenomegaly
- Portal hypertension
- Edema, third spacing (accumulation of fluid in tissue or body cavities), and ascites
- Paraneoplastic syndrome (manifestations and diseases that result from cancer)
- Diaphoresis
- Weight loss

Treatment strategies vary depending on the primary site and progression of the cancer. Chemotherapy is used systemically when metastasis is evident or may be injected directly into localized tumors. If the tumor is small, a section of the liver may be surgically removed (a procedure called a hepatectomy). If the cancer has spread throughout the liver or has caused significant damage, a liver transplant will be the best option if metastasis has not occurred. Several nontraditional cancer treatment procedures are also available to treat liver cancer. Cryoablation is a procedure that uses extreme cold to destroy cancer cells by injecting liquid nitrogen into the tumor. Radiofrequency ablation uses electric current to heat and destroy cancer cells. Pure alcohol can also be injected into the tumor to dry and eventually kill the cancer cells.

Pancreatic Cancer

Pancreatic cancer is an aggressive malignancy (most commonly adenocarcinoma) that can quickly spread to nearby structures (e.g., stomach, intestines, spleen, liver, and kidneys). Its incidence and mortality rates have remained steady since 1980. According to the American Cancer Society (2016), pancreatic cancer is the ninth most common cancer in women, and it is the fourth leading cause of cancer deaths in men and women.

Pancreatic cancer occurs most frequently in men and African Americans. Other risk factors include family history, obesity, chronic pancreatitis, long-standing diabetes mellitus, cirrhosis, alcohol abuse, and tobacco use.

The overall 5-year survival rate for this disease is a mere 7%. This dismal prognosis is due largely to the asymptomatic nature of pancreatic cancer and the lack of a reliable early detection method. Clinical manifestations do not generally develop until the cancer is well advanced and has metastasized,

delaying diagnosis and treatment. These manifestations may include the following signs and symptoms:

- Upper abdominal pain that may radiate to the back (pain worsens as cancer progresses)
- Jaundice
- Dark urine and clay-colored stools
- Indigestion
- Anorexia
- Weight loss
- Depression
- Malnutrition
- Hyperglycemia
- Increased clotting tendencies

No effective treatment has been developed for pancreatic cancer. Surgical removal of the tumor (called a Whipple procedure) is recommended, but few pancreatic tumors can be surgically removed. Chemotherapy and radiation are often used as palliative treatment or in combination with surgery. Any biliary blockages that develop will require repair through surgery or endoscopy.

Colorectal Cancer

Colorectal cancer most often develops from an adenomatous polyp. According to WHO (2015), colorectal cancer is the fourth most common cancer worldwide. According to the American Cancer Society (2016), colorectal cancer is the third most common and most fatal cancer in men and women in the United States, although its rates have been declining since 1980. Incidence and mortality rates are the highest among men and African Americans. The 5-year survival rate for colorectal cancer is a robust 65%.

Dietary factors that have been associated with colorectal cancer include excessive intake of fat, calories, red meat, processed meat, and alcohol as well as deficient intake of fiber. Other risk factors involve family history, advancing age, obesity, tobacco use, physical inactivity, and IBD.

Like many other GI cancers, colorectal cancer remains asymptomatic until it is well advanced. When present, clinical manifestations may include the following symptoms:

- Lower abdominal pain and tenderness
- Blood in the stool (occult or frank)
- Diarrhea, constipation, or other change in bowel habits
- Intestinal obstruction

- Narrow stools
- Unexplained anemia (usually iron-deficiency anemia)
- Unintentional weight loss

Routine screening can dramatically improve prognosis. The 5-year survival rate for colorectal cancer if detected when it is localized to the large intestine is approximately 90%. The U.S. Preventive Services Task Force (2016) and American Cancer Society (2016) recommend regular colorectal screening beginning at 50 years of age for both sexes (earlier if risk factors are present). The screening tests and recommended intervals are identified here:

- A high-sensitivity fecal occult blood test (which checks for hidden blood in three consecutive stool samples) should be administered every year.
- A fecal immunochemical test (which is more accurate than the fecal occult blood test) should be administered every year.

- Flexible sigmoidoscopy should be administered every 5 years.
- Colonoscopy should be administered every 10 years.

Colonoscopy is also used as a diagnostic test when symptoms are present, and it can be used as a follow-up test when the results of another colorectal cancer screening test are unclear or abnormal. Additionally, early (stage 0) cancer cells can be removed during the colonoscopy.

Cancers stage I through III require extensive surgery (colon resection). Chemotherapy and radiation use varies depending on the cancer stage. The patient may require a colostomy (a colon diversionary procedure in which the colon is brought to the abdominal wall to drain into an externally attached pouch) because of the colon resection. Because colorectal cancer often reoccurs, lifestyle changes (e.g., diet and physical activity) and follow-up screenings are crucial to long-term survival.

Myth Busters

Several myths regarding the gastrointestinal system merit discussion.

Myth 1: Smoking a cigarette helps relieve heartburn.

Actually, cigarette smoking may contribute to heartburn. Heartburn occurs when the lower esophageal sphincter relaxes, allowing the acidic contents of the stomach to reflux into the esophagus. Esophagitis is more frequent in people who smoke, presumably as a result of increased acid reflux. The increased reflux is thought to occur because cigarette smoking relaxes the LES.

Myth 2: After ostomy surgery, men have erectile dysfunction and women have impaired sexual function and are unable to become pregnant.

Ostomy surgery does not, in general, interfere with a person's sexual or reproductive capabilities. Ostomy surgery is a procedure in which the diseased part of the small or large intestine is removed, and the remaining intestine is attached to an opening in the abdomen. Stool is collected in a bag taped to the skin over the opening or in an internal pouch. Although some men who have had radical ostomy surgery lose the ability to achieve and sustain an erection, most do not. Temporary erectile dysfunction may be experienced because of damage to the nerves innervating the penis. In women, ostomy surgery does not damage sexual or reproductive organs, so it is not a direct cause of sexual problems or sterility. Factors such as pain and the adjustment to a new body image may create temporary sexual problems, but these problems can usually be resolved with time and, in some cases, counseling. Unless a woman has undergone a hysterectomy, she can still bear children.

Myth 3: Bowel regularity means a bowel movement every day.

The frequency of bowel movements among normal, healthy people varies from three a day to three a week, and some perfectly healthy people fall outside both ends of this range. Nevertheless, even three bowel movements a day can be abnormal in someone who usually has one bowel movement a day. The key to determining normality is comparing current bowel activities to the individual's usual patterns.

application to practice

Now that we have discussed conditions of the GI system, let's put that knowledge into practice. While working in the clinic, you encounter the following patients. Which patient would be at greatest risk for developing an intestinal obstruction?

- An adult diagnosed with cirrhosis of the liver
- An individual eating a low-fiber, high-fat diet
- A Jewish patient who smokes and consumes large amounts of caffeine

- An elderly patient who is on bed rest because of postoperative abdominal surgery

When determining who is at greatest risk, just start counting risk factors—the patient with the most risk factors "wins." Here, we start with the adult with cirrhosis. This patient has no risk factors for developing an intestinal obstruction. The patient with a low-fiber, high-fat diet may be at risk because consuming low-fiber diet can put individuals at risk for constipation. Keep this patient on the short list. Next, consider the Jewish patient. This patient does not have any risk factors, so eliminate this individual. Finally, the elderly patient has three risk factors—advancing age, immobility, and abdominal surgery. With three risk factors, the elderly patient is at the most risk for developing an intestinal obstruction.

CHAPTER SUMMARY

The GI system is responsible for ingestion, absorption, and removal of food. These functions obtain the essential nutrients, water, and electrolytes the body needs to maintain many physiologic activities and homeostasis. Disorders of the GI tract range in severity from harmless to life threatening. These disorders can be congenital, infectious, structural, or cancerous in nature. Regardless of the pathogenesis, GI disorders often create short- or long-term nutritional deficits or elimination issues that can affect the individual's overall health. Promoting GI health focuses primarily on dietary strategies that include following a well-balanced diet.

REFERENCES

American Cancer Society. (2016). Cancer facts and figures 2016. Retrieved from http://www.cancer.org/acs/groups /content/@research/documents/document/acspc-047079.pdf

Anand, B. (2015). Peptic ulcer disease. *Medscape*. Retrieved from http://emedicine.medscape.com/article/181753 -overview#a3

Buggs, A., & Dronen, S. (2014). Viral hepatitis. *Medscape*. Retrieved from http://emedicine.medscape.com/article /775507-overview

Centers for Disease Control and Prevention (CDC). (2015a). Facts about cleft lip and cleft palate. Retrieved from http://www .cdc.gov/ncbddd/birthdefects/CleftLip.html

Centers for Disease Control and Prevention (CDC). (2015b). Viral hepatitis surveillance, United States 2014. Retrieved from https://www.cdc.gov/hepatitis/statistics/2014 surveillance/pdfs/2014hepsurveillancerpt.pdf

Chiras, D. (2011). *Human biology* (7th ed.). Burlington, MA: Jones & Bartlett Learning.

Crowley, L. V. (2012). *An introduction to human disease* (9th ed.). Burlington, MA: Jones & Bartlett Learning.

Elling, B., Elling, K., & Rothenberg, M. (2004). *Anatomy and physiology*. Sudbury, MA: Jones and Bartlett.

Gould, B. (2015). *Pathophysiology for the health professions* (5th ed.). Philadelphia, PA: Elsevier.

Heuman, D., Allen, J., & Mihas, A. (2016). Gallstones (cholelithiasis). *Medscape*. Retrieved from http://emedicine.medscape .com/article/175667-overview#a1

Madara, B., & Pomarico-Denino, V. (2008). *Quick look nursing: Pathophysiology* (2nd ed.). Sudbury, MA: Jones and Bartlett.

Professional guide to pathophysiology (3rd ed.). (2010). Philadelphia, PA: Lippincott Williams & Wilkins.

Singh, J., & Sinert, R. (2015). Pediatric pyloric stenosis. *Medscape*. Retrieved from http://emedicine.medscape.com/article /803489-overview#a6

U.S. Preventive Services Task Force. (2016). Colorectal cancer: Screening recommendations. Retrieved from http://www .uspreventiveservicestaskforce.org/Page/Document /UpdateSummaryFinal/colorectal-cancer-screening2?ds=1 &s=colorectal

Wolf, D. (2015). Cirrhosis. *Medscape*. Retrieved from http: //emedicine.medscape.com/article/185856-overview#a1

World Health Organization (WHO). (2015). Cancer fact sheet. Retrieved from http://www.who.int/mediacentre/factsheets /fs297/en/

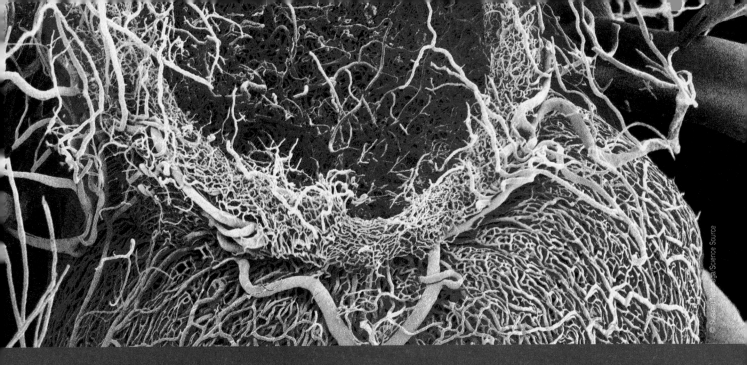

CHAPTER 10

Endocrine Function

LEARNING OBJECTIVES

- Discuss normal endocrine anatomy and physiology.
- Compare and contrast disorders of the parathyroid gland.

- Describe and differentiate the types of diabetes mellitus.
- Compare and contrast disorders of the thyroid gland.
- Compare and contrast disorders of the adrenal glands.

KEY TERMS

acromegaly
Addison's disease
adrenal gland
aldosterone
alpha cell
amylin
beta cell
calcitonin
cortex
cortisol
Cushing's syndrome
delta cell
diabetes insipidus
diabetes mellitus (DM)
diabetic ketoacidosis
dwarfism
epinephrine
epsilon cell
exophthalmos

follicles
gestational diabetes
ghrelin
gigantism
glucagon
glucocorticoid
goiter
gonadocorticoid
Graves' disease
Hashimoto's thyroiditis
hyperglycemia
hyperparathyroidism
hyperpituitarism
hyperprolactinemia
hyperthyroidism
hypoglycemia
hypoparathyroidism
hypopituitarism
hypothalamic–pituitary axis

hypothalamus
hypothyroidism
insulin
islets of Langerhans
isthmus
medulla
metabolic syndrome
mineralocorticoid
myxedema
negative feedback system
norepinephrine
pancreas
pancreatic polypeptide
panhypopituitarism
parathyroid gland
parathyroid hormone (PTH)
pheochromocytoma
pituitary gland
polydipsia

polyphagia
polyuria
positive feedback system
PP cell
somatostatin
syndrome of inappropriate antidiuretic hormone (SIADH)
T_3
T_4
thyroid gland
thyroid-stimulating hormone (TSH)
thyrotoxicosis
type 1 diabetes
type 2 diabetes

The endocrine system consists of glands located throughout the body (**FIGURE 10-1**) that are responsible for producing and secreting a wide range of hormones and chemical transmitters. These hormones serve as chemical messengers, traveling to various sites to regulate several processes, including (1) growth and development, (2) metabolism, (3) sexual function, (4) reproduction, and (5) mood stability. Hormones influence these processes by binding to receptors on the surface or within their target cells. Only small amounts of these potent substances are required to make a significant impact at the cellular and organism levels. Consequently, subtle fluctuations in hormone levels can disrupt the body's delicate balance. Disorders of the endocrine system can result from insufficient or excessive amounts of these hormones that alter their specific function. Causes of these disorders vary, but include genetic alterations, lifestyle behaviors, and tumors. The severity of these endocrine disorders can range from mild conditions that are easily managed to life-shortening or life-threatening conditions.

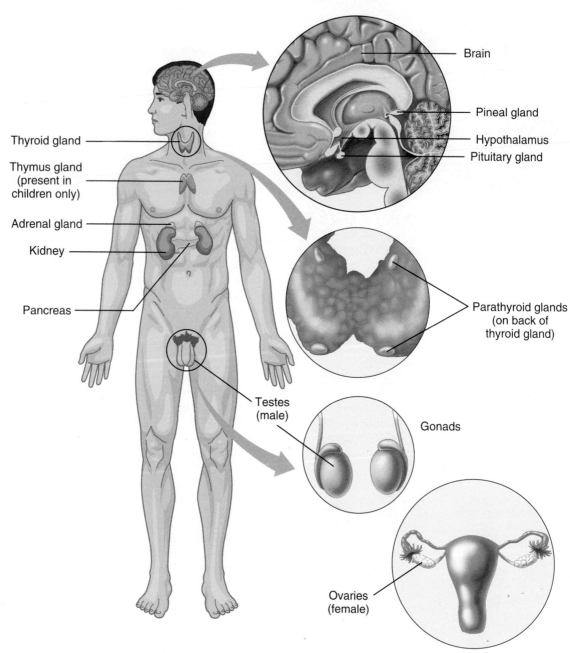

FIGURE 10-1 The human endocrine system.

Anatomy and Physiology

The endocrine system is a complex messaging and control system that interacts with several body functions. It uses hormones to orchestrate these multifaceted communication and control operations. Endocrine glands located throughout the body produce and secrete these hormones. The term *endocrine* refers to the act of secreting substances directly into the bloodstream (**FIGURE 10-2**) rather than in a duct (like the exocrine glands of the gastrointestinal tract; see the *Gastrointestinal Function* chapter). In addition to these structures, reproductive glands (e.g., testes and ovaries) produce hormones (see the *Reproductive Function* chapter).

Hormones can be classified or described in regard to their action (e.g., altering serum and glucose levels), source (e.g., anterior pituitary gland), or chemical structure. They can also be divided into four categories based on chemical composition: (1) steroids (e.g., androgens, glucocorticoids, and thyroid hormones), which are lipid soluble; (2) proteins or polypeptides (e.g., insulin and growth hormone), which are water soluble; (3) amines and amino acids (e.g., epinephrine), which are water soluble; and (4) fatty acid derivatives (e.g., prostaglandins).

Release of these hormones from their respective glands is primarily controlled by a **negative feedback system**, but may occasionally be controlled by a **positive feedback system** (see the *Cellular Function* chapter). The nervous system, other substances, and circadian rhythm can all influence these systems. In a negative feedback loop, the end product (in this case, hormones) of a biochemical process inhibits its own production—the hormone is released only when its levels decline, and production stops when its levels rise (e.g., insulin is released in response to serum glucose levels). In the endocrine system, a positive feedback loop is rare and occurs when one hormone product stimulates the production of another (e.g., release of oxytocin during childbirth). Tropic hormones

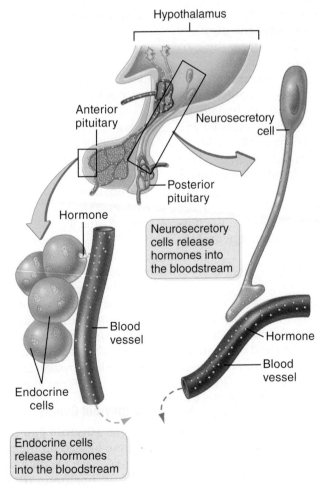

Hypothalamus

Anterior pituitary

Neurosecretory cell

Posterior pituitary

Hormone

Neurosecretory cells release hormones into the bloodstream

Blood vessel

Hormone

Blood vessel

Endocrine cells

Endocrine cells release hormones into the bloodstream

FIGURE 10-2 Endocrine release of hormones.

regulate endocrine glands to produce other hormones (e.g., thyroid-stimulating hormone). Nontropic hormones directly stimulate cellular metabolism and other activities.

Once released from the gland, hormones travel through the circulatory system to their target cells in other glands and tissues. Multiple hormone signals continuously interact with these target cells, but these cells respond only to their specific hormone. This selective response is due to protein receptors located in the cell membrane or the cytoplasm. Once the hormone has acted on the target cells, the liver metabolizes the hormone and the kidneys excrete it to prevent an accumulative effect.

Pituitary Gland and Hypothalamus

Roughly the size of a pea, the **pituitary gland** is located at the base of the brain. This gland can be divided into two parts—the anterior and posterior pituitary gland. The pituitary gland is often referred to as the master gland. Despite its small size, this gland secretes several hormones that influence many different body functions (**FIGURE 10-3**; **TABLE 10-1**). The **hypothalamus**, which is the basal (bottom) portion of the diencephalon, regulates the pituitary gland. The hypothalamus connects the nervous and endocrine systems. It contains receptors that monitor hormone, nutrient, and ion levels. When activated, these receptors stimulate neurosecretory neurons in the hypothalamus to secrete various types of releasing and inhibiting hormones (Figure 10-2). These hypothalamus hormones, in turn, regulate the hormones produced by the anterior pituitary gland (a relationship known as the **hypothalamic–pituitary axis**). In contrast to the anterior pituitary, the brain controls the posterior pituitary gland by producing neurohormones in this region.

Pancreas

The **pancreas** is an organ with both exocrine digestive functions (see the *Gastrointestinal Function* chapter) and endocrine functions. The pancreas lies underneath the liver and between the two kidneys in the retroperitoneum (the space behind the peritoneum) (**FIGURE 10-4**). Its endocrine functions are carried out by the **islets of Langerhans**, which are situated among the many small acini (cell clusters that produce digestive enzymes) in the pancreas. The human pancreas contains approximately 1 million islets of Langerhans, and each islet of Langerhans contains five types of cells: (1) **alpha cells**, which secrete glucagon; (2) **beta cells**, which secrete insulin; (3) **delta cells**, which secrete somatostatin; (4) **PP cells**, which secrete a pancreatic polypeptide; and (5) **epsilon cells**, which secrete ghrelin. **Glucagon** is released when serum glucose levels fall. Glucagon stimulates the breakdown of glycogen to glucose, which raises serum glucose levels. **Insulin** is released when serum glucose levels increase. Insulin stimulates cellular uptake of glucose, which in turn decreases serum glucose levels. **Amylin** is released from the beta cells along with insulin. Amylin has a synergistic relationship with insulin in controlling glucose. **Somatostatin** in the pancreas regulates insulin and glucagon. **Pancreatic polypeptide** is thought to regulate some of the other pancreatic activities. Finally, **ghrelin** stimulates hunger.

Thyroid Gland

The **thyroid gland** (**FIGURE 10-5**) is located at the base of the neck below the larynx. This gland consists of two lobes, one on either side of the trachea, which are connected by a thin band of tissue (**isthmus**) that extends across the anterior aspect of the trachea. The thyroid is a highly vascular gland that contains several functional units called **follicles**. These follicles produce three hormones: (1) thyroxine, or T_4; (2) triiodothyronine, or T_3; and (3) thyrocalcitonin, or calcitonin.

Together, T_3 and T_4 account for 95% of circulating thyroid hormones; they regulate cellular metabolism as well as growth and development. The hypothalamus stimulates the pituitary gland to produce **thyroid-stimulating hormone (TSH)** using a negative feedback system. TSH, in turn, drives the thyroid to produce T_3 and T_4. The thyroid requires iodine to synthesize these hormones.

Calcitonin, along with parathyroid hormone, regulates serum calcium levels. Calcitonin alters serum calcium levels by inhibiting osteoclast activity (which decreases calcium release from the bone) and stimulating osteoblast activity (which increases calcium deposits in the bone). Calcitonin is also regulated with a negative feedback system and is secreted when serum calcium levels are high.

Parathyroid Glands

The **parathyroid glands**, usually four in number, are located on the posterior surface of the thyroid. Each parathyroid gland secretes **parathyroid hormone (PTH)**. PTH works in the opposite way to calcitonin to regulate serum

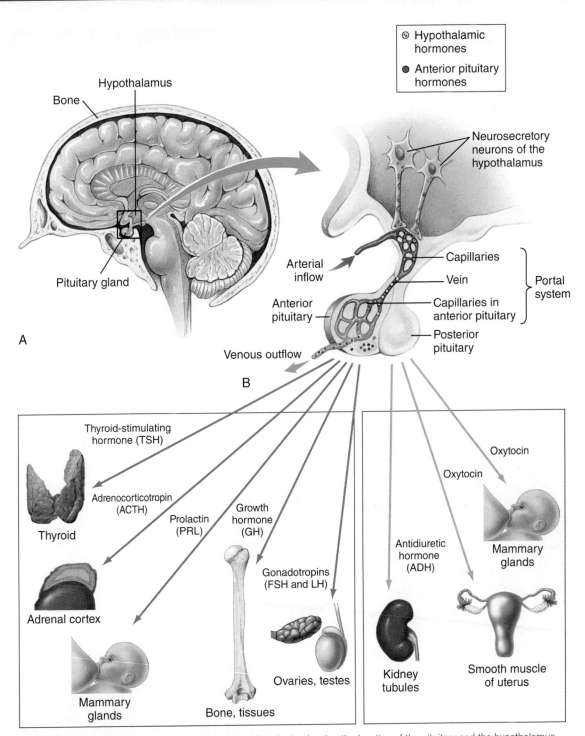

⊗ Hypothalamic hormones
● Anterior pituitary hormones

Bone

Hypothalamus

Pituitary gland

A

Neurosecretory neurons of the hypothalamus

Arterial inflow

Anterior pituitary

Venous outflow

B

Capillaries

Vein

Capillaries in anterior pituitary

Posterior pituitary

} Portal system

Thyroid-stimulating hormone (TSH)

Adrenocorticotropin (ACTH)

Prolactin (PRL)

Growth hormone (GH)

Gonadotropins (FSH and LH)

Thyroid

Adrenal cortex

Mammary glands

Bone, tissues

Ovaries, testes

Oxytocin

Oxytocin

Antidiuretic hormone (ADH)

Mammary glands

Kidney tubules

Smooth muscle of uterus

FIGURE 10-3 The pituitary gland. (a) A cross section of the brain showing the location of the pituitary and the hypothalamus. (b) The structure of the pituitary gland. Releasing and inhibiting hormones travel via the portal system from the hypothalamus to the anterior pituitary, where they affect hormone secretion.

TABLE 10-1	Hormones Secreted by the Pituitary Gland

Hormone	Function
Anterior Pituitary	
Growth hormone (GH)	Stimulates cell growth and fat breakdown. Primary targets are muscle and bone, where GH stimulates amino acid uptake and protein synthesis.
Thyroid-stimulating hormone (TSH)	Stimulates release of thyroxine and triiodothyronine.
Adrenocorticotropic hormone (ACTH)	Stimulates secretion of hormones by the adrenal cortex, especially glucocorticoids.
Gonadotropins: follicle-stimulating hormone (FSH) and luteinizing hormone (LH)	Stimulate gamete production and hormone production by the gonads.
Prolactin	Stimulates milk production by the breast.
Melanocyte-stimulating hormone (MSH)	Function in humans is unknown.
Posterior Pituitary	
Antidiuretic hormone (ADH)	Stimulates water reabsorption by nephrons of the kidney.
Oxytocin	Stimulates breast to release milk and uterine contractions during birth.

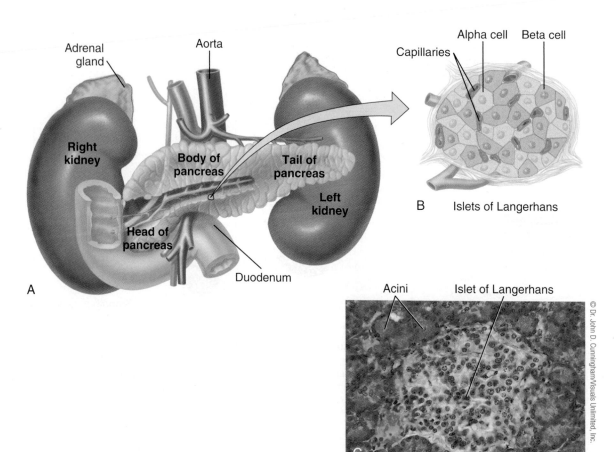

FIGURE 10-4 The pancreas. (a) The pancreas produces two hormones, insulin and glucagon, as well as digestive enzymes. (b) Hormones are produced by specialized cells within the islets of Langerhans. (c) The islets of Langerhans are located among the acini, very small groups of digestive enzyme–producing cells of the pancreas.

© Dr. John D. Cunningham/Visuals Unlimited, Inc.

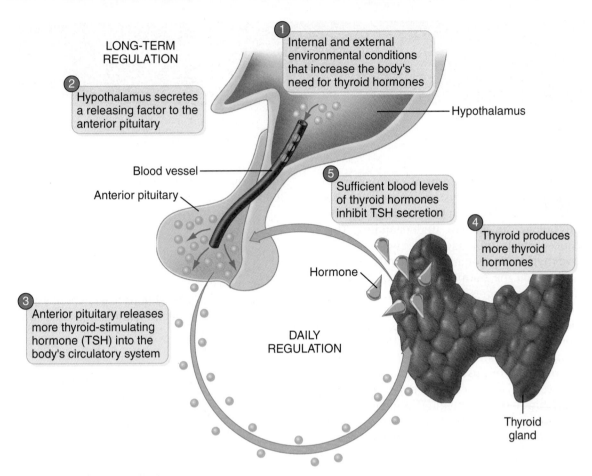

LONG-TERM
REGULATION

1 Internal and external environmental conditions that increase the body's need for thyroid hormones

2 Hypothalamus secretes a releasing factor to the anterior pituitary

Hypothalamus

Blood vessel

Anterior pituitary

5 Sufficient blood levels of thyroid hormones inhibit TSH secretion

4 Thyroid produces more thyroid hormones

Hormone

3 Anterior pituitary releases more thyroid-stimulating hormone (TSH) into the body's circulatory system

DAILY REGULATION

Thyroid gland

FIGURE 10-5 The thyroid gland.

calcium levels. Specifically, PTH is secreted when serum calcium levels drop. This hormone increases serum calcium levels by increasing osteoclast activity (which increases calcium release from the bone) as well as by increasing absorption of calcium in the gastrointestinal tract and kidneys.

Adrenal Glands

The **adrenal glands** are located on each kidney. Each adrenal gland has an inner portion, or **medulla**, and an outer portion, or **cortex**. The hypothalamus influences both portions of the adrenal glands, albeit by different mechanisms.

The adrenal cortex is regulated by negative feedback involving the hypothalamus and adrenocorticotropic hormones; the medulla is regulated by nerve impulses from the hypothalamus. The medulla produces **epinephrine** and **norepinephrine** during times of stress. Epinephrine and norepinephrine

mediate the fight-or-flight response of the sympathetic nervous system (see the *Immunity* chapter).

The cortex has three separate regions that produce different steroids. The outermost region of the adrenal cortex secretes **mineralocorticoids**. The principal mineralocorticoid is **aldosterone**, which acts to conserve sodium and water in the body. The middle region of the adrenal cortex secretes **glucocorticoids**. The principal glucocorticoid is **cortisol**, which increases serum glucose levels. Lastly, the innermost region of the cortex secretes **gonadocorticoids**, or sex hormones. Male hormones (e.g., androgen) and female hormones (e.g., estrogen) are secreted in minimal amounts in both sexes by the adrenal cortex, but the hormones from the testes and ovaries usually mask their effect. In females, the masculinization effect of androgen secretion may become evident after menopause, when estrogen levels from the ovaries decrease.

UNDERSTANDING CONDITIONS THAT AFFECT THE ENDOCRINE SYSTEM

When considering alterations in the endocrine system, organizing them based on their basic underlying pathophysiology can increase understanding. These concepts focus on inadequate (hypo) or excessive (hyper) functioning of the glands. Once you understand the normal function of the glands and the hormones they produce, it becomes clear that those functions can be either insufficient or exaggerated. In most cases of hypofunctioning, something has destroyed the gland (e.g., aging or autoimmune conditions). Treatment for hypofunctioning usually centers on hormone replacement. In most cases of hyperfunctioning, something is overstimulating the gland or secreting hormone-like substances (e.g., tumors). Treatment for hyperfunctioning usually centers on giving medications to block hormone production, removing the cause (e.g., tumor), or removing part or all of the gland.

Disorders of the Pituitary Gland

Disorders of the pituitary gland can have significant consequences because of the many hormones and processes this gland influences. Like most endocrine disorders, pituitary gland disorders result in either increased or decreased levels of hormones associated with the gland (Table 10-1). These conditions can be caused by tumors (most common), infection, trauma, and necrosis.

Hypopituitarism

Hypopituitarism is a rare, complex condition in which the pituitary gland does not produce sufficient amounts of some or all (**panhypopituitarism**) of its hormones (e.g., TSH, growth hormone, adrenocorticotropic hormone [ACTH], follicle-stimulating hormone, luteinizing hormone, prolactin melanocyte-stimulating hormone, antidiuretic hormone, and oxytocin). As a result, the gland or process that the hormone controls is impaired. Hypopituitarism may result from primary or secondary causes, including the following:

- Congenital defects (e.g., pituitary hypoplasia or aplasia)
- Cerebral or pituitary trauma (may be a result of surgery, infections, stroke, radiation, or injury)
- Autoimmune conditions (e.g., hypophysitis)
- Infections of the brain and tissues that support the brain
- Tuberculosis
- Pituitary tumors
- Hemochromatosis (a condition resulting in excessive iron absorption)
- Histiocytosis X (an abnormal immune condition that results in tissue damage)
- Sarcoidosis (an abnormal inflammatory condition that results in tissue damage)
- Hypothalamic dysfunction (the only secondary cause)

Hypopituitarism can result in several conditions depending on the hormones involved. The severity of these conditions reflects the degree of hormone deficit. Two of these conditions are noted here:

- **Dwarfism**—short stature caused by deficient levels of growth hormone, somatotropin, or somatotropin-releasing hormone (**FIGURE 10-6**)
- **Diabetes insipidus**—excessive fluid excretion in the kidneys caused by deficient antidiuretic hormone levels

Hypopituitarism is a progressive disorder that can occur suddenly but usually develops slowly. Clinical manifestations vary greatly depending on the hormones affected and the severity of those alterations. These manifestations may include the following signs and symptoms:

- Fatigue
- Headache

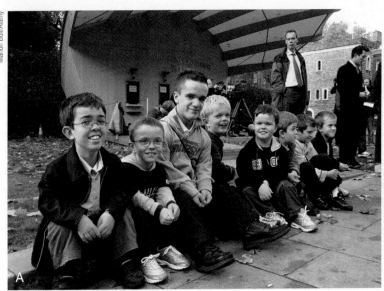
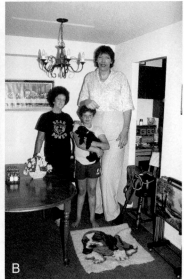

FIGURE 10-6 (a) Dwarfism and (b) gigantism.

- Cessation of menstruation
- Infertility (in women)
- Decreased libido
- Low tolerance for stress
- Hypotension
- Muscle weakness
- Nausea
- Constipation
- Weight loss or gain
- Anorexia
- Abdominal discomfort
- Cold sensitivity
- Visual disturbances
- Loss of body or facial hair
- Joint stiffness
- Hoarseness
- Facial edema
- Thirst
- Excessive urination
- Short stature
- Delayed growth and development

Diagnosis of hypopituitarism is often delayed because of its variable presentation. Diagnostic procedures usually include a history, physical examination, serum hormone levels, brain computed tomography (CT), pituitary magnetic resonance imaging (MRI), vision testing, and X-rays (to identify any bone abnormalities).

Lifelong hormone replacement therapy is the cornerstone of treatment. Resolving the underlying cause is also important when possible (e.g., cancer treatment). Additional strategies depend on the specific hormones affected (e.g., infertility treatments and counseling). The patient will likely require monitoring by an endocrinologist and will need to wear a medical alert bracelet.

Hyperpituitarism

Hyperpituitarism is a condition in which the pituitary gland secretes excessive amounts of one or all of the pituitary hormones. It is most commonly caused by tumors that secrete hormones or hormone-like substances. Hyperpituitarism can result in several conditions depending on the hormones involved. The severity of these conditions reflects the degree of hormone excess. Some of these conditions are highlighted here:

- **Gigantism**—tall stature caused by excessive growth hormone levels prior to puberty (Figure 10-6)
- **Acromegaly**—increased bone size caused by excessive growth hormone levels in adulthood (**FIGURE 10-7**)
- **Syndrome of inappropriate antidiuretic hormone (SIADH)**—increased renal water retention caused by excessive antidiuretic hormone levels
- **Hyperprolactinemia**—excessive prolactin levels that result in menstrual dysfunction and galactorrhea (inappropriate lactation)
- **Cushing's syndrome**—excessive cortisol levels that result from the increased ACTH levels

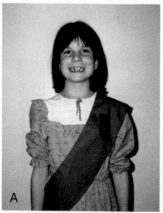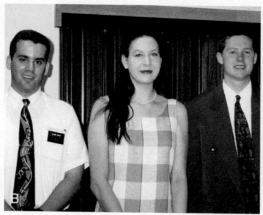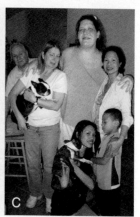

FIGURE 10-7 A woman with acromegaly (a) as a child, (b) as a teenager, and (c) as an adult.

Courtesy of Tanya Angus and Karen Strutynsky (www.tanyaangus.com)

- **Hyperthyroidism**—a hypermetabolic state caused by excessive thyroid hormones that result from increased TSH levels

Hyperpituitarism is a progressive disorder that can occur suddenly but usually develops slowly. Clinical manifestations vary greatly depending on the hormones affected and the severity of those alterations. These manifestations are similar to those noted with hypopituitarism:

- Headache
- Visual field loss or double vision
- Excessive sweating
- Hoarseness
- Galactorrhea (spontaneous lactation unassociated with childbirth or nursing)
- Sleep apnea
- Carpal tunnel syndrome
- Joint pain and stiffness
- Muscle weakness
- Paresthesia

Diagnosis of hyperpituitarism is often delayed because of its varying presentation. Diagnostic procedures usually include a history, physical examination, serum hormone levels, brain CT, pituitary MRI, vision testing, and X-rays (to identify any bone abnormalities).

Treatment strategies depend on the underlying etiology and the hormone affected. Tumors will likely require surgery, radiation, and chemotherapy, but often reoccur. Additionally, analogues that inhibit hormone production may be given.

Diabetes Mellitus

Diabetes mellitus (DM) refers to a group of conditions characterized by hyperglycemia (high serum glucose levels) resulting from defects in insulin production, insulin action, or both. Glucose is a vital energy source for the body, but insulin is required for glucose to travel into the cell, where it can be used. Insulin acts like a key that unlocks the cell membrane and allows the glucose to enter. Impaired insulin production or action results in abnormal carbohydrate, protein, and fat metabolism because of the glucose transportation issue. Some cells, such as those in the brain, digestive tract, and skeletal muscles, can use glucose without insulin to some degree. DM can occur in three forms—type 1, type 2, and gestational diabetes—each with its own pathogenesis.

An estimated 422 million people worldwide have DM (World Health Organization, 2016). DM is extremely common in the United States—approximately 29.1 million Americans have diabetes and another 86 million have prediabetes (1 out of 3 adults) (Centers for Disease Control and Prevention [CDC], 2015). Nevertheless, DM prevalence rates have begun to fall in the United States. DM incidence is relatively equal across genders, but it is most common in people older than 65 years of age, with nearly 27% of this population having DM. DM is most frequent among Native Americans, African Americans, and Hispanics. In 2014, DM accounted for $245 billion in medical costs in the United States.

Although DM was only the seventh most common listed cause of death on U.S. death certificates in 2015, it likely played a role in many more deaths because this disease contributes to several complications (e.g., heart disease, stroke, and kidney disease). According to the CDC (2015), the risk of death for persons with DM is twice that of persons without DM.

DM can result in an array of acute and chronic complications. Acute complications may include the following conditions:

- **Hyperglycemia**—may be a result of excessive dietary carbohydrate intake as well as insufficient or inappropriate diabetic pharmacologic therapy.
- **Diabetic ketoacidosis**—pH imbalance characterized by increased ketones in the urine caused by insufficient insulin; if cells are starved for energy, the body may begin to break down fat-producing toxic acids (ketones).
- **Hypoglycemia** (low serum glucose level)—may result from insufficient dietary intake, increased physical activity, and excessive diabetic pharmacologic therapy.

Chronic complications are a direct result of long-term excessive glucose levels, especially when DM is not adequately managed. Over time, increased glucose levels contribute to thickening and hardening of vessel walls (much in the same way that the sugar in icing hardens on a cake), causing diffuse ischemia and necrosis. DM complications reflect these circulatory changes. Adequate DM management is the best strategy to prevent chronic complications, which include the following problems:

- Heart disease—heart disease death rates are 2 to 4 times higher in people with DM.
- Stroke—occurrence rates are 2 to 4 times higher in people with DM.
- Hypertension—75% of people with DM also have hypertension.
- Hypercholesterolemia.
- Diabetic retinopathy.
- Blindness—DM, as a result of diabetic retinopathy, is the leading cause of blindness.
- Kidney disease—DM is the leading cause of kidney disease.
- Diabetic neuropathy—approximately 70% of people with DM have neuropathy (pain and numbness in the hands and feet).
- Amputations—approximately 60% of nontraumatic amputations occur in persons with DM.
- Periodontal disease—occurrence rates are approximately 2 times higher in people with DM.
- Pregnancy complications (e.g., birth defects and high birth weights).
- Increased susceptibility to infections and delayed healing.
- Erectile dysfunction.

- Depression—occurrence rates are 2 times higher in people with DM.

Clinical manifestations of DM may vary depending on the type. These manifestations, which include the following symptoms, are a direct result of the excess glucose levels:

- Hyperglycemia
- Glucosuria (glucose is excreted in the urine in an attempt to lower serum levels)
- Polyuria (increased urine output because of the osmotic effects of the glucosuria)
- Polydipsia (increased thirst because of the dehydration caused by the increased urine output)
- Polyphagia (increased appetite because of the energy loss as glucose is excreted)
- Weight loss (from increased fat catabolism)
- Blurred vision (excessive glucose changes the shape and flexibility of the lens of the eye, distorting the ability to focus and causing blurred vision)
- Fatigue (because of a lack of an energy source)
- Nausea, vomiting, and abdominal pain (associated with sudden onset of type 1 diabetes)

Diagnostic procedures for DM are complex. These procedures are used for diagnosing DM and complications as well as for assessing the effectiveness of DM management (**TABLE 10-2**). Diagnostic procedures include a history, physical examination, urinalysis (to detect the presence of glucose), fasting blood glucose test, oral glucose tolerance test, random blood glucose test, hemoglobin A_{1c} ($HgbA_{1c}$; an average of glucose control for the previous 2–3 months), blood pressure measurement, and cholesterol panel.

Learning Points

The classic clinical manifestations of diabetes mellitus are referred to as the *three P's*: **polyuria**, **polydipsia**, and **polyphagia**. As the levels of glucose increase in the bloodstream, the kidneys try to compensate by increasing urinary excretion. Normally, glucose is not found in the urine, so the presence of any glucose in the urine is an abnormal finding. Glucose has a relationship with water similar to the one between sodium and water (see the *Fluid, Electrolyte, and Acid–Base Homeostasis* chapter): *Wherever glucose is, water will follow it*. Because glucose is being excreted in the urine, more water is excreted (polyuria). The excess water loss creates a fluid volume deficit, which triggers the thirst sensation in an attempt to replace the fluid (polydipsia). Additionally, the loss of glucose creates an energy deficit, which triggers the hunger sensation (polyphagia).

TABLE 10-2	Diagnostic Procedures and Treatment Goals for Diabetes Mellitus

Criteria for Diagnosis of Prediabetes

$HgbA_{1c}$ 5.7–6.4%

OR

Impaired fasting glucose 100–125 mg/dL (fasting plasma glucose)

OR

Impaired glucose tolerance 140–199 mg/dL (2-hour post 75 g glucose challenge)

Criteria for Diagnosis of Diabetes

$HgbA_{1c} \geq 6.5\%$

OR

Fasting plasma glucose ≥ 126 mg/dL[a]

OR

2-hour plasma glucose ≥ 200 mg/dL[a] post 75 g glucose challenge

OR

Random plasma glucose ≥ 200 mg/dL with symptoms (polyuria, polydipsia, and unexplained weight loss)

Treatment Goals for the ABCs of Diabetes

$HgbA_{1c}$

Should be less than 7% for patients in general.

Preprandial capillary plasma glucose 70–130 mg/dL.

Peak postprandial capillary plasma glucose < 180 mg/dL (usually 1–2 hours after the start of a meal). Be alert to the impact of hemoglobin variants on $HgbA_{1c}$ values.

Blood Pressure

Systolic < 130 mm Hg

Diastolic < 80 mm Hg

Cholesterol: Lipid Profile

LDL cholesterol < 100 mg/dL

HDL cholesterol

- Men > 40 mg/dL
- Women > 50 mg/dL

Triglycerides < 150 mg/dL

[a] Repeat to confirm on subsequent day unless symptoms are present

Data from American Diabetes Association. (2016). American Diabetes Association standards of medical care. *Diabetes Care, 39* (Suppl. 1), S1–S112.

Treatment strategies for DM vary depending on the type, but dietary changes (American Diabetic Association recommendations) and exercise are the first line of treatment. Management also includes glucose self-monitoring, weight loss (if the patient is overweight), oral hyperglycemia medications, supplemental insulin, and complication management. In addition, bariatric and metabolic surgeries have shown promise as potential cures for DM.

Type 1 Diabetes

Type 1 diabetes was previously called insulin-dependent DM and juvenile-onset DM

TABLE 10-3	Comparison of Type 1 and Type 2 Diabetes	
	Type 1	**Type 2**
Age	Usually in children or young adults	Usually after age 40, and incidence increases with age
Onset	Generally abrupt	More often insidious
	Often diagnosed after infection	Patients often obese
	Diabetic ketoacidosis	Nonketotic coma resulting from dehydration
Treatment	Insulin	Diet, exercise, oral medication
		Insulin may be required in severe cases
Complications	Occur early, often severe	Full range of complications may be present at diagnosis
Insulin levels	Low or absent	Frequently normal or high

(**TABLE 10-3**). Type 1 DM develops when the body's immune system destroys pancreatic beta cells. To survive, people with type 1 DM must obtain insulin delivered by injection or a pump. This form of DM usually strikes children and young adults, although its onset can occur at any age. In adults, type 1 DM accounts for 5–10% of all diagnosed cases. The exact cause of type 1 diabetes is unknown, but most likely a viral or environmental trigger in genetically susceptible people causes an autoimmune reaction. Type 1 DM cannot be prevented.

Type 2 Diabetes

Type 2 diabetes was previously called noninsulin-dependent DM and adult-onset DM. In adults, type 2 DM accounts for approximately 90–95% of all newly diagnosed DM cases. This form of diabetes usually begins as insulin resistance, a disorder in which the body's cells do not use insulin properly. As the need for insulin rises, the pancreas gradually loses its ability to produce this hormone. Type 2 DM is associated with advancing age, obesity, family history of DM, history of gestational DM, impaired glucose metabolism, and physical inactivity. African Americans, Hispanics, Native Americans, Asians, Native Hawaiians, and other Pacific Islanders are at particularly high risk for type 2 DM and its complications. Type 2 DM in children and adolescents, although still rare, is being diagnosed more frequently among Native Americans, African Americans, Hispanics, Asians, and Pacific Islanders.

Type 2 DM is usually managed initially with oral antidiabetic medications that increase insulin production and action. As the condition progresses, supplemental insulin often becomes necessary as pancreatic production declines.

Additionally, type 2 DM has been associated with depression and schizophrenia.

Gestational Diabetes

Gestational diabetes is a form of glucose intolerance diagnosed during pregnancy. Gestational DM occurs most frequently among African Americans, Hispanics, and Native Americans. Other risk factors include obesity and a family history of DM. During pregnancy, gestational DM requires treatment (usually lifestyle changes and insulin) to normalize maternal blood glucose levels to avoid fetal complications. Immediately after pregnancy, 5–10% of women with gestational DM are diagnosed with DM, usually type 2. Women who have had gestational DM have a 40–60% chance of developing DM within 5–10 years.

Metabolic Syndrome

Metabolic syndrome is a cluster of risk factors that occur together—specifically, hyperglycemia, high blood pressure, hypercholesterolemia, and increased waist circumference. Metabolic syndrome is not a form of DM, but is related to DM because metabolic syndrome increases the risk of cardiovascular disease, DM, and stroke. The diagnostic criteria for metabolic syndrome include the presence of three or more of those risk factors. Treatment strategies focus on lifestyle changes (e.g., weight loss, dietary changes, and physical activity) to prevent development of complications.

Disorders of the Thyroid

Because of the thyroid hormones' responsibilities, disorders of the thyroid have a significant impact on metabolic activities. These disorders result in either an increase or a decrease in the thyroid

Myth Busters

Several myths regarding diabetes mellitus (DM) in the community merit discussion.

Myth 1: People with diabetes cannot eat sweets or chocolate.

If chocolate and other sweets are eaten as part of a healthy meal plan, or combined with exercise, people with DM can eat them. They are no more off-limit foods for people with DM than they are for people without DM.

Myth 2: Eating too much sugar causes diabetes.

DM is caused by a combination of genetic and lifestyle factors, not by eating too much sugar. However, being overweight does increase your risk for developing type 2 DM. If there is a family history of DM, following a healthy meal plan and getting regular exercise are recommended to manage weight.

Myth 3: Pills for DM provide oral insulin.

Oral medications for DM affect the ability of the body to produce insulin and use insulin better—they are not oral insulin. Going through the gastrointestinal system would destroy the insulin; therefore, insulin is injected.

Myth 4: Drinking water can excrete the extra sugar in the blood.

Extra glucose in the blood cannot be excreted by drinking extra water. However, DM can be controlled by eating healthy food, being physically active, managing weight, routine examinations, taking prescribed medications, and monitoring blood glucose often.

Myth 5: Fruit is a healthy food, so it is acceptable to eat large quantities of it.

Fruit is a healthy food, containing fiber and lots of vitamins and minerals. Because fruit contains carbohydrates that break down quickly into simple sugars, it needs to be included in a healthy meal plan, but amounts should be controlled because fruit will raise blood glucose levels.

Myth 6: When taking oral diabetic medications or insulin, people with DM can eat anything they want.

The oral medications or insulin taken for DM are more effective when they do not have to work as hard to lower blood glucose. Combining medicines with a healthy meal plan and physical activity gives better glucose control.

Myth 7: Once a person begins taking oral diabetic medications or insulin for type 2 diabetes, they must be taken for life.

Sometimes, temporary circumstances may cause elevated glucose levels (e.g., glucocorticoid therapy and total parenteral nutrition administration), and diabetic medications will be needed only during those events. Some people who have been started on oral diabetic medications and/or insulin find that they can control their blood glucose without medications with weight loss, exercise, and healthy dieting.

Data from American Diabetes Association. (2015). Diabetes myths. Retrieved from http://www.diabetes.org/diabetes-basics/myths/

---

hormones. Several etiologies can give rise to these conditions, including tumors, congenital defects, damage (e.g., from surgery, radiation, or infections), and aging. These conditions are usually easily managed with medications and surgery.

Goiter

A **goiter** refers to a visible enlargement of the thyroid gland (**FIGURE 10-8**). This enlargement is usually painless but may affect the respiratory and gastrointestinal systems. The enlargement is not necessarily malignant. Goiters can occur in hyperthyroidism, hypothyroidism, and normal thyroid states.

Iodine deficiency is the most common cause of goiters in the United States. Iodine deficiency leads to decreased T_3 and T_4 production, and TSH production increases in an attempt to compensate for the low levels of these thyroid hormones. Increased levels of TSH lead to thyroid hyperplasia and hypertrophy. A similar reaction occurs in both hyperthyroidism and hypothyroidism states.

Hypothyroidism

Hypothyroidism refers to a condition in which the thyroid does not produce sufficient amounts of the thyroid hormones. This endocrine disorder is relatively common (affecting 1 out of 500 Americans) and may be a result of hypothalamus, pituitary, or thyroid (the most common) dysfunction. Several conditions can result in hypothyroidism. Hypothyroidism risk increases with age (especially in persons older than 50 years).

In many cases, a previous or current inflammation of the thyroid gland leaves a large percentage of thyroid cells damaged and incapable of producing sufficient hormone amounts. The most common cause of this kind of thyroid gland failure is called autoimmune thyroiditis (also called **Hashimoto's thyroiditis**).

The second major cause of hypothyroidism is iatrogenic (resulting from medical treatments). The treatment of many thyroid conditions, such as hyperthyroidism, warrants partial or complete surgical removal of the thyroid gland. If the total remaining thyroid hormone–producing cells are not able to meet the needs of the body, hypothyroidism develops. This result is often the goal of surgery for thyroid cancer. Similarly, goiters and some other thyroid conditions can be treated with radioactive iodine therapy. The aim of the radioactive iodine therapy (for benign conditions) is to kill a

portion of the thyroid to prevent goiters from growing larger or developing into hyperthyroidism. Occasionally, the radioactive iodine treatment can damage too many cells, but this consequence is usually preferred over the original problem. Hypothyroidism can also result from use of certain medications (e.g., lithium and amiodarone).

The clinical manifestations of hypothyroidism vary widely, depending on the severity of the hormone deficiency. Generally, clinical manifestations tend to be insidious and develop slowly, often over a number of years. These clinical manifestations reflect the decreased thyroid activity (e.g., metabolism):

- Fatigue
- Sluggishness
- Increased sensitivity to cold
- Constipation
- Pale, dry skin
- Edema in the face, hands, and feet
- Hoarseness
- Hypercholesterolemia
- Unexplained weight gain
- Myalgia
- Arthralgia

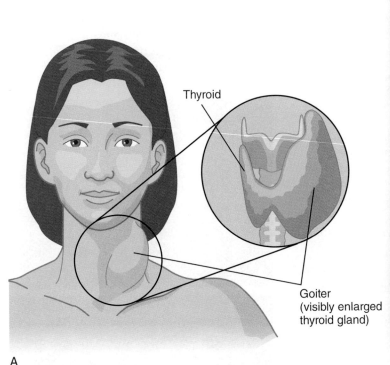

Thyroid

Goiter
(visibly enlarged
thyroid gland)

A

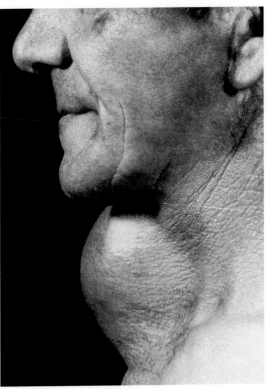

B

© Biophoto Associates/Science Source

FIGURE 10-8 Goiter.

- Muscle weakness
- Heavier than normal menstrual periods
- Infertility
- Brittle fingernails
- Hair loss or thinning
- Bradycardia
- Hypotension
- Depression
- Goiter

Advanced hypothyroidism, known as **myxedema**, is rare. When it occurs, however, myxedema can be life threatening. Clinical manifestations include marked hypotension, respiratory depression, hypothermia, lethargy, and coma.

Diagnostic procedures for hypothyroidism include a history, physical examination, serum thyroid hormone levels, serum TSH, liver function tests, complete blood counts (CBC), cholesterol panel, and electrocardiogram (EKG). Hypothyroidism is easily managed with thyroid hormone replacement (e.g., levothyroxine [Synthroid]). Additional strategies are implemented to manage symptoms and may include weight management (e.g., a low-calorie diet and increased physical activity), constipation measures (e.g., stool softener and increase in dietary fiber and fluid intake), and avoidance of cold temperatures.

Hyperthyroidism

Hyperthyroidism refers to a condition of excessive levels of thyroid hormones. This overabundance of thyroid hormones results in a hypermetabolic state. Hyperthyroidism can result from a variety of conditions, including the following:

- Excessive iodine
- **Graves' disease** (an autoimmune condition that stimulates thyroid hormone production)
- Nonmalignant thyroid tumors (which produce thyroid or thyroidlike hormones)
- Thyroid inflammation (increased capillary permeability resulting from the inflammatory process causes additional thyroid hormones to be released in the bloodstream)
- Taking large amounts of thyroid hormone replacement

Hyperthyroidism can mimic other health problems, and its clinical manifestations can vary, making diagnosis difficult. These clinical manifestations reflect increased thyroid activity:

- Sudden weight loss
- Tachycardia
- Dysrhythmias (especially atrial fibrillation)
- Hypertension

- Increased appetite
- Nervousness, anxiety or anxiety attacks, and irritability
- Difficulty concentrating
- Tremor (usually a fine trembling in the hands)
- Diaphoresis
- Changes in menstrual patterns
- Increased sensitivity to heat
- Diarrhea
- Goiter
- Difficulty sleeping
- **Exophthalmos** (protruding eyes with decreased blinking and movement) (**FIGURE 10-9**)

Thyroid crisis (storm), also called **thyrotoxicosis**, is a sudden worsening of hyperthyroidism symptoms that may occur with infection or stress. This medical emergency is characterized by fever, decreased mental alertness, and abdominal pain. Additional complications of hyperthyroidism include cardiomyopathy, heart failure, and osteoporosis.

Diagnostic procedures for hyperthyroidism include a history, physical examination, serum thyroid hormone levels, serum TSH, radioactive iodine uptake test, liver function tests, EKG, and thyroid scan. Hyperthyroidism can usually be easily managed with medication and surgery. Pharmacologic treatment usually includes radioactive iodine (which shrinks the gland), antithyroid agents (to decrease hormone production), and beta blockers (to treat cardiac symptoms). Surgical removal of the thyroid (thyroidectomy) with subsequent hormone replacement is warranted when the patient does not respond to or tolerate medications. Even with treatment, exophthalmos

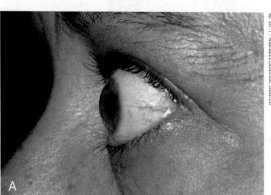
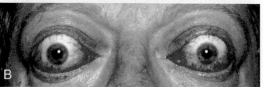

FIGURE 10-9 Exophthalmos.

usually remains. Strategies to improve the discomfort associated with exophthalmos include cool compresses, wearing sunglasses, eye lubricants, and elevating the head of the bed. Increasing caloric and calcium intake is crucial to maintain weight and prevent bone loss.

Learning Points

Hypothyroidism and hyperthyroidism present very differently. When considering the clinical manifestations of these disorders, think about what increasing or decreasing thyroid hormones would do in the body. With hypothyroidism, the hormone levels are decreased, and so are all the clinical manifestations (e.g., bradycardia, hypotension, depression, and constipation), with the exception of weight. With hyperthyroidism, the hormone levels are increased, and so are all the clinical manifestations (e.g., tachycardia, hypertension, anxiety, and diarrhea) with the exception of weight.

Disorders of the Parathyroid

Parathyroid disorders result in an increase or decrease in PTH. Because of PTH's responsibilities, disorders of the parathyroid have a significant impact on calcium balance that has a domino effect on other electrolytes (phosphorus and magnesium; see the *Fluid, Electrolyte, and Acid–Base Homeostasis* chapter). Several etiologies can result in these conditions, including tumors, congenital defects, damage (e.g., from surgery, radiation, or infections), and renal failure. These conditions are usually easily managed with medications and surgery.

Hypoparathyroidism

Hypoparathyroidism refers to a condition in which the parathyroid gland does not produce sufficient amounts of PTH. Hypoparathyroidism, which is uncommon, can be caused by congenital defects (a lack of one or more of the four parathyroid glands) as well as by damage following surgery, radiation, autoimmune conditions, hypomagnesemia, or metabolic alkalosis. This hormone deficiency results in hypocalcemia and a subsequent increase in phosphorus levels. Its clinical manifestations reflect these electrolyte and pH imbalances:

- Paresthesias of the fingertips, toes, and lips
- Muscle twitching or spasms (tetany)
- Seizures
- Fatigue or weakness
- Dysrhythmias
- Hypotension
- Abdominal cramping
- Diarrhea
- Painful menstruation

- Patchy hair loss
- Dry, coarse skin
- Brittle nails
- Anxiety or nervousness
- Headaches
- Depression or mood swings
- Memory loss

Diagnostic procedures for hypoparathyroidism include a history, physical examination, serum PTH check, blood chemistry, EKG, X-rays, and bone density studies. Treatment regimens rarely include PTH replacement. Strategies generally focus on correcting electrolyte and pH imbalances (see the *Fluid, Electrolyte, and Acid–Base Homeostasis* chapter).

Hyperparathyroidism

Hyperparathyroidism refers to a condition of excessive PTH production by the parathyroid gland. This imbalance may be caused by tumors, hyperplasia, or chronic hypocalcemia (kidney disease). Hyperparathyroidism will result in hypercalcemia. The excessive calcium levels can lead to decreases in phosphorus levels, increases in magnesium levels, and metabolic acidosis (see the *Fluid, Electrolyte, and Acid–Base Homeostasis* chapter). The clinical manifestations of hyperparathyroidism reflect these electrolyte and pH imbalances:

- Osteoporosis
- Bone pain
- Pathological fractures
- Renal calculi
- Polyuria
- Abdominal pain
- Constipation
- Fatigue or weakness
- Flaccid muscles
- Dysrhythmias
- Hypertension
- Depression or forgetfulness
- Nausea and vomiting
- Anorexia

Diagnostic procedures for hyperparathyroidism include a history, physical examination, serum PTH check, blood chemistry, EKG, X-rays, and bone density studies. Treatment varies depending on the underlying etiology. Tumors will likely require surgery and radiation. Calcitonin may be administered to shift the calcium from the bloodstream to the bones. Calcimimetics may be administered to mimic calcium circulating in the blood and, in turn, may lead to decreased PTH production. Bisphosphates can decrease the loss of calcium from the bone and lessen osteoporosis. Phosphates may be administered to correct phosphorus deficits, which will decrease calcium levels (see the *Fluid, Electrolyte, and Acid–Base Homeostasis* chapter). Increasing fluid intake (either oral or intravenous) will increase renal excretion of calcium. Additionally, magnesium and pH imbalances may need correction (see the *Fluid, Electrolyte, and Acid–Base Homeostasis* chapter).

Disorders of the Adrenal Gland

Adrenal gland disorders may affect one or both areas of the adrenal gland. These disorders result in an increase or a decrease in one or more adrenal hormones. Depending on the hormone affected and the severity of the condition, adrenal gland disorders can have serious consequences. Several etiologies can result in these conditions, including tumors, congenital defects, medications (e.g., corticosteroids), and damage (e.g., from surgery, radiation, or infections). These disorders are usually easily managed with medications and surgery, but they can become life threatening if not managed promptly.

Pheochromocytoma

Pheochromocytoma is a rare tumor of the adrenal medulla. The tumor excretes epinephrine and norepinephrine and can be life threatening because of the effects of these hormones (e.g., increased blood pressure and tachycardia). Pheochromocytoma can occur as a single tumor or as multiple tumors in one or both adrenal glands, but is rarely malignant (10% of cases). The exact cause is unknown. The tumors can occur at any age, but are more common in early to middle adulthood. Clinical manifestations reflect the fight-or-flight response and occur in unpredictable attacks that usually last 15 to 20 minutes. These manifestations include the following symptoms:

- Hypertension
- Tachycardia
- Dysrhythmias
- Forceful heartbeat
- Chest pain
- Profound diaphoresis
- Hyperglycemia
- Abdominal pain
- Sudden onset of severe headaches
- Anxiety
- Feeling of extreme fright
- Pallor
- Weight loss
- Difficulty sleeping

Diagnostic procedures for pheochromocytoma include a history, physical examination, serum catecholamines and metanephrines, serum glucose, urine catecholamines and metanephrines, EKG, abdominal CT, abdominal MRI, *m*-iodobenzylguanidine scintiscan (a nuclear scan to confirm pheochromocytoma), and biopsy. If not promptly treated, pheochromocytoma can lead to hypertensive crisis, stroke, kidney disease, psychosis, and seizures. Surgical removal of the tumor or adrenal gland is the cornerstone of treatment. Administration of antihypertensive medications (e.g., alpha blockers and beta blockers) is often necessary until surgery can be performed.

Cushing's Syndrome

Cushing's syndrome, also referred to as Cushing's disease, is a condition characterized by excessive amounts of glucocorticoids. The most common cause of this excess is iatrogenic, resulting from ingestion of glucocorticoid medications. When these medications are ingested, they mimic the body's own hormones. Cushing's syndrome can also be caused by adrenal tumors that secrete glucocorticoids or by pituitary tumors that secrete ACTH and cortisol. Paraneoplastic syndrome resulting from cancers outside the endocrine system can also cause Cushing's syndrome by increasing production of ACTH and cortisol.

Glucocorticoids are essential for life but can produce serious effects when present in excessive amounts (**FIGURE 10-10**). The clinical manifestations of Cushing's syndrome are a direct result of the excessive amounts of glucocorticoids:

- Obesity (especially around the trunk) (**FIGURE 10-11**)
- Round, full, red face ("moon" face) (**FIGURE 10-12**)
- Fatty pad between shoulders ("buffalo hump")
- Muscle weakness
- Delayed growth and development
- Acne
- Broad purple striae (marks) on the abdomen, thighs, and breast
- Thin skin that bruises easily
- Delayed wound healing
- Osteoporosis
- Hirsutism (abnormal hair growth)
- Changes in menstruation
- Decreased libido
- Erectile dysfunction
- Insulin resistance
- Hypertension

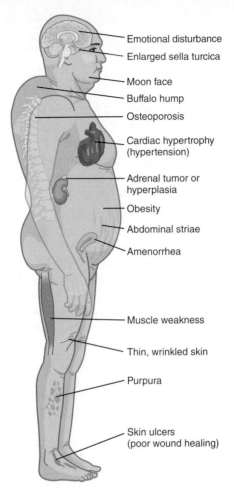

- Emotional disturbance
- Enlarged sella turcica
- Moon face
- Buffalo hump
- Osteoporosis
- Cardiac hypertrophy (hypertension)
- Adrenal tumor or hyperplasia
- Obesity
- Abdominal striae
- Amenorrhea
- Muscle weakness
- Thin, wrinkled skin
- Purpura
- Skin ulcers (poor wound healing)

FIGURE 10-10 Signs and symptoms of Cushing's syndrome.

- Edema
- Hypokalemia
- Mood changes and psychosis

Diagnostic procedures for Cushing's syndrome include a history, physical examination, serum hormone levels (e.g., cortisol and ACTH), serum glucose, CBC, blood chemistry, urine cortisol, bone density studies, adrenal and pituitary CT and MRI, and biopsy. Treatment varies depending on the underlying cause. Gradual tapering of any glucocorticoids being administered is crucial. If these medications are suddenly discontinued, the adrenal gland does not have the opportunity to initiate its own production of hormones, leading to an adrenal crisis. Tumors will likely require surgical removal and radiation. Medications can be used to control cortisol production (e.g., ketoconazole [Nizoral], mitotane [Lysodren], metyrapone [Metopirone]), control the effects of cortisol (e.g., mifepristone [Korlym]), and decrease ACTH production (e.g., pasireotide [Signifor]). Interventions may be necessary to manage specific complications as they develop (e.g., osteoporosis, DM, and hypertension).

Addison's Disease

Addison's disease refers to a deficiency of adrenal cortex hormones (glucocorticoids, mineralocorticoids, and androgens). It can be caused

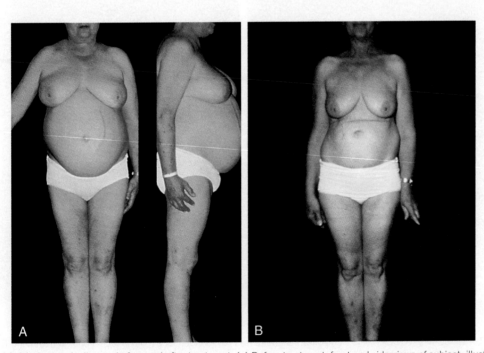

FIGURE 10-11 Cushing's disease before and after treatment. (a) Before treatment, front and side views of subject, illustrating trunk obesity with relatively thin extremities. (b) After treatment, illustrating normal body configuration.

Courtesy of Leonard V. Crowley, MD, Century College

A 68-year-old woman with an 8-year history of diabetes mellitus presents to the clinic for worsening dyspnea and cough. She has had chronic obstructive pulmonary disease (COPD; see the *Respiratory Function* chapter) since age 55. She now has dyspnea from walking one-third of a block, as well as a persistent cough. She has managed her type 2 DM with diet and exercise. Her last glycosylated hemoglobin (HgbA$_{1c}$), which was measured 1 month ago, was 6.8% (normal range is 4–6%). Physical examination reveals an anxious woman with blood pressure of 134/70 mm Hg, pulse of 116, respiratory rate of 24 breaths per minute, and weight of 190 pounds. Expiratory wheezing is present bilaterally. No accessory muscles are being used. No cyanosis is present. The lab evaluation results are as follows: arterial blood gas (ABG) 7.46; PaO$_2$ 60; PaCO$_2$ 40;

O$_2$ sat 88% (see the *Fluid, Electrolyte, and Acid–Base Homeostasis* chapter).

The patient is started on albuterol (bronchodilator) and a course of prednisone (glucocorticoid) at 40 mg/day for 3 days, then tapering over 2 weeks. On day 3, she calls back to the clinic to report that her blood glucose level is 358 mg/dL at 4:00 p.m.

1. Which of the following is the most likely cause of this patient's acute loss of glucose control?

    A. An acid–base imbalance
    B. Prednisone therapy
    C. COPD exacerbation
    D. Albuterol

2. All of the following actions are important for this patient to learn regarding glucocorticoid therapy, but which is the most important?

    A. Monitor cuts for healing
    B. Take the medication with food

    C. Do not stop taking the medication abruptly
    D. Contact her healthcare provider if she has any manifestations of infection

3. Which of the following endocrine conditions is this patient at risk of developing?

    A. Hyperthyroidism
    B. Pheochromocytoma
    C. Addison's disease
    D. Cushing's syndrome

4. Given this patient's acute loss of glucose control, which of the following interventions would the nurse expect to be ordered for this patient?

    A. Insulin as needed per routine sliding scale (dosing based on blood glucose levels)
    B. Increase exercise
    C. Decrease caloric intake
    D. Decrease prednisone dose

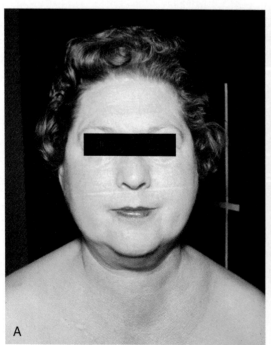 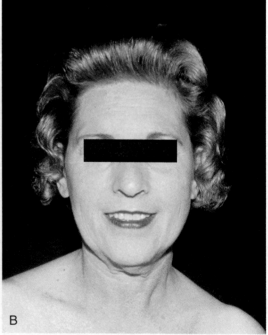

FIGURE 10-12 Cushing's disease before and after treatment. (a) Full, rounded face ("moon face") prior to treatment. (b) Normal facial appearance after treatment.

Now that we have discussed conditions of the endocrine system, let's put that knowledge into practice. While working in a clinic, you have the following patient messages. Which patient would you call back first?

- A 58-year-old male diagnosed with diabetes, reporting a fasting blood glucose of 112 and requesting prescription refills for his diabetic medication
- A 64-year-old female diagnosed with Cushing's syndrome, reporting a pulse of 74, blood pressure of 150/90 mm Hg, and blood glucose of 290
- A 72-year-old female diagnosed with hypothyroidism, reporting a pulse of 78 and blood pressure of 128/70 mm Hg, and requesting prescription refills for her thyroid medication
- A 45-year-old female diagnosed with hyperthyroidism, reporting a pulse of 89 and blood pressure of 130/78 mm Hg

You will want to treat these callbacks in the same way you treat other priority questions like "who you see first"—that is, by considering who would die first, acute versus chronic conditions, Maslow's hierarchy of needs, and patient safety. Start with the 58-year-old man diagnosed with diabetes. The fasting blood glucose is not alarming; the prescription refills are important but can wait. Now move on to the 64-year-old woman diagnosed with Cushing's syndrome. Her pulse is normal, but her blood pressure and glucose readings are high. Keep this patient on the short list. Now consider the 72-year-old woman diagnosed with hypothyroidism. Her pulse and blood pressure are normal, and the prescription refills can wait. Finally, look at the 45-year-old woman diagnosed with hyperthyroidism. Her pulse and blood pressure are on the high end of normal, but they are still normal. After considering all the patients, the 64-year-old patient with Cushing's syndrome should be called back first.

by damage resulting from autoimmune conditions (the most common cause), infections (e.g., tuberculosis, human immunodeficiency virus, fungal infections, and meningitis), hemorrhage, and tumors. Additionally, Addison's disease may result from pituitary dysfunction that results in insufficient ACTH levels. Clinical manifestations reflect the deficiency of the hormones and usually develop slowly over weeks to months:

- Hypotension
- Changes in heart rate
- Hypoglycemia
- Chronic diarrhea
- Patchy hyperpigmentation
- Pallor
- Extreme weakness and fatigue
- Anorexia
- Mouth lesions on the inside of a cheek (buccal mucosa)
- Nausea and vomiting
- Salt craving
- Slow, sluggish movement
- Unintentional weight loss
- Mood changes and depression
- Electrolyte disturbances (particularly hyperkalemia, hyponatremia, and hypochloremia)

Diagnostic procedures for Addison's disease include a history, physical examination, serum hormone levels (e.g., cortisol, ACTH, and androgens), serum glucose levels, CBC, blood chemistry, urine cortisol, adrenal and pituitary CT and MRI, and biopsy. Treatment of this disease requires lifelong hormone replacement therapy. Increases in hormone doses may be required during times of infections, stress, and trauma. The patient should wear a medical alert bracelet and carry extra medication at all times.

CHAPTER SUMMARY

The endocrine system is responsible for producing a wide range of hormones necessary for a variety of processes. Endocrine disorders are often caused by congenital defects, tumors, or gland damage. These conditions vary from harmless to life threatening, and most are managed easily with medications and surgery. Clinical manifestations of these conditions reflect the hormones affected and the degree of deviation. Regardless of the disorder and the severity, lifelong management is necessary to prevent significant complications or death.

REFERENCES

AAOS. (2004). *Paramedic: Anatomy and physiology*. Sudbury, MA: Jones and Bartlett.

American Diabetes Association. (2016). American Diabetes Association standards of medical care. *Diabetes Care, 39*(suppl 1), S1–S112.

Centers for Disease Control and Prevention (CDC). (2015). Diabetes. Retrieved from http://www.cdc.gov/diabetes /data/national.html

Chiras, D. (2011). *Human biology* (7th ed.). Burlington, MA: Jones & Bartlett Learning.

Elling, B., Elling, K., & Rothenberg, M. (2004). *Anatomy and physiology*. Sudbury, MA: Jones and Bartlett.

Gould, B. (2015). *Pathophysiology for the health professions* (5th ed.). Philadelphia, PA: Elsevier.

Hart, M., & Loeffler, A. (2015). *Introduction to human disease: Pathophysiology for health professionals* (6th ed.). Burlington, MA: Jones & Bartlett Learning.

Madara, B., & Pomarico-Denino, V. (2008). *Pathophysiology* (2nd ed.). Sudbury, MA: Jones and Bartlett.

Professional guide to pathophysiology (3rd ed.). (2010). Philadelphia, PA: Lippincott Williams & Wilkins.

World Health Organization. (2016). Diabetes. Retrieved from http://www.who.int/mediacentre/factsheets/fs312/en /index.html

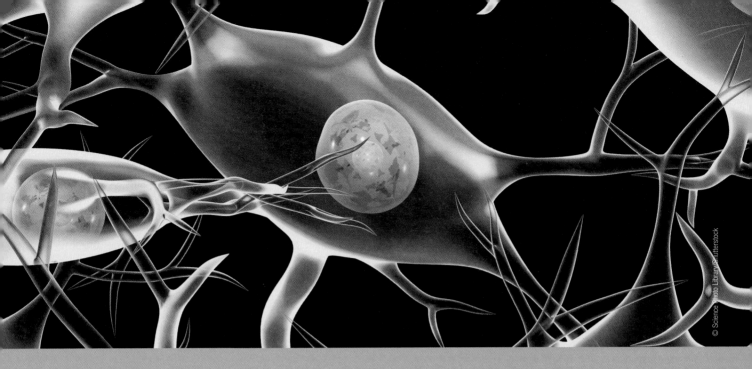

CHAPTER 11
Neural Function

LEARNING OBJECTIVES

- Discuss normal neural anatomy and physiology.
- Describe and compare congenital neurologic disorders.
- Compare and contrast traumatic neurologic disorders.
- Compare and contrast infectious neurologic disorders.

- Describe and compare vascular neurologic disorders.
- Compare and contrast types of seizure disorders.
- Compare and contrast chronic degenerative neurologic disorders.
- Compare and contrast types of dementia.
- Describe and compare cancers of the nervous system.

KEY TERMS

action potential
afferent nerve
afferent tracts
AIDS dementia complex
Alzheimer's disease (AD)
amyotrophic lateral
  sclerosis (ALS)
arachnoid layer
ascending fibers
aura
automatism
autonomic hyperreflexia
autonomic nervous system
autoregulation
axon
basal ganglia
basilar skull fracture

brain
brain stem
cauda equina
cauda equina syndrome
central nervous system (CNS)
cerebellum
cerebral aneurysm
cerebral contusion
cerebral palsy (CP)
cerebral vascular
  accident (CVA)
cerebrospinal fluid (CSF)
cerebrum
chorea
comminuted skull fracture
compound skull fracture
concussion

contrecoup
coup
cranial nerves
Creutzfeldt-Jakob
  disease (CJD)
Cushing's reflex
Cushing's triad
dementia
dendrite
depolarization
depressed skull fracture
dermatome
descending fibers
diencephalon
dorsal root
dura mater
efferent nerve

efferent tracts
encephalitis
epidural hematoma
epilepsy
epithalamus
flexor reflex
focal seizure
foramen magnum
frontal lobe
generalized seizure
gyrus
hematoma
hemorrhagic stroke
herniation
Huntington's disease
hydrocephalus
hypothalamus

increased intracranial pressure	nerve	postsynaptic cell membrane	substantia nigra
interneuron	neuroglia	presynaptic terminal	subthalamus
intracerebral hematoma	neuromelanin	prion	sulcus
ischemic stroke	neuron	quadriplegia	sympathetic nervous system (SNS)
linear skull fracture	neurotransmitter	resting potential	synapse
lobe	node of Ranvier	reticular activation system	synaptic cleft
longitudinal fissure	occipital lobe	reticular formation	temporal lobe
medulla	paralysis	rootlet	terminal bouton
meninges	paraplegia	Schwann cell	thalamus
meningitis	parasympathetic nervous system	seizure	transient ischemic attack (TIA)
meningocele	parietal lobe	sensory nerve	traumatic brain injury (TBI)
midbrain	Parkinson's disease	spina bifida	ventral root
Monro-Kellie hypothesis	peripheral nerve	spina bifida occulta	ventricle
motor nerve	peripheral nervous system (PNS)	spinal cord	vertebral canal
multiple sclerosis (MS)	pia mater	spinal cord injury (SCI)	white matter
myasthenia gravis	plexus	spinal reflex arc	Zika virus disease
myasthenic crisis	pons	spinal shock	
myelin sheath	postictal period	status epilepticus	
myelomeningocele		subarachnoid hemorrhage	
		subdural hematoma	

The nervous system consists of complex structures that control many body functions and cognition. The functions this system manages include (1) structures such as muscles, glands, and organs; (2) heart rate; (3) blood flow; (4) breathing; (5) digestion; (6) urination; and (7) defecation. The nervous system works with other systems to maintain homeostasis by receiving and responding to input from the environment. Disorders of the nervous system may be acute or chronic; regardless of their severity, these conditions often have grave or life-altering effects on the body. Causes of these disorders include congenital defects, trauma, infections, tumors, chemical imbalances, and vascular changes.

Anatomy and Physiology

The nervous system is an intricate network of specialized cells and tissue that receive and react to environmental stimuli on physiologic and cognitive levels. To communicate this input, these structures conduct electric impulses between the brain and the rest of the body. The nervous system consists of three main components: the brain, the spinal cord, and the nerves. The brain and spinal cord make up the **central nervous system (CNS)**, and the nerves make up the **peripheral nervous system (PNS)**.

Central Nervous System

The skull and vertebral column house and protect the brain and spinal cord. Additionally, a set of three tough membranes, called the **meninges**, encase the CNS (FIGURE 11-1). The **dura mater** is the outer and toughest layer. The **arachnoid layer** is the middle layer, named for its spider web–like vascular system. The **pia mater** is the innermost layer that rests directly on the brain and spinal cord. **Cerebrospinal fluid (CSF)** is a plasmalike liquid that fills the space between the arachnoid and pia mater layers to provide additional cushioning and support to the CNS. The choroid plexus cells in the brain's ventricles continuously produce the CSF. The **ventricles** are interconnected, hollow areas of the brain that the CSF fills and where it flows freely between them. Excess CSF drains into the bloodstream.

The **brain** is located within the skull and contains billions of neurons. Neural tissue consists of two basic types of cells—neuroglia and neurons. **Neuroglia** cells play several important supportive roles in the nervous system. In particular, these cells scaffold neural tissue as well as isolate and protect neuron cell membranes. Additionally, neuroglia cells regulate interstitial fluid, defend the neurons against pathogens, and assist with neural repair.

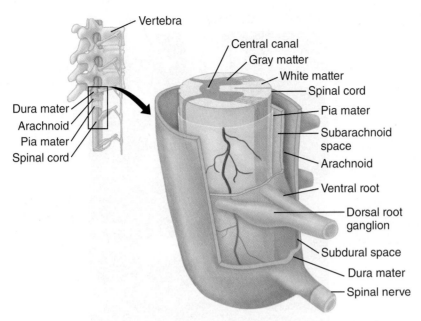

FIGURE 11-1 The meninges enclose the brain and the spinal cord.

Neurons are the fundamental unit of the nervous system; they generate bioelectrical impulses and transmit these signals from one area of the body to another. Neurons occur in several sizes and shapes, but all share similar characteristics. Neurons do not have the ability to divide; thus, when these cells are lost due to aging or injury, they cannot be replaced. Not all cell death results in loss of functioning, however. For example, if neurons become damaged in one area of the brain, neurons in other areas can eventually assume responsibility for those functions. In the PNS, severed nerves can regenerate to a point to reestablish connections with the tissue they once supplied. In the brain or spinal cord, in contrast, severed axons cannot be repaired. Severed spinal cord nerves result in paralysis and loss of sensation below the area of damage. In addition to being unable to divide, nerve cells require a constant supply of oxygen and glucose. This characteristic makes neurons vulnerable to the effects of hypoxia and hypoglycemia. Neurons can begin dying within minutes of these events.

Most neurons have a spherical cell body that houses the nucleus, most of the cytoplasm, and organelles. Neurons contain projections called **axons** and **dendrites** that make connections with nearby cells (FIGURE 11-2). Axons transmit impulses away from the cell body, whereas dendrites transmit impulses toward the cell body. When the axon reaches its destination, it often branches into several small fibers that terminate into miniscule bulges, called **terminal boutons**. These terminal boutons communicate with neurons, muscle fibers, or glands. Axons may be surrounded by a **myelin sheath**, which increases the rate of impulse transmission to approximately 400 times faster than is possible in unmyelinated nerves (FIGURE 11-3). **Schwann cells** produce the myelin sheath; these cells are separated by **nodes of Ranvier**. Because of the myelin, impulses move at greater speeds down the axon, jumping from one node to the next, much like stones skipping across water. Bundles of these myelinated nerves are referred to as **white matter**. Impulses move in a slow, wavelike pattern in unmyelinated nerves. Gaps between the neurons are referred to as **synapses**. Each of these gaps includes a **presynaptic terminal** (e.g., a terminal bouton or some similar structure), a **synaptic cleft** (the space between neurons), and a **postsynaptic cell membrane** (FIGURE 11-4). The presynaptic and postsynaptic terminals are opposite ends of the nerve.

Electrical impulses of the nervous system are not like the electrical current that powers appliances, which is formed by the flow of electrons. Instead, small ionic changes (e.g., potassium and sodium moving across cell membranes) generate neural impulses. The creation of this charge is referred to as an **action potential** (FIGURE 11-5). The plasma side of the neuron membrane has a slight charge at rest, or **resting potential**, because of the sodium ions concentrated on the outside of the cell. When the

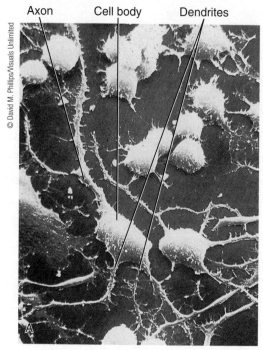

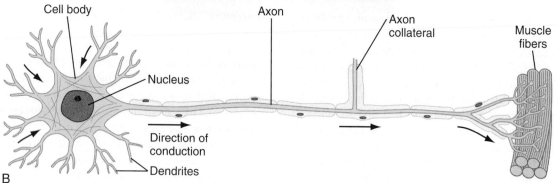

FIGURE 11-2 A neuron. (a) A scanning electron micrograph of the cell body and dendrites. (b) Collateral branches may occur along the length of the axon. In motor neurons, when the axon terminates, it branches many times, ending in individual muscle fibers.

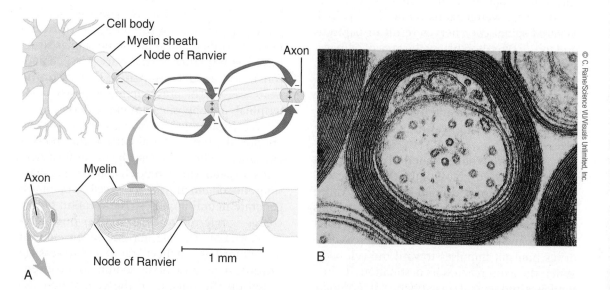

FIGURE 11-3 A myelinated nerve. (a) The myelin sheath allows impulses to "jump" from node to node, greatly accelerating the rate of transmission. (b) A transmission electron micrograph of an axon in the cross section, showing a myelin sheath.

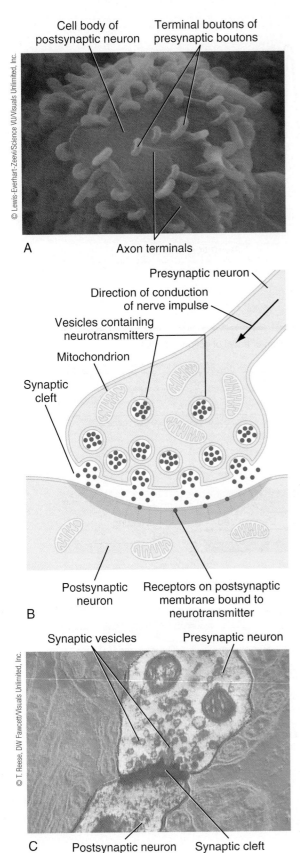

A

Cell body of postsynaptic neuron

Terminal boutons of presynaptic boutons

Axon terminals

© Lewis-Everhart-Zeevi/Science VU/Visuals Unlimited, Inc.

B

Presynaptic neuron

Direction of conduction of nerve impulse

Vesicles containing neurotransmitters

Mitochondrion

Synaptic cleft

Postsynaptic neuron

Receptors on postsynaptic membrane bound to neurotransmitter

C

Synaptic vesicles

Presynaptic neuron

Postsynaptic neuron

Synaptic cleft

© T. Reese, DW Fawcett/Visuals Unlimited, Inc.

neuron is stimulated, protein gates open and sodium flows into the cell. The rapid inflow of positively charged sodium ions increases the charge—a process called **depolarization**. Immediately following depolarization, the cell membrane returns to its resting state through the rapid outflow of the positively charged potassium ions. When generated, these impulses travel down the nerve to trigger the release of **neurotransmitters** from the presynaptic terminal. The neurotransmitters cross the synaptic cleft, albeit only in one direction, to stimulate an electrical reaction in nearby neurons. Synaptic transmission of the impulse takes a mere millisecond. This electrical reaction passes through those neurons to the next synapse, where the process is repeated. At each synaptic transmission, a small burst of neurotransmitters is released and then removed. Neurotransmitters are either destroyed by enzymes or reabsorbed by the postsynaptic membrane to be recycled for the next transmission. Whereas some neurotransmitters stimulate the action potentials of neurons, other neurotransmitters inhibit action potentials.

The brain is responsible for a variety of physiologically vital functions and cognitive activities. It accomplishes these functions in part through the set of cranial nerves. Twelve pairs of **cranial nerves** branch directly from the base of the brain (FIGURE 11-6). Some of the cranial nerves carry only sensory fibers (I, II, and VIII), others carry only motor fibers (III, IV, VI, XI, and XII), and a few carry both types of fibers (V, VII, IX, and X). Each nerve travels from the brain through the foramen to its destination.

The major regions of the brain include the cerebrum (including the cerebral cortex), diencephalon (thalamus and hypothalamus), brain stem (pons, midbrain, and medulla), and

FIGURE 11-4 The function of neurotransmitters in the synaptic cleft. (a) A scanning electron micrograph showing the terminal boutons of an axon ending on the cell body of another neuron. (b) The arrival of the impulse stimulates the release of neurotransmitters held in synaptic vesicles in the axon terminals. Neurotransmitter diffuses across the synaptic cleft and binds to the postsynaptic membrane, where it elicits another action potential that travels down the dendrite to the cell body. (c) A transmission electron micrograph showing the details of the synapse.

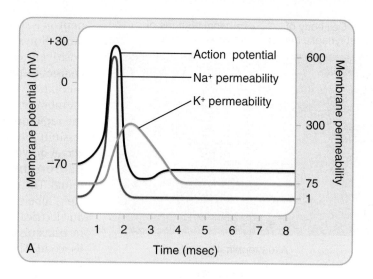

A

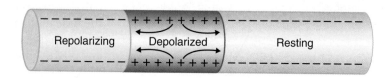

Direction of travel of action potential

B. The end of the axon away from the neuron's body becomes depolarized in response to a signal.

C. Depolarization extends through the axon as the initial part of the membrane repolarizes.

D. Action potential spreads across the axon.

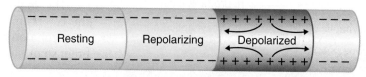

FIGURE 11-5 Action potential. (a) Stimulating the neuron creates a bioelectric impulse, which is recorded as an action potential. The resulting potential shifts from 270 millivolts to 130 millivolts. The membrane is said to be depolarized. This graph shows the shift in potential and the change in the permeability of sodium (Na⁺) and potassium (K⁺) ions, which is largely responsible for the action potential. (b) The influx of sodium ions and the depolarization that occur at the point of stimulation. (c) The impulse travels along the membrane as a wave of depolarization. (d) The efflux of potassium ions restores the resting potential, allowing the neuron to transmit additional impulses almost immediately.

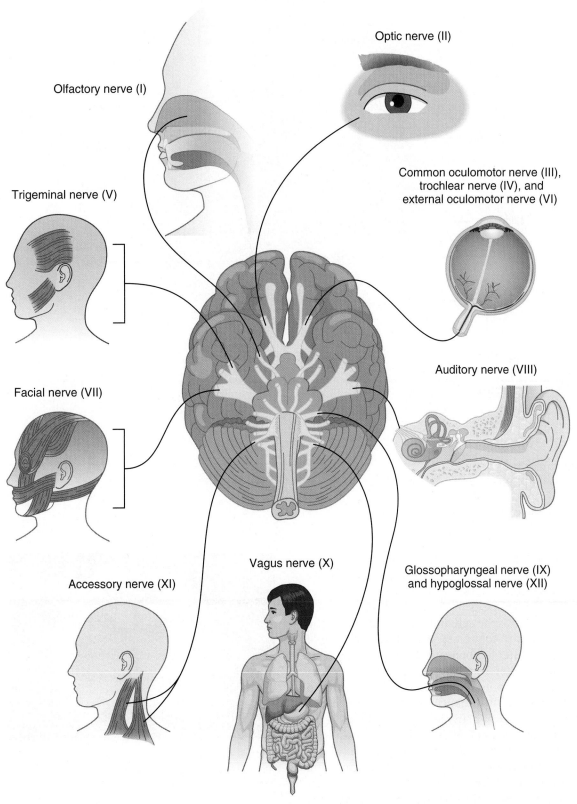

Optic nerve (II)

Olfactory nerve (I)

Common oculomotor nerve (III), trochlear nerve (IV), and external oculomotor nerve (VI)

Trigeminal nerve (V)

Auditory nerve (VIII)

Facial nerve (VII)

Vagus nerve (X)

Accessory nerve (XI)

Glossopharyngeal nerve (IX) and hypoglossal nerve (XII)

FIGURE 11-6 The cranial nerves.

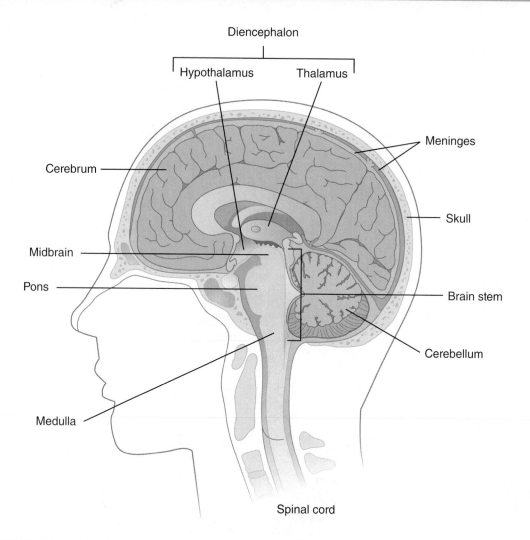

Diencephalon

Hypothalamus   Thalamus

Meninges

Cerebrum

Skull

Midbrain

Pons

Brain stem

Cerebellum

Medulla

Spinal cord

FIGURE 11-7 The major regions of the brain.

cerebellum (**FIGURE 11-7**). The **cerebrum** is the largest of the regions (accounting for 80% of the brain's total mass) and controls the higher thought processes. A thin layer of gray matter, referred to as the cerebral cortex, surrounds the cerebrum (**FIGURE 11-8**). A thick central core of white matter lies beneath the gray matter. This white matter contains bundles of axons that transmit impulses from the cerebral cortex to the spinal cord, enhancing communication and coordination of activities. The cerebrum is divided into right and left hemispheres by a **longitudinal fissure**. Although minor shifts of one hemisphere into the other may occur, impinging of one hemisphere on the other can have significant—even life-threatening—effects. Numerous folds, or **gyri**, increase the surface area of the cerebrum. The grooves in between the gyri are called **sulci**. At birth, only a minimal set of gyri is present, but these folds increase as the brain develops into adulthood.

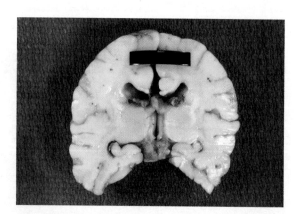

FIGURE 11-8 The cerebrum.
© University of Alabama at Birmingham Department of Pathology PEIR Digital Library (http://peir.net)

Within each hemisphere of the brain are subdivisions called **lobes**; each lobe is named for the bone of the skull that covers it (**FIGURE 11-9**). The **frontal lobe** facilitates voluntary motor activity and plays a role in

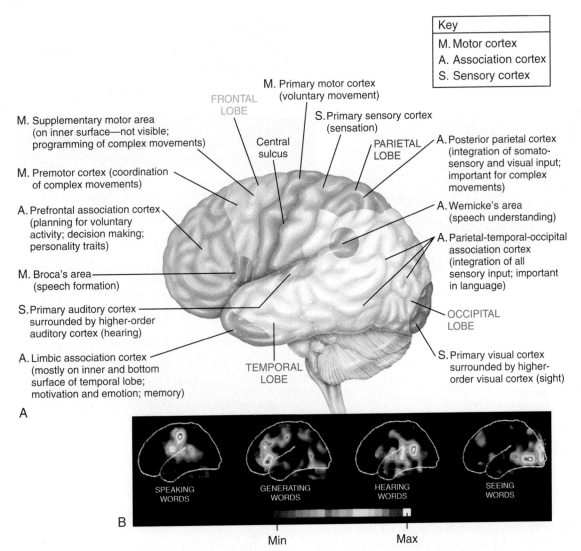

Key
M. Motor cortex
A. Association cortex
S. Sensory cortex

M. Primary motor cortex (voluntary movement)

FRONTAL LOBE

S. Primary sensory cortex (sensation)

M. Supplementary motor area (on inner surface—not visible; programming of complex movements)

Central sulcus

PARIETAL LOBE

A. Posterior parietal cortex (integration of somato-sensory and visual input; important for complex movements)

M. Premotor cortex (coordination of complex movements)

A. Prefrontal association cortex (planning for voluntary activity; decision making; personality traits)

A. Wernicke's area (speech understanding)

A. Parietal-temporal-occipital association cortex (integration of all sensory input; important in language)

M. Broca's area (speech formation)

S. Primary auditory cortex surrounded by higher-order auditory cortex (hearing)

OCCIPITAL LOBE

A. Limbic association cortex (mostly on inner and bottom surface of temporal lobe; motivation and emotion; memory)

TEMPORAL LOBE

S. Primary visual cortex surrounded by higher-order visual cortex (sight)

A

SPEAKING WORDS   GENERATING WORDS   HEARING WORDS   SEEING WORDS

B

Min   Max

FIGURE 11-9 The lobes of the cerebrum. (a) The cerebral cortex has three principal functions: receiving sensory input, integrating sensory information, and generating motor responses. Special sensory areas handle vision, smell, taste, and hearing. (b) A PET scan reveals the locations of increased blood flow in the brain during performance of certain tasks.

Photo: Courtesy of Marcus Raichle, MD, Mallinckrodt Institute of Radiology, Washington University in St. Louis School of Medicine

personality traits. The **parietal lobe** receives and interprets sensory input, with the exception of smell, hearing, and vision stimuli. The **occipital lobe** processes visual information. The **temporal lobe** plays an essential role in hearing and memory. Areas within and across these lobes can be classified as three types—motor (which stimulates muscle activity), sensory (which receives sensory information), and association (which integrates information and initiates coordinated responses).

The **diencephalon** includes the thalamus and hypothalamus (FIGURE 11-10). The **thalamus** receives and relays most of the sensory input, affects mood, and initiates body movements (especially those associated with fear or anger). The **subthalamus** participates in motor activities, but the functions of the **epithalamus**—especially the pineal body—are unclear. The **hypothalamus** is the most inferior portion of the diencephalon; it regulates many bodily functions (see the *Endocrine Function* chapter).

The **brain stem** (including the pons, cerebellum, and medulla) connects the brain to the spinal cord. This structure is crucial for many basic body functions (e.g., maintaining heart rate, blood pressure, and respiration), and injury to the brain stem can easily result in death. The brain stem collaborates with the hypothalamus to regulate these vital activities. In addition to containing control regions, the brain stem serves

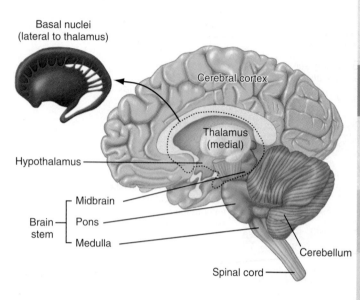

Cerebral cortex
- Receives sensory information from skin, muscles, glands, and organs
- Sends messages to move skeletal muscles
- Integrates incoming and outgoing nerve impulses
- Performs associative activities such as thinking, learning, and remembering

Basal nuclei
- Play a role in the coordination of slow, sustained movements
- Suppress useless patterns of movement

Thalamus
- Relays most sensory information from the spinal cord and certain parts of the brain to the cerebral cortex
- Interprets certain sensory messages such as those of pain, temperature, and pressure

Hypothalamus
- Controls various homeostatic functions such as body temperature, respiration, and heart rate
- Directs hormone secretions of the pituitary

Cerebellum
- Coordinates subconscious movements of skeletal muscles
- Contributes to muscle tone, posture, balance, and equilibrium

Brain stem
- Origin of many cranial nerves
- Reflex center for movements of eyeballs, head, and trunk
- Regulates heart rate and breathing
- Plays a role in consciousness
- Transmits impulses between brain and spinal cord

Labels on figure: Basal nuclei (lateral to thalamus); Cerebral cortex; Thalamus (medial); Hypothalamus; Brain stem — Midbrain, Pons, Medulla; Cerebellum; Spinal cord

FIGURE 11-10 The regions of the brain and their functions.

as the main thoroughfare for information traveling to and from the brain. Of the 12 cranial nerves, 10 exit from the brain stem. The **pons** contains nerves that regulate sleep and breathing. The **midbrain**, which is the smallest region of the brain, acts as a sort of relay station for auditory and visual information. It controls the visual and auditory systems as well as eye movement. The **medulla** is a conduction pathway for ascending and descending nerve tracts. It coordinates heart rate, peripheral vascular resistance, breathing, swallowing, vomiting, coughing, and sneezing.

Most of the many nerve fibers passing through the brain stem have branches that terminate in a region of the brain stem called the **reticular formation**. The reticular formation acts like a gatekeeper, receiving all incoming and outgoing information. It sends impulses to the cerebral cortex through specialized nerve fibers. These fibers, in turn, make up the **reticular activation system** (FIGURE 11-11). The reticular formation and the reticular activation system are responsible for alertness during the day, and

their ongoing activation can prevent sleeping at night.

The **cerebellum** communicates with other regions of the brain to coordinate the synergistic motion of muscle movement and balance as well as cognition. Deep within the cerebrum, diencephalon, and midbrain is a set of key structures called the **basal ganglia**. The basal ganglia play a pivotal role in coordination, motor movement, and posture. Portions of the cerebrum and diencephalon constitute the limbic system (FIGURE 11-12). The limbic system works in conjunction with the hypothalamus to influence instinctive behavior, emotions, motivation, mood, pain, and pleasure.

The **spinal cord** exits the skull through the large (and only) opening in the skull, called the **foramen magnum**. The spinal cord extends through the **vertebral canal** to the second lumbar vertebra. At this point, the spinal cord transitions into individual nerve roots referred to as the **cauda equina**. The spinal cord consists of 31 pairs of spinal nerves that branch off at regular intervals (FIGURE 11-13).

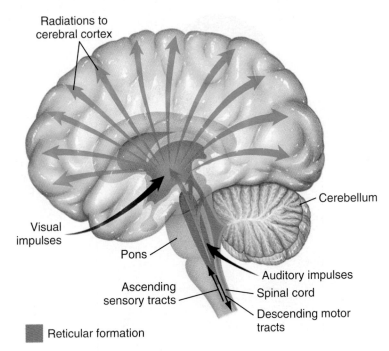

FIGURE 11-11 The reticular activation system.

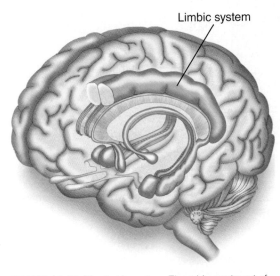

FIGURE 11-12 The limbic system. The odd assortment of structures shown in blue is the limbic system. The limbic system is the seat of emotions, such as joy, and instincts; it is home to other functions as well.

The central portion of the spinal cord is an H-shaped area of gray matter, which contains nerve cell bodies. White matter consisting of nerve fiber tracts, or pathways, surrounds the gray matter (FIGURE 11-14). **Ascending fibers**, also known as **afferent tracts**, carry sensory information in the form of action potentials from the periphery back to the brain. **Descending fibers**, also known as **efferent tracts**, carry

motor impulses in the form of action potentials from the brain to the PNS. The ascending fibers contain a variety of tracts that communicate specific sensory input:

- Anterior spinothalamic tracts permit sensations of light touch, pressure, tickling, and itching.
- Lateral spinothalamic tracts allow the sensations of pain and temperature.
- Spinocerebellar tracts establish the body's position in relation to the cerebellum.
- Corticospinal tracts coordinate movements, especially in the hands.
- Vestibulospinal tracts are responsible for involuntary movements.
- Reticulospinal tracts are also responsible for involuntary movements.

The **spinal reflex arcs** refer to the process that creates an unconscious response to stimuli (FIGURE 11-15). An example of this arc can be seen when the patella is gently tapped with a reflex hammer. The tendon stretch reflex is elicited when the patella is tapped, causing the lower leg to sharply move first forward (called extension) and then backward (called flexion). The **flexor reflex** is a withdrawal reflex that occurs in response to touching an unpleasant stimulus (e.g., extreme heat). This reflex causes the muscles of a limb to withdraw the limb from the source of the stimulus without any

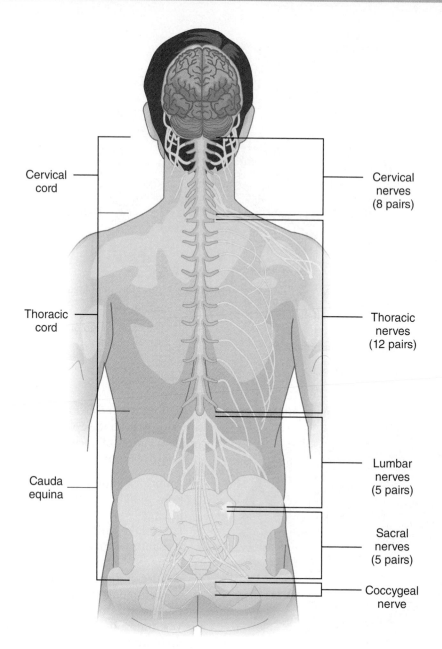

Cervical cord

Thoracic cord

Cauda equina

Cervical nerves (8 pairs)

Thoracic nerves (12 pairs)

Lumbar nerves (5 pairs)

Sacral nerves (5 pairs)

Coccygeal nerve

FIGURE 11-13 The spinal cord.

conscious action. The tracts of the spinal cord and brain regulate these impulses.

Peripheral Nervous System

The **nerves** of the PNS consist of bundles of nerve fibers, with each fiber being part of the neuron. These nerves transport messages to and from the CNS. The nerves end on receptors that respond to a variety of internal and external stimuli. The 31 spinal nerve pairs (8 cervical, 12 thoracic, 5 lumbar, 5 sacral, and 1 coccygeal) branch directly off the spinal cord to make up

the PNS. Each spinal nerve pair is named for the vertebral level at which it exits the spinal cord (e.g., C3 is the 3rd cervical nerve and T12 is the 12th thoracic nerve) and innervates specific areas of the body (FIGURE 11-16). Ganglia comprise collections of nerve cell bodies outside the CNS. Spinal nerves arise from several small nerves called **rootlets** along the dorsal and ventral surfaces of the spinal cord (FIGURE 11-17). Approximately 6–8 rootlets combine to form each **dorsal root** and **ventral root**. These roots, in turn, come together to form the spinal nerve.

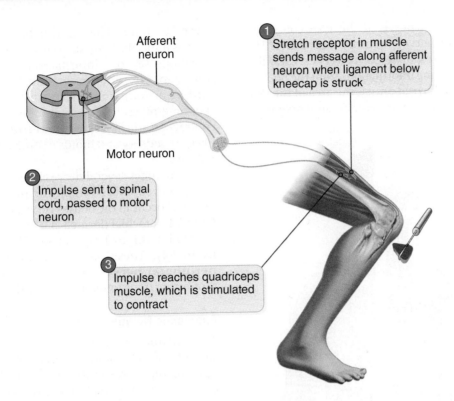

Afferent neuron

Motor neuron

① Stretch receptor in muscle sends message along afferent neuron when ligament below kneecap is struck

② Impulse sent to spinal cord, passed to motor neuron

③ Impulse reaches quadriceps muscle, which is stimulated to contract

FIGURE 11-14 Spinal cord nerve tracts.

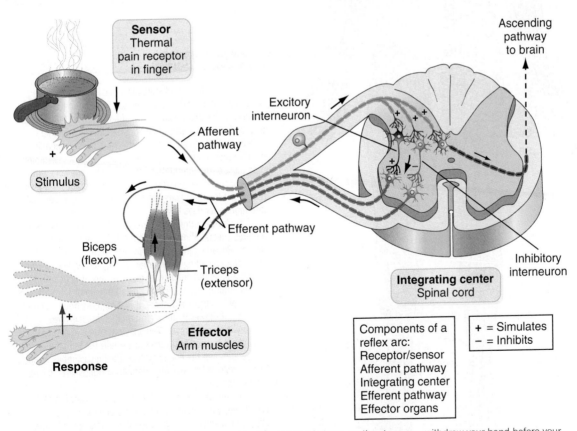

Sensor
Thermal pain receptor in finger

Stimulus

Afferent pathway

Excitory interneuron

Ascending pathway to brain

Efferent pathway

Biceps (flexor)

Triceps (extensor)

Inhibitory interneuron

Integrating center
Spinal cord

Effector
Arm muscles

Response

Components of a reflex arc:
Receptor/sensor
Afferent pathway
Integrating center
Efferent pathway
Effector organs

+ = Simulates
− = Inhibits

FIGURE 11-15 The spinal reflex arc. When you accidentally touch a hot pan on the stove, you withdraw your hand before your brain even knows what is happening. This reaction occurs because of a reflex arc. Sensory fibers send impulses to the spinal cord. The sensory impulses stimulate motor neurons in the spinal cord. This stimulation (1) causes muscle contraction in the flexor muscles and (2) inhibits muscle contraction in the extensor muscles, allowing you to withdraw your hand. Nerve impulses also ascend to the brain to let it know what is happening.

Each spinal nerve of the PNS comprises two types of nerves—sensory and motor. The **sensory nerves**, or **afferent nerves**, carry impulses (regarding information) from the body to the brain. A **dermatome** is the area of the skin innervated by a given pair of spinal sensory nerves. Each spinal nerve, with the exception of C1, has a specific body surface area from which it obtains sensory information. The **motor nerves**, or **efferent nerves**, carry impulses (regarding action) from the brain to the corresponding muscle receptor, resulting in muscle contraction and movement. **Interneurons** connect the sensory and motor neurons in the spinal cord.

Sometimes several nerves intersect to form an organized collaboration, or **plexus**. Four plexuses occur in the body—cervical (located at C1 to C4), brachial (located at C5 to T1), lumbar (located at L1 to L4), and sacral (located at L4 to S4). These plexuses branch into the **peripheral nerves** that supply sensory and motor functions to many areas of the body.

Autonomic Nervous System

The **autonomic nervous system** controls smooth muscles and is responsible for the fight-or-flight response (see the *Immunity* chapter). The autonomic nervous system, which is not under conscious control, affects such activities as heart rate, blood pressure, and

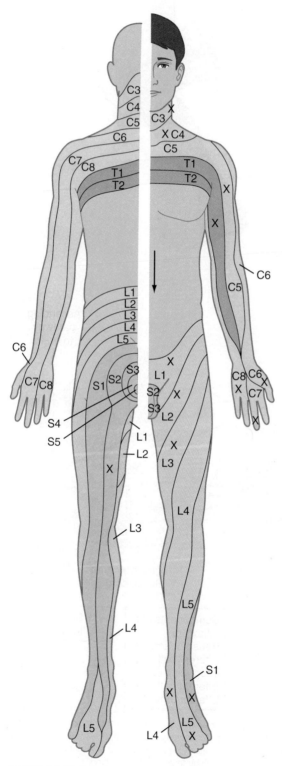

FIGURE 11-16 Spinal nerve innervation.

Learning Points

How do we learn and store memories? Learning is the acquisition and retention of new information, and memory is the storage and recall of information. Both depend on proper nutrition and adequate sleep. Newly acquired memory is first stored in the short-term memory, where it is held for seconds to hours. Cramming for tests, for example, puts most of the information into short-term memory. Unfortunately, soon after the test, the information fades—a good reason not to cram! Long-term memory, by comparison, holds information for days to years.

Transferring information from short- to long-term memory requires special efforts such as repetition, mnemonics, and rhymes. Recalling information in short-term memory is often faster than recalling information in long-term memory. When information is lost from short-term memory, it is usually lost forever. Information you cannot recall from long-term memory, in contrast, is often still there; it just requires time or stimuli to extract it. However, not all information in long-term memory is stored forever. Memories are stored in neurons throughout the cerebral cortex (especially the temporal lobe), cerebellum, and the limbic system. The hippocampus seems to be crucial in transferring information from short- to long-term memory.

You can use this knowledge to help you study by not cramming, but instead moving information from short- to long-term memory by paying attention, making the information memorable, and relating new information with facts you already know. But do not forget that you still have to get plenty of rest and eat a balanced diet to optimize your learning potential!

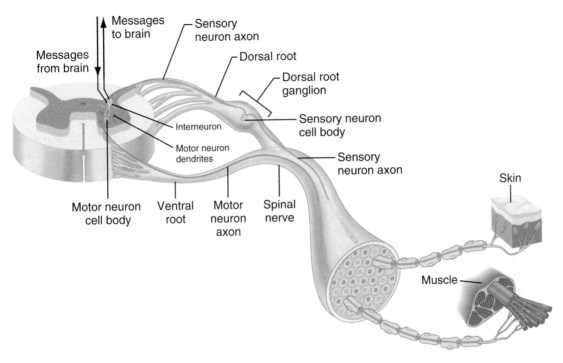

Messages to brain

Messages from brain

Sensory neuron axon

Dorsal root

Dorsal root ganglion

Sensory neuron cell body

Sensory neuron axon

Interneuron

Motor neuron dendrites

Motor neuron cell body

Ventral root

Motor neuron axon

Spinal nerve

Skin

Muscle

FIGURE 11-17 The dorsal root ganglion.

intestinal motility. This system has two subdivisions—sympathetic and parasympathetic. The two divisions have an antagonistic effect on each other that aids in maintaining homeostasis (FIGURE 11-18). The **sympathetic nervous system (SNS)** is responsible for the fight-or-flight response; this response is initiated when a person is startled or faced with danger and is augmented by secretions of the adrenal medulla. In contrast, the **parasympathetic nervous system** is responsible for the rest-and-digest response. Neurotransmitters and receptors are important in the autonomic nervous system because the SNS and the parasympathetic nervous system will stimulate or inhibit these sites, leading to the physiologic response (**TABLE 11-1**). The SNS stimulates the adrenergic receptors, while the parasympathetic nervous system stimulates the cholinergic receptors. Some medications can also stimulate or inhibit these receptors.

UNDERSTANDING CONDITIONS THAT AFFECT THE NERVOUS SYSTEM

When considering alterations in the nervous system, organizing them based on their basic underlying pathophysiology can increase understanding. Conditions of the nervous system are usually complex, affecting many areas of function. For example, these disorders may lead to impaired physical mobility, chronic pain, impaired social interaction, incontinence, risk for injury, and self-care deficit, just to name a few possibilities. Each of these nursing diagnoses presents its own set of interventions. Patients experiencing these

Myth Busters

Some myths surrounding the brain warrant discussion.

Myth 1: The brain is gray.

The living, pulsing brain currently residing in your skull is not just a dull, bland, gray organ like the image often depicted in movies; instead, the brain is also white, black, and red. Like many myths, this one has a grain of truth, because much of the brain *is* gray. Sometimes the entire brain is referred to as gray matter. However, the brain also contains white matter, which comprises nerve fibers that connect the gray matter. The black component is called **substantia nigra**, which is Latin for "black substance." The substantia nigra has a black color because of **neuromelanin**, a specialized type of pigment. Finally, the brain is red in some areas because of the many blood vessels it contains.

Myth 2: Listening to classical music, especially by Mozart, increases intelligence.

How did this myth get started? In the 1950s, a physician named Albert Tomatis claimed he had successfully used Mozart's music to help people with speech and auditory disorders. In the 1990s, 36 students in a study at the University of California at Irvine listened to 10 minutes of a Mozart sonata before taking an IQ test. The study reported that the students' IQ scores went up by about 8 points—and thus the "Mozart effect" was born. Multiple products have been sold based on this assumption. However, the original University of California at Irvine study remains controversial within the scientific community. Other scientists have been unable to replicate the original results, and current scientific evidence does not support the contention that listening to Mozart—or any other classical music, for that matter—increases intelligence. However, some evidence indicates that learning an instrument improves concentration, self-confidence, and coordination. Mozart's music certainly cannot hurt you, and you might even enjoy it if you try listening to this music; however, you will not get any smarter because of this activity.

Myth 3: You use only 10% of your brain.

This myth is probably one of the most well-known legend about the brain. This assumption seems puzzling at first glance. We have the biggest brain in proportion to our bodies of any animal, so why would we not use all of it? Many people have jumped on this idea, writing books and selling products that claim to tap into the other 90%. Believers in psychic abilities use this claim as proof, suggesting that people with these abilities have tapped into the rest of their brains.

In fact, this myth is false. In addition to 100 billion neurons, the brain is full of other types of cells that are continually in use. Significant neurologic deficits can occur from even minor damage depending on the location, so it is highly unlikely that we could function with only 10% of our brain in use. Brain scans have shown that no matter what we are doing, our brains are always active. Some areas are more active at any one time than others, but unless we have brain damage, no one part of the brain is completely turned off. Thus there is no hidden, extra potential you can tap into, in terms of actual brain space.

Myth 4: Games like Sudoku and brain age keep your brain young.

There is some truth to this myth! Continued mental engagement has benefits, and puzzles can help you get good at a specific skill, such as memorizing grocery lists or hand–eye coordination. Most evidence, however, suggests practicing a task helps you get better only at that particular task. Far better for mental function is physical exercise. Regular fitness exercise is especially effective in the elderly, who may suffer from gradual problems with cognitive function such as planning ahead and abstract thinking.

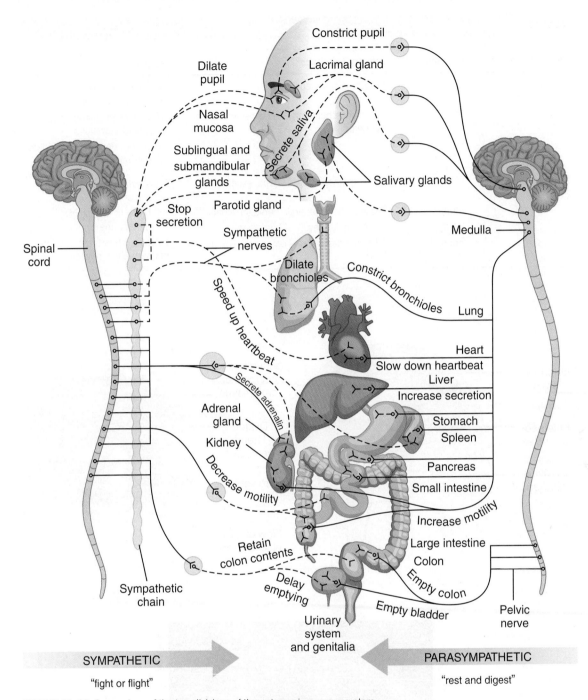

FIGURE 11-18 Comparison of the two divisions of the autonomic nervous system.

neurologic conditions often require vigilance to manage the complexity of the situation.

Congenital Neurologic Disorders

Congenital defects of the nervous system are often serious, with lifelong consequences. These disorders often have limited treatment options and require long-term management of complications.

Hydrocephalus

Hydrocephalus is a condition in which excess CSF accumulates within the skull, which dilates the ventricles and compresses the brain and blood vessels (FIGURE 11-19). The pressure from the excess CSF thins the cortex, causing severe brain damage. The CSF accumulates when the flow of this fluid is disrupted (referred to as noncommunicating or an obstructive

TABLE 11-1   Types of Autonomic Receptors

Neurotransmitter	Receptor	Primary Locations	Responses
Acetylcholine (cholinergic)	Nicotinic	Postganglionic neurons	Stimulation of smooth muscle and gland secretions
	Muscarinic	Parasympathetic target: organs other than the heart	Stimulation of smooth muscle and gland secretions
		Heart	Decreased heart rate and force of contraction
Norepinephrine (adrenergic)	Alpha$_1$	All sympathetic target organs except the heart	Constriction of blood vessels, dilation of pupils
	Alpha$_2$	Presynaptic adrenergic nerve terminals	Inhibition of release of norepinephrine
	Beta$_1$	Heart and kidneys	
	Beta$_2$	All sympathetic target organs except the heart	Increased heart rate and force of contraction; release of renin

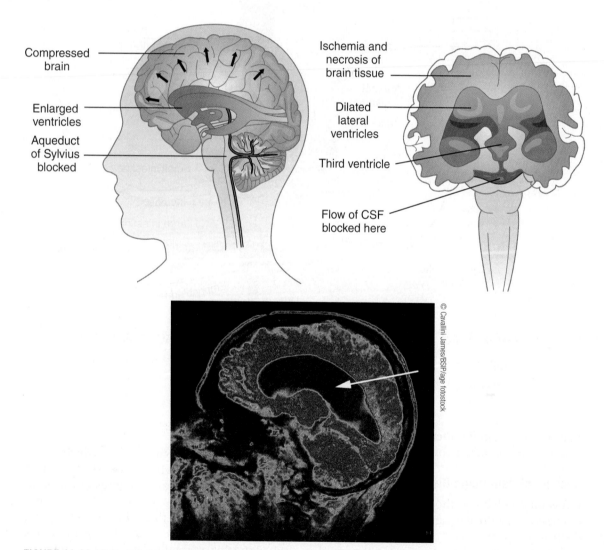

FIGURE 11-19 Hydrocephalus development.

hydrocephalus) or when too much CSF is made or not properly absorbed by the bloodstream (referred to as communicating hydrocephalus). Hydrocephalus is a common condition that may be present at birth (in an estimated 1 out of 500 births) or develop later in life (another 6,000 children younger than 2 years of age develop it each year) (National Hydrocephalus Foundation, 2014). Risk factors for hydrocephalus at any age include prematurity, pregnancy complications, other congenital defects (especially nervous system defects such as spina bifida), nervous system tumors, CNS infections, cerebral hemorrhage, and severe head injuries. If left untreated, hydrocephalus is often fatal (60% mortality rate). The prognosis depends on early treatment and comorbidity.

Clinical manifestations of hydrocephalus reflect the increased intracranial pressure (ICP). These manifestations vary by age group, underlying etiology, and disease progression. In infants, clinical manifestations often include the following:

- An unusually large head (FIGURE 11-20)
- A rapid increase in the head size
- A bulging fontanelle, or soft spot, on the top of the head
- Vomiting (often projectile)
- Lethargy
- Irritability
- High-pitched cry
- Feeding difficulties
- Seizures
- Eyes that gaze downward (setting-sun appearance)
- Developmental delays

In older children and adults, the head cannot enlarge because the sutures have closed. Clinical manifestations in these groups may include the following signs and symptoms:

- Headache followed by vomiting
- Nausea
- Blurred vision or diplopia (double vision)
- Sluggish pupil response to light; eyes that gaze downward (setting-sun appearance)
- Problems with balance, coordination, or gait
- Extreme fatigue
- Slowing or regression of development
- Memory loss
- Confusion
- Urinary incontinence
- Irritability
- Personality, memory, or cognition changes
- Impaired performance in school or work

Diagnostic procedures for hydrocephalus may be performed during pregnancy or after birth. These procedures consist of a history, physical examination (including head circumference measurement and a neurologic assessment), head computed tomography (CT), head magnetic resonance imaging (MRI), skull X-ray, cranial ultrasound, and prenatal ultrasound.

The goal of treatment is to minimize brain damage by reducing CSF. Blockages are surgically removed, if possible. If the blockage cannot be removed, a shunt (flexible tube) may be placed within the brain to allow CSF to flow around the blocked area. The shunt tubing travels to another part of the body, such as the peritoneal cavity (ventriculoperitoneal) or right atrium (ventriculoatrial), where the extra CSF can be drained and absorbed. Shunt replacement may be needed periodically as a child grows or if it becomes blocked or infected. Antibiotic therapy will treat hydrocephalus caused by an infection or if a shunt infection develops. An endoscopic third ventriculostomy can also be performed to relieve pressure without replacing the shunt. Additionally, the area producing too much CSF may be cauterized. Follow-up examinations generally continue throughout a child's life to monitor developmental progress and to manage any intellectual, neurologic, or physical problems. A multidisciplinary team (e.g., nurses, occupational therapists, educational specialists, social services personnel, and support groups) can provide emotional support and assistance with the care of those patients who have significant brain damage.

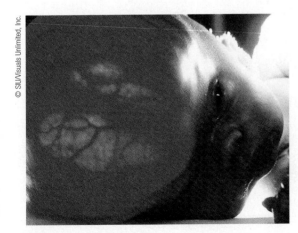

© SIU/Visuals Unlimited, Inc.

FIGURE 11-20 Hydrocephalus.

Spina Bifida

Although rates have been declining over the last 15 years, **spina bifida** remains the second most common birth defect in the United States, affecting approximately 1 child in every 1,500 births each year (Centers for Disease Control and Prevention [CDC], 2015c). Spina bifida is a neural tube defect that can vary in severity from mild to debilitating. Neural tube development begins early in pregnancy, starting at the cervical area and progressing toward the lumbar area, and the neural tube usually closes by the fourth week of gestation. In spina bifida, the posterior spinous processes on the vertebrae fail to fuse. This opening permits the meninges and spinal cord to herniate, resulting in neurologic impairment. The lumbar area of the vertebrae is most commonly the site of the defect.

The exact cause of spina bifida is unknown, but it is thought to result from genetic and environmental influences. Spina bifida is most common in Hispanic and Caucasian populations, with females being more affected than males. Additional maternal risk factors for development of this defect in a child include family history of neural defects, folate deficiency (thought to be a key factor), certain medications (e.g., antiseizure agents), diabetes mellitus, prepregnancy obesity, and increased body temperature (e.g., from fever, hot tubs, saunas, and tanning beds).

Complications of spina bifida include physical and neurologic impairments as well as hydrocephalus and meningitis. Children with spina bifida are usually of normal intelligence, but they may have learning problems because of the chronic nature of the condition.

Spina bifida occurs in three forms, each varying in severity (FIGURE 11-21):

- **Spina bifida occulta** is the mildest and most common form. It results in a small gap in one or more of the vertebrae. The spinal nerves and meninges do not usually protrude through the opening, so most children with this form have no clinical manifestations and experience no neurologic deficits. The defect may not be evident other than as a dimple, birthmark, or tuft of hair over the site.

- **Meningocele** is a rare form that involves the same bony defect as in spina bifida occulta, but the meninges protrude through the vertebral opening. The meninges and CSF form a sac on the surface of the infant's back. Transillumination (shining light through the tissue) can confirm the absence of nerve tissue in the sac. Because the spinal cord develops normally, neurologic impairment is usually not present, and these membranes can be removed by surgery with little or no damage to nerve pathways. However, infection or rupture of the sac can lead to neurologic impairment.

- **Myelomeningocele**, also known as open spina bifida, is the most severe form. In this variant, the spinal canal remains open along several vertebrae in the lower or middle back. The meninges, spinal cord, spinal nerves, and CSF protrude through this large opening at birth and form a sac on the infant's back (FIGURE 11-22). Skin covers the sac in some cases. However, tissues and nerves are exposed in most cases, making the infant vulnerable to life-threatening infections. Neurologic impairment (often including paralysis), bowel and bladder

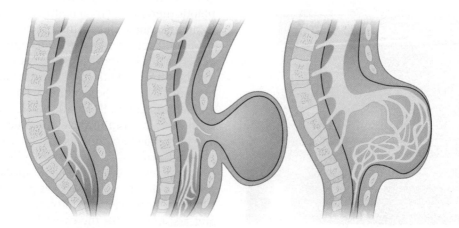

Spina bifida occulta   Meningocele   Myelomeningocele

FIGURE 11-21 Most common types of spina bifida.

M.S. is a 26-year-old woman pregnant who is with her first child. Her husband accompanied her to all her prenatal visits. An ultrasound during a routine visit at 34 weeks' gestation revealed that the baby had hydrocephalus and a myelomeningocele. The parents were initially devastated but remained very excited about the birth of their first child. M.S. was scheduled for a cesarean section at 38 weeks' gestation, and the couple was anxious about their child's condition and care following birth.

M.S. delivered a baby boy by cesarean section; he was transferred to the pediatric intensive care unit. On admission to the nursery, the baby's vital signs and weight were within normal limits, but his head circumference was large. He had bulging fontanelles and a high-pitched cry. The nurse noted a saclike projection in the lumbar region of his spine.

1. Discuss the rationale for delivering the infant by cesarean section.
2. Discuss the significance of the infant's clinical manifestations.
3. Discuss the complications associated with myelomeningocele.

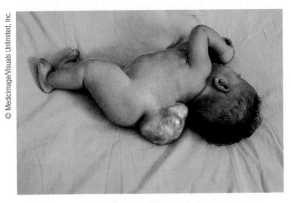

FIGURE 11-22 Myelomeningocele.

problems (e.g., incontinence, urinary tract infections, and constipation), seizures, and other medical complications (e.g., skin conditions and latex allergies) are common.

Clinical manifestations depend on the type and severity of spina bifida. Diagnostic procedures may be performed during pregnancy or after birth. These procedures may include a history, physical examination, check of maternal serum and amniotic fluid alpha-fetoprotein levels (high levels indicate a possible neural tube or other congenital defect), prenatal ultrasound, spinal X-ray, spinal CT, and spinal MRI.

Treatment strategies vary depending on the type and severity. For instance, spina bifida occulta often requires no treatment. Surgery is the mainstay of treatment for the other two types; however, the appropriate timing of the surgery (in utero, immediately after birth, or delayed) remains a topic of debate. Surgery usually includes replacing the meninges and closing the vertebral opening. A shunt may be placed during surgery to control hydrocephalus. Performing the surgical repair in utero may enhance outcomes but will not restore lost neurologic functioning. Additional risk may be incurred with this procedure, including premature delivery and death. If spina bifida is diagnosed before birth, cesarean delivery is preferred to prevent rupture of the sac or damage to any exposed nerves. Long-term support from a multidisciplinary team (e.g., a nurse, physical therapist, social worker, and an education specialist) will be necessary to limit complications and promote positive outcomes.

Cerebral Palsy

Cerebral palsy (CP) refers to a group of nonprogressive disorders that appear in infancy or early childhood and permanently affect motor movement and muscle coordination. In addition to motor dysfunction, other cerebral functioning may be affected (e.g., cognition and communication). CP usually results from damage to the cerebellum during the prenatal period (often during childbirth), but it can also occur at any time during the first 3 years of life, when the brain is developing. In addition, this disorder can occur because of brain abnormalities. In the United States, CP is the leading cause of childhood disability, affecting approximately 3–4 out of 1,000 births (CDC, 2016a). CP is more common in males, in African Americans, and in persons of lower socioeconomic status.

Although CP is not curable, the right treatment can make a significant impact on the child's prognosis. These therapies are costly, however. According to the CDC (2016a), the average lifetime costs (direct and indirect) for one person with CP are estimated to be $921,000 (in 2003 dollars). The estimated lifetime costs (direct and indirect) for all people with CP who were born in 2000 will total $11.5 billion (in 2003 dollars).

The following factors contribute to the development of CP:

- Prematurity
- Low birth weight
- Breech births (feet first rather than head first)
- Multiple fetuses
- Hypoxia
- Hypoglycemia (in either the mother or the child)
- Cerebral hemorrhage
- Neurologic infections (e.g., meningitis and encephalitis)
- Head injury
- Maternal infections during pregnancy (e.g., rubella and varicella)
- Maternal exposure to toxins during pregnancy (e.g., mercury)
- Severe jaundice

CP is classified according to the movement disorder involved, which reflects the area of the brain affected: spasticity (stiff muscles), dyskinesia (uncontrolled movements), or ataxia (poor balance and coordination). Spasticity is present in 80% of cases. In most patients, one or more movement disorders are present.

Clinical manifestations of CP may or may not be evident at birth. These manifestations vary from mild to severe in their effects. CP may affect the entire body (resulting in quadriplegia) or just one area (resulting in diplegia); it may affect one side or both sides of the body. Manifestations may include the following signs and symptoms:

- Persistence of early reflexes (e.g., Moro reflex)
- Developmental delays
- Ataxia
- Spasticity
- Flaccidity (weak, limp muscles)
- Hyperreflexia (exaggerated reflexes)
- Asymmetrical walking gait, with one foot or leg dragging
- Unusual positioning of limbs when resting or when held up (e.g., scissors position of the legs)
- Excessive drooling
- Difficulties swallowing, sucking, or speaking
- Facial grimaces
- Tremors
- Difficulty with precise motions (e.g., writing and buttoning a shirt)

Complications of CP result because of these clinical manifestations:

- Balance and coordination issues
- Contractures (shortening of a muscle causing severe limitation in movement)
- Scoliosis
- Malnutrition
- Communication issues and speech delays
- Learning or cognition difficulties
- Seizures (occur in approximately 50% of patients)
- Vision and hearing issues
- Urinary incontinence
- Constipation
- Osteoporosis
- Chronic pain
- Injury

Diagnostic procedures for CP include a history, physical examination, head CT, head MRI, and electroencephalogram (EEG) as well as hearing and vision screening. Treatment strategies focus on maximizing functioning and minimizing complications. Management is long term in nature and requires a multidisciplinary team (e.g., the primary care provider, nurses, a social worker, a physical therapist, an occupational therapist, a speech therapist, a dietitian, and education specialists). Therapeutic strategies often include the following measures:

- Muscle relaxants
- Botulinum toxin type A (Botox) injections directly into spastic muscles
- Antiseizure medications
- Pain management (e.g., massage therapy and analgesics)
- Physical therapy
- Occupational therapy
- Speech therapy
- Nutritional support
- Home safety (e.g., remove rugs)
- Braces and orthopedic devices (e.g., splints)
- Ambulation devices (e.g., walker and wheelchair)
- Constipation prevention (e.g., high-fiber diet, adequate water intake, and stool softeners)
- Glasses and hearing aids
- Surgical procedures to relieve contractures or to sever nerves of spastic muscles
- Support groups (especially for caregivers)
- Individualized education program

Infectious Neurologic Disorders

Nervous system infections can have serious effects by triggering the infectious and inflammatory response (see the *Immunity* chapter). These infections can be caused by a number of bacterial, viral, and fungal pathogens. Regardless of the causative agent, neurologic compromise (either temporary or permanent) can result. Early diagnosis and treatment is imperative for positive outcomes.

Meningitis

Meningitis refers to an inflammation of the meninges, usually resulting from an infection. The CSF may also become affected. Any number of bacteria (e.g., *Neisseria meningitidis*, *Streptococcus pneumoniae*, and *Haemophilus influenzae*) and viruses (most common; e.g., enterovirus, West Nile virus, influenza, HIV, and herpes) can cause this infection. These infectious agents invade the meninges through the blood or nearby structures or by direct access (e.g., wounds). Additional causes of meningitis include chemical irritants, tumors, fungi, parasites, and allergens. The infection or irritant triggers the inflammatory process, leading to swelling of the meninges and increased ICP.

Risk factors for developing meningitis include age younger than 25 years, living in a community setting (e.g., a college dormitory), pregnancy, working with animals, and immunodeficiency. Depending on the cause of the infection, meningitis can be self-limiting (as with viral meningitis) or life-threatening (as with acute bacterial meningitis). Complications of meningitis may include permanent neurologic damage, seizures, hearing loss, blindness, speech difficulties, learning disabilities, behavior problems, paralysis, acute renal failure, adrenal gland failure, cerebral edema, shock, and death.

Clinical manifestations of meningitis result from the inflammation of the meninges. Initially, these manifestations mimic those associated with an influenza infection (e.g., fever, chills, and malaise). The clinical manifestations, which usually arise suddenly, include the following signs and symptoms:

- Fever and chills
- Mental status changes (e.g., confusion and lethargy)
- Nausea and vomiting
- Photophobia
- Severe headache
- Stiff neck (meningismus)
- Agitation
- Bulging fontanelle
- Decreased consciousness
- Opisthotonos (abnormal positioning that involves rigidity and severe arching of the back with the head thrown backward)

- Poor feeding or irritability in children
- Tachypnea (increased breathing)
- Tachycardia (increased heart rate)
- Rash

Diagnostic procedures for meningitis include a history, physical examination, throat cultures, lumbar puncture with CSF analysis, polymerase chain reaction test, and head CT. Treatment varies depending on the underlying etiology. Strategies may include antibiotics (if the infection is bacterial in origin), antivirals (usually reserved for those cases caused by a herpes virus), hydration, and fever management. Additional strategies are geared toward managing complications as they develop (e.g., seizures, cerebral edema, and shock). Vaccinations, including those for *H. influenzae*, pneumococcal, and meningococcal infections, are the cornerstone of meningitis prevention.

Encephalitis

Encephalitis refers to an inflammation of the brain and spinal cord, usually resulting from an infection. A virus (e.g., coxsackievirus, echovirus, poliovirus, adenovirus, herpes virus, cytomegalovirus, Eastern equine encephalitis virus, West Nile virus, St. Louis virus, measles, or mumps) most frequently causes this infection. Viral exposure occurs through respiratory inhalation of droplets, ingestion of contaminated food or beverages, insect bites (especially mosquitoes and parasites), and skin contact. Encephalitis can also result from bacterial infections such as Lyme disease, tuberculosis, and syphilis. Noninfectious causes of encephalitis include allergic reactions (especially to vaccinations) and autoimmune conditions. The infection or other etiologic process triggers the inflammatory response, which causes vasodilation, increased capillary permeability, and leukocyte infiltration. This inflammatory process can cause nerve cell degeneration and diffuse brain destruction.

Encephalitis is classified as either primary or secondary. Primary encephalitis involves a direct infection of the brain and spinal cord. In secondary encephalitis, an infection first occurs elsewhere in the body and then travels to the brain.

Most cases of encephalitis are mild and self-limiting, but in rare cases this condition can be severe and life threatening. Those individuals who are particularly vulnerable to more severe progression of encephalitis include immunocompromised persons (e.g., those with AIDS), young children, older adults, persons living in high-incidence areas, and persons who are frequently outdoors. Complications of encephalitis include cerebral edema, cerebral hemorrhage, and brain damage.

Clinical manifestations of encephalitis result from the meningeal irritation and neurologic damage associated with the inflammatory response. These manifestations are similar to those noted in meningitis but have a more gradual onset. In most cases, clinical manifestations are mild and go undetected. When present, manifestations of encephalitis may include the following signs and symptoms:

- Flulike symptoms (e.g., fever, lethargy, and joint pain)
- Headache
- Neck rigidity
- Confusion and hallucinations
- Personality changes (e.g., flat affect, impaired judgment, and withdrawal from social interactions)
- Diplopia and photophobia
- Seizures
- Muscle weakness
- Ataxia
- Paresthesia or paralysis
- Loss of consciousness
- Tremors
- Abnormal deep tendon reflexes
- Rash
- Bulging fontanelle (in infants)

Diagnostic procedures for encephalitis include a history, physical examination, head CT, head MRI, EEG, lumbar puncture with CSF analysis, polymerase chain reaction test, and serum viral antibodies. Encephalitis is usually self-limiting, so treatment is largely supportive. Treatment strategies often include the following measures:

- Rest
- Adequate nutrition, including plenty of fluids
- Respiratory support (e.g., oxygen therapy or endotracheal intubation with mechanical ventilation) (for severe cases)
- Reorientation and emotional support
- Analgesics and antipyretics to relieve headaches and fever
- Antiviral agents (if viral)
- Antibiotic therapy (if bacterial)
- Corticosteroids to reduce cerebral edema
- Antiseizure agents
- Sedatives to treat irritability and restlessness
- Physical, speech, and occupational therapy as necessary for any residual neurologic dysfunction

Infection by many of the encephalitis-causative organisms can be prevented. Prevention strategies include vaccinations, wearing protective clothing when outside (e.g., long-sleeve shirts), using mosquito repellant, and eliminating water sources around the home (e.g., standing water in containers).

Zika Virus Disease

A growing worldwide health concern, **Zika virus disease** is a condition caused by a flavivirus that is transmitted primarily by mosquitos (Navalkele, Chandrasekar, & Levine, 2016). In 1952, this virus was first discovered in Uganda and the United Republic of Tanzania (World Health Organization [WHO], 2016). Since then, several outbreaks—usually involving a mild illness—have been recorded in Africa, the Americas, Asia, and the Pacific. In 2015, Brazil reported a large outbreak causing more severe neurologic complications. Within a short period of time, cases of Zika virus disease were noted in Florida (tracked to foreign travel to Zika-affected regions), and then the virus spread across the southeast United States. As of September 2016, nearly 3,000 cases of Zika had been diagnosed in the United States. Transmission of the infection in these cases has been attributed to foreign travel (most common), local mosquito spread, sexual transmission, and laboratory exposure (CDC, 2016d). In addition to being carried by mosquitos, the Zika virus can be transmitted from mother to fetus, through sexual contact, and via blood transfusions.

In most cases, Zika virus infection causes a mild, self-limiting illness. In fact, more than 80% of the cases go unnoticed. The incubation period is thought to be 3–12 days. Most individuals will not experience any manifestations, but even when they do, manifestations are usually mild. Manifestations may include the following signs and symptoms:

- Flulike symptoms (e.g., fever, lethargy, and joint pain)
- Rash
- Conjunctivitis
- Muscle pain
- Headache

In rare cases, complications of Zika infection can be severe. The most severe complications occur with maternal–fetal transmission, and may include miscarriage and microcephaly (FIGURE 11-23). Additionally, the Zika virus can cause Guillain-Barré syndrome.

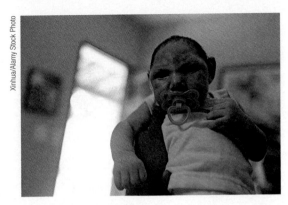

Xinhua/Alamy Stock Photo

FIGURE 11-23 Microcephaly.

Diagnostic procedures for Zika virus disease include a history, physical examination, and body fluid examination (e.g., blood, urine, saliva, and semen). Treatment is primarily supportive and includes rest, hydration, analgesics, and antipyretics. Prevention is paramount. It includes wearing protective covering, minimizing outdoor exposure, using an insect repellant containing DEET (*N,N*-diethyl-meta-toluamide), using condoms, and abstaining from sex while pregnant.

Traumatic Neurologic Disorders

Traumatic neurologic disorders vary significantly in severity and presentation depending on the location and extent of damage. Even minor injuries to the nervous system can have substantial effects on neurologic functioning. Traumatic injuries to the nervous system can result from a number of events that cause physical damage (e.g., motor vehicle accidents, gunshot wounds, and falls). Commonly, a number of these traumatic conditions overlap and occur concurrently (e.g., subdural hematoma and increased intracranial pressure).

Brain Injuries

A **traumatic brain injury (TBI)** is usually caused by a sudden and violent blow or jolt to the head (called a closed injury) or a penetrating head wound (known as an open injury) that disrupts the normal brain function. However, not all blows or jolts to the head result in a TBI. With such injuries, the brain collides with the skull (**FIGURE 11-24**) and any penetrating objects (**FIGURE 11-25**). These events can bruise the brain, damage nerve fibers, and cause hemorrhaging.

According to the CDC (2016c), the main causes of TBI are falls (41%), motor vehicle accidents (14%), penetration of an object (16%), and assaults (11%). TBIs range from mild (e.g., a brief change in mental status or consciousness) to severe (e.g., an extended period of unconsciousness or amnesia after the injury). Such injuries contribute to a substantial number of deaths and cases of permanent disability annually. According to the CDC (2016c), 2.5 million Americans sustain a TBI each year—50,000 of whom die from this cause. Persons at highest risk for experiencing a TBI include the following groups:

- Males (nearly three times as likely as females to have a TBI)
- Young children (0- to 4-year-olds) and 15- to 19-year-olds
- Adults 65 years of age or older
- Certain military personnel (e.g., paratroopers)
- African Americans (highest death rates)
- Individuals with a history of substance abuse

Many TBIs result in a wide range of long-term and potentially life-altering complications such as changes in thinking, sensation, language, or emotions. These injuries can increase the risk for seizures, migraine headaches, Alzheimer's disease, and Parkinson's disease. Multiple mild TBIs can have an accumulative effect and result in neurologic dysfunction, cognitive deficits, and death. This damage can be seen in a study of professional football players (Schwenk, Gorenflo, Dopp, & Hipple, 2007) and the growing body of evidence related to long-term effects of TBIs experienced by members of this group. These athletes, especially those who encounter routine impacts (e.g., linemen), have higher rates of cognitive deficits (e.g., memory impairment) and neurologic diseases (e.g., Alzheimer's disease, Parkinson's disease, and depression).

Closed TBIs often result in a variety of conditions. **Concussion** describes a momentary interruption of brain function. Concussions usually result from a mild blow to the head that causes sudden movement of the brain, disrupting neurologic functioning. They may or may not lead to a loss of consciousness. Amnesia, confusion, sleep disturbances, and headaches may follow a concussion for weeks or months. **Cerebral contusion** refers to a bruising of the brain accompanied by rupture of small blood vessels and edema. Most contusions result from a blunt blow to the head that causes the brain to make sudden impact with the skull. The initial area where the brain impacts the skull is

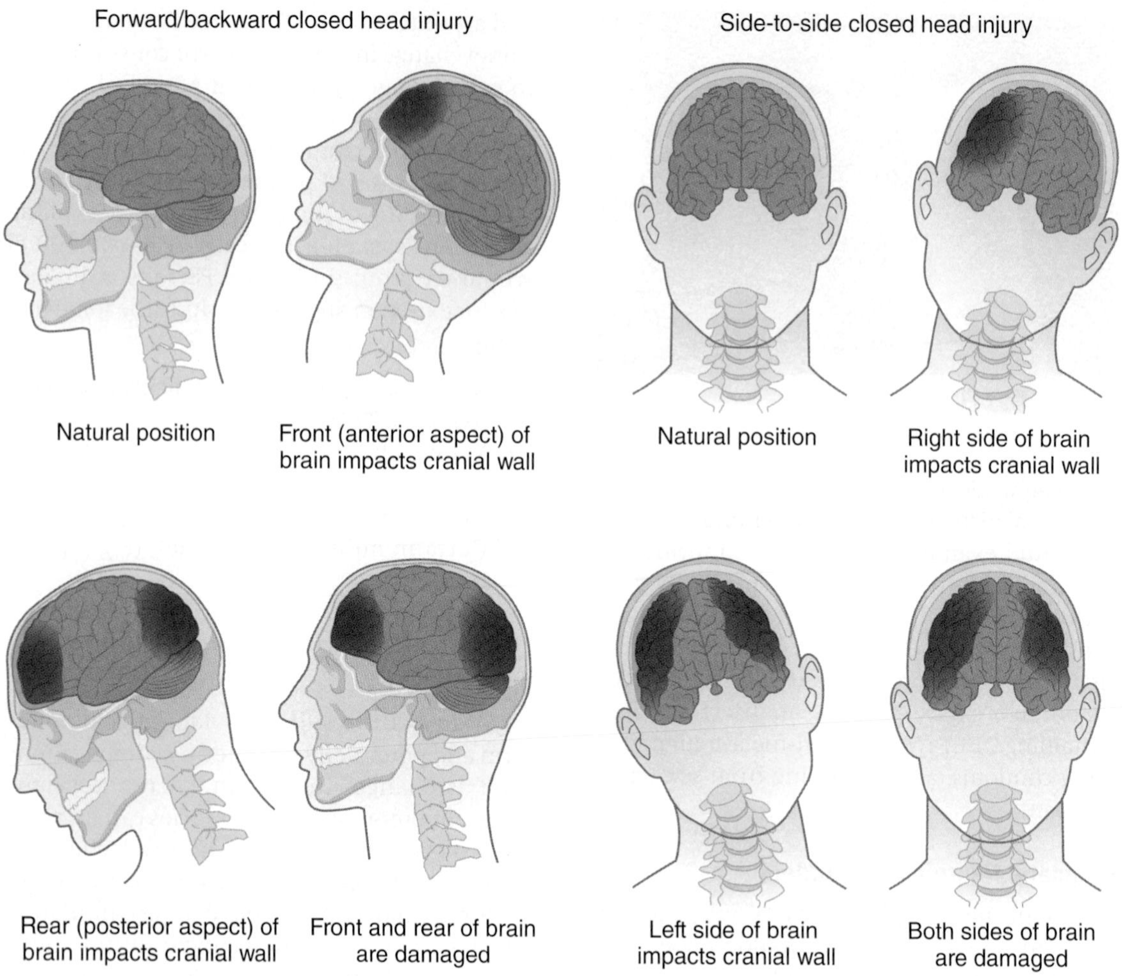

Forward/backward closed head injury

Side-to-side closed head injury

Natural position

Front (anterior aspect) of brain impacts cranial wall

Natural position

Right side of brain impacts cranial wall

Rear (posterior aspect) of brain impacts cranial wall

Front and rear of brain are damaged

Left side of brain impacts cranial wall

Both sides of brain are damaged

FIGURE 11-24 Closed traumatic brain injury.

referred to as the **coup**. The brain then rebounds and impacts the opposite side of the skull, causing another area of damage referred to as the **contrecoup** (Figure 11-24). Contusions vary in severity depending on the extent of damage and the amount of bleeding. The presence and severity of residual effects depend on these factors.

Open TBIs can result in serious issues. In addition to the tissue damage from the impact of the brain with the skull, such injuries can cause damage owing to the penetrating object and skull fragments. The skull fractures as the object breaches it. Much like when an egg is broken, the skull usually ends up in multiple pieces when it is struck by an external force. The resulting fracture may take the form of a **linear skull fracture** (a simple crack), a **comminuted skull fracture** (several fracture lines), a **compound skull fracture** (a fracture where the brain tissue is exposed), a **depressed skull fracture** (displacement of the bone fragments into the brain), or a **basilar skull fracture** (located at the base of the skull and usually accompanied by CSF leakage). In addition to the brain damage from impact and penetrating objects, open TBIs carry a higher risk for developing infections because they permit direct access to the brain by infectious organisms (see the *Immunity* chapter). As discussed in previous sections, infections of the nervous system can have serious consequences.

Clinical manifestations of TBIs may be vague and develop slowly, or they may be sudden and severe. Symptoms may improve and then suddenly worsen. The outward appearance of the head is not an indication of the injury severity—serious injuries can occur even while the skin and the skull remain intact. When a TBI is suspected, the individual should be asked to give an account of the accident. Not being able to recall details is an indication

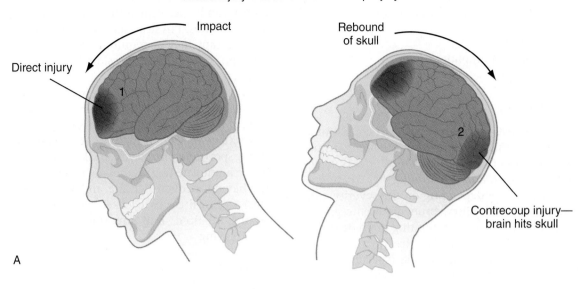

Closed injury—direct and contrecoup injury

Impact

Rebound of skull

Direct injury

1

2

Contrecoup injury—
brain hits skull

A

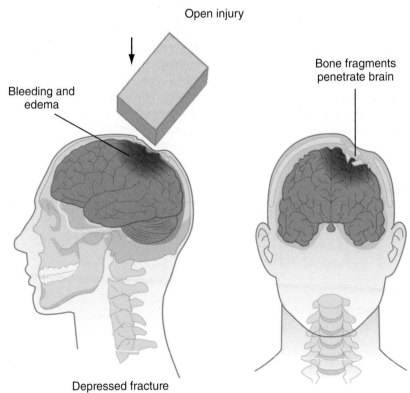

Open injury

Bone fragments
penetrate brain

Bleeding and
edema

B   Depressed fracture

FIGURE 11-25 Comparison of closed and open traumatic brain injury.

of a TBI. Additional clinical manifestations may include the following signs and symptoms:

- Indications of a concussion (e.g., amnesia, confusion, and headache)
- Changes in or unequal size of pupils
- Seizures
- Asymmetrical facial features

- Fluid draining from the nose, mouth, or ears (may be clear or bloody; likely CSF)
- Fracture in the skull or face, bruising of the face, swelling at the site of the injury, or scalp wound
- Impaired hearing, smell, taste, speech, or vision
- Inability to move one or more limbs
- Irritability (especially in children), personality changes, or unusual behavior

- Loss of consciousness
- Bradypnea (slowed breathing)
- Hypotension
- Restlessness
- Lack of coordination
- Lethargy
- Stiff neck
- Vomiting

Diagnostic procedures for TBI consist of a history, physical examination (including using the Glasgow Coma Scale [FIGURE 11-26]), head CT, head MRI, and ICP monitoring. Treatment strategies vary depending on the severity and the time since injury. Immediate emergency care for TBI focuses on limiting brain damage. Mild injuries usually require no treatment other than rest and analgesics (specifically acetaminophen [Tylenol]) if headache is present. Nonsteroidal anti-inflammatory drugs (NSAIDs), such as aspirin and ibuprofen (Motrin), should be avoided because they can increase bleeding risk. Cold compresses can be applied to any outward edema. Severe brain injuries usually require hospitalization, and patients with such damage often need intensive care. Osmotic diuretics (e.g., mannitol) may be given to reduce cerebral edema. Additionally,

antiseizure agents and sedatives may be needed. Surgery can be performed to remove blood or repair fractures. Physical, speech, and occupational therapy may be required after the acute injury phase to minimize residual neurologic dysfunction.

Prevention strategies for TBIs include wearing a seat belt when driving or riding in a motor vehicle, using appropriate child safety seats, wearing a helmet when appropriate (e.g., when playing sports, riding a bicycle, or skating), making the home safe (e.g., removing tripping hazards, having adequate lighting, and using safety gates), storing firearms in locked cabinets, never driving impaired, and supervising children when playing.

Increased Intracranial Pressure

Increased intracranial pressure describes increased volume in the limited space of the cranial cavity. Increased ICP may occur because of a TBI as well as other conditions that would increase the volume in the skull (e.g., tumor, hydrocephalus, cerebral edema, and hemorrhage). The delicate pressure–volume relationship among ICP; volume of CSF, blood, and brain tissue; and cerebral perfusion is explained by the

Parameter	Score	Response
Eye opening	Spontaneous	4
	To voice	3
	To pain	2
	No response	1
Best verbal response	Oriented, converses	5
	Disoriented, converses	4
	Inappropriate words	3
	Incomprehensible sounds	2
	No response or intubated	1
Best motor response	Follows commands	6
	Localizes response (pushes away stimulus)	5
	Withdraws	4
	Abnormal flexion (decorticate)	3
	Abnormal extension (decerebrate)	2
	No response	1

FIGURE 11-26 Glasgow Coma Scale.

Monro-Kellie hypothesis (FIGURE 11-27). The Monro-Kellie hypothesis states that the cranial cavity cannot be compressed, and the volume inside the cavity is fixed (normal ICP is 60–200 mm H_2O or 4–15 mm Hg). The skull and its components (blood, CSF, and brain tissue) create a state of volume equilibrium, such that any increase in the volume of one component must be compensated by a decrease in the volume of another component. This compensation is primarily accomplished by shifts in the CSF and, to a lesser extent, blood volume. These fluids respond to increases in the volume of the remaining components. For example, an area of bleeding into the brain tissue (e.g., epidural hematoma) will be compensated for by the downward displacement of CSF and venous blood. Transient increases in ICP routinely occur with position changes, coughing, or sneezing. These compensatory mechanisms are able to maintain a normal ICP for changes in volume up to a point (approximately 100–120 mL of volume increases).

In addition to shifting volumes, the brain has two other compensatory mechanisms to maintain tissue perfusion—autoregulation and Cushing's reflex. With **autoregulation**, the blood vessels dilate to increase blood flow and constrict if the ICP is increased. **Cushing's reflex** is a complex cascade of events that results in increased blood pressure. When the mean arterial pressure (average blood pressure) drops below the ICP, the hypothalamus increases sympathetic stimulation. This stimulation causes vasoconstriction, increased cardiac contractility, and increased cardiac output. If unresolved, the increased ICP eventually leads to a trio of effects known as **Cushing's triad**—increased blood pressure, bradycardia, and changes in respiratory pattern (FIGURE 11-28).

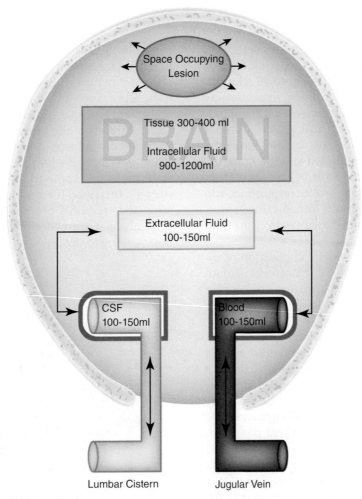

FIGURE 11-27 Monro-Kellie hypothesis.

Reproduced from Leffert, L.R., & Schwamm, L.H. (2013). Neuraxial anesthesia in parturients with intracranial pathology: A comprehensive review and reassessment of risk. *Anesthesiology, 119,* 703–718. http://anesthesiology.pubs.asahq.org/journal.aspx

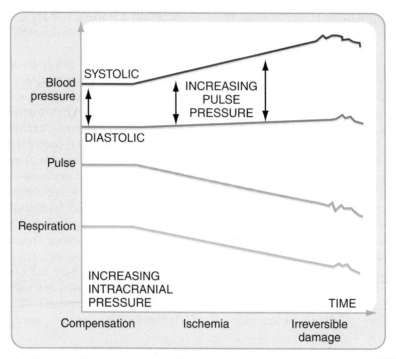

FIGURE 11-28 Vital sign changes with increased intracranial pressure.

Baroreceptors in the carotid arteries detect the increase in blood pressure, triggering a parasympathetic response through vagal stimulation that induces bradycardia. Bradycardia may also be stimulated by the increased ICP impinging on the vagal nerve, causing a parasympathetic response. As pressure increases inside the skull, space becomes limited and the brain tissue shifts downward. An irregular respiratory pattern, called Cheyne-Stokes respiration, and bradypnea typically result from increased pressure on the brain stem due to swelling, or from brain stem herniation.

Herniation—a feared complication of increased ICP—involves the displacement of brain tissue. Several types of herniation are possible (FIGURE 11-29). In transtentorial (central) herniation, the cerebral hemispheres, diencephalon, and midbrain are displaced downward. The pressure created by this type of herniation impairs the cerebral blood flow, CSF, reticular activation system, and respirations. Uncal (uncinate) herniation occurs when the uncus (the hooklike anterior end of the hippocampal gyrus) of the temporal lobe shifts downward past the tentorium cerebelli (the extension of the dura mater that separates the cerebellum from the inferior portion of the occipital lobes). This type of herniation creates pressure on cranial nerve III, the posterior cerebral artery, and the reticular activation system. Cerebellar, or tonsillar (intrafratentorial), herniation occurs when the cerebellar tonsils (the rounded lobules on the undersurface of each cerebellar hemisphere) are pushed downward through the foramen magnum. This type of herniation compresses the brain stem and vital centers, causing death.

Regardless of the cause, increased ICP past the point of compensation compresses cerebral blood vessels and other structures as well as shifts the brain's contents. Eventually, brain tissue dies. Increased ICP is a life-threatening situation that requires prompt treatment. If left unresolved, it causes declining neurologic function, leading to death.

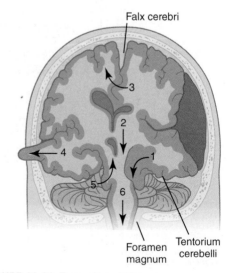

FIGURE 11-29 Types of herniation.

The clinical manifestations of increased ICP vary depending on the patient's age and reflect the effects of the rising pressures:

- Decreasing level of consciousness (results from pressure on the brain stem and cerebral cortex)
- Vomiting, often projectile (results from pressure on the medulla)
- Increasing blood pressure with increasing pulse pressure (the difference between systolic and diastolic pressure) (results from Cushing's reflex)
- Bradycardia (response to the increasing blood pressure)
- Papilledema (results from increased pressure exerted by CSF, which causes swelling around the optic disk)
- Fixed and dilated pupils (results from pressure on cranial nerve III)
- Posturing (FIGURE 11-30)

Two manifestations of increased ICP are unique to infants:

- Separated sutures
- Bulging fontanelle

Manifestations in older children and adults include the following symptoms:

- Behavior changes
- Severe headache (results from stretching of the dura and walls of the large blood vessels)
- Lethargy
- Neurologic deficits
- Seizures

Diagnostic procedures for increased ICP consist of a history, physical examination (including completing the Glasgow Coma Scale), head CT, head MRI, and ICP monitoring. Increased ICP requires prompt diagnosis and treatment for optimal patient outcomes. Treatment strategies vary depending on the underlying etiology, and attempts should be made to resolve the source of the increased pressure if possible (e.g., remove the tumor or blood). Additional strategies are similar to those for TBIs and may include respiratory support (e.g., oxygen therapy or endotracheal intubation with mechanical ventilation), semi-Fowler's positioning, draining excess CSF, osmotic diuretics, corticosteroids, seizure precautions (e.g., low lighting and minimal stimulation), antiseizure agents, sedatives, stool softeners (because straining increases ICP), antiulcer agents (for those patients at high risk for stress ulcers), thermoregulation, and glucose management. Rarely, surgical removal of a skull segment may be performed.

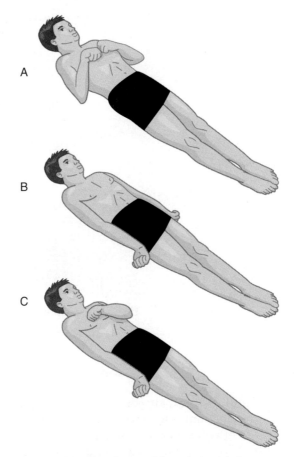

FIGURE 11-30 Decorticate and decerebrate posturing. (a) Decorticate response: flexion of the arms, wrists, and fingers with adduction in the upper extremities; extension, internal rotation, and plantar flexion in the lower extremities. (b) Decerebrate response: all four extremities in rigid extension with hyperpronation of the forearms and plantar extension of the feet. (c) Decorticate response on the left side of the body and decerebrate response on the right side of the body.

Hematomas

Secondary brain damage can be caused by additional injurious factors such as hemorrhaging. A **hematoma** is a collection of blood in the tissue that develops from ruptured blood vessels. Hematomas, which can develop immediately or slowly because of a TBI or surgery, are classified by their location (FIGURE 11-31).

- **Epidural hematomas** result from bleeding between the dura and skull, usually caused by an arterial tear. Clinical manifestations of epidural hematomas include marked neurologic dysfunction that usually develops within a few hours of injury. The typical symptom pattern of an epidural hematoma is a brief loss of consciousness, followed by a short period of alertness, then loss of consciousness again. This pattern may not appear in all people.

TYPES OF INTRACRANIAL HEMATOMAS

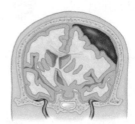

A   Subdural

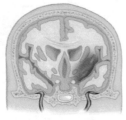

B   Intracerebral

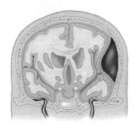

C   Epidural

FIGURE 11-31 Types of hematomas. (a) Beneath the dura but outside the brain (subdural hematoma). (b) Within the substance of the brain tissue (intracerebral hematoma). (c) Outside the dura and under the skull (epidural hematoma).

- **Subdural hematomas** develop between the dura and the arachnoid, and are frequently caused by a small venous tear (**FIGURE 11-32**). Because they are the result of a venous tear, these types of hematomas generally develop slowly. Subdural hematomas follow several patterns. With acute subdural hematomas, manifestations of neurologic deficits present within 24 hours of an injury. This type of hematoma progresses rapidly and has a high mortality. With subacute subdural hematomas, ICP increases over a period of about a week after the injury. With chronic subdural hematomas, manifestations develop several weeks after the injury because of a slow leak. Chronic subdural hematomas are more common in elderly adults because of the brain atrophy that occurs with age, which gives the hematoma more space to develop.
- **Intracerebral hematomas** result from bleeding in the brain tissue itself. These types of hematomas are caused by contusion or shearing injuries, but can also result from hypertension, cerebral vascular accidents (strokes), aneurysms, or vascular abnormalities.
- A **subarachnoid hemorrhage** results from bleeding in the space between the arachnoid and the pia. Its primary clinical presentation is a severe headache that has a sudden onset and is worse near the back of the head.

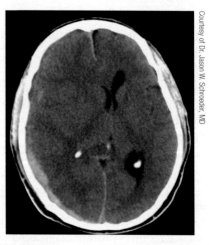

Courtesy of Dr. Jason W. Schroeder, MD

FIGURE 11-32 Midline shift associated with right-sided subdural hematoma.

In all types of hematomas, the bleeding leads to localized pressure on nearby tissue and increases ICP. Blood may coagulate and form a solid mass. The hematoma becomes encapsulated by fibroblasts, and blood cells within the capsule lyse. The fluid from the hemolysis exerts osmotic pressure, drawing more fluid into the capsule. This edema increases the size of the mass, applying pressure on the surrounding tissue and increasing ICP. Bleeding can trigger vasospasms, worsening ischemia. Additionally, increasing ICP can result in herniation.

Diagnostic procedures for all types of hematomas and hemorrhaging consist of a history, physical examination (including completing the Glasgow Coma Scale), head CT, head MRI, cerebral angiogram, and intracranial pressure monitor. Treatment strategies depend on the location and bleeding severity. No treatment may be required in mild cases in which the volume is small and the bleeding has ceased. For many patients, surgical removal of the blood through a burr hole or a craniotomy is required. In some cases, however, removal of the blood may not be possible. In these situations, patients may experience significant residual neurologic deficits that require physical, speech, and occupational therapy. Additionally, strategies similar to those used for TBIs and increased ICP (e.g., respiratory management, seizure precautions, and thermoregulation) may be required.

Learning Points

Immediately following a head injury, some key actions should be avoided:

- Do *not* apply direct pressure to a bleeding site; cover the wound with sterile gauze.
- Do *not* wash a head wound that is deep or bleeding profusely.
- Do *not* remove any object sticking out of a wound.
- Do *not* move the person unless it is absolutely necessary.
- Do *not* shake the person if he or she seems dazed.
- Do *not* remove a helmet if you suspect a serious head injury.
- Do *not* pick up a fallen child with any sign of a head injury.
- Do *not* drink alcohol within 48 hours of a serious head injury.

Spinal Cord Injuries

Spinal cord injuries (SCIs) result from direct injury to the spinal cord or indirectly from damage to surrounding bones, tissues, or blood vessels. SCIs are often caused by motor vehicle accidents, falls, violence, and sports injuries. Minor injuries to the spinal cord can occur because of weakening vertebral structures (e.g., rheumatoid arthritis or osteoporosis). Direct damage can occur if the spinal cord is pulled, pressed sideways, or compressed (FIGURE 11-33). Such damage may occur, for example, if the head, neck, or back twists abnormally during an accident or injury. As this result of such an injury, hemorrhage, fluid accumulation, and edema can occur inside or outside the spinal cord (but within the spinal canal). The accumulation of blood or fluid can compress the spinal cord and damage it. **Spinal shock** refers to a temporary suppression of

neurologic function because of spinal cord compression. In spinal shock, neurologic function gradually returns.

SCIs are most common in Caucasians and in males (National Spinal Cord Injury Statistical Center, 2016). The average age for experiencing SCI has increased from 29 years in the 1970s to 42 years today.

SCIs result in a significant loss of neurologic functioning, often requiring extensive, long-term management. SCIs can also result in death, either immediately or because of complications (e.g., pneumonia, embolism, or septicemia). The degree of dysfunction depends on the severity of the injury and its location (Figure 11-16). The injury may result in a partial or complete disruption of the neurons and neural tracts anywhere along the spinal cord. SCIs are classified based on the location of damage (e.g., C4, T12) and the degree of function lost. An injury to one of the eight cervical segments of the spinal cord causes **quadriplegia** (tetraplegia)—loss of all or most function in all four limbs. Injury to the thoracic, lumbar, or sacral regions causes **paraplegia**—loss of lower extremity function. The individual may experience complete **paralysis** (no voluntary use of the affected limbs) or incomplete paralysis (some voluntary use of the affected limbs). Incomplete quadriplegia is the most frequently occurring injury, accounting for approximately 30% of SCIs. The spinal cord does not extend beyond the first lumbar vertebra, so injuries at and below this level do not cause SCIs. However, they may cause **cauda equina syndrome** (injury to the nerve roots in the area of the cauda equina).

Complications of SCIs are numerous and can contribute to the mortality associated with SCIs:

- **Autonomic hyperreflexia** (a massive sympathetic response that can cause headaches, hypertension, tachycardia, seizures, stroke, and death; most commonly associated with injuries above T6 and triggered by noxious stimuli)
- Neurogenic shock (an abnormal vasomotor response secondary to disruption of sympathetic impulses)
- Respiratory failure (caused by paralysis of the respiratory muscles)
- Effects of immobility (e.g., constipation, pulmonary infections, urinary infections, thrombus, impaired skin integrity, and contractures)

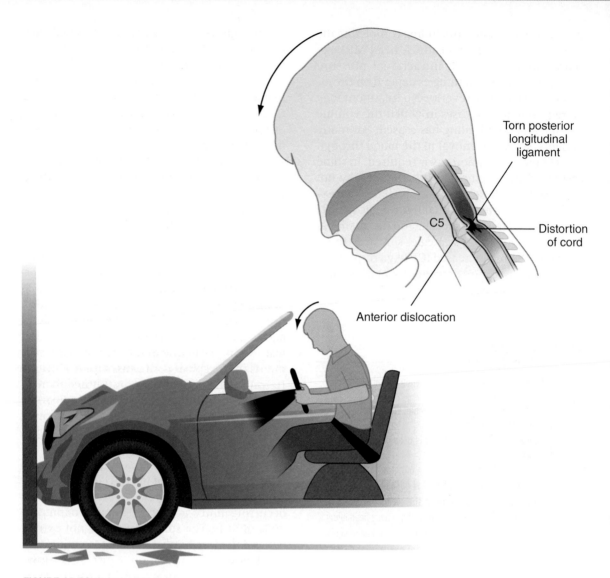

Torn posterior
longitudinal
ligament

Distortion
of cord

C5

Anterior dislocation

FIGURE 11-33 Spinal cord injuries.

- Changes in bowel and bladder function (e.g., urinary retention, incontinence, and constipation)
- Sexual dysfunction (e.g., erectile dysfunction)
- Chronic pain

Clinical manifestations of SCIs depend on the level of injury. Cervical injuries can affect both the upper and lower extremities. Manifestations of such injuries include the following symptoms:

- Breathing difficulties resulting from paralysis of the respiratory muscles
- Loss of normal bowel and bladder control (e.g., constipation, incontinence, and bladder spasms)
- Paresthesia
- Sensory changes

- Spasticity
- Pain
- Weakness or paralysis
- Blood pressure instability
- Temperature fluctuations
- Diaphoresis

Thoracic injuries affect the lower extremities, and the symptoms can be similar to those for cervical injuries. Lumbar sacral injuries can affect the lower extremities in varying degrees. Manifestations of lumbar sacral injuries are similar to those of cervical injuries, with the exception of breathing difficulties.

Diagnostic procedures for SCIs consist of a history, physical examination (including a neurologic assessment), spinal CT, spinal MRI, spinal X-ray, somatosensory evoked potential testing or magnetic stimulation, and spinal myelogram (X-ray using contrast dye). These injuries are always medical emergencies requiring immediate treatment. Therapeutic strategies include both immediate interventions to minimize residual effects and long-term interventions to limit complications. Immediate strategies may include the following measures:

- Immobilization of the spine
- Corticosteroid agents to reduce swelling
- Spinal traction to reduce fractures and immobilize the spine
- Surgical repair of vertebral fractures or surgical removal of the fluid compressing the spinal cord (decompression laminectomy)
- Respiratory management (e.g., oxygen therapy and endotracheal intubation with mechanical ventilation)
- Bed rest

Long-term strategies may include the following interventions:

- Physical, occupational, and speech therapy
- Mobility assistive devices (e.g., a wheelchair, walking assistance system)
- Electronic devices (e.g., brain–computer interface, functional electronic stimulation systems, and electronic aids for daily living)
- Long-term respiratory management (e.g., mechanical ventilation)
- Meticulous skin care
- Bowel and bladder training or management (e.g., catheterization and stool softeners)
- Antispasmotic agents and botulinum toxin type A (Botox) injections to treat muscle spasms
- Pain management
- Nutritional support
- Prompt treatment of infections (pneumonia is the leading cause of death)

Vascular Neurologic Disorders

Vascular neurologic disorders generally involve ischemic injuries to the brain resulting from occlusion of blood flow or hemorrhage. These disorders vary significantly in their severity and presentation depending on the location and extent of damage. Often they result in some degree of neurologic dysfunction. These conditions may occur due to congenital abnormalities or chronic diseases such as hypertension, hypercholesterolemia, and atherosclerosis.

Transient Ischemic Attack

A **transient ischemic attack (TIA)** is a temporary episode of cerebral ischemia that results in symptoms of neurologic deficits. TIAs are often called ministrokes because these neurologic deficits mimic a cerebral vascular accident (CVA) or stroke except that the deficits resolve within 24 hours (1–2 hours in most cases). TIAs may occur singly or in a series. They serve as warning signs that a CVA may be impending; approximately 1 in 3 people who experiences a TIA will eventually have a stroke, with about half of these CVAs occurring within one year of the TIA. However, not all CVAs are preceded by a TIA.

This type of ischemia can occur because of a cerebral artery occlusion (e.g., thrombus, embolus, or plaque), cerebral arterial narrowing (e.g., atherosclerosis or spasms), or cerebral artery injury (e.g., inflammation or hypertension). Additional risk factors for TIAs include migraines, smoking, diabetes mellitus, advancing age, inadequate nutrition, hypercholesterolemia, oral contraceptive usage, excessive alcohol consumption, and illicit drug use. Complications of TIAs include permanent brain damage from the lack of oxygen and glucose, injury from falls, and CVA from the ischemia.

Clinical manifestations of TIAs begin suddenly and last for a short period. Within 24 hours, symptoms disappear completely. Although TIAs are not strokes, they have the same manifestations as CVAs. These manifestations reflect the location of the ischemia and may include the following symptoms:

- Muscle weakness or paralysis of the face, arm, or leg (usually unilateral)
- Paresthesia on one side of the body
- Aphasia (difficulty speaking) or receptive aphasia (difficulty understanding spoken language)
- Dysphagia (difficulty swallowing)
- Dysgraphia (difficulty writing)
- Difficulty reading
- Vision issues (e.g., diplopia, nystagmus, and partial or complete loss of vision)
- Changes in sensation (e.g., touch, pain, temperature, pressure, hearing, and taste)
- Change in levels of consciousness (e.g., lethargy, unconscious, or coma)
- Personality, mood, or emotional changes
- Confusion
- Agnosia (inability to recognize or identify sensory stimuli)
- Ataxia
- Vertigo (abnormal sensation of movement) or dizziness
- Bowel or bladder incontinence

Because these clinical manifestations often resolve prior to the patient reaching a healthcare facility, diagnosis may be made based on a history alone. Additional diagnostic procedures consist of a physical examination (including a neurologic assessment and blood pressure), head CT, head computed tomography angiography (CTA), head MRI, head magnetic resonance angiography (MRA), carotid ultrasound, cerebral arteriogram, EEG, serum clotting studies, blood chemistry, complete blood count (CBC), erythrocyte sedimentation rate test (can identify inflammatory process), and serum lipids test.

Treatment strategies for TIAs focus on preventing the occurrence of a CVA. These strategies typically include managing any underlying conditions (e.g., hypertension, atherosclerosis, and diabetes mellitus). Medications, such as antiplatelet aggregation agents (e.g., aspirin and clopidogrel [Plavix]) or anticoagulants (e.g., warfarin [Coumadin]), may be used to prevent clotting. Angioplasty (balloon dilation) can be undertaken to open narrowed arteries, or a carotid endarterectomy (surgical removal of plaque) may be performed to increase cerebral blood flow. Lifestyle management includes smoking cessation, minimizing dietary cholesterol and fat, increasing dietary fruits and vegetables, exercising regularly, limiting alcohol consumption, and eliminating illicit drug use.

Cerebral Vascular Accident

Much like a TIA, a **cerebral vascular accident (CVA)**, or stroke, refers to an interruption of cerebral blood supply (FIGURE 11-34). The chief difference between a CVA and a TIA is that CVA damage is permanent. A CVA is an infarction of the brain, so it is often referred to as a brain attack. This kind of interruption in the brain's blood flow may result from a total vessel occlusion (e.g., thrombus, embolus, or plaque) or cerebral vessel rupture (e.g., cerebral aneurysm, arteriovenous malformation, or hypertension). Thus there are two major types of CVA—ischemic and hemorrhagic. **Ischemic strokes** are the most common (87%), but **hemorrhagic strokes** are the most deadly. Even five minutes (sometimes less) of altered tissue perfusion can lead to irreversible cell damage from the lack of oxygen and glucose. CVA can result in significant neurologic dysfunction and death; in fact, it is the chief cause of long-term disability and fifth leading cause of death in the United States (CDC, 2015d).

CVA incidence and mortality rates are highest in the southeastern United States, often referred to as the "Stroke Belt." In the United States, someone experiences a CVA every 40 seconds and dies from a CVA every 4 minutes. The costs associated with this widespread problem and its extensive consequences are estimated at $34 billion annually in the United States (CDC, 2015d). In this country, CVA prevalence and mortality are highest among African Americans. Additional risk factors include physical inactivity, obesity, hypertension, smoking, hypercholesterolemia, diabetes mellitus, atherosclerosis, oral contraceptive usage, excessive alcohol consumption, and illicit drug use.

Clinical manifestations of CVA are similar to those of a TIA, except that CVA symptoms do not resolve in the same way as TIA symptoms. TIA symptoms disappear in less than 24 hours; in contrast, CVA manifestations may improve with time and therapy, but they may also persist, creating complications. In addition to the manifestations of neurologic impairment associated with TIAs, headaches may be present with hemorrhagic strokes because of increasing ICP.

Diagnostic procedures for CVA consist of a history, physical examination (including a neurologic assessment), head CT, head MRI, carotid ultrasound, cerebral arteriogram, serum clotting studies, blood chemistry, and CBC. A CVA is a medical emergency that requires prompt treatment to minimize brain damage. Determining whether the CVA is ischemic or hemorrhagic in origin prior to treatment is crucial because the interventions vary depending on the type. Additionally, some interventions for ischemic strokes can worsen hemorrhagic strokes (e.g., thrombolytic agents). The differential diagnosis should be made as soon as possible because early treatment will improve outcomes. Optimally, treatment should be delivered within 3 hours of symptom onset; therefore, persons or family

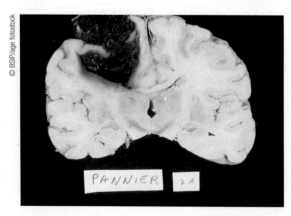

© BSIP/age fotostock

FIGURE 11-34 Cerebral vascular accident (CVA), or stroke.

Anna Bryant, an 88-year-old Caucasian female, is brought to the emergency room by her daughter, Pat. Ms. Bryant complains of right-sided weakness, a severe headache, and not feeling well for the last couple of days. Upon assessment, she is alert, but has trouble answering questions. Her speech is slurred, and she appears frightened.

1. Which additional clinical manifestations would the nurse expect to find if Ms. Bryant's symptoms have been caused by a stroke?

A. A carotid bruit
B. Hypotension
C. Increased deep tendon reflexes
D. Decreased bowel sounds

2. While assessing Ms. Bryant every 15 minutes, which of the following findings warrants immediate action?

A. Glasgow Coma Scale score increasing from 11 to 14
B. Bilateral grip strength is unequal
C. Responding only to painful stimuli
D. Negative Babinski's reflex

3. Due to her deteriorating condition, Ms. Bryant is immediately referred to the neurologist. This patient has likely suffered a left-sided brain attack. Which clinical manifestation further supports this conclusion?

A. Visual field deficit on the left side
B. Spatial-perceptual deficits
C. Paresthesia of the left side
D. Global aphasia

members of persons who seem to be experiencing a CVA should make note of when the symptoms began.

Ischemic strokes are treated with thrombolytic agents (to dissolve any clots) and aspirin (to limit platelet activity). This treatment is contraindicated in persons with a recent history of bleeding issues. Additionally, procedures such as angioplasty or carotid endarterectomy may be necessary in patients with ischemic strokes. Surgical repair of aneurysms or arteriovenous malformations as well as blood removal may be required in patients with hemorrhagic strokes. Corticosteroids may also be administered with either type of CVA to reduce cerebral edema, and antihypertensive agents may be used cautiously to reduce blood pressure. A multidisciplinary approach (using a team consisting of a nurse, physical therapist, speech therapist, occupational therapist, dietitian, and social worker) should be initiated as soon as the patient is stable and may be required on a long-term basis to minimize or prevent complications. Depending on the degree of dysfunction, strategies may be necessary to prevent complications of immobility (e.g., constipation, impaired skin integrity, contractures, and infections).

Cerebral Aneurysm

A **cerebral aneurysm** is a localized outpouching of a cerebral artery (see the *Cardiovascular Function* chapter). This weakening of the artery may occur as a congenital defect, or it may develop later in life because of conditions such as hypertension, connective tissue disease (e.g., Marfan syndrome), TBI, and arterial wall infection (FIGURE 11-35; FIGURE 11-36). The bulging artery segment can put pressure on surrounding tissue. Additionally, the aneurysm may leak or rupture, causing a CVA or death. Several types of aneurysms are possible, but most cerebral aneurysms are berry or saccular forms. Cerebral

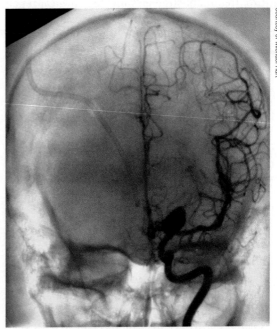

FIGURE 11-35 Cerebral aneurysm.

Courtesy of Michael Hart

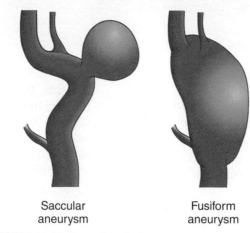

Saccular   Fusiform
aneurysm   aneurysm

FIGURE 11-36 Types of cerebral aneurysms.

aneurysms most frequently occur as multiple aneurysms on the circle of Willis.

Many cerebral aneurysms remain asymptomatic until they grow large enough to compress surrounding structures or they rupture. Clinical manifestations that may appear as the aneurysm compresses nearby structures include vision issues (e.g., diplopia and loss of vision), headache, eye pain, or neck pain. A sudden, severe headache is an indication that the aneurysm has ruptured. Additional manifestations resemble those associated with increased ICP and CVA.

Often diagnosis occurs inadvertently with a head CT or MRI. Additional diagnostic procedures include a history, physical examination, cerebral arteriography, and EEG. If discovered prior to rupture, treatment strategies include surgical repair (if possible) and managing contributing factors (e.g., hypertension). Rupture is a medical emergency that requires immediate surgical repair. Additional strategies are similar to those for a CVA and subarachnoid hemorrhage.

Seizure Disorders

A **seizure** is a transient physical or behavior alteration that results from abnormal electrical activity in the brain. Mechanisms that may be responsible for this abnormal electrical activity include altered membrane ion channels, altered extracellular electrolytes, and imbalances in excitatory and inhibitory neurotransmitters. Some neurons are hypersensitive or remain in a partial state of depolarization, increasing excitability. Trauma, hypoglycemia, electrolyte disorders, acidosis, infection, tumors, and chemical ingestion (e.g., medications, illicit drugs, and alcohol) can all provoke isolated seizure activity. Additionally, seizures can occur as a disorder referred to as **epilepsy**.

Epilepsy results from spontaneous firing of abnormal neurons and is characterized by recurrent seizures for which there is no underlying or correctable cause. According to the CDC (2016b), epilepsy affects approximately 2.9 million Americans. Complications of seizures may include brain damage, TBIs, aspiration, mood disorders, and **status epilepticus** (seizures that last longer than 20 minutes or subsequent seizures that occur before the individual has fully regained consciousness).

Seizures can be classified into two broad categories—focal and generalized. **Focal seizures**, also called partial seizures, occur in just one part of the brain. Approximately 60% of people with epilepsy have focal seizures. These seizures vary depending on the area of the brain affected, and they are frequently described by the area of the brain in which they originate (**FIGURE 11-37**). In a simple focal seizure, the individual having the seizure remains conscious but experiences unusual feelings or sensations that can take many forms. The person may experience sudden and unexplainable feelings of joy, anger, sadness, or nausea. Additionally, he or she may hear, smell, taste, see, or feel things that are not real. In a complex focal seizure, the individual has changes in or loss of consciousness and memory, producing a dreamlike experience. People having a complex focal seizure may display strange, repetitious behaviors (e.g., blinking, twitching, moving one's mouth, walking in a circle) called **automatisms**. These seizures usually last just a few seconds. Some people with focal seizures, especially complex focal seizures, experience **auras** (unusual sensations just prior to an impending seizure). An aura is actually a simple focal seizure in which the person maintains consciousness. The symptoms an individual has and the progression of those symptoms tend to be similar with every seizure. Because the symptoms of focal seizures can easily be confused with other disorders (e.g., migraine headaches, narcolepsy, syncope, and psychiatric disorders), those disorders should be ruled out as part of the differential diagnosis.

Generalized seizures are a result of abnormal neuronal activity on both sides of the brain. These seizures may cause loss of consciousness, falls, or massive muscle spasms. Many kinds of generalized seizures are possible. A person having an absence seizure (previously called a petit mal seizure) may appear to be staring into space and/or have jerking or twitching muscles (**FIGURE 11-38**). These seizures usually are brief,

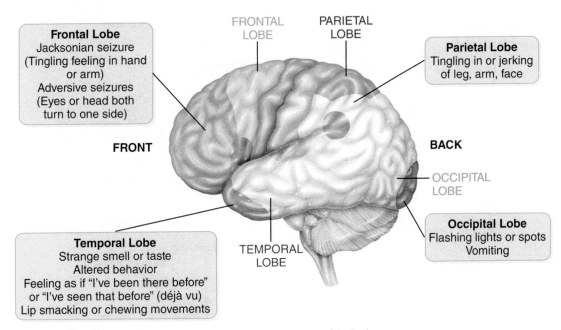

Frontal Lobe
Jacksonian seizure
(Tingling feeling in hand
or arm)
Adversive seizures
(Eyes or head both
turn to one side)

FRONTAL LOBE

PARIETAL LOBE

Parietal Lobe
Tingling in or jerking
of leg, arm, face

FRONT

BACK

OCCIPITAL LOBE

Occipital Lobe
Flashing lights or spots
Vomiting

Temporal Lobe
Strange smell or taste
Altered behavior
Feeling as if "I've been there before"
or "I've seen that before" (déjà vu)
Lip smacking or chewing movements

TEMPORAL LOBE

FIGURE 11-37 Manifestations of focal seizures depending on the region of the brain.

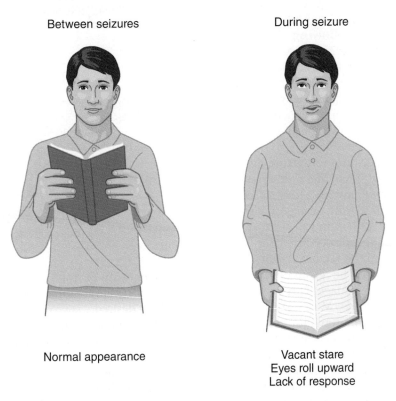

Between seizures

During seizure

Normal appearance

Vacant stare
Eyes roll upward
Lack of response

FIGURE 11-38 Absence seizures.

lasting less than 15 seconds. Tonic seizures cause stiffening of muscles of the body, generally those in the back and extremities. Clonic seizures cause repeated jerking movements of muscles on both sides of the body. Myoclonic seizures cause jerks or twitches of the upper body, arms, or legs (FIGURE 11-39). Atonic seizures cause a loss of normal muscle tone, such that the affected person will fall down or may drop his or her head involuntarily. Tonic–clonic seizures (previously called grand mal seizures) cause a mixture of symptoms, including stiffening of the body and repeated jerks of the arms and/or legs as well as loss of consciousness (FIGURE 11-40).

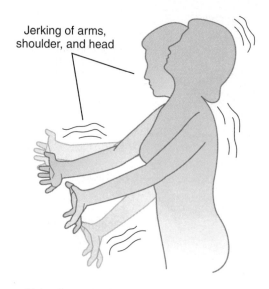

Jerking of arms, shoulder, and head

Episodes typically occur soon after awakening

FIGURE 11-39 Myoclonic seizures.

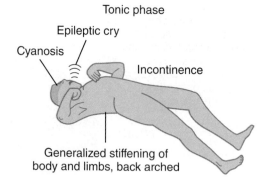

Tonic phase

Epileptic cry

Cyanosis

Incontinence

Generalized stiffening of body and limbs, back arched

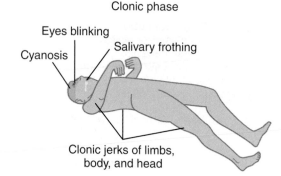

Clonic phase

Eyes blinking

Salivary frothing

Cyanosis

Clonic jerks of limbs, body, and head

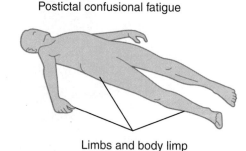

Postictal confusional fatigue

Limbs and body limp

FIGURE 11-40 Tonic–clonic seizures.

The individual having a generalized seizure may be confused, be fatigued, and fall into a deep sleep in the period following the seizure, referred to as the **postictal period**.

Not all seizures can be easily defined as either focal or generalized. Some people have seizures that begin as focal seizures but then spread to the entire brain. Other people may have both types of seizures but with no clear pattern.

Diagnostic procedures for seizure disorders consist of a history (including a description of the seizure activity if possible), physical examination, head CT, head MRI, head positron emission tomography (PET), and EEG. Treatment focuses on preventing the occurrence and limiting the duration of the seizure activity. Treatment strategies can be grouped into two categories—those to manage acute seizures and those to prevent seizures. Most seizures resolve spontaneously within a few minutes, but employing safety precautions can prevent injury. During a seizure, positioning the individual on his or her side can prevent aspiration (vomiting is common). Additionally, the head should be protected. Items should not be forced in between the individual's teeth; doing so is more likely to cause harm than to help. Attempts should not be made to restrain the individual; this also is more likely to cause injury. Airway management and oxygen therapy may be necessary to minimize hypoxia. If status epilepticus develops, medication (e.g., muscle relaxants or antiseizure agents) will often be administered intravenously to stop the seizure. Following a seizure, the individual should be allowed to sleep as desired.

For epilepsy, antiseizure agents will be administered daily to minimize the frequency and duration of seizure activity. These medications require close monitoring and accurate administration to ensure therapeutic dosing and limit side effects. If medications are not successful in controlling seizure activity, surgical resection or transaction of the region in which the abnormal electrical activity originates might be necessary. Additionally, persons with seizure disorders should wear a medical alert bracelet and avoid precipitating factors (e.g., sleep deprivation, alcohol, illicit drugs, and excessive stimuli).

Chronic Degenerative Disorders

Chronic degenerative disorders of the nervous system include those conditions in which neurologic function deteriorates over time. These conditions usually result in significant neurologic dysfunction that requires lifelong management. Such disorders are not usually preventable, and often treatment options are limited.

Multiple Sclerosis

Multiple sclerosis (MS) is a debilitating autoimmune condition that involves a progressive and irreversible demyelination of brain, spinal cord, and cranial nerve neurons as a result of inflammation. This damage occurs in diffuse patches throughout the nervous system and slows or stops nerve impulses. As the disease progresses, the brain's cortex atrophies and scar tissue (plaques) develops throughout the white matter (FIGURE 11-41). The progression of this damage varies from person to person. As is true with most autoimmune disorders, the underlying cause of MS is unknown.

According to the National Institutes of Health (NIH, 2016c), approximately 300,000 Americans have MS. The prevalence rates are the highest among women, Caucasians, and persons living in temperate climates. MS is the most common disabling neurologic disease among young adults, often presenting in persons between 20 and 40 years of age. Some evidence suggests that smoking increases risk, whereas increased sun exposure may decrease risk.

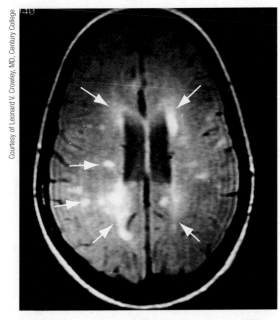

FIGURE 11-41 Multiple sclerosis demonstrated by MRI.

The course of MS is unpredictable. Some patients will have a mild course with little to no disability, whereas others will experience a steady deterioration with increasing disability. Clinical manifestations of MS vary depending on the degree of damage and the specific nerves affected; however, the disease is typically characterized by remissions and exacerbations. Exacerbations may last for days to months. Fever, hot baths, sun exposure, and stress can trigger or worsen these episodes. Although remissions and exacerbations are common, the disease may continue to progress in some individuals without remissions. Clinical manifestations include the following symptoms:

- Fatigue
- Ataxia
- Muscle spasms
- Paresthesia or abnormal sensation in any area
- Difficulty moving arms or legs
- Weakness in one or more arms or legs
- Unsteady gait
- Lack of coordination
- Tremor in one or more arms or legs
- Constipation and stool leakage
- Urinary frequency, urgency, hesitancy, or incontinence
- Vision issues (e.g., diplopia and vision loss)
- Decreased attention span, poor judgment, and memory loss
- Difficulty reasoning and solving problems
- Dizziness
- Hearing loss
- Sexual dysfunction
- Slurred speech
- Dysphagia

Some patients may experience transverse myelitis, a condition caused by inflammation of the spinal cord that causes a loss of cord functioning that can last several hours to several weeks. Transverse myelitis usually begins as a sudden onset of lower back pain, muscle weakness, or paresthesia of the toes and feet, and can rapidly progress to more severe symptoms, including paralysis. In most cases of transverse myelitis, people recover at least some function within the first 12 weeks after an attack begins. Transverse myelitis is also associated with neuromyelitis optica, a type of optic nerve inflammation. Other complications of MS include epilepsy, paralysis (most often the legs), and depression.

There is no definitive test for MS, which can delay diagnosis of this condition. Diagnostic procedures for MS may consist of a history, physical examination (including a neurologic assessment), MRI studies (brain and spinal cord), lumbar puncture with CSF analysis (this often shows high levels of protein, gamma globulin, and lymphocytes), nerve conduction studies, and autoimmune testing (e.g., erythrocyte sedimentation rate, antimyelin titers, and antinuclear antibody).

No cure for MS exists, but treatment can often slow its progression. Treatment strategies focus on minimizing symptoms and maximizing quality of life. These strategies include medications such as corticosteroids (treat exacerbations), interferons (slow damage), plasmapheresis (used for unresponsive exacerbations), disease-modifying agents, and immunomodulators (suppress immune response). Other medications may be used to manage symptoms (e.g., antispasmodics, cholinergics, laxatives, and antidepressants). Additionally, physical and occupational therapy, along with assistive devices (e.g., wheelchairs, walkers, and handrails), can maximize functioning. Coping strategies, support, proper nutrition, and adequate rest can promote and maintain overall health.

Parkinson's Disease

Parkinson's disease is a progressive condition involving the destruction of the substantia nigra in the brain. This destruction results in a lack of dopamine, a chemical messenger that allows smooth, coordinated muscle movement. When approximately 80% of the dopamine-producing cells are destroyed, movement issues develop—which typically include tremors (involuntary shaking) of the hands and head. These tremors may disappear or decrease when the body part is moved intentionally. Recent evidence suggests that norepinephrine-producing cells may also be destroyed, explaining the issues with blood pressure regulation noted in Parkinson's disease. Additionally, Lewy bodies (unusual deposits of the alpha-synuclein protein) have been identified in many cases, but their role in the disease is not yet understood. The cause of Parkinson's disease is unknown, but genetic vulnerability that has been activated by an environmental trigger (e.g., a virus) is thought to be a strong possibility.

According to the NIH (2016d), approximately 50,000 Americans are diagnosed with Parkinson's disease each year. Parkinson's disease is the most common nervous system disorder of the elderly. For unknown reasons, prevalence rates are twice as high in men as in women, and some evidence suggests that rates are higher in persons living in rural areas.

Clinical manifestations of Parkinson's disease vary depending on the degree of dopamine deficit. These manifestations often include the following signs and symptoms (FIGURE 11-42):

- Slowing or stopping of automatic movements (e.g., blinking)
- Constipation
- Dysphagia
- Drooling
- Unsteady gait
- Masklike appearance to face
- Myalgia
- Problems with movement, including the following:
  - Difficulty initiating or continuing movement (e.g., walking or getting out of a chair)
  - Loss of fine hand movements (writing may become small and difficult to read; eating can become more difficult)
  - Shuffling gait
  - Bradykinesia (slowed movements)
  - Rigid or stiff muscles (often beginning in the legs)
- Tremors
  - Usually occur in the limbs at rest or when the arm or leg is held out
  - Stop during purposeful movement

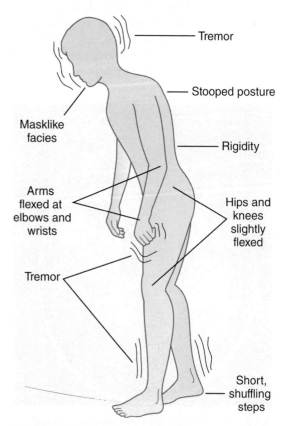

FIGURE 11-42 Clinical presentation of Parkinson's disease.

- Eventually, can be seen in the head, lips, tongue, and feet
- May be worse when the affected individual is tired, excited, or stressed
- Finger-thumb rubbing (called "pill-rolling" tremor) may be present
- Slowed, quieter speech with monotone voice
- Stooped position
- Anxiety, stress, and tension
- Confusion
- Dementia
- Depression
- Syncope
- Hallucinations
- Memory loss
- Seborrhea (oily skin)
- Orthostatic hypotension

Much like MS, Parkinson's disease does not have a definitive test available for its diagnosis. Diagnostic procedures consist of a history, physical examination (including neurologic assessment), and other tests to rule out other conditions.

There is no cure for Parkinson's disease; instead, the goal of treatment is to control symptoms. Medications (e.g., levodopa, dopamine agonists, and monoamine oxidase B [MAO-B] inhibitors) can increase the levels of dopamine, but the effects of the medications often diminish over time, requiring increased doses to maintain effectiveness. Medications may eventually reach maximum dosing, and symptom control will be lost. Deep brain stimulation is a common surgical treatment for Parkinson's disease. Additionally, physical and occupational therapy, along with assistive devices (e.g., wheelchairs, walkers, and handrails), can maximize functioning. Coping strategies, support, proper nutrition, and adequate rest can promote and maintain overall health.

Amyotrophic Lateral Sclerosis

Amyotrophic lateral sclerosis (ALS)—also called Lou Gehrig's disease, after the famous baseball player who died from this condition—is a disease that involves damage to the upper motor neurons of the cerebral cortex and lower motor neurons of the brain stem and spinal cord (FIGURE 11-43). Sensory neurons, cognitive function, and cranial nerves III, IV, and VI are not affected. The nerves lose their ability to trigger muscle movement, resulting in muscle weakness, disability, paralysis, and eventually death (usually within 3 years of onset of symptoms). ALS may also increase the risk for dementia. In most cases,

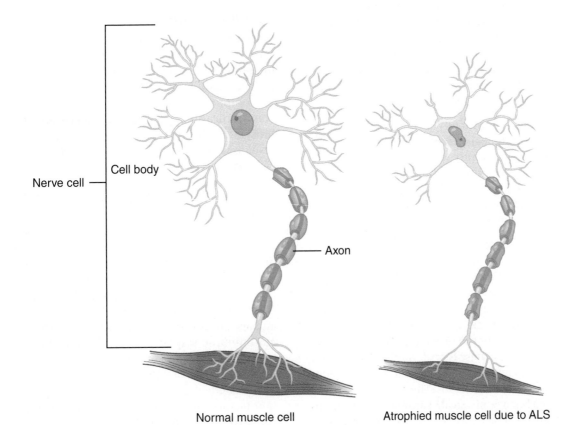

FIGURE 11-43 Effects of amyotrophic lateral sclerosis.

the cause of ALS is undetermined, but genetics plays a role in 10% of cases.

Researchers are exploring several possible etiologies of ALS. The first possible cause is free radical damage (see the *Cellular Function* chapter). The inherited form of ALS often involves a mutation in a gene responsible for producing a strong antioxidant enzyme that protects cells from damage caused by free radicals. The second possible cause being explored is glutamate's influence. People who have ALS typically have higher than normal levels of glutamate, a chemical messenger in the brain, in their CSF. Too much glutamate is toxic to some nerve cells. Finally, possible autoimmune responses are being studied as a possible trigger for ALS.

The exact number of cases in the United States is unknown, but the NIH (2016a) estimates that 12,000 Americans have ALS. Although this condition is not necessarily common, it is a public concern because there is no way to prevent the continuous and rapid decline in motor function. In 2010, a National ALS registry was launched to collect, manage, and analyze data about people with ALS. This registry is intended to provide information that will illuminate the scope and epidemiology of the problem as well as guide practice and research.

Clinical manifestations of ALS become progressively worse as more motor neurons are damaged. The loss of upper motor neurons results in spastic paralysis and hyperreflexia, and the loss of lower motor neurons results in flaccid paralysis. Early manifestations of ALS include the following symptoms:

- Footdrop (difficulty lifting the front of the foot and toes)
- Lower-extremity weakness
- Hand weakness or clumsiness
- Slurred speech or dysphagia
- Muscle cramps and twitching in the upper extremities and the tongue

The disease frequently begins in the upper or lower extremities and then spreads to other parts of the body. As it advances, muscles become progressively weaker until they are paralyzed. ALS eventually affects chewing, swallowing, speaking, and breathing.

As is true for the other degenerative neurologic disorders, there is no definitive test for ALS. Instead, diagnostic procedures are often used to rule out other conditions. These procedures consist of a history, physical examination (including a neurologic assessment), electromyogram (in which an electrode is inserted into the muscles to measure electrical activity), nerve conduction studies, MRI studies (head and spinal cord), lumbar puncture with CSF analysis, and muscle biopsy.

ALS has no cure. Treatment strategies focus on slowing the progression and controlling symptoms. Riluzole (Rilutek), a benzothiazole, is the only medication approved by the Food and Drug Administration for slowing ALS. This drug appears to slow the disease's progression in some people, perhaps by reducing levels of glutamate. Additionally, stem cell therapy is being explored as a possible treatment. Antispasmodic agents may be given to treat muscle spasms. Physical, occupational, and speech therapy, along with assistive devices (e.g., wheelchairs and braces), can maximize muscle function. Because of risk for aspiration and dysphagia, nutritional support including high-caloric foods, soft or pureed foods, thickened liquids, and parenteral feedings becomes critical to maintaining optimal health as the patient's muscles weaken. Respiratory management (e.g., oxygen therapy, pulmonary hygiene, respiratory treatments, and mechanical ventilation) also becomes necessary as muscle weakness progresses. Coping strategies and support for the patient and caregivers can be helpful as the condition worsens.

Myasthenia Gravis

Myasthenia gravis is an autoimmune condition in which acetylcholine receptors are impaired or destroyed by immunoglobulin G (IgG) autoantibodies. This acetylcholine receptor compromise leads to a disruption of normal communication between the nerve and the muscle at the neuromuscular junction. The result is weakness of the voluntary skeletal muscles because of inadequate nerve stimulation. Muscle weakness typically increases during periods of activity and improves after periods of rest. Muscles that control eye and eyelid movement, facial expression, chewing, talking, and swallowing are often, but not always, involved in the disorder. Muscles that control breathing and neck and limb movements may also be affected.

Myasthenia gravis is common (2–3 cases per 10,000 people) and affects all gender, ethnic, and age groups equally. The exact trigger for the autoimmune response is unclear, but the thymus gland is thought to play a role. Persons with myasthenia gravis often have a thymus gland abnormality (e.g., hyperplasia and tumors). Certain factors can worsen myasthenia gravis and cause **myasthenic crisis**, including fatigue, illness, stress, extreme heat, alcohol consumption, and certain medications (e.g., beta blockers, calcium-channel blockers, quinine, and some antibiotics). Myasthenic crisis is a potentially life-threatening complication, which occurs when the muscles become too weak to maintain adequate ventilation.

Clinical manifestations of myasthenia gravis reflect the muscle weakness that is characteristic of this disease:

- Breathing difficulty
- Dysphagia
- Difficulty climbing stairs, lifting objects, or rising from a seated position
- Dysarthria
- Drooping head
- Facial paralysis or weakness
- Fatigue
- Hoarseness or changing voice
- Eye and vision issues (e.g., diplopia, ptosis, blurred vision, and difficulty maintaining gaze)

Diagnosis of myasthenia gravis is primarily made based on the clinical presentation. Diagnostic procedures consist of a history, physical examination (including a neurologic assessment), edrophonium test (a short-acting anticholinesterase inhibitor called edrophonium is injected, and a sudden, albeit temporary, improvement in muscle strength indicates possible myasthenia gravis), serum antibody levels, nerve conduction study, electromyogram, thymus CT or MRI, and autoimmune testing (e.g., erythrocyte sedimentation rate, acetylcholine receptor antibodies, and antinuclear antibody).

There is no cure for myasthenia gravis, but treatment strategies can be employed to manage its symptoms. Medications used to treat this disorder include anticholinesterase agents, which improve neuromuscular transmission and increase muscle strength. Immunosuppressive drugs may improve muscle strength by suppressing the production of abnormal antibodies. Other therapies include thymectomy, plasmapheresis (removal of abnormal antibodies from the blood), and high doses of immunoglobulins. Additional self-care strategies to maximize health and functioning include proper nutrition, adequate rest, assistive devices, coping strategies, and support.

Huntington's Disease

Huntington's disease (HD), or Huntington's chorea, is a condition caused by a genetically programmed degeneration of neurons in the brain. HD is an autosomal dominant disorder (see the *Cellular Function* chapter) involving a defect on chromosome 4. This defect causes a segment of DNA, called a CAG repeat, to occur many more times than usual. Normally, this section of DNA is repeated 10–35 times within the DNA coding sequence, but it is repeated 36–120 times in persons with HD. This defect leads to progressive atrophy of the brain, particularly in the basal ganglia and the frontal cortex (FIGURE 11-44). The ventricles dilate, gamma-aminobutyric acid levels diminish, and acetylcholine levels fall. As the gene is transmitted from one generation to the next, the number of repeats (called CAG repeat expansion) tends to increase. With a larger number of repeats, the chance of developing symptoms at an earlier age increases. As the disease is transmitted in families, it becomes evident at younger and younger ages. The earlier HD symptoms appear, the faster the disease progresses. Most cases of HD appear in persons between 30 and 40 years of age, but HD may appear in childhood or adolescence in a small number of cases. In general, the duration of the illness ranges from 10 to 30 years. The most common causes of death for persons with HD are infection (most often pneumonia), injuries related to a fall, or other complications (e.g., suicide).

According to the NIH (2016b), more than 15,000 Americans have HD. At least 150,000 others have a 50% risk of developing the disease, and thousands more of their family members live with the possibility of developing HD.

Clinical manifestations of HD reflect the cerebral atrophy caused by neural degeneration. Initially, manifestations are insidious and vary from person to person. Family members may first notice that the individual experiences mood swings or becomes uncharacteristically irritable, apathetic, passive, depressed, or angry. Other behavioral symptoms may include antisocial behavior, hallucinations, paranoia, and psychosis. These symptoms may lessen as the disease progresses or, in some individuals, may persist and

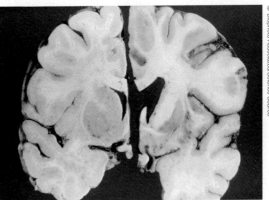

FIGURE 11-44 Neurologic changes of Huntington's disease.

expand to include aggression or severe depression. HD may produce dementia as the individual's judgment, memory, and other cognitive functions become affected. Early signs often include having trouble driving, learning new things, remembering facts, answering questions, or making decisions. Some people may even display changes in handwriting. As the disease progresses, concentration on intellectual tasks becomes increasingly difficult.

In some people, the disease may initially manifest with uncontrolled, rapid, jerky movements (**chorea**, Greek for "dance")—for example, tremors, grimaces, and twitching—in the fingers, feet, face, or trunk. These movements often intensify when the person is anxious. HD can also begin with mild clumsiness, unsteady gait, and rigidity. Some people develop chorea manifestations later, after the disease has progressed. Chorea often creates serious problems with ambulation, increasing the likelihood of falls. As the disease progresses, speech becomes slurred and other functions (e.g., swallowing, eating, speaking, and walking) continue to decline. Many people with HD remain aware of their environment and are able to express emotions, but some cannot recognize their family members.

Because of its psychological manifestations, HD is often mistaken for various psychiatric disorders. Diagnostic procedures for this disease include a history, physical examination, psychiatric evaluation, genetic testing for the defective gene (either before or after the onset of symptoms), head CT, head MRI, and head PET.

There is no cure for HD, and no treatment to stop its progression. Treatment strategies focus on slowing the progression and managing symptoms to maximize functioning. Tetrabenazine (Xenazine) is the first medication specifically approved by the Food and Drug Administration for the treatment of HD signs and symptoms. This agent reduces the jerky, involuntary movements associated with HD by increasing the amount of dopamine available in the brain. Tranquilizers and antipsychotic agents can control movements, violent outbursts, and hallucinations. Antidepressant agents can control depression and the obsessive–compulsive rituals that some people with HD develop. Some evidence suggests that coenzyme Q10 may also slow the course of the disease. Physical, occupational, and speech therapy can maximize function. Coping strategies, support, adequate hydration, proper nutrition, and regular exercise for both the patient and caregivers can support optimal health. New therapies are currently under investigation, including stem cell therapy, new medications, and new combinations of existing medications.

Dementia

Dementia refers to a group of conditions in which cortical function is decreased, impairing cognitive skills (e.g., language, logical thinking, judgment, and learning) and motor coordination. Issues with memory are common with dementia and include short-term memory losses as well as confusion of historical events. Behavioral and personality changes may interfere with relationships, work, and activities of daily living. Vascular disease (e.g., atherosclerosis), infections, toxins, and genetic conditions may cause dementia.

Several types of dementia have been identified, each of which has only limited treatment options. Although great strides have been made in recent years, most types of dementia remain poorly understood.

Alzheimer's Disease

Alzheimer's disease (AD) is the most common form of dementia among older adults. In AD, healthy brain tissue degenerates and atrophies (**FIGURE 11-45**). This atrophy causes a steady decline in memory and mental abilities. The exact etiology of AD is unknown, but three pathologic characteristics are associated with AD. First, amyloid plaques, which contain fragments of a protein called beta-amyloid peptide, mix with a collection of additional proteins, neuron remnants, and other nerve cell pieces. Second, neurofibrillary tangles, found inside neurons, form as abnormal collections of a protein called tau. Normal tau is required for healthy neurons; however, in AD, tau clumps together. As a result, neurons fail to function normally and eventually die. Third, connections among the neurons responsible for memory and learning are lost. Neurons cannot survive when their connections to other neurons are lost. As neurons die throughout the brain, the affected regions begin to atrophy, or shrink. By the final stage of AD, damage is widespread and brain tissue has shrunk significantly.

Although AD is not a part of normal aging, risk for developing this disease does increase with age (onset usually occurs after 60 years of age). Prevalence rates are higher in women, in part because of their longer life expectancy relative to men. Some evidence suggests that AD rates are higher in those persons with less education, but the precise reason for this association remains unknown. Some researchers

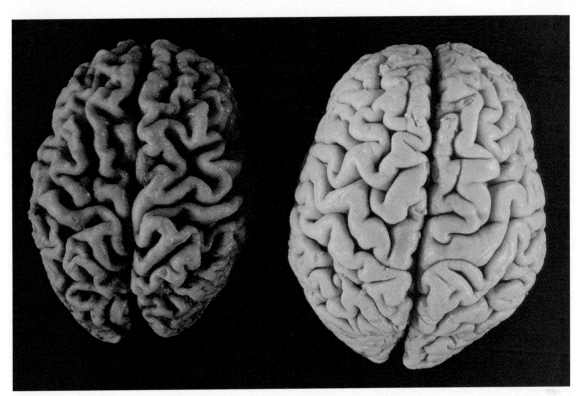

FIGURE 11-45 Alzheimer's disease (left) compared to a normal brain (right).

Courtesy of Michael Hart

theorize that the more the brain is used, the more synapses are created, which provides a greater reserve with aging. Additional risk factors include family history, hypertension, hypercholesterolemia, diabetes mellitus, and history of TBI. According to the CDC (2015a), as many as 5 million Americans have AD; this prevalence is double the prevalence in 1980. AD has recently surpassed diabetes mellitus as the sixth leading cause of death among U.S. adults. Notably, mortality rates for AD are on the rise—unlike heart disease and cancer death rates, which continue to decline. Complications such as infections (primarily pneumonia and urinary tract infections), injuries related to falls, malnutrition, dehydration, and decubitus ulcers contribute to the mortality associated with AD.

The onset of AD tends to be insidious. Clinical manifestations may start with mild memory loss and confusion, but AD eventually leads to irreversible mental impairment that destroys a person's ability to remember, reason, learn, and imagine. This course may extend 10–20 years. Clinical manifestations may include the following symptoms:

- Memory loss (e.g., the person might repeat things, forget conversations or appointments, misplace things, and eventually forget the names of family members and everyday objects)

- Problems with abstract thinking (e.g., trouble balancing a checkbook, a problem that progresses to trouble recognizing and dealing with numbers)
- Difficulty finding the right word to express thoughts or even follow conversations
- Difficulty reading and writing
- Disorientation, even in familiar surroundings
- Loss of judgment (e.g., not knowing what to do if food on the stove is burning)
- Difficulty performing familiar tasks (e.g., driving, cooking, bathing, dressing, and eating)
- Personality changes (e.g., mood swings, paranoia, stubbornness, withdrawal, depression, anxiety, and aggression)
- Hallucinations
- Bowel or bladder incontinence

Diagnosis of AD is often difficult and involves ruling out other conditions. Diagnostic procedures consist of a history, physical examination (including a neurologic assessment and mental status evaluation), head CT, head MRI, and head PET.

There is no cure for AD, nor are there any therapies that will slow its progression. Medications can, however, manage symptoms and maximize functioning. Cholinesterase inhibitors (e.g., donepezil [Aricept], rivastigmine [Exelon], and galantamine [Razadyne]) can improve neurotransmitter levels in the brain in some cases.

Memantine (Namenda) is specifically approved to treat AD. It blocks *N*-methyl-D-aspartic acid receptors, which are glutamate receptors. Memantine may be given in combination with a cholinesterase inhibitor. Other medications may be given to control aggression. Alternative therapies that may improve symptoms include vitamin B₆, vitamin B₁₂, vitamin E, ginkgo, and Huperzine A, although the research evidence is mixed regarding their efficacy. Other strategies may include memory aids (e.g., calendars), nutritional support, physical exercise, cognitive activities, safety precautions (e.g., supervision and removing clutter), maintaining a calm environment, and social interactions (e.g., adult day care). Coping strategies and support for both the patient and the caregiver can decrease stress and anxiety.

Creutzfeldt-Jakob Disease

Creutzfeldt-Jakob disease (CJD) is a rare, but rapidly progressive form of dementia caused by an infectious prion. A **prion** is an abnormal protein particle that causes proteins to fold abnormally, especially in nervous tissue. The prion renders the protein dysfunctional, creating plaques and vacuoles (empty spaces) (FIGURE 11-46).

CJD may be classified into two types (classic and variant) and three main categories (sporadic, hereditary, and acquired). Although also caused by a prion, classic CJD is *not* related to bovine spongiform encephalopathy (commonly known as mad cow disease). However, the new variant *is* related to bovine spongiform encephalopathy. The most common form of classic CJD occurs sporadically, caused by the spontaneous transformation of normal prion proteins into abnormal prions. This sporadic disease occurs worldwide, including in the United States, at an annual rate of approximately 1 case per 1 million people (CDC, 2015b). Hereditary CJD is rare and occurs when the

abnormal protein is inherited. Finally, acquired CJD is rare (accounting for fewer than 1% of cases worldwide) and occurs when the individual is exposed to infected materials (e.g., via tissue transplants and ingestion). The prion is resistant to common methods of sterilization and disinfection.

CJD has a long incubation period (up to 40 years) after being introduced into the brain; however, it is rapidly progressing and always fatal (usually within 1 year of onset). Clinical manifestations develop rapidly and include the following symptoms:

* Blurred vision
* Ataxia
* Hallucinations
* Lack of coordination
* Muscle twitching
* Myoclonic jerks or seizures
* Spasticity
* Anxiety
* Personality changes
* Profound confusion or disorientation
* Lethargy
* Speech impairment

Diagnostic procedures for CJD consist of a history, physical examination (including a neurologic assessment and mental status evaluation), EEG, head MRI, and other tests to rule out other forms of dementia (e.g., lumbar puncture and serum tests). There is no known cure for CJD, although interleukins and other immunomodulator agents may slow the progression of the disease. Custodial care (nonmedical care that assists with activities of daily living) may be required early in the course of the disease. Medications may be needed to control aggressive behaviors, spasticity, pain, and seizure activity. Providing a safe environment, controlling

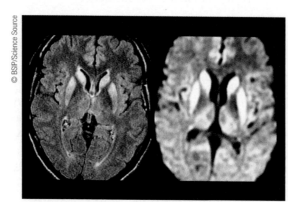
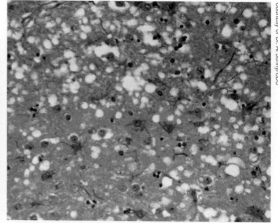

FIGURE 11-46 Creutzfeldt-Jakob disease.

aggressive or agitated behavior, and meeting physiologic needs may require monitoring and assistance in the home or in an institutionalized setting. Family counseling may help in coping with the changes required for home care.

AIDS Dementia Complex

Dementia is common in later stages of AIDS (see the *Immunity* chapter), a condition that is referred to as **AIDS dementia complex**, or human immunodeficiency virus (HIV)–associated encephalopathy. When HIV invades the brain tissue, its effects may be exacerbated by the other infections and tumors that are frequently associated with AIDS. Clinical manifestations include encephalitis, behavioral changes, and a gradual decline in cognitive function (e.g., trouble with concentration, memory, and attention). Persons with AIDS dementia complex also show progressive slowing of motor function with a loss of dexterity and coordination. In children with congenital HIV infection, the brain is often affected, causing mental retardation and delayed motor development.

A staging system is used to describe the condition's progression. The staging system ranges from 0 (normal) to 4 (nearly vegetative).

Diagnostic procedures for AIDS dementia complex consist of a history, physical examination (including a neurologic assessment and mental status evaluation), head CT, head MRI, and biopsy. When left untreated, AIDS dementia complex can be fatal. Aggressive antiretroviral therapy is the cornerstone of treatment.

Cancers of the Nervous System

Nervous system malignancies can originate in the brain or spinal cord, or they may spread there from other sites. Regardless of the etiology, these cancers can result in significant neurologic dysfunction and death. Typical cancer diagnosis, staging, and treatments are usually utilized in such cases (see the *Cellular Function* chapter).

Brain Tumors

Brain tumors, whether malignant or benign, can be life threatening because they often increase ICP and are difficult to access (FIGURE 11-47). Brain tumors may be primary, but most are secondary tumors. Any cancer can spread to the brain, but the types that most commonly do so include breast cancer, colon cancer, kidney cancer, lung cancer, melanoma, and sarcoma. Primary tumors are thought to arise from genetic mutations. The risk for such mutations increases with age and exposure to radiation and occupational chemicals. In the

United States, prevalence and mortality rates of brain tumors are highest among Caucasians and males (National Cancer Institute, 2016). Complications of brain tumors include neurologic deficits, seizures, personality changes, and death. The 5-year survival rate for brain tumors is nearly 34%.

Clinical manifestations of brain tumors vary depending on their size and location. These manifestations reflect the increased ICP associated with such tumors:

* New onset or change in pattern of headaches
* Headaches that gradually become more frequent and more severe
* Unexplained nausea or vomiting
* Vision problems (e.g., blurred vision, diplopia, or loss of peripheral vision)
* Gradual loss of sensation or movement in an extremity
* Balance difficulties
* Speech difficulties
* Confusion
* Hearing problems
* Hormonal (endocrine) disorders

Diagnostic procedures consist of a history, physical examination (including a neurologic assessment), head MRI, biopsy, and other tests to determine cancer histology. Treatment of brain tumors depends on the size and location of the originating cancer, if any. If possible, surgical removal of the tumor is recommended. Additional treatment options include radiation (external and radiosurgery), chemotherapy (e.g., temozolomide [Temodar]), and targeted drug therapy (e.g., bevacizumab [Avastin]). Regardless of the strategy, rehabilitation will be necessary to minimize residual neurologic dysfunction. Rehabilitation will likely require physical, occupational, and speech therapy.

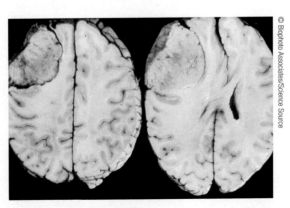

FIGURE 11-47 Brain tumor.

© Biophoto Associates/Science Source

application to practice

Now that we have discussed conditions of the nervous system, let's put that knowledge into practice. While working in the clinic, you encounter the following patients. Which patient would be at greatest risk for developing Alzheimer's disease?

- A young Caucasian woman with rheumatic heart disease
- A middle-aged African American woman with a history of several head injuries
- A middle-aged Hispanic man with diabetes mellitus
- An older Caucasian man who consumes a diet high in red meat

When determining who is at greatest risk, remember to start by counting risk factors, with the patient with the most risk factors being the "winner." First, consider the young woman. Ethnicity does not increase risk for Alzheimer's disease. Women are at greater risk of AD, but rheumatic heart disease does not further increase this risk. Thus this patient has one risk factor. Now consider the middle-aged African American woman. She is reaching the age at which AD is more likely to appear, and TBIs increase the risk for developing AD. Including gender, this patient has three risk factors. Moving on to the middle-aged Hispanic man, his risk factors include age and diabetes. Finally, consider the older Caucasian man. Red meat is high in cholesterol, which can be a contributing factor in AD development. Including his age, he has two risk factors. After considering all the patients, the middle-aged African American woman is at the highest risk for AD owing to her three risk factors.

CHAPTER SUMMARY

The nervous system is a complex network that receives, organizes, and responds to internal and external stimuli—functions that are vital for achieving and maintaining homeostasis. The nervous system controls all sensory and motor functions. Damage to this system—even when minor—can result in significant neurologic deficits. The nature and severity of those deficits depend on the location and extent of damage. Such damage can result from trauma, infections, tumors, chemical imbalances, or genetic conditions. Regardless of the neurologic disorder, the individual may face significant neurologic dysfunction and even death. Supporting neurologic health involves strategies such as observing safety precautions (e.g., wearing safety equipment), avoiding illicit drug use, minimizing alcohol consumption, getting vaccinations, and maintaining adequate nutrition.

REFERENCES

AAOS. (2004). *Paramedic: Anatomy & physiology*. Sudbury, MA: Jones & Bartlett.

Centers for Disease Control and Prevention (CDC). (2015a). Alzheimer's disease. Retrieved from http://www.cdc.gov/aging/aginginfo/alzheimers.htm

Centers for Disease Control and Prevention (CDC). (2015b). Creutzfeldt-Jakob disease. Retrieved from http://www.cdc.gov/prions/cjd/index.html

Centers for Disease Control and Prevention (CDC). (2015c). Spina bifida. Retrieved from http://www.cdc.gov/ncbddd/spinabifida/data.html

Centers for Disease Control and Prevention (CDC). (2015d). Stroke. Retrieved from http://www.cdc.gov/stroke/facts.htm

Centers for Disease Control and Prevention (CDC). (2016a). Data and statistics for cerebral palsy. Retrieved from http://www.cdc.gov/ncbddd/cp/data.html

Centers for Disease Control and Prevention (CDC). (2016b). Epilepsy fast facts. Retrieved from http://www.cdc.gov/epilepsy/basics/fast-facts.htm

Centers for Disease Control and Prevention (CDC). (2016c). Traumatic brain injury. Retrieved from http://www.cdc.gov/TraumaticBrainInjury/get_the_facts.html

Centers for Disease Control and Prevention (CDC). (2016d). Zika virus. Retrieved from http://www.cdc.gov/zika/geo/index.html

Chiras, D. (2011). *Human biology* (7th ed.). Burlington, MA: Jones & Bartlett Learning.

Elling, B., Elling, K., & Rothenberg, M. (2004). *Anatomy and physiology*. Sudbury, MA: Jones and Bartlett.

Gould, B. (2015). *Pathophysiology for the health professions* (5th ed.). Philadelphia, PA: Elsevier.

Hart, M., & Loeffler, A. (2012). *Introduction to human disease: Pathophysiology for health professionals*. Burlington, MA: Jones & Bartlett Learning.

Madara, B., & Pomarico-Denino, V. (2008). *Quick look nursing: Pathophysiology* (2nd ed.). Sudbury, MA: Jones and Bartlett.

National Cancer Institute. (2016). Brain cancer. Retrieved from http://seer.cancer.gov/statfacts/html/brain.html#incidence-mortality

National Hydrocephalus Foundation. (2014). Facts about hydrocephalus. Retrieved from http://nhfonline.org/facts-about-hydrocephalus.htm

National Institutes of Health (NIH). (2016a). Amyotrophic lateral sclerosis. Retrieved from https://www.ninds.nih.gov/Disorders/All-Disorders/Amyotrophic-Lateral-Sclerosis-ALS-Information-Page

National Institutes of Health (NIH). (2016b). Huntington's disease. Retrieved from https://www.ninds.nih.gov/Disorders/All-Disorders/Huntingtons-Disease-Information-Page

National Institutes of Health (NIH). (2016c). Multiple sclerosis. Retrieved from https://www.ninds.nih.gov/Disorders/All-Disorders/Multiple-Sclerosis-Information-Page

National Institutes of Health (NIH). (2016d). Parkinson's disease. Retrieved from https://www.ninds.nih.gov/Disorders/All-Disorders/Parkinsons-Disease-Information-Page

National Spinal Cord Injury Statistical Center (NSCISC). (2016). Spinal cord injury facts and figures at a glance. Retrieved from https://www.nscisc.uab.edu/Public/Facts%202016.pdf

Navalkele, B., Chandrasekar, P., & Levine, M. (2016). Zika virus. *Medscape*. Retrieved from http://emedicine.medscape.com/article/2500035-overview#a2

Professional guide to pathophysiology (3rd ed.). (2010). Philadelphia, PA: Lippincott Williams & Wilkins.

Schwenk, T., Gorenflo, D., Dopp, R., & Hipple, E. (2007). Depression and pain in retired professional football players. *Medicine & Science in Sports & Exercise, 39*(4), 599–605.

World Health Organization (WHO). (2016). Zika virus. Retrieved from http://www.who.int/mediacentre/factsheets/zika/en/

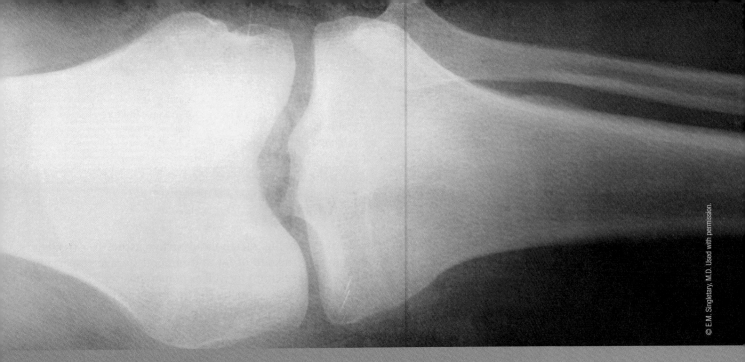

© E.M. Singletary, M.D. Used with permission.

CHAPTER 12
Musculoskeletal Function

LEARNING OBJECTIVES

- Discuss normal musculoskeletal anatomy and physiology.
- Compare and contrast congenital musculoskeletal disorders.
- Compare and contrast traumatic musculoskeletal disorders.
- Compare and contrast metabolic bone disorders.
- Compare and contrast inflammatory joint disorders.
- Describe and discuss chronic muscle disorders.
- Describe and discuss bone cancers.

KEY TERMS

actin	depressed fracture	kyphosis	osteomyelitis
amphiarthrose	diaphysis	lamella	osteonecrosis
ankylosing spondylitis	dislocation	ligament	osteopenia
ankylosis	epiphysis	long bone	osteoporosis
appendicular skeleton	Ewing's sarcoma	lordosis	osteosarcoma
axial skeleton	fascia	matrix	Paget's disease
bone	fat embolism	muscle fiber	pathologic fracture
bone marrow	fibromyalgia	muscular dystrophy (MD)	periosteum
callus	flat bone	myofibril	red marrow
cardiac muscle	fracture	myofilament	reduce
cartilage	gout	myosin	rheumatoid arthritis (RA)
chondrosarcoma	greenstick fracture	oblique fracture	rickets
closed fracture	herniated intervertebral disk	open fracture	sarcomere
comminuted fracture	hyaline cartilage	osteoarthritis (OA)	sciatica
compact bone	impacted fracture	osteoblast	scoliosis
compartment syndrome	incomplete fracture	osteochondroma	sesamoid bone
complete fracture	irregular bone	osteoclast	short bone
compression fracture	joint	osteocyte	simple fracture
crepitus	joint capsule	osteomalacia	skeletal muscle

skeleton	sprain	synarthrose	tophus
smooth muscle	strain	synovial fluid	transverse fracture
spiral fracture	stress fracture	synovial joint	yellow marrow
spongy bone	suture	tendon	

The musculoskeletal system consists of bones, joints, muscles, ligaments, tendons, and other connective tissue that provide support for the body and protection of organs. The musculoskeletal system collaborates with the nervous system to make movement possible. It plays a role in homeostasis by storing calcium and other minerals that can be mobilized when needed. Additionally, hematopoiesis occurs in the bones (see the *Hematopoietic Function* chapter).

Disorders of the musculoskeletal system may be either acute or chronic. Many of these conditions are easily treatable and leave no lasting effects (e.g., fractures). Other conditions can leave the individual with chronic pain or significant disability (e.g., fibromyalgia). These disorders may have congenital, genetic, autoimmune, trauma, nutritional deficits, and excessive use causes.

Anatomy and Physiology

The structures of the musculoskeletal system are essential for standing erect and locomotion. This system also gives the human body form and stability while protecting the body's vital organs. As noted earlier, it plays a role in homeostasis and is the site for hematopoiesis. The musculoskeletal system consists of bones, joints, muscles, ligaments, tendons, and other connective tissues that work together to accomplish these functions. Connective tissues are the biologic material that supports and binds tissues and organs together. The chief components of connective tissue include elastic fibers and collagen (a protein substance).

Bones

Bone is a specialized form of connective tissue. At first glance, the bone appears to be a dry, dead material. In fact, the word *skeleton* is derived from a Greek word that means "dried-up body." Looks can be deceiving, however, because nothing could be further from the truth. Bone is a living, metabolically active tissue. This tissue is the site of fat and mineral storage (especially calcium) as well as hematopoiesis. The human body contains 206 bones of varying shapes and sizes that make up the **skeleton** (FIGURE 12-1). The skeleton provides support and protection for vital organs such as the heart, lungs, and brain. It is organized into two divisions—axial and appendicular. The **axial skeleton** forms the long axis of the body and includes the skull, vertebral column, and rib cage. The **appendicular skeleton** consists of the bones that form the arms, shoulders, pelvis, and legs.

Five types of bone are found within the skeleton—long, short, flat, irregular, and sesamoid bones (FIGURE 12-2). **Long bones** (FIGURE 12-3) have bodies (**diaphyses**) that are longer than they are wide, growth plates (**epiphyses**) at either end, hard outer surfaces (**compact bone**), and inner regions (**spongy bone**) that are less dense than the outer regions and contain bone marrow. Both ends of long bones are covered in hyaline cartilage to help protect the bone by reducing friction and absorbing shock. Long bones include some of the longest bones in the body (e.g., femur, humerus, and tibia) as well as some of the smallest (e.g., metacarpals, metatarsals, and phalanges). **Short bones** are approximately as wide as they are long; their primary function is providing support and stability with little movement. Short bones consist of only a thin layer of compact bone along with spongy bone but contain relatively large amounts of bone marrow. Examples of short bones include the carpals and tarsals.

Flat bones are strong, level plates of bone that provide protection to the body's vital organs and serve as a base for muscular attachment. The anterior and posterior surfaces of flat bones are formed from compact bone to provide strength, and the center consists of spongy bone and varying amounts of bone marrow. In adults, most red blood cells are formed in flat bones. Examples of flat bones include the scapula, sternum, skull, pelvis, and ribs.

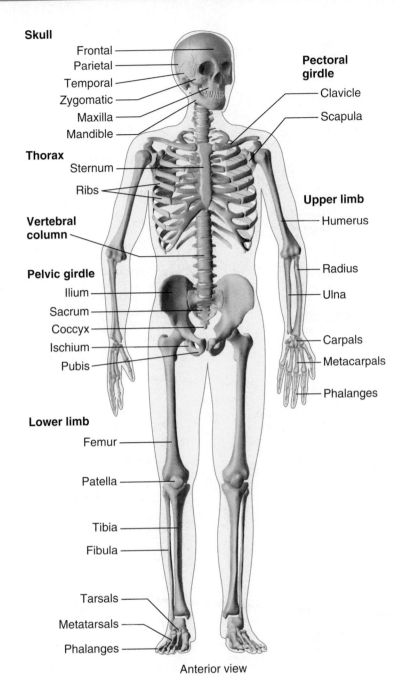

Skull
Frontal
Parietal
Temporal
Zygomatic
Maxilla
Mandible

Thorax
Sternum
Ribs

Vertebral column

Pelvic girdle
Ilium
Sacrum
Coccyx
Ischium
Pubis

Lower limb
Femur
Patella
Tibia
Fibula
Tarsals
Metatarsals
Phalanges

Pectoral girdle
Clavicle
Scapula

Upper limb
Humerus
Radius
Ulna
Carpals
Metacarpals
Phalanges

Anterior view

FIGURE 12-1 The human skeleton.

Irregular bones include bones that do not fall into any other category, due to their non-uniform shape. They primarily consist of spongy bone, with a thin outer layer of compact bone. Examples of irregular bones include the vertebrae, sacrum, and mandible.

Sesamoid bones are usually short or irregular bones embedded in a tendon. Sesamoid bones are often present in a tendon where it passes over a joint, and serve to protect the tendon. Examples of sesamoid bones include the patella, pisiform (smallest of the carpals), and

the two small bones at the base of the first metatarsal.

A layer of connective tissue called the **periosteum** covers compact bone surfaces. The periosteum serves as the site of muscle attachment (via tendons). The outer surface of the periosteum contains cells that aid in remodeling and repair (**osteoblasts**). The periosteum is richly supplied with blood vessels that enter the bone at numerous sites (**FIGURE 12-4**). These vessels travel through small tubes (Haversian canals) in the compact bone and flow through the spongy

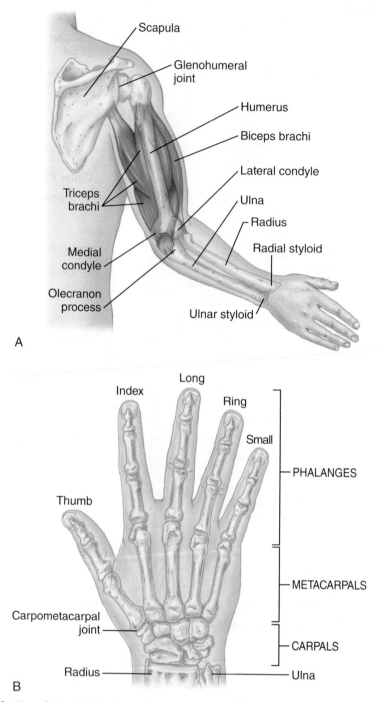

FIGURE 12-2 Classifications of bones. (a) The scapula is a flat bone, and the humerus, ulna, and radius are long bones. (b) The carpals, or wrist bones, are short bones.

bone, providing nutrients and oxygen while removing waste products. The periosteum is also richly supplied with nerve fibers.

Inside the shaft of long bones is a large cavity for **bone marrow**. The marrow cavities in most bones of a fetus or newborn contain red marrow. **Red marrow**, so named because of its color, serves as a blood-cell factory (hematopoiesis). As humans age, this red marrow is slowly replaced by fat, creating **yellow marrow**. Yellow marrow begins to form during adolescence and is present in most bones by adulthood. At this point, hematopoiesis continues in the vertebrae, pelvis, and a few other sites. The yellow marrow can be reactivated to produce blood cells under certain circumstances (e.g., after an injury).

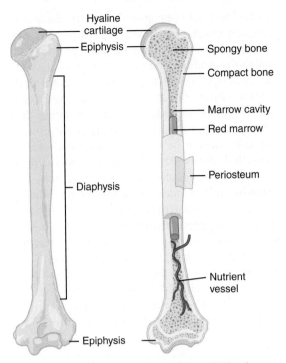

FIGURE 12-3 Long bones. (a) The humerus. Notice the long shaft and dilated ends. (b) Longitudinal section of the humerus showing compact bone, spongy bone, and marrow.

Bone is a dynamic tissue that is constantly undergoing remodeling to repair aging bone or to adjust for factors such as changes in activity. For example, spongy bone is remodeled to increase bone strength when a person's activity level increases after periods of inactivity. During remodeling, cells called **osteoclasts** break down some spongy bone, while osteoblasts rebuild new compact bone to increase bone strength (**TABLE 12-1**). Osteoblasts lay down new bone during the remodeling process; when these osteoblasts become surrounded by calcified extracellular material, the complex is referred to as an **osteocyte**. Bone tissue contains many of these osteocytes organized into thin layers called **lamellae** (**FIGURE 12-5**). The osteocytes are embedded in an extracellular material referred to as the **matrix**. The matrix consists of calcium phosphate crystals (hydroxyapatite) that make the bones hard and strong. It also contains collagen fibers that reinforce the bone, giving it flexible strength. Balance between the mineral components and collagen is necessary for optimal bone function. Bone without adequate

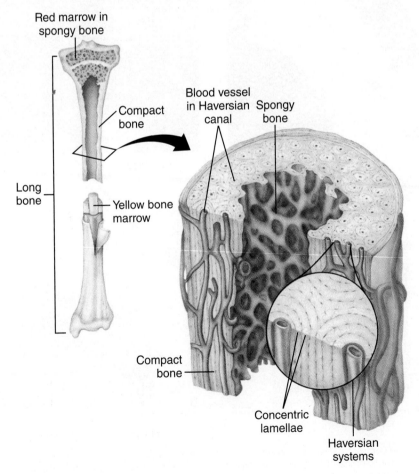

FIGURE 12-4 Shaft of the bone.

TABLE 12-1 Structural Elements of Bone

Bone Cells	Function
Osteoblasts	Build bone through collagen
Osteoclasts	Enable the matrix to be absorbed and assist with the release of calcium and phosphate
Osteocytes	Mature cells that help maintain the bone matrix; also play a major role in the release of calcium into blood

mineral quantities is too flexible; bone without adequate collagen amounts is extremely brittle.

Several hormones influence bone structure. Growth hormone produced by the anterior pituitary gland works with thyroid hormones to control normal bone growth (see the *Endocrine Function* chapter). Growth hormone increases the rate of growth by causing cartilage and bone cells to reproduce and lay down their intercellular matrix as well as by stimulating mineralization within the matrix. Bones grow in two ways—appositional growth and endochondral growth. In appositional growth, new bone forms on the surface of a bone. In endochondral growth, bone eventually replaces new cartilage growth in the epiphyseal plate. Calcitonin and parathyroid hormone regulate bone remodeling and mineralization of calcium (see the *Endocrine Function* chapter). Estrogen inhibits formation of osteoclasts in women, whereas testosterone increases bone length and density in men.

Vitamin D also plays a critical role in bone metabolism. This fat-soluble vitamin controls the absorption of calcium from the intestine as well as increases calcium and phosphate

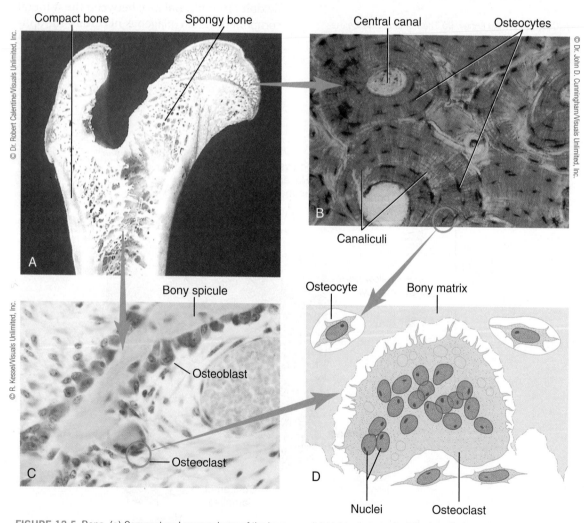

FIGURE 12-5 Bone. (a) Compact and spongy bone of the humerus. (b) Light micrograph of the lamella (concentric circles) showing the osteocytes and canaliculi. (c) Photomicrograph of spongy bone showing osteoblasts and osteoclasts. (d) An osteoclast digesting the surface of a bony spicule (sharp body or spike).

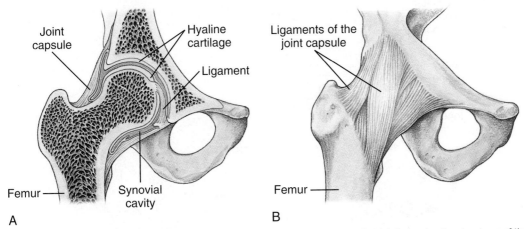

FIGURE 12-6 A synovial joint. (a) A cross section through the hip joint (a ball-and-socket joint) showing the structures of the synovial joint. (b) Ligaments in the outer portion of the joint capsule help support the joint.

reabsorption in the kidneys. Proper nutrition (including adequate intake of dietary calcium and vitamin D) and physical activity from childhood onward are essential for the development and maintenance of healthy bone.

During fetal development, the skeleton forms from hyaline cartilage. **Cartilage** is a shiny connective tissue that is tough and flexible. Although several types of cartilage can be found throughout the body in the ears, nose, and joints, **hyaline cartilage** is the type most closely associated with bone. This cartilage is often found in **joints**—structures that connect bones of the skeleton. Joints are classified based on their degree of movement as moveable, slightly moveable, or immoveable.

The most common type of joint is the freely moveable, or synovial, joint (**FIGURE 12-6**). **Synovial joints** are complex and vary significantly, but they all share similar features. Synovial joints contain cartilage that is lubricated by a transparent viscous fluid (**synovial fluid**) secreted by the synovial membrane (a soft tissue that lines the noncartilaginous surfaces within joints). This lubricated cartilage reduces friction by providing a slippery surface that enables bones to move freely. In addition to lubrication, synovial fluid contains leukocytes that fight infections in the joints and delivers nutrients to the cartilage. The second commonality among synovial joints is the presence of a **joint capsule**, a structure that joins one bone to another. The outer layer of the synovial joint capsule consists of dense connective tissue that is attached to the periosteum of adjacent bones. Many of these joints contain parallel bundles of dense connective tissue called **ligaments**. Ligaments connect bones to bones in a joint and provide support to the joint.

Slightly moveable joints, or **amphiarthroses**, can be seen in the vertebral column (**FIGURE 12-7**). An intervertebral disk unites the components of each vertebra. The inner portion of this disk serves as a cushion, absorbing the impact of walking and running. The outer, fibrous portion holds the disk in place and joins one vertebra to the next.

The skull is an example of an immoveable joint, or **synarthrose** (**FIGURE 12-8**). In the skull, the bones interlock together to form immoveable joints called **sutures**. Fibrous connective tissue extends the space between the interlocking bones, holding them together. Another immoveable joint is the pubic symphysis, where the two pubic bones come together and are held in position by fibrocartilage.

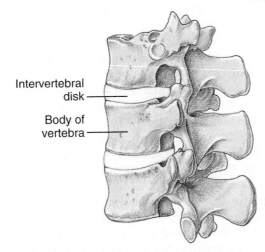

FIGURE 12-7 A slightly movable joint. The intervertebral disks allow for some movement, giving the vertebral column flexibility.

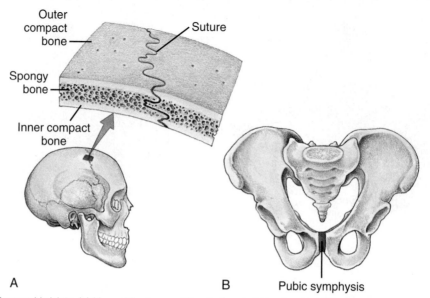

FIGURE 12-8 Immovable joints. (a) Many of the bones of the skull are held in place by joints called sutures. These bones are linked by fibrous tissue, and the joints are immovable. (b) The pubic symphysis is another immovable joint. During childbirth, it softens and expands to permit delivery.

Muscles

Motion requires a skeleton with moveable joints as well as muscles acting on the bones. There are three types of muscles: skeletal, smooth, and cardiac. **Skeletal muscles** connect to bone. They are the most frequently occurring muscle type, making up approximately 40% of the body's weight. The more than 350 skeletal muscles are under the voluntary control of the brain (**FIGURE 12-9**). **Smooth muscles** line the walls of hollow organs and tubes; they are also found in the eyes, skin, and glands. Smooth muscles are involuntary, meaning they work without conscious control by the brain. **Cardiac muscle** makes up the heart and is under involuntary control.

Almost every muscle in the body attaches to bones through structures such as **tendons**. Tendons are specialized tough cords or bands of dense connective tissue that are continuous extensions of the periosteum.

In addition, most muscles cross one or more joints. Muscles contract to produce movement of the bones at the joints. They work in groups to produce smooth movements (**FIGURE 12-10**). When one muscle contracts to produce a movement, the antagonistic (opposing) muscles relax to allow the movement. Muscles contract in response to nerve stimulation (see the *Neural Function* chapter). Because muscle fibers are elastic, the fibers return to their normal length after contracting. Not all skeletal muscles make bones move. Some muscles steady joints, allowing other muscles to act. These muscles assist with posture, permitting the body to sit or stand upright against gravitational pull. Like nerve cells, muscle fibers are excitable cells with high action potential, allowing them to respond to stimulation rapidly.

Skeletal muscles are composed of muscle fibers, connective tissue, blood vessels, and nerves (**FIGURE 12-11**). Each skeletal **muscle fiber** or cell is a cylinder with multiple nuclei. Within each fiber are **myofibrils**, threadlike structures extending for the entire length of the muscle fiber. Myofibrils contain two types of **myofilaments** (protein fibers)—actin and myosin. **Actin** myofilaments are involved in muscular contractions, cellular movement, and cell shape maintenance. **Myosin** myofilaments are darker and thicker than their actin counterparts. Myosin myofilaments are fibrous globulins (a type of protein) that work with actin to form actomyosin. The alignment of these two kinds of myofilaments gives the skeletal muscle its striated appearance (alternating light and dark bands) (**FIGURE 12-12**). Myofilaments are organized into repeated structural units called **sarcomeres** (Figure 12-11).

Muscle fibers contract when actin filaments slide over myosin filaments. In this process, the myosin filament pulls the actin filament. The myosin attaches to the actin when calcium is released from inside the muscle fibers. Calcium is stored in the smooth endoplasmic reticulum (see the *Cellular Function* chapter), which forms an extensive network inside muscle fibers.

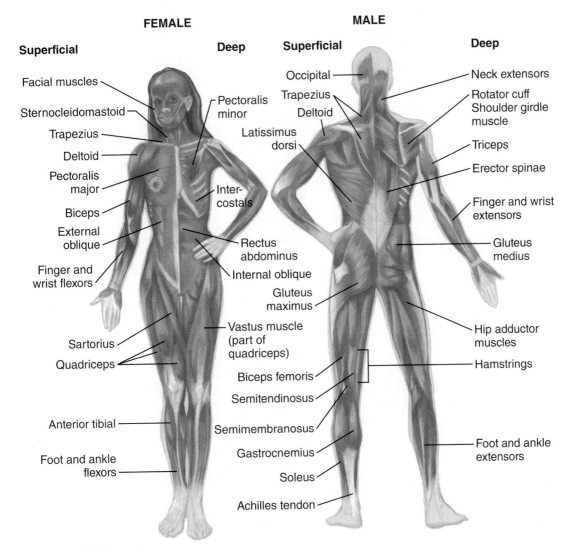

FEMALE

Superficial — Deep

MALE

Superficial — Deep

- Facial muscles
- Sternocleidomastoid
- Trapezius
- Deltoid
- Pectoralis major
- Biceps
- External oblique
- Finger and wrist flexors
- Sartorius
- Quadriceps
- Anterior tibial
- Foot and ankle flexors

- Pectoralis minor
- Latissimus dorsi
- Intercostals
- Rectus abdominus
- Internal oblique
- Gluteus maximus
- Vastus muscle (part of quadriceps)
- Biceps femoris
- Semitendinosus
- Semimembranosus
- Gastrocnemius
- Soleus
- Achilles tendon

- Occipital
- Trapezius
- Deltoid

- Neck extensors
- Rotator cuff Shoulder girdle muscle
- Triceps
- Erector spinae
- Finger and wrist extensors
- Gluteus medius
- Hip adductor muscles
- Hamstrings
- Foot and ankle extensors

FIGURE 12-9 Skeletal muscles.

Impulses from nerve cells—specifically, motor neurons—trigger this release of calcium. Once the calcium causes the head of the myosin to attach to the actin filament, adenosine triphosphate in the muscle provides the energy needed to pull the actin filament inward. To meet the muscle cell's high energy needs, adenosine triphosphate is recycled repeatedly in rapid succession. During vigorous activity, adenosine triphosphate stores become depleted, oxygen levels drop sharply, glucose production ceases, and lactic acid accumulates.

Each muscle fiber is enclosed by a cell membrane (sarcolemma) (**FIGURE 12-13**). Numerous muscle fibers are bundled together and surrounded by connective tissue called endomysium. Additional connective tissue called perimysium surrounds several of these bundles,

grouping them together to form a muscle. Yet another layer of connective tissue called epimysium and fibrous connective tissue (**fascia**) surround these muscles. This fascia may also surround muscle groups.

In addition to stimulating bone growth, growth hormone causes muscle growth. The number of muscle fibers or cells in a muscle remains relatively constant throughout the life span. Thus, increases in muscle sizes reflect increases in individual muscle fibers, rather than greater numbers of fibers. When muscles work harder, they respond by becoming larger and stronger. This increase in size and strength results from an increase in the amount of contractile protein inside the muscle fiber. Unfortunately, muscle protein is produced and destroyed quickly. In fact, approximately

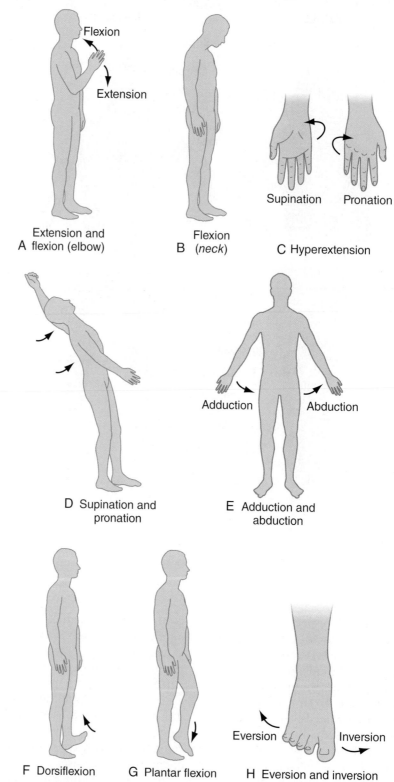

FIGURE 12-10 Common body movements.

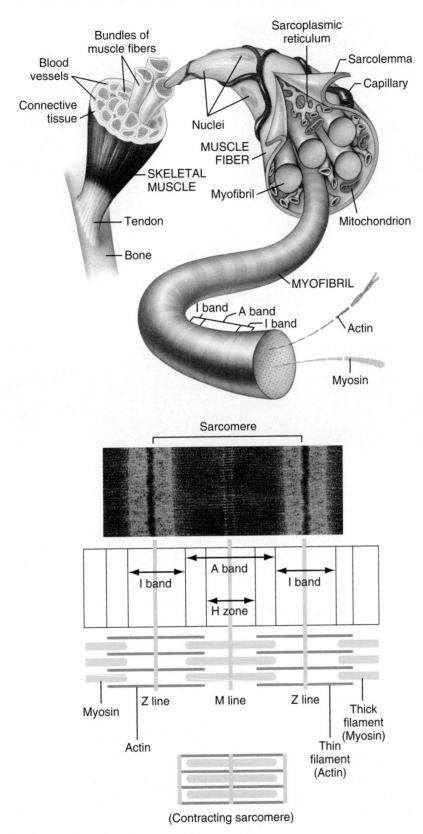

FIGURE 12-11 Structure of a skeletal muscle.

Photo: © Don W. Fawcett/Visuals Unlimited, Inc.

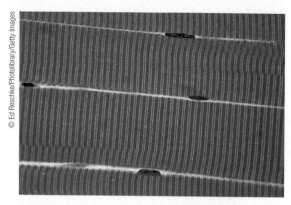

FIGURE 12-12 Striated pattern of skeletal muscle.

half of the muscle gained in a weight-lifting program is broken down 2 weeks after ceasing the activity. The only way to maintain the muscle gain is to continue the weight-lifting program.

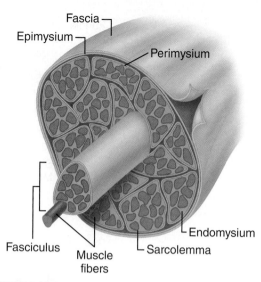

FIGURE 12-13 Muscle group.

UNDERSTANDING CONDITIONS THAT AFFECT THE MUSCULOSKELETAL SYSTEM

When considering alterations of the musculoskeletal system, organizing them based on their basic underlying pathophysiology can increase understanding. In patients with musculoskeletal system disorders, the primary nursing diagnosis is impaired physical mobility, in recognition of the fact that the primary function of this system is movement. Interventions are specifically selected to prevent complications of immobility (e.g., osteoporosis, renal calculi, thrombus, constipation, and decubiti). Depending on the condition, other nursing diagnoses that may come into play are chronic pain, risk for injury, and self-care deficit.

Congenital Musculoskeletal Disorders

Some musculoskeletal disorders are congenital in nature and primarily affect posture. These conditions may be apparent at birth or, alternatively, they may materialize as the child grows. During growth spurts in affected individuals, muscular development lags behind skeletal growth; this lag results in inadequate skeletal support. Additionally, comorbidity of developmental abnormalities (e.g., Down syndrome and cerebral palsy) may become aggravated during these growth periods. These postural deformities require early treatment to prevent progression and complications.

Kyphosis

Kyphosis refers to an increase in the curvature of the thoracic spine outward (**FIGURE 12-14**). Often called hunchback, kyphosis is rarely present at birth. Instead, it usually appears during the adolescent growth spurts and can appear as poor posture (referred to as Scheuermann's disease). In adults, kyphosis usually develops secondary to osteoporosis, degenerative spine disease (e.g., arthritis or disk degeneration), or injury. Severe kyphosis can impair lung expansion and ventilation. Additionally, patients with this disorder are at increased risk for injury because of alterations in their center of gravity. Other manifestations may include fatigue, back pain, and spine stiffness.

Diagnostic procedures for kyphosis include a history, physical examination, spine X-ray,

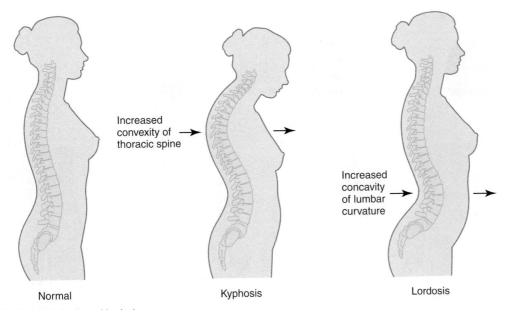

Increased
convexity of
thoracic spine

Increased
concavity
of lumbar
curvature

Normal   Kyphosis   Lordosis

FIGURE 12-14 Kyphosis and lordosis.

computed tomography (CT), and magnetic resonance imaging (MRI). Exercises (including back strengthening) and proper posture can usually reverse mild deformities. Bracing and surgical correction may be necessary for more severe cases.

Lordosis

Lordosis refers to an exaggerated concave of the lumbar spine (Figure 12-14). Often called swayback, lordosis may develop during adolescent growth spurts or because of poor posture. Obesity can increase the tendency toward this posture because of an altered center of gravity and postural compensation. Lordosis is also commonly associated with dwarfism.

Diagnostic procedures for lordosis include a history, physical examination, spine X-ray, CT, and MRI. Much as with kyphosis, treatment for lordosis includes exercises, proper posture, bracing, and surgery.

Scoliosis

Scoliosis refers to a lateral deviation of the spine (FIGURE 12-15). This lateral curvature may affect the thoracic area, the lumbar area, or both. Scoliosis may also include a rotation of the vertebrae on their axis. Stress on the vertebrae causes an imbalance in osteoclast activity; therefore, the curvature increases during growth spurts. Scoliosis may also be associated with kyphosis and lordosis.

Scoliosis varies in severity and is more common in females. Most cases are idiopathic, but known causes may include genetic influences (autosomal dominant), embryonic developmental deformities (usually involving the hemivertebrae), degenerative diseases (e.g., osteoporosis and osteoarthritis), unequal leg lengths, spinal nerve compression, and asymmetrical muscle support (e.g., partial paralysis, muscular dystrophy, cerebral palsy, poliomyelitis, trauma, or spinal tumors). Complications of scoliosis include pulmonary compromise, chronic pain, degenerative arthritis of the spine, intervertebral disk disease, and sciatica.

Clinical manifestations vary depending on the degree of curvature and are exaggerated when an affected person bends over. These manifestations may include the following symptoms:

- Asymmetrical hip and shoulder alignment
- Asymmetrical thoracic cage
- Asymmetrical gait
- Back pain or discomfort
- Fatigue
- Indications of respiratory compromise (e.g., dyspnea and reduced chest expansion)

Because of the prevalence of scoliosis in adolescent females, schools often conduct periodic scoliosis screening. Diagnostic procedures consist of a history, physical examination (including the "forward bending" test), spinal X-rays, use of a scoliometer (which measures the angle of trunk rotation), CT, and MRI.

Without treatment, the curvature associated with scoliosis often progresses in adulthood.

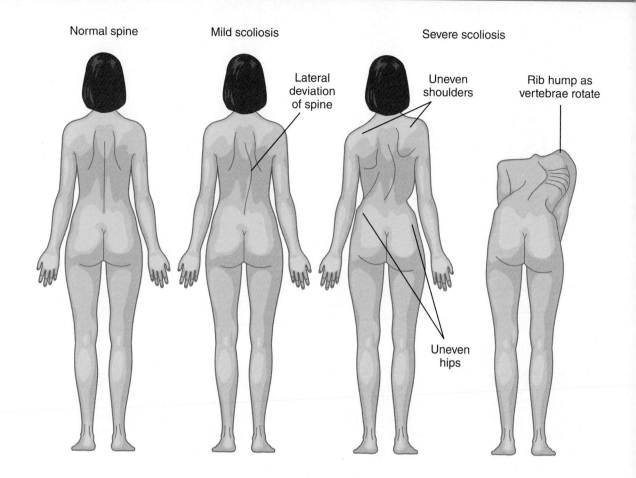

Normal spine   Mild scoliosis   Severe scoliosis

Lateral deviation of spine

Uneven shoulders

Rib hump as vertebrae rotate

Uneven hips

Rotation of vertebra and rib deformity

Wedge vertebra   Fused vertebra   Fused ribs

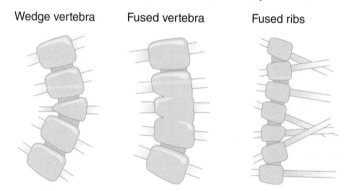

FIGURE 12-15 Scoliosis.

Patient outcomes improve with early treatment. Treatment strategies may include exercises (including back strengthening), bracing, and surgical correction (with instrumentation or fusion).

Traumatic Musculoskeletal Disorders

Traumatic musculoskeletal disorders are usually mild and easily treated; however, occasionally these conditions can result in life-threatening complications (e.g., fat embolism and osteomyelitis). Many of these conditions are caused by events similar to the ones that lead to traumatic neurologic disorders (e.g., falls, motor vehicle accidents, and sports-related injuries). Additionally, neurologic dysfunction may occur in conjunction with the musculoskeletal injury. These traumatic conditions are on the rise because of increasing numbers of children and adults participating in fitness, recreation, and sport activities. Factors contributing to these injuries include inappropriate or inadequate equipment, training, or warm-up techniques; more aggressive approaches to sports; and failure to allow minor injuries to heal.

Fractures

A **fracture** is a break in the rigid structure of the bone (FIGURE 12-16). Fractures are the most common type of traumatic musculoskeletal disorders. They mainly occur as a primary condition because of falls, motor vehicle accidents, and sports-related injuries. Additionally, fractures can occur secondary to conditions that weaken the bone (e.g., osteoporosis, Paget's disease, and bone cancer). Fractures are classified based on characteristics such as the direction of the fracture line, the number of fracture lines, or other characteristics (FIGURE 12-17). Fracture types include the following:

- **Simple fracture**—a fracture with a single break in the bone and in which bone

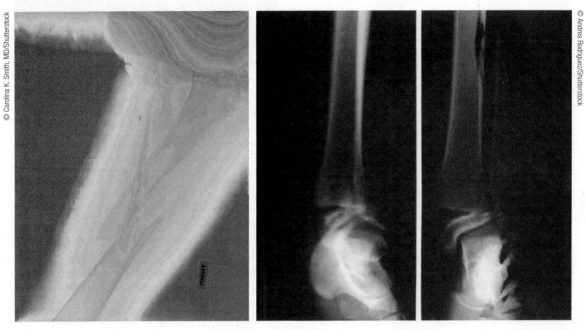

FIGURE 12-16 Fractures.

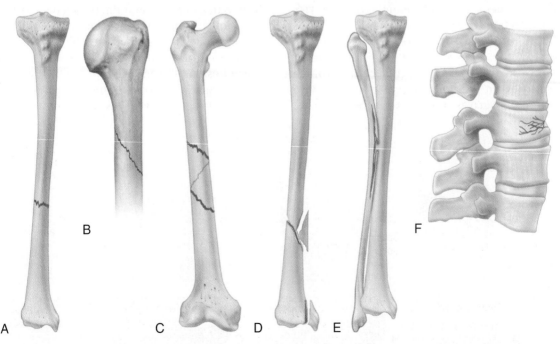

FIGURE 12-17 Classifications of fractures. (a) Transverse fracture of the tibia. (b) Oblique fracture of the humerus. (c) Spiral fracture of the femur. (d) Comminuted fracture of the tibia. (e) Greenstick fracture of the fibula. (f) Compression fracture of a vertebral body.

ends maintain their alignment and position:

- **Transverse fracture**—a fracture straight across the bone shaft
- **Oblique fracture**—a fracture at an angle to the bone shaft
- **Spiral fracture**—a fracture that twists around the bone shaft
- **Comminuted fracture**—a fracture characterized by multiple fracture lines and bone pieces
- **Greenstick fracture**—an incomplete fracture in which the bone is bent and only the outer curve of the bend is broken; commonly occurs in children because of minimal calcification and often heals quickly
- **Compression fracture**—a fracture in which the bone is crushed or collapses into small pieces

A variety of other terms may be used to describe a fracture. For example, fractures may be described based on the degree of break. **Complete fractures** occur when the bone is broken into two or more separate pieces; in contrast, in **incomplete fractures**, the bone is partially broken (e.g., greenstick fracture). Additionally, fractures may be described as open or closed. In **open fractures**, or compound fractures, the skin is broken (**FIGURE 12-18**). The bone fragments or edges may be angled and protrude out of the skin. Open fractures are characterized by more damage to soft tissue and are at risk for infection. In **closed fractures**, the skin is intact. **Impacted fractures** occur when one end of the bone is forced into the adjacent bone. **Pathologic fractures** result from a weakness in the bone structure secondary to conditions such as bone tumors or osteoporosis.

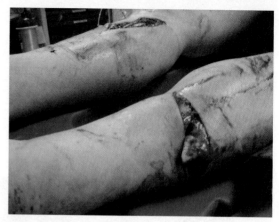

FIGURE 12-18 Open fracture.
Courtesy of Rhonda Hunt

Stress fractures, or fatigue fractures, occur from repeated excessive stress. These fractures are common in the tibia, femur, and metatarsals. Finally, **depressed fractures** occur in the skull when the broken piece is forced inward on the brain.

When a bone breaks, blood from damaged vessels in the periosteum and bone marrow pours into the fracture and forms a hematoma, or blood clot (**FIGURE 12-19**). Necrosis occurs to the broken ends of the bone because of the blood vessel damage. Over time, the necrotic tissue is reabsorbed and replaced by new bone. Within a few days of the fracture, fibroblasts (connective tissue from the periosteum) invade the clot. These fibroblasts secrete collagen fibers, which form a mass of cells and fibers called a **callus**. The callus bridges the broken bone ends together inside and outside. The callus takes 2–6 weeks to form. At that point, osteoblasts from the periosteum invade the callus, which slowly convert the callus to bone. This ossification process can take from 3 weeks to several months

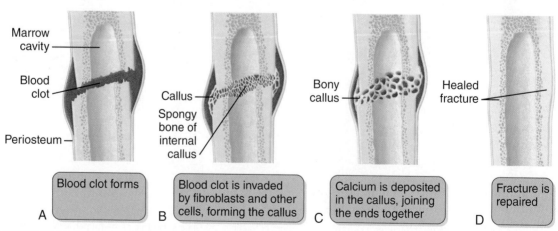

FIGURE 12-19 Stages of fracture repair.

(usually 4–6 weeks) to reach completion. Healing time can vary depending on age, nutritional status, blood supply, and fracture type and location. The callus is initially a large, often palpable structure, but osteoclasts gradually remodel the bone by removing the excess bone. This remodeling process leaves little to no evidence that the fracture occurred and may take as long as a year.

Multiple complications can result from fractures. Delayed union, malunion, or nonunion, for example, may occur due to poor nutrition, inadequate blood supply, malalignment, and premature weight bearing. Other fracture complications may include compartment syndrome, fat embolism, osteomyelitis, and osteonecrosis:

- **Compartment syndrome** is a serious condition that results from increased pressure in a compartment, usually the muscle fascia in the case of fractures. This pressure impinges on the nerves and blood vessels present within the compartment, potentially compromising the distal extremity. Compartment syndrome requires prompt identification and treatment to prevent permanent tissue damage. Clinical manifestations usually include excruciating pain beyond what would be expected given the injury. Compartment syndrome can be diagnosed by measuring pressures inside the muscle fascia. Treatment usually includes removing the cast (if present) and performing an immediate fasciotomy to relieve the pressure.
- A **fat embolism** occurs when fat has an opportunity to enter the bloodstream (e.g., during surgery). Fatty marrow can enter the bloodstream after a fracture to one of the long bones. The outcome can be fatal if the emboli travel to vital organs such as the lungs, brain, or heart. Fat embolism can be prevented with early immobilization of the fracture.
- **Osteomyelitis** refers to an infection of the bone tissue. It is a serious complication because it often goes undetected, can take months to resolve, and can result in bone or tissue necrosis. Osteomyelitis is treated with potent antibiotic therapy (often delivered on a long-term basis) and surgery (e.g., debridement).
- **Osteonecrosis**, or avascular necrosis, is death of bone tissue due to a loss of the blood supply to that tissue. It can result from displaced fractures or dislocations. Osteonecrosis often requires surgical replacement of the necrotic bone and/or joint.

Clinical manifestations of a fracture reflect the tissue trauma caused by the bone fragments as well as the disruption of function:

- Deformity (e.g., angulation, shortening, and rotation)
- Swelling at the site (due to the inflammatory process triggered by the tissue trauma)
- Inability to move the affected limb
- **Crepitus** (grating sound or sensation, usually occurring with movement)
- Pain (results from tissue trauma and muscle spasms triggered by the bone fragments)
- Paresthesia
- Muscle flaccidity progressing to spasms

Diagnostic procedures for fractures consist of a history, physical examination (including neurovascular assessment), and X-rays. Treatment strategies include immediate immobilization with devices such as splints or traction (application of a force or weight pulling a limb). The fracture is **reduced** to restore the bone to its normal position. Reduction can be accomplished with closed manipulation by applying pressure or traction (pulling force) or with open manipulation via surgery. During surgery, devices such as pins, plates, rods, or screws may be placed to secure the bone fragments in position. These instruments may be either internal and permanent, or externally fixated and gradually retracted. Any necrotic tissue or foreign material is also removed in a process called debridement. When a fracture is suspected, the individual with the injury should not consume anything by mouth in the event that surgery is deemed necessary. Surgical repair may be delayed up to a few days after the injury to allow the edema secondary to the inflammatory response to resolve. Immobilization of the fracture during this time is crucial to prevent complications. Long-term immobilization that permits bone healing to occur is accomplished with casts, splints, or traction. Traction maintains bone alignment and prevents muscle spasms. As the fracture is healing, exercise is helpful to limit muscle atrophy, joint stiffness, and contracture formation as well as to maintain adequate circulation.

Dislocation

Dislocation refers to the separation of two bones where they meet at a joint (**FIGURE 12-20**). With this type of injury, the two bones are no longer in their normal position. The dislocation may involve a complete or partial (subluxation) loss of contact. Such an injury causes deformity

Gina Dickerson is a 34-year-old woman who is being admitted to the orthopedic unit following a motor vehicle accident. She was driving her car through an intersection when someone ran a stop sign and hit her vehicle. Ms. Dickerson was diagnosed in the emergency room with a compound fracture of tihe left femur and a comminuted fracture of the left ankle.

When this patient arrived in the orthopedic unit at 1600, her left leg was immobilized with an air cast and ice bags were applied. She was medicated in the emergency room with morphine sulfate, 2 mg intravenously at 1200. The nursing admission assessment data revealed that Ms. Dickerson had no significant medical problems. Her vital signs on admission to the unit were as follows: temperature, 99.2°F; pulse, 90 beats per minute; respirations, 24 breaths per minute; oxygen saturation, 95% on room air; and blood pressure, 140/80 mm Hg. She was scheduled for surgery in the morning to repair both fractures.

1. Explain the type of fractures this patient has incurred.
2. List the top three priority nursing interventions for this patient upon admission.
3. What are some complications that this patient is at high risk for developing?
4. What is the significance of the patient's vital signs?

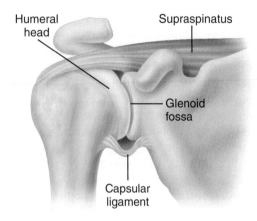

Normal

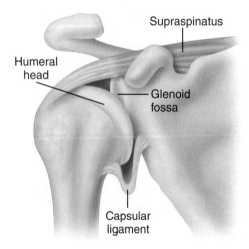

Anterior dislocation

FIGURE 12-20 Anterior dislocation of the shoulder.

and immobility of the joints, and it may damage nearby ligaments and nerves. Dislocations usually result from a sudden impact to the joint (e.g., blow, fall, or other trauma), but they may also be congenital (e.g., congenital hip dysplasia) or pathologic (e.g., arthritis, ligament injuries, paralysis, or neuromuscular disease). Any joint can be affected, but dislocations are especially common in the shoulder and clavicle joints.

Clinical manifestations of a dislocated joint may include the following signs and symptoms:

- Visibly out-of-place, discolored, or deformed joint
- Limited movement
- Swelling or bruising
- Intense pain, especially with movement or weight bearing
- Paresthesia near the injury (often distal to the injury)

Diagnostic procedures for dislocations consist of a history, physical examination, X-rays, and MRI. Immediately following the injury, treatment strategies focus on limiting tissue damage:

- Immobilize the area above and below the joint with a splint or sling in the position that the joint was found.
- Do not attempt to straighten or move the joint.
- Assess for tissue perfusion (e.g., perform a blanch test on skin in the affected area) and report any suspected tissue perfusion impairment immediately.
- Apply ice to ease pain and swelling.
- Do not move the person unless the injury has been completely immobilized.
- Do not move a person with an injury to any weight-bearing joint (e.g., hip, pelvis, or knees) unless it is absolutely necessary.
- Do not give the person anything by mouth (in case surgery is needed).

After the injury has been stabilized, treatment depends on the site and severity of the injury. Reduction may occur spontaneously, or gentle manipulation may be used to return the bones to their usual position (closed reduction). Depending on the amount of pain and swelling, a local anesthetic or even a general anesthetic may be administered before a closed reduction is performed. Pain usually subsides after the joint is reduced. Surgical reduction (open reduction) may be necessary if blood vessels or nerves are damaged or if the dislocation is reoccurring (common with dislocations of the shoulder).

After the reduction, the joint will need to be immobilized with a splint or sling for several weeks. Analgesics and muscle relaxants may be required during this recovery period. After the splint or sling is removed, a gradual rehabilitation program (primarily physical therapy) designed to restore the joint's range of motion and strength is often needed. Strenuous activity involving the injured joint should be avoided until full movement, normal strength, and stability have been regained.

Some dislocations, such as those involving the hip, may need up to several months to heal. Healing of dislocations is also slowed when ligament or soft-tissue damage is present. Preinjury function is usually restored, but some residual deficits may occur in more severe injuries.

Sprains

A **sprain** is an injury to a ligament that often involves stretching or tearing of the ligament. Sprains are caused when a joint is forced to move into an unnatural position (e.g., twisting one's ankle). The severity of the sprain is described using a grading scale (**TABLE 12-2**; FIGURE 12-21). Of all sprains, ankle and knee sprains occur most often. Such an injury triggers the inflammatory process, resulting in edema and pain at the site. Additionally, blood vessels may be damaged, resulting in bleeding and bruising. Bleeding into the joint capsule can delay healing. If a tear occurs, granulation tissue develops along with the inflammation. Collagen fibers form to create a link between the torn ligament fragments, and eventually fibrous tissue binds them together. Sprained ligaments swell rapidly and are painful. Generally, the degree of pain reflects the severity of injury. Other clinical manifestations may include joint stiffness, limited function, disability, and discoloration (usually bruising).

Diagnostic procedures for sprains may consist of a history, physical examination, X-rays, and MRI. Most sprains can be managed at home. Treatment strategies include the following measures:

- Apply ice immediately to reduce pain and swelling. Wrap the ice in a cloth—do not place ice directly on the skin because it can worsen tissue damage.
- Immobilize the joint with a splint or an elastic wrap or bandage (e.g., ACE bandage).
- Elevate the swollen joint above the level of the heart.
- Rest the affected joint for several days and gradually increase activity.
- Provide nonsteroidal anti-inflammatory drugs (NSAIDs; e.g., aspirin and ibuprofen [Motrin]) to relieve pain and inflammation.
- Keep pressure off the injured area until pain subsides (usually 7–10 days for mild sprains and 3–5 weeks for severe sprains). The injured person may require crutches when walking.
- Repair ligament tears surgically.
- Rehabilitate the injured area (usually including physical therapy) to regain joint motion and strength, beginning within 1 week.

TABLE 12-2	Sprain Grading System	
Grade	**Degree of Damage**	**Clinical Findings and Implications**
Grade I	Minimal damage or disruption	Tender without swelling No bruising Active and passive range of motion are painful Prognosis is good, with no expectation of instability or functional loss
Grade II	Moderate damage	Moderate swelling and bruising Very tender, with more diffuse tenderness than grade I Range of motion is very painful and restricted Joint may be unstable, and functional loss may result
Grade III	Complete disruption of the ligament	Prognosis is variable (injury may require surgery) Requires a prolonged healing/rehabilitation period

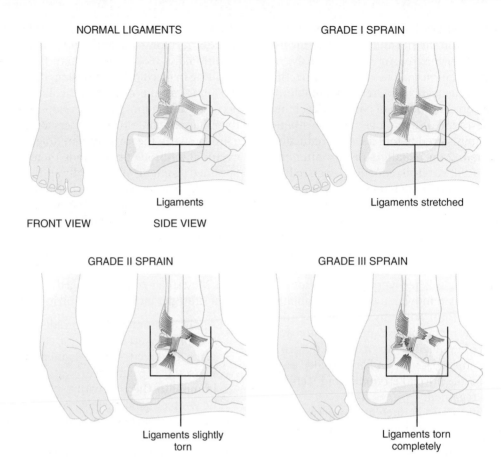

FIGURE 12-21 Sprain grading system.

Treatment strategies for soft-tissue injuries such as sprains and strains can be remembered using the acronym PRICE.

P = Protect the injured limb from further injury by not using the joint. The patient may need crutches or splints to accomplish this.

R = Rest the injured limb, but do not avoid all activity; exercise other muscles to minimize deconditioning.

I = Ice the affected area (e.g., cold pack, a slush bath, or a compression sleeve filled with cold water) as soon as possible after injury to limit swelling, and continue to ice the area for 10–15 minutes (any longer than that may cause tissue damage) 4 times a day for 48 hours.

C = Compress the area with an elastic wrap or bandage; compressive wraps or sleeves made from elastic or neoprene are best.

E = Elevate the injured limb above the level of the heart whenever possible to help prevent or limit swelling.

Strains

A **strain** is an injury to a muscle or tendon that often involves stretching or tearing of the muscle or tendon (**FIGURE 12-22**). Strains may occur suddenly or develop over time. Also called a pulled muscle, a strain results from an awkward muscle movement or excess force that can be caused by

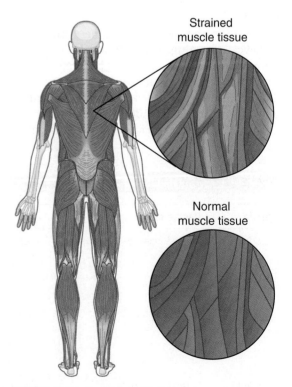

FIGURE 12-22 Strained muscle tissue.

an accident, improper use of a muscle, or overuse of a muscle. Excessive physical activity, improper stretching prior to activity, and poor flexibility can contribute to this injury. The lower back is the most common site for strains. The severity of the strain is described using a grading scale similar to that used for sprains (Table 12-2).

Strains follow the same pathogenesis pathway as sprains (e.g., inflammation, granulation, and bleeding). Scar tissue may be present as the tissue heals. Clinical manifestations of a strain include pain, stiffness, difficulty moving the affected muscle, skin discoloration (often bruising), and edema.

Diagnostic procedures for strains may consist of a history, physical examination, X-rays, and MRIs. Treatment strategies for strains are similar to those for sprains:

- Apply ice immediately to reduce pain and swelling; wrap the ice in cloth and do not place ice directly on the skin because it can worsen tissue damage.
- Use ice for the first 3 days; after then, either heat or ice may be helpful.
- Rest the affected muscle for at least a day.
- Keep the affected muscle elevated above the level of the heart (if possible).
- Avoid using the affected muscle until pain subsides; then, advance activity slowly and in moderation.
- Use NSAIDs to relieve pain and inflammation.
- Use muscle relaxants to relieve muscle stiffness.
- Repair severe tendon tears surgically.
- Rehabilitate the injured area (usually including physical therapy) to regain muscle movement and strength as necessary.

Herniated Intervertebral Disk

A **herniated intervertebral disk** describes a state in which the nucleus pulposus (the inner gelatinous component of the intervertebral disk) protrudes through the annulus fibrosus (the tough outer covering of the disk) (**FIGURE 12-23**). This condition may also be called a slipped disk or ruptured disk. The tear in the capsule may occur suddenly or gradually. Such a condition may be considered either an orthopedic or a neurologic problem because protrusions into the extradural space can exert pressure on the spinal cord, interfering with nerve conduction (**FIGURE 12-24**). Sensory, motor, or autonomic function may be impaired depending on the location of injury. The most frequently involved vertebrae are in the lumbosacral region, but some injuries may involve the cervical disks. If pressure

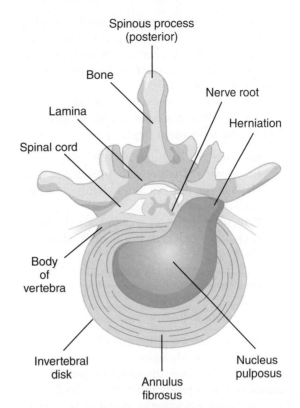

FIGURE 12-23 Herniated vertebral disk.

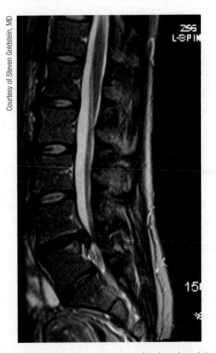

Courtesy of Steven Goldstein, MD

FIGURE 12-24 Spinal cord compression by a herniated disk.

on nerve tissue or blood supply is prolonged or severe, permanent neurologic damage may result.

A herniated intervertebral disk often occurs due to improper body mechanics, lifting heavy objects, repetitive use, or trauma (e.g., a fall or a blow to the back). Additional contributing factors include vertebral stress secondary to obesity, degenerative changes secondary to aging, and demineralization secondary to metabolic conditions (e.g., osteoporosis).

Herniated intervertebral disks may be asymptomatic. When present, manifestations may include the following symptoms:

- **Sciatica** (a radiating, aching pain, sometimes with tingling and numbness, that starts in the buttock and extends down the back or side of one leg)
- Pain, paresthesia, or weakness in the lower back and one leg, or in the neck, shoulder, chest, or arm
- Low back pain or leg pain that is worsened by sitting, coughing, sneezing, laughing, bending, or walking
- Limited mobility

Spinal tumors and herniated intervertebral disks may present similarly, so a differential diagnosis should be made. Diagnostic procedures may consist of a history, physical examination (including neurologic assessment), spinal X-rays, spinal CT, spinal MRI, nerve conduction study, myelogram (injection of contrast medium into the spinal fluid, followed by X-rays), and electromyography.

Immediate treatment for herniated intervertebral disks may include a short period of rest, analgesics, NSAIDs, muscle relaxants, physical therapy (including back-strengthening exercises), heat/cold application, and traction. Most people will recover with such treatment and return to their normal functioning, but a small number of patients will need further treatment such as injections (e.g., corticosteroid and chemonucleolysis) into the site or surgical repair (e.g., diskectomy, laminectomy, and spinal fusion). Weight loss may be beneficial if the patient is overweight.

Metabolic Bone Disorders

Metabolic bone disorders refer to a variety of bone conditions associated with mineral abnormalities. These abnormalities may be caused by genetic factors or dietary deficits. Metabolic bone disorders are usually treated easily once identified, but they can lead to significant complications if left untreated (e.g., electrolyte disturbances and fractures).

Osteoporosis

Osteoporosis is a condition characterized by a progressive loss of bone calcium that leaves the bones brittle (**FIGURE 12-25**). This loss can occur due to multiple pathogenetic mechanisms that

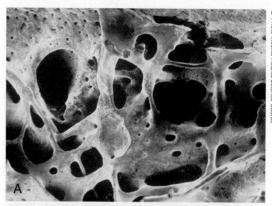
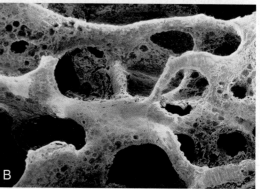

FIGURE 12-25 Osteoporosis. The loss of estrogen or prolonged immobilization weakens bone. In these situations, bone is dissolved and becomes brittle and easily breakable. (a) Normal bone. (b) Bone weakened by osteoporosis.

interact to cause either a decrease in osteoblast activity or an increase in osteoclast activity. The spongy bone becomes porous, particularly in the vertebrae and wrist, and the compact bone becomes thin (**FIGURE 12-26**). Osteoporosis can occur as a primary or secondary condition. The incidence of this common disease is affected by factors including genetic, dietary, and hormonal influences. Approximately 54 million Americans have osteoporosis and low bone density, putting them at risk for osteoporosis (National Osteoporosis Foundation, 2016).

By age 20, the average woman has acquired most of her skeletal mass. Subsequently, a large decline in bone mass occurs with advanced age, increasing the risk of osteoporosis. For women, this decrease occurs around the time of menopause because of hormonal changes. A person with high bone mass as a young adult is more likely to have a higher bone mass later in life; therefore, achieving maximum bone mass in young adulthood is important for maintaining bone health throughout the life span. In particular, adequate calcium consumption and physical activity (including weight-bearing exercises) early in life are vital to achieve maximum bone mass in adulthood.

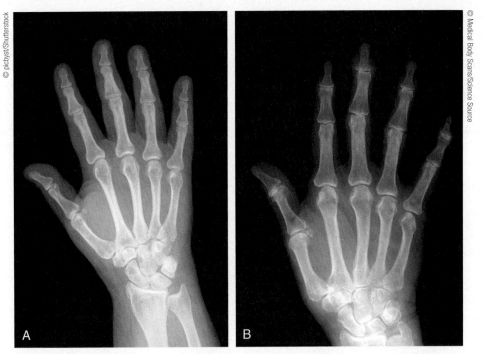

FIGURE 12-26 Bone changes of osteoporosis. (a) An X-ray of normal bones. (b) An X-ray of bones affected by osteoporosis.

Deficient intake of protein, vitamin C, and vitamin D as well as excessive intake of phosphorus (which is present in high levels in soda) also increase the risk of osteoporosis. Individuals who have had gastrointestinal procedures such as a gastrectomy or gastrointestinal bypass are at particular risk of developing osteoporosis because of the nutritional deficits that often occur as a result of these surgeries. In addition, Caucasians (especially those with fair skin tone) and Asians are at higher risk for developing osteoporosis because of their (genetically determined) smaller bones. Other risk factors include smoking, excessive alcohol or caffeine consumption, use of certain medications (e.g., corticosteroids, chemotherapy, thyroid replacements, heparin, and antacids), specific health conditions (e.g., Cushing's disease, thyroid dysfunction, hyperparathyroidism, bone tumors, malabsorption, and anorexia nervosa), being underweight, and family history.

Osteoporosis increases an individual's risk of bone fractures, especially in the wrist, hip, and spine. An estimated one in two women and one in four men age 50 or older will experience a fracture secondary to osteoporosis. This risk for fractures significantly increases mortality rates in the elderly, particularly in individuals who experience hip fractures (20% of whom will die within a year of the fracture).

Osteoporosis is often asymptomatic in its early stages, and a fracture may be the first indication of its presence. As the disease progresses, clinical manifestations may include the following signs and symptoms:

- **Osteopenia** (bone mass that is less than expected for age, ethnicity, or gender)
- Bone pain or tenderness
- Fractures with little or no trauma
- Low back and neck pain
- Kyphosis (**FIGURE 12-27**)
- Height reduction (as much as 6 inches) over time

Because of the high prevalence rates of this disease, screening for osteoporosis should be conducted periodically on those persons at risk. Diagnostic procedures include a history, physical examinations, bone mineral density scans (e.g., dual energy X-ray absorptiometry), X-rays, spinal CT, and serum test (e.g., calcium, thyroid hormones, parathyroid hormone, estrogen, and vitamin D).

Treatment strategies focus on minimizing further bone loss and, in some cases, restoring bone density. These strategies may include the following measures:

- Proper nutrition (especially increasing dietary calcium and vitamin D intake)
- Increasing physical activity (including weight-bearing activities)
- Eliminating modifiable risk factors (e.g., smoking cessation and limited alcohol and caffeine consumption)

- Pharmacologic therapies, including the following:
  - Bisphosphonates (which inhibit bone breakdown, preserve bone mass, and increase bone density)
  - Estrogen receptor modulators (which mimic estrogen)
  - Calcitonin (which increases calcium and phosphate deposits in the bone)

- Safety measures (e.g., assistive devices, handrails, and removal of clutter)
- Pain management (e.g., analgesics, heat and cold application, and relaxation techniques)
- Surgical repair of fractures or weakened bones

Rickets and Osteomalacia

Rickets is a softening and weakening of bones in children, usually because of an extreme and

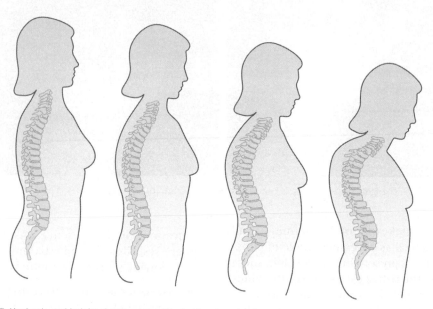

FIGURE 12-27 Kyphosis and height changes associated with osteoporosis.

Myth Busters

Osteoporosis is a common condition associated with several myths that warrant discussion.

Myth 1: People with osteoporosis can feel their bones getting weaker.

Osteoporosis often has no apparent symptoms. In fact, breaking a bone may be the first clue that someone has osteoporosis. Some people may learn they have osteoporosis after they lose height from one or more vertebral fractures. These fractures can even occur without any noticeable pain. Thus, individuals at risk should be screened for this often "silent" disease.

Myth 2: Children and teens do not need ot worry about their bone health.

While it is true that osteoporosis typically appears in older populations, building strong bones and preventing osteoporosis begins in youth. Bone mass peaks around the third decade of life. Being physically active and getting enough calcium and vitamin D early, and maintaining these habits throughout life, can build strong bones for later in life.

Myth 3: Osteoporosis isn't serious.

This is an important myth to dispel. The fractures that can result from osteoporosis can be very painful and have serious complications. Older individuals are at particular risk for life-altering and life-threatening effects from these fractures. These individuals tend to be immobile for longer periods of time because of their extended healing time, which puts them at risk for problems associated with immobility (e.g., renal calculi, thrombus, constipation, decubiti, and incontinence).

Data from National Osteoporosis Foundation. (2016). What is osteoporosis and what causes it? Retrieved from https://www.nof.org/patients/what-is-osteoporosis/

prolonged vitamin D, calcium, or phosphate deficiency. When this condition occurs in adults, it is called **osteomalacia**. If the blood levels of these minerals become too low, calcium and phosphate are released from the bones to maintain homeostasis. This shift of minerals out of the bone leads to weak and soft bones.

Vitamin D plays an essential role in promoting absorption of calcium and phosphorus from the gastrointestinal tract. This vitamin is absorbed from food or produced by the skin when exposed to sunlight. Lack of vitamin D production by the skin may occur in people who live in climates with little exposure to sunlight, must stay indoors (e.g., bedbound or institutionalized persons), work indoors during the daylight hours, or have dark skin. Dietary deficiency may occur with persons who are lactose intolerant, do not drink milk products, or follow a vegetarian diet. Infants who are only breastfed may also develop vitamin D deficiency because human milk does not supply the proper amount of vitamin D. Using very strong sunscreen and limiting sun exposure to minimize skin cancer risk may also increase the risk for vitamin D deficiency. Conditions that reduce the digestion or absorption of fats will make it more difficult for vitamin D to be absorbed into the body (e.g., celiac disease, cystic fibrosis, and undergoing a gastrectomy).

Insufficient dietary calcium and phosphorus intake can also lead to rickets, but this condition is rare in developed countries because calcium and phosphorus are found in both milk and green vegetables. Rickets may also occur because of genetic influences. Hereditary rickets occurs when the kidneys are unable to reabsorb phosphate. For this reason, rickets may occur in some individuals with renal disease. Occasionally, this metabolic bone disorder may occur in children who have liver disorders or who cannot convert vitamin D to its active form.

Clinical manifestations of rickets and osteomalacia develop slowly, as the bones weaken over time. Rickets may become apparent as the soft bones cannot support the growing child. Manifestations in adults and children usually include the following signs and symptoms:

- Skeletal deformities (e.g., bowed legs, asymmetrical skull, scoliosis, kyphosis, pelvic deformities, sternum projection) **(FIGURE 12-28)**
- Fractures
- Delayed growth in height or limbs
- Dental problems (e.g., defects in tooth structure, dental caries, poor enamel, delayed teeth formation)

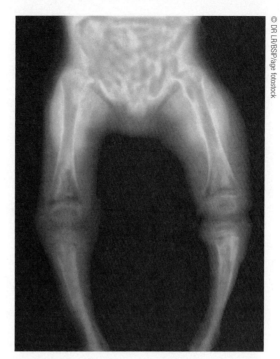

FIGURE 12-28 Rickets.

- Bone pain (usually a dull, aching pain or tenderness in the spine, pelvis, and legs)
- Muscle cramps or weakness

Diagnostic procedures for rickets and osteomalacia include a history, physical examination, serum mineral levels, serum parathyroid hormone levels, serum alkaline phosphatase, X-rays, and bone density study. Treatment focuses on correcting or managing the underlying cause. Providing calcium, phosphorus, or vitamin D that is lacking will eliminate most symptoms. The body's vitamin D levels can be increased through dietary intake (e.g., fish, liver, and processed milk), exposure to moderate amounts of sunlight, or administration of vitamin D supplements. Calcium levels can be increased through dietary intake (e.g., dairy products; dark green, leafy vegetables; and nuts). Positioning or bracing may be used to reduce or prevent deformities associated with rickets and osteomalacia, although some skeletal deformities may require corrective surgery.

Paget's Disease

Paget's disease is a progressive condition characterized by abnormal bone destruction and remodeling, which results in bone deformities **(FIGURE 12-29)**. In the usual bone metabolism process, old bone is recycled into new bone throughout the life span. In Paget's disease,

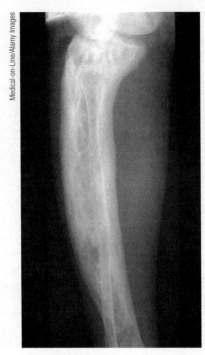

FIGURE 12-29 Paget's disease.

however, the rate at which old bone is broken down and new bone forms is distorted. Notably, bone turnover proceeds at 20 times the normal rate. Excessive bone destruction occurs, along with the replacement of bone by fibrous tissue and abnormal bone. The new bone is bigger but weakened and filled with new blood vessels (FIGURE 12-30). Over time, Paget's disease results in fragile, misshapen bones. This disease may be present in only one or two areas of the skeleton, or it may occur throughout the body. Paget's disease often involves the pelvis, long bones, skull, and vertebrae.

The exact cause of Paget's disease is unknown, but it is thought be caused by a virus capable of increasing osteoclast activity or genetic defects that produce an increase in interferon-6. An estimated 1 to 3 million people are affected by Paget's disease, but the actual numbers may be higher because this condition is often asymptomatic (Alikhan, Lohr, & Driver, 2015). Paget's disease is more common in men, those of central European descent, and persons with a family history.

Paget's disease proceeds through three phases (lytic, mixed lytic, and blastic), and at any point, multiple stages may be present in different regions of the body. The disease begins with the lytic phase, in which normal bone is resorbed by osteoclasts that are more numerous, are larger, and have more nuclei. These abnormal osteoclasts increase bone turnover. The mixed lytic phase is characterized by rapid increases in bone formation from the numerous osteoblasts present. Although increased in number, these osteoblasts remain morphologically normal. In contrast, the new bone formed by them is abnormal, with collagen fibers being haphazardly deposited throughout the bone structure. In the final blastic phase, the bones formed are weak and deformed. The bone marrow becomes infiltrated by excessive fibrous connective tissue and blood vessels, leading to a hypervascular bone state (Alikhan et al., 2015).

The clinical manifestations of Paget's disease vary depending on the area affected. This condition is often insidious in onset and may be asymptomatic early. When present, clinical manifestations may include the following signs and symptoms:

- Bone pain (may be severe and persistent)
- Skeletal deformities (e.g., bowing of the legs, asymmetrical skull, and enlarged head)
- Fractures
- Headache
- Hearing and vision loss
- Joint pain or stiffness
- Neck pain
- Reduced height
- Warmth over the affected bone
- Paresthesia or radiating pain in the affected region (due to nerve compression)
- Hypercalcemia

Complications of Paget's disease may include pathologic fractures, osteoarthritis, heart failure (related to hypercalcemia and increased cardiac workload, as the body must pump more blood to the affected areas), osteosarcoma (bone cancer), and nerve compression.

Diagnostic procedures for Paget's disease consist of a history, physical examination, bone scan, X-rays, serum alkaline phosphatase, and serum calcium. Mild cases may require just periodic monitoring—no treatment. Treatment strategies focus on reducing fractures and

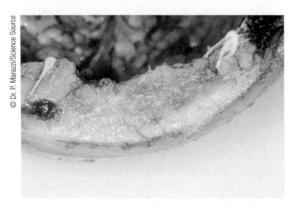

FIGURE 12-30 Paget's disease.

deformities. Pharmacologic therapies may include bisphosphonates (which increase bone density), calcitonin (which increases bone density), NSAIDs (to alleviate pain and inflammation), and analgesics (to relieve pain). Surgery may be required to correct severe bone deformities.

Inflammatory Joint Disorders

Inflammatory joint disorders encompass a group of arthritic conditions that are often degenerative in nature. These conditions involve inflammation that can be triggered by an autoimmune response, excessive use, increased physical stress, or injury. Complications of these conditions often include chronic pain and disability. Treatment strategies focus on slowing the progression, managing pain, and promoting independence.

Osteoarthritis

Osteoarthritis (OA), also known as wear-and-tear arthritis and degenerative joint disease, is a localized joint disease characterized by deterioration of articulating cartilage and its underlying bone as well as bony overgrowth (**FIGURE 12-31**; **TABLE 12-3**). The surface of the cartilage becomes rough and worn, interfering with joint movement. Tissue damage triggers the release of enzymes from local cells that accelerate cartilage disintegration. Eventually, the subchondral bone is exposed and damaged, and cysts and osteophytes (bone spurs) develop as the bone attempts to remold itself. Pieces of the osteophytes and cartilage break off into the synovial cavity, which further increases irritation. Additionally, nearby muscles and ligaments may become weakened and loose. These changes collectively cause narrowing of the joint space, joint instability, stiffness, and pain. The joints most commonly affected by OA are the knees, hips, and joints in the hands and spine. OA is not inflammatory in origin, but inflammation results from the tissue irritation. Erosion of the cartilage usually occurs secondary to excessive mechanical stress on the joint (e.g., aging, obesity, overuse, injury, and congenital musculoskeletal conditions). Additionally, OA may occur as a primary condition in which the cause is idiopathic.

The Centers for Disease Control and Prevention (CDC, 2015b) estimates that nearly 27 million Americans have OA, with women having higher prevalence rates than men. OA is a significant contributor of disability, healthcare costs, and job loss in the United States.

Disease onset is gradual and usually begins after the age of 40. The following clinical manifestations often develop slowly and worsen over time:

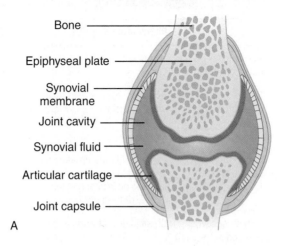

Normal synovial joint

Bone
Epiphyseal plate
Synovial membrane
Joint cavity
Synovial fluid
Articular cartilage
Joint capsule

A

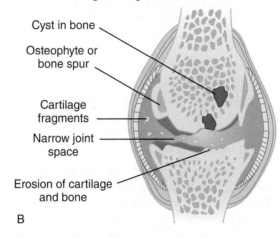

Pathologic changes in osteoarthritis

Cyst in bone
Osteophyte or bone spur
Cartilage fragments
Narrow joint space
Erosion of cartilage and bone

B

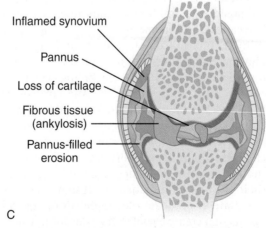

Pathologic changes in rheumatoid arthritis

Inflamed synovium
Pannus
Loss of cartilage
Fibrous tissue (ankylosis)
Pannus-filled erosion

C

FIGURE 12-31 Pathological changes associated with osteoarthritis and rheumatoid arthritis.

- Joint pain that is exacerbated during or after movement or weight bearing
- Joint tenderness with light pressure
- Joint stiffness, especially upon rising in the morning or after a period of inactivity

TABLE 12-3 | Comparison of Major Features of Common Types of Arthritis

	Rheumatoid Arthritis	Osteoarthritis	Gout
Age and sex of usual patient	Young and middle-aged, female	Adult, older persons, both sexes	Middle-aged, male
Major characteristic	Systemic disease with major effects in joints; causes chronic synovitis	"Wear and tear"; degeneration of articular cartilage	Disturbance of purine metabolism; acute episodes caused by crystals of uric acid in joints
Secondary effects of disease	Ingrowth of inflammatory tissue over cartilage destroys cartilage, leads to destruction of joint space; deformities common	Overgrowth of bone; thickening of periarticular soft tissues	Deposits of uric acid in joints with damage to joints (gouty arthritis); soft tissue tophi
Joints usually affected	Small joints of hands and feet	Major weight-bearing joints	Small joints; joint at base of great toe often affected
Special features	Autoantibody against gamma globulin (rheumatoid factor)	No systemic symptoms or biochemical abnormalities	High blood level of uric acid

- Enlarged, hard joints
- Joint swelling
- Limited joint range of motion
- Crepitus
- Hard nodules around the affected joint (bone spurs)

Diagnostic procedures for OA consist of a history, physical examination, X-rays, and MRI. There is currently no cure for OA. The goals of treatment are to increase joint strength, maintain joint mobility, reduce disability, and relieve pain. Treatment strategies may include a combination of physical therapy, weight loss/management, ambulatory aids (e.g., walkers and canes), orthopedic devices (e.g., braces and splints), pharmacologic agents, and surgery. Pharmacologic therapies may involve oral and topical analgesics, NSAIDs (including cyclooxygenase 2 [COX-2] inhibitors), and corticosteroids. Additionally, synthetic synovial fluid and corticosteroids may be injected directly into the joint. Herbal therapies that may be helpful include glucosamine, chondroitin, and ginger, although research evidence is mixed regarding their efficacy. Pain management may focus on adequate rest, heat/cold application, topical agents that create a cool or hot sensation, water therapy (e.g., whirlpool, water aerobics), acupuncture, tai chi, and yoga.

In some cases, surgery may be necessary to repair or replace damaged joints. These procedures may include arthroscopy to trim torn and damaged cartilage, osteotomy to change the alignment of a bone and relieve stress on the bone or joint, surgical fusion, and arthroplasty to completely or partially replace the damaged joint with an artificial joint.

Rheumatoid Arthritis

Rheumatoid arthritis (RA) is a systemic, autoimmune condition involving multiple joints. In RA, the inflammatory process primarily affects the synovial membrane, but it can also affect other organs (e.g., heart, skin, and eyes). Most cases of RA follow a typical autoimmune pattern of remissions and exacerbations. This type of arthritis usually starts with an initial acute inflammatory episode, after which the joint may appear to recover. The process is repeated with each exacerbation and includes synovitis, pannus formation (granulation tissue), cartilage erosion (due to enzymes from the pannus), fibrosis, and **ankylosis** (joint fixation and deformity) (Figure 12-31; Table 12-3). Over time, the recurring inflammation has a cumulative effect: it thickens the synovium, which can eventually invade and destroy the cartilage and bone within the joint. In addition, the muscles, tendons, and ligaments that hold the joint together weaken and stretch. Gradually, the joint loses its shape and alignment.

The course and the severity of this illness can vary considerably. Nevertheless, RA usually affects joints on both sides of the body equally. Wrists, fingers, knees, feet, and ankles are the most commonly affected.

The exact cause of RA is unknown, but it is thought to be caused by a genetic vulnerability that permits a virus or bacterium to trigger the disease. Risk factors include family history, advancing age (although a juvenile form also exists), and smoking. RA is more common in women, and research is being conducted to explore the potential role that hormones might play in its etiology. RA rates in the United States have declined since 1990. According to the CDC (2016b), an estimated 1.5 million Americans have RA.

Like other autoimmune disorders, RA is typically characterized by remissions and exacerbations. The disease onset is usually insidious, with vague manifestations that can mimic other conditions. Clinical manifestations are progressive and may include the following signs and symptoms:

- Fatigue
- Anorexia
- Low-grade fever
- Lymphadenopathy
- Malaise
- Muscle spasms
- Morning stiffness lasting longer than 1 hour
- Warmth, tenderness, and stiffness in the joints when not used for as little as 1 hour
- Bilateral joint pain
- Swollen and boggy joints
- Limited joint range of motion
- Contractures and joint deformity (e.g., boutonniere deformity and swan neck deformity) (FIGURE 12-32)
- Unsteady gait
- Depression
- Anemia

Diagnostic procedures for RA may consist of a history, physical examination, serum rheumatoid factor test, serum anticyclic citrullinated peptide antibodies test, erythrocyte sedimentation rate test, serum C-reactive protein, serum antinuclear antibody, synovial fluid analysis (rheumatoid factor is usually present), joint X-rays, joint MRI, and joint ultrasounds. There is no cure for RA, so treatment focuses on slowing the progression, managing the pain, and promoting independence. Early, aggressive treatment for RA can delay joint destruction. Treatment strategies are complex and often require the support of a multidisciplinary team (made up of a rheumatologist, nurse, and a wide

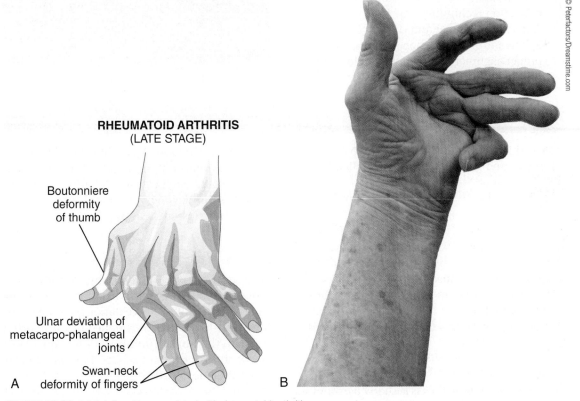

RHEUMATOID ARTHRITIS
(LATE STAGE)

Boutonniere deformity of thumb

Ulnar deviation of metacarpo-phalangeal joints

Swan-neck deformity of fingers

A   B

© Peterfactors/Dreamstime.com

FIGURE 12-32 Joint deformities associated with rheumatoid arthritis.

range of therapists). Strategies may include the following measures:

- Adequate rest and pacing activities
- Physical and occupational therapy (including therapy directed at maintaining or increasing range of motion)
- Regular exercise
- Pharmacologic therapies, including the following:
  - NSAIDs (to relieve pain and inflammation)
  - Corticosteroids (either orally or as an intra-articular injection to decrease inflammation)
  - Disease-modifying antirheumatic drugs (to decrease inflammatory response), including the following:
    - Gold compounds
    - Immunosuppressant agents (e.g., methotrexate)
    - Antimalarial agents (e.g., hydroxy-chloroquine [Plaquenil])
  - Biologic response–modifying agents (e.g., infliximab [Remicade]) (which block tumor necrosis factor, an inflammatory cytokine associated with RA)
  - Herbal therapies, including thunder god vine, plant oils, and fish oil
- Nonpharmacologic pain management (e.g., relaxation techniques, tai chi)
- Application of heat and cold
- Splints and braces (to support joints, maintain proper alignment, and prevent deformities)
- Assistive devices (e.g., walkers and rails)
- Coping strategies and support
- Surgical repair (e.g., synovectomy and arthroplasty)

Gout

Gout is an inflammatory disease resulting from deposits of uric acid crystals (monosodium urate) in tissues and fluids within the body (**FIGURE 12-33**; Table 12-3). The body produces uric acid when it breaks down purines, a substance naturally found in the body as well as in certain foods (e.g., organ meats, shellfish, anchovies, herring, asparagus, and mushrooms). Normally, uric acid dissolves in the blood and is excreted by the kidneys. Gout results from an overproduction or underexcretion (most common) of uric acid (urate), although not all people with hyperuricemia have gout.

Gout affects approximately 8.3 million people in the United States, but is most common in

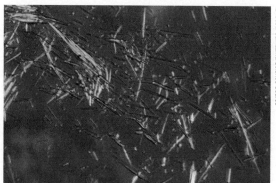

FIGURE 12-33 Uric acid crystals in the synovial fluid.

© Scott Camazine/Science Source

Myth Busters

Arthritis is a common condition associated with several myths that should be dispelled.

Myth 1: Cracking your joints causes arthritis.

As arthritis myths go, this one is a biggie. When you crack a joint, you are actually either snapping the ligament over the joint or pulling on the joint, which causes a negative nitrogen bubble. You are not cracking the bone—just manipulating the joint to make it feel better—so cracking your joints does *not* cause arthritis.

Myth 2: Being double-jointed increases your risk for arthritis.

The term *double-jointed* is actually a misnomer. No one has two joints where there should be

one. Some people have hypermobility (or extra flexibility) in their joints, but there is no evidence to suggest this condition causes arthritis. However, hypermobility could cause other injuries such as sprains, strains, and tears.

Myth 3: Vaccinations can cause arthritis.

This notion is a hot topic, but the Arthritis Foundation's position is that immunizations (particularly rubella vaccinations) do not cause arthritis. No research evidence has supported this myth. Some immunizations can cause some short-term joint aching, but that effect is not the same as arthritis.

males and African Americans (CDC, 2016a). It may occur as a primary inborn error in metabolism or secondary to some contributing factor. Factors contributing to its development include being overweight or obese, having certain diseases (e.g., hypertension, diabetes mellitus, renal disease, and sickle cell anemia), consuming alcohol (beer and spirits more so than wine), using certain medications (e.g., diuretics), and eating a diet rich in meat and seafood.

Gout typically follows four phases. Initially, the individual with gout is asymptomatic, though uric levels are climbing in the bloodstream and uric acid crystals are being deposited in the tissues (FIGURE 12-34). Over time, these crystals accumulate, damaging tissues. This damage triggers an acute inflammation that characterizes the second phase of gout, referred to as acute flares or attacks. A flare is distinguished by pain, burning, redness, swelling, and warmth at the affected joint lasting days to weeks. Pain may be mild or excruciating. Most initial attacks occur in the lower extremities. The metatarsophalangeal joint of the big toe is the presenting joint for 50% of people with gout. After the acute attack subsides, the person may enter intercritical periods in which the disease remains clinically inactive until the next flare (the third phase). The person with gout continues to have hyperuricemia, which results in continued deposits of uric acid crystals in tissues that causes damage. These intercritical periods become shorter as the disease progresses. Reoccurring attacks are often precipitated by sudden increases in serum uric acid. In the final phase,

chronic gout is characterized by chronic arthritis, associated with soreness and aching of joints. People with gout may also develop tophi (large, hard nodules composed of uric acid crystals deposited in soft tissue), usually in cooler areas of the body (e.g., toes, elbows, ears, and distal finger joints). Because some renal calculi (kidney stones) are made of uric acid, renal calculi may also be associated with gout (see the *Urinary Function* chapter).

Clinical manifestations of gout vary depending on the phase that the individual is experiencing. Manifestations of acute gout attacks include the following symptoms:

- Intense pain at the affected joint (usually the big toe) that frequently starts during the night and is often described as throbbing, crushing, burning, or excruciating
- Joint warmth, redness, swelling, and tenderness (even to light touch)
- Fever

After a first gout attack, patients may have no symptoms for varying lengths of time. Some people may go months or even years between gout attacks. Although some individuals develop chronic gouty arthritis, others have no further attacks. Those patients with chronic arthritis develop joint deformities and limited joint mobility. With chronic gout, joint pain and other symptoms will be present most of the time. Tophi may form below the skin around joints or in other places with chronic gout. Tophi can cause a local inflammatory response, and draining them may reveal the presence of a chalky material.

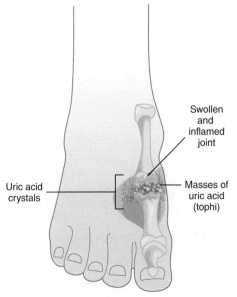

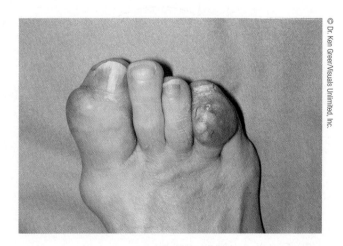

© Dr. Ken Greer/Visuals Unlimited, Inc.

Uric acid crystals

Swollen and inflamed joint

Masses of uric acid (tophi)

FIGURE 12-34 Gout.

Diagnostic procedures for gout include a history, physical examination, serum uric acid levels, urine uric acid levels (will be low in those with gout caused by underexcretion), synovial fluid analysis (presence of uric acid crystals), and joint X-rays. Treatment strategies focus on lowering uric acid levels, usually with medications and dietary changes. Medications often vary depending on the current phase of gout the patient is experiencing. Treatment strategies may include the following measures:

- Pharmacologic therapy for acute gout attacks, including the following:
  - NSAIDs to control inflammation and pain; higher doses may be used to stop an acute attack
  - Colchicine, an analgesic that is particularly effective in reducing gout pain
  - Corticosteroids to relieve inflammation and pain
- Pharmacologic therapies to prevent the complications associated with frequent gout attacks, including the following:

- Xanthine oxidase inhibitors (e.g., allopurinol [Zyloprim]) to block uric acid production
- Probenecid (Probalan) to improve renal excretion of uric acid
- Avoiding triggers (e.g., stress, high protein intake, and alcohol intake)

Ankylosing Spondylitis

Ankylosing spondylitis is a progressive inflammatory disorder affecting the sacroiliac joints, intervertebral spaces, and costovertebral joints. The inflammation associated with this condition starts in the vertebral joints. As the inflammation persists, new bone forms in an attempt to remodel the damage. Fibrosis and calcification, or fusion, of the joints follows. The vertebral joints become fixed, or ankylosed, and lose mobility. Inflammation begins in the lower back at the sacroiliac joints and progresses up the spine. The vertebrae appear square, and the vertebral column becomes rigid and loses curvature (**FIGURE 12-35**).

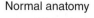

Normal anatomy

Ankylosing spondylitis

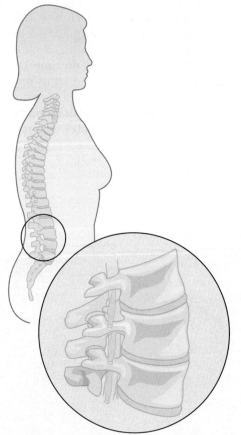

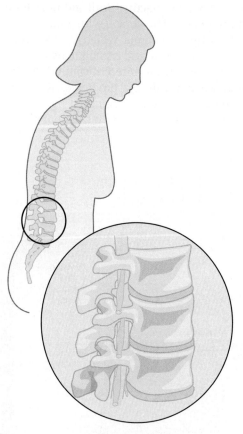

Normal S-curve of spine

Loss of normal curvature

FIGURE 12-35 Ankylosing spondylitis.

The exact cause of ankylosing spondylitis is unknown, although genetic factors seem to be involved. In particular, people who have a gene called *HLA-B27* are at significantly increased risk of this condition. Ankylosing spondylitis is more common in males than in females and typically appears between 20 and 40 years of age. Complications include kyphosis, osteoporosis, respiratory compromise (due to reduced lung expansion resulting from fusion of the rib cage), endocarditis (inflammation of the internal cardiac structures), and uveitis (inflammation of the eye).

Clinical manifestations of ankylosing spondylitis reflect the decreased joint mobility. The individual may experience periods of remission and exacerbation. The following manifestations may worsen as the disease progresses:

- Intermittent lower back pain (early)
- Pain and stiffness that typically worsens with inactivity (e.g., when sleeping) and improves after activity
- Lower back pain that evolves to include the entire back
- Pain in other joints (especially the shoulders, hips, or lower extremities)
- Muscle spasms
- Fatigue
- Low-grade fever
- Weight loss
- Kyphosis

Diagnostic procedures for ankylosing spondylitis may consist of a history, physical examination, test for serum presence of the *HLA-B27* gene, erythrocyte sedimentation rate, C-reactive protein, spine X-rays, spine CT, and spine MRI. The goal of treatment is to relieve pain and stiffness as well as prevent or delay complications and spinal deformity. Treatment of ankylosing spondylitis is most successful when it is initiated before the disease causes irreversible damage (e.g., fusion), especially in positions that limit function. Treatment strategies may include the following measures:

- NSAIDs, disease-modifying antirheumatic drugs, corticosteroids, and tumor necrosis factor blockers to relieve inflammation, pain, and stiffness
- Muscle relaxants to treat muscle spasms
- Physical therapy (including range-of-motion exercises and positioning)
- Surgical repair
- Health-promoting lifestyle behaviors (e.g., proper nutrition, adequate rest, stress management, and smoking cessation)
- Coping strategies and support

Chronic Muscle Disorders

Chronic muscle disorders include conditions that result from a wide range of causes (e.g., genetic predisposition, trauma, and infection). These conditions may lead to chronic pain, weakness, and paralysis. Chronic muscle disorders may be progressive, requiring lifelong treatment. Because most of these conditions have no known cure, treatment is often aimed at managing symptoms.

Muscular Dystrophy

Muscular dystrophy (MD) refers to a group of inherited, non-inflammatory disorders characterized by degeneration of skeletal muscle. Muscles become weaker as damage from these disorders worsens. Nine different forms of MD are distinguished (including Becker's MD, Duchenne MD, myotonic MD, and limb-girdle MD), each with its own pattern of inheritance (e.g., X-linked recessive, autosomal dominant, and autosomal recessive) and pathogenesis (e.g., age of onset and progression). The commonality across all types is the presence of a muscle protein abnormality (dystrophin). This defect causes muscle dysfunction, weakness, muscle fiber loss, and inflammation, and it may involve other tissues (e.g., cardiac and smooth muscle tissues). Over time, fat and fibrosis connective tissues eventually replace skeletal muscle fibers in persons with MD.

Some types of MD are rare, while others are relatively common. Most types of MD are inherited, but some may occur because of a genetic mutation (often spontaneously). Some types cause tremendous disability and rapid decline, whereas others are associated with minimal symptoms and hardly noticeable progression. Some types present in childhood, while others present in late adulthood. Duchenne MD is the most common and severe type, affecting only males (X-linked recessive). Complications of MD may include cardiomyopathy, recurrent respiratory infections, respiratory compromise, and death.

Clinical manifestations of MD vary depending on the type. All of the muscles may be affected or just a selected group. In general, manifestations may include the following signs and symptoms:

- Intellectual disability (in some types)
- Muscle weakness that slowly worsens to hypotonia
- Muscle spasms
- Delayed development of muscle motor skills

- Difficulty using one or more muscle groups
- Poor coordination
- Drooling
- Ptosis (eyelid drooping)
- Frequent falls
- Problems walking (e.g., delayed walking)
- Gower's maneuver (an affected child pushes to an erect position by using his or her hands to climb the legs)
- Progressive loss of joint mobility and contractures (e.g., clubfoot and foot drop)
- Unilateral calf hypertrophy
- Scoliosis or lordosis

Diagnostic procedures for MD may consist of a history, physical examination, muscle biopsy, electromyography, electrocardiogram, serum creatine kinase levels, test for serum presence of defective dystrophin, and genetic testing. Additionally, fetal chorionic villus testing can be performed prenatally at 12 weeks' gestation.

There is no cure for MD; however, gene therapy may potentially be feasible. Currently, the goal of treatment is to maintain motor function and prevent deformities as long as possible. Treatment strategies may include physical therapy, proper nutrition, muscle relaxants, immunosuppressant agents, assistive devices (e.g., walker, braces, and splints), and surgical contracture release. Additionally, coping strategies and support for the patient and caregivers may be beneficial.

Fibromyalgia

Fibromyalgia is a syndrome predominately characterized by widespread muscular pains and fatigue. This disorder affects joints, muscles, tendons, and surrounding tissues. Eighteen fibromyalgia-specific pressure points (**FIGURE 12-36**), where pain or tenderness may be stimulated, have been identified in the neck, shoulder, trunk, and limbs. No apparent inflammation or degeneration is associated with fibromyalgia. Its cause remains uncertain, but fibromyalgia may be related to an altered pattern of central neurotransmission that results in sensitivity to substance P (a neurotransmitter responsible for pain sensation). Other pain-processing abnormalities that have been identified in patients with fibromyalgia include decreased levels of inhibitory neurotransmitters (e.g., serotonin and norepinephrine), enhanced temporal summation of second pain (delayed, longer-lasting pain), altered endogenous opioid analgesic activity,

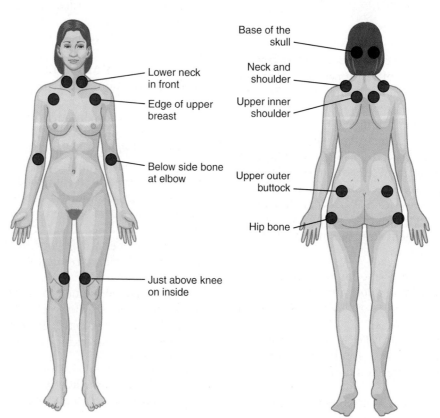

FIGURE 12-36 Fibromyalgia-specific pressure points.

and dopamine dysregulation. In fibromyalgia, the brain's pain receptors seem to develop a sort of pain memory and become more sensitive to pain signals (i.e., lowered pain threshold). Additional postulated causes include physical or emotional trauma, sleep disturbances, altered skeletal muscle metabolism, infections, and genetic predisposition. The CDC (2015a) estimates that approximately 5 million Americans have fibromyalgia, with the prevalence rates being highest among women.

Clinical manifestations may vary depending on the weather, stress, fatigue, physical activity, and time of day. In general, fibromyalgia is characterized by widespread pain, typically described as a constant, dull muscle ache. Fatigue, sleep disturbances, depression, irritable bowel syndrome, headaches, and memory problems may also occur with this chronic disorder. Conditions often associated with fibromyalgia include RA, systemic lupus erythematosus, and ankylosing spondylitis.

Diagnostic procedures for fibromyalgia center on the 18 identified pressure points. Diagnosis is based on the presence of widespread pain (at least 3 months' duration) and tenderness on 11 of 18 pressure points. Additional diagnostic procedures consist of a history, physical examination, and other tests to rule out other conditions.

Treatment strategies focus on minimizing symptoms and improving overall health. These strategies may include stress reduction, regular exercise, adequate rest, proper nutrition, heat application, massage therapy, acupuncture, physical therapy, analgesics, NSAIDs, antidepressant agents, muscle relaxants, and antiseizure agents (specifically, pregabalin [Lyrica]). Coping strategies, counseling, and support may be helpful as well.

Bone Tumors

Tumors of the musculoskeletal system typically arise from the bone. The majority of bone tumors are malignant and occur as secondary tumors stemming from other cancers (e.g., breast, lung, and prostate). Bone tumors rarely occur as primary tumors. The exact cause of these primary tumors is unknown, but they are more common in men and Caucasians (National Cancer Institute, 2016). Paget's disease increases the risk of developing primary bone cancer. The overall 5-year survival rate for bone cancer is approximately 67%.

Bone cancer usually occurs in areas of rapid bone growth and is described based on the type of cell in which the cancer originates. Bone cancer types include the following:

- **Osteochondroma**—a tumor that develops adjacent to growth plates. The most common benign bone tumor, it occurs most often in persons between 10 and 20 years of age.
- **Osteosarcoma**—an aggressive tumor that begins in the bone cells, usually in the femur, tibia, or fibula (**FIGURE 12-37**). It occurs most often in children and young adults.
- **Chondrosarcoma**—a slow-growing tumor that begins in the cartilage cells that are

Myth Busters

Fibromyalgia remains a mysterious condition, and two myths about fibromyalgia deserve discussion.

Myth 1: Fibromyalgia is an autoimmune disease.

Fibromyalgia is *not* an autoimmune disease. An autoimmune disease results from the body's overactive and inappropriate immune response. There is no evidence that fibromyalgia follows this path. However, people with fibromyalgia also commonly have one or more autoimmune diseases.

Myth 2: Fibromyalgia is a psychological problem.

Fibromyalgia is a physical disorder with real, measurable, biological abnormalities. This myth probably causes the most frustration for patients with fibromyalgia. After years of being told, "It is all in your head," patients finally have proof that fibromyalgia is a very real, physical illness— research studies have revealed a number of biological abnormalities associated with its development. Nevertheless, despite the scientific evidence, fibromyalgia continues to be dismissed as a psychological problem by many in the medical community, who continue to insist that the symptoms are caused by depression.

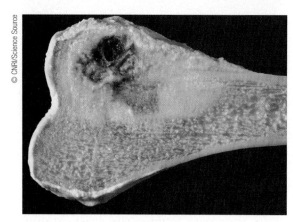

FIGURE 12-37 Osteosarcoma.

commonly found on the ends of bones. It most frequently affects older adults.

- **Ewing's sarcoma**—an aggressive tumor whose origin is unknown. This type of bone tumor may begin in nerve tissue within the bone. Ewing's sarcoma occurs most frequently in children and young adults, and it is 10 times more common in Caucasians as compared to other ethnic groups.

Bone tumors are often asymptomatic in their early stages. When present, clinical manifestations usually include pathologic fractures, bone pain, a palpable mass, fatigue, and unintended weight loss.

Diagnostic procedures for bone tumors may consist of a history, physical examination, X-rays, CT, MRI, positron emission tomography, bone scan, and biopsy. Treatment varies depending on the type and stage of the cancer. Surgical excision or amputation is often the treatment of choice. Radiation and chemotherapy may be used following surgery, if the tumor is inoperable, or in the presence of metastasis.

application to practice

Now that we have discussed conditions of the musculoskeletal system, let's put that knowledge into practice. After receiving the change-of-shift report on the following patients being treated in the orthopedic unit, which patient would you assess first?

- A patient who had an open reduction and internal fixation and casting of a tibia fracture 3 days ago and is complaining of nausea
- A patient who is being discharged with an upper-extremity external fixation device and needs teaching about pin care
- A patient who had an open reduction and internal fixation of a left femoral fracture 6 hours ago and states, "I can't feel my left foot"
- A patient who developed a deep vein thrombosis in the right leg

4 days postoperatively following a hip replacement and has a heparin infusion

Once again, you go through the usual thought process—who would die first, acute versus chronic conditions, Maslow's hierarchy of needs, and patient safety. The patient with the tibia repair is 3 days post surgery and probably has stabilized. This patient is not exhibiting any signs of distress. Nausea is unpleasant but not life threatening. Next, consider the patient who needs pin care education. Education is important and necessary prior to discharge; however, this need is not life threatening or pressing. Now think about the patient who is 6 hours post femoral fracture repair. With the repair being recent and the patient complaining of numbness, this patient may be experiencing some negative effects from the procedure. The numbness may be merely a residual effect of the anesthesia, but it could also be the result of nerve damage. This patient should stay on the short list. Finally, consider the patient with the deep vein thrombosis. Although the thrombosis is a new development, it is being treated with heparin, and the patient is not exhibiting any clinical manifestations indicating any other issues.

After weighing all the options, the patient 6 hours post femoral repair surgery should be assessed first. This assessment would start by evaluating the neurovascular integrity of the patient's left foot and leg. This neurovascular assessment focuses on the five P's—pain, pulse, paralysis, paresthesia, and pallor.

CHAPTER SUMMARY

The musculoskeletal system forms the framework for the body, provides support and protection, and allows for movement. Damage to this system is likely to cause issues with mobility. Musculoskeletal disorders vary from short lived and mild to long term and debilitating in nature. Although most are not life threatening, many of these disorders can result in life-altering effects.

Musculoskeletal damage may be caused by trauma, genetic defects, metabolic imbalances, as well as daily wear and tear. Supporting musculoskeletal health involves strategies such as weight management, proper nutrition, regular exercise, abstaining from smoking, and observing safety precautions (e.g., wearing safety equipment).

REFERENCES

AAOS. (2004). *Paramedic: Anatomy and physiology*. Sudbury, MA: Jones & Bartlett.

Alikhan, M., Lohr, K., & Driver, K. (2015). Paget disease. *Medscape*. Retrieved from http://emedicine.medscape.com /article/334607-overview#a3

Centers for Disease Control and Prevention (CDC). (2015a). Fibromyalgia. Retrieved from http://www.cdc.gov/arthritis /basics/fibromyalgia.htm

Centers for Disease Control and Prevention (CDC). (2015b). Osteoarthritis. Retrieved from http://www.cdc.gov/arthritis /basics/osteoarthritis.htm

Centers for Disease Control and Prevention (CDC). (2016a). Gout. Retrieved from http://www.cdc.gov/arthritis/basics /gout.html

Centers for Disease Control and Prevention (CDC). (2016b). Rheumatoid arthritis. Retrieved from http://www.cdc.gov /arthritis/basics/rheumatoid.htm

Chiras, D. (2011). *Human biology* (7th ed.). Burlington, MA: Jones & Bartlett Learning.

Crowley, L. V. (2017). *An introduction to human disease* (10th ed.). Burlington, MA: Jones & Bartlett Learning.

Elling, B., Elling, K., & Rothenberg, M. (2004). *Anatomy and physiology*. Sudbury, MA: Jones and Bartlett.

Gould, B. (2015). *Pathophysiology for the health professions* (5th ed.). Philadelphia, PA: Elsevier.

Madara, B., & Pomarico-Denino, V. (2008). *Quick look nursing: Pathophysiology* (2nd ed.). Sudbury, MA: Jones and Bartlett.

National Cancer Institute. (2016). Bone and joint cancer. Retrieved from http://seer.cancer.gov/statfacts/html/bones.html

National Osteoporosis Foundation. (2016). What is osteoporosis and what causes it? Retrieved from https://www.nof .org/patients/what-is-osteoporosis/

Professional guide to pathophysiology (3rd ed.). (2010). Philadelphia, PA: Lippincott Williams & Wilkins.

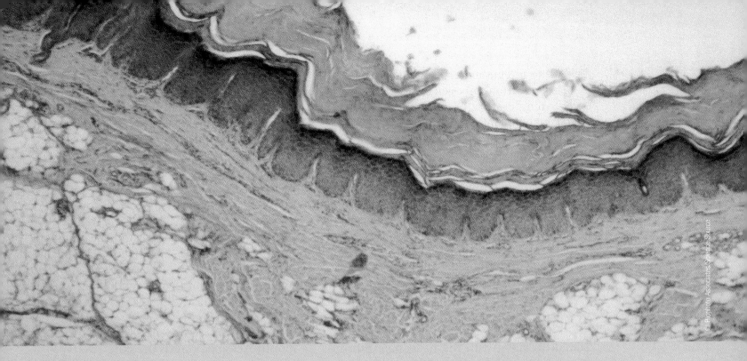

CHAPTER 13
Integumentary Function

LEARNING OBJECTIVES

- Discuss normal integumentary anatomy and physiology.
- Compare and contrast congenital integumentary disorders.
- Describe and discuss integumentary changes and conditions associated with aging.
- Compare and contrast inflammatory integumentary disorders.

- Compare and contrast infectious integumentary disorders.
- Describe and discuss traumatic integumentary disorders.
- Describe and discuss chronic integumentary disorders.
- Describe and discuss integumentary cancers.

KEY TERMS

acne vulgaris	epidermis	mole	skin
albinism	folliculitis	Mongolian spot	skin cancer
apocrine gland	furuncle	necrotizing fasciitis	skin tag
atopic dermatitis	hemangioma	papule	tinea
birthmark	herpes simplex type 1	pediculosis	urticaria
burn	herpes zoster	pigmented birthmark	vascular birthmark
café au lait spot	hypodermis	port-wine stain	verruca
carbuncle	impetigo	psoriasis	vesicle
cellulitis	keratin	rosacea	vitiligo
contact dermatitis	lentigo	scabies	welt
dermis	macular stain	sebaceous gland	
eccrine gland	melanin	sebum	

The integumentary system protects the body from pathogen invasions, regulates temperature, senses environmental changes, and maintains water balance. This system comprises the skin, nails, hair, mucous membranes, and glands. Disorders of the integumentary structures can result in numerous issues because of the extensive functions of this system. Such disorders can stem from a wide range of causes, including congenital defects, advancing age, inflammation, infections, and cancers. Many of these conditions are mild and may not require treatment (e.g., birthmarks), whereas others can be life threatening (e.g., skin cancer).

Anatomy and Physiology

The **skin**, along with the nails, hair, mucous membranes, and glands, constitutes the integumentary system. In addition to participating in sensory functions, the integumentary system plays a key role in immunity (see the *Immunity* chapter), temperature regulation, and water balance. Moreover, this system excretes a small amount of waste products. The integumentary system is the body's largest organ system, covering all external surfaces and accounting for approximately 15% of the body's weight.

The skin consists of three layers—the hypodermis, the dermis, and the epidermis (FIGURE 13-1). The **hypodermis**, or subcutaneous tissue, is the innermost layer of the skin, consisting of soft, fatty tissue as well as blood

vessels, nerves, and immune cells (e.g., macrophages). The **dermis**, the middle layer, is composed of dense, irregular connective tissue and very little fatty tissue. The dermis includes nerves, hair follicles, smooth muscle, glands, blood vessels, and lymphatic vessels. The **epidermis**, or outermost layer of the skin, comprises squamous epithelia, or flat sheets of cells. The epidermis consists of five distinct layers (FIGURE 13-2). New cells proliferate from the innermost layer and push upward. The outer layers often contain 25 sheets of dead cells that are continuously shed. Most of these cells produce **keratin**, a protein that strengthens skin, and **melanin**, a pigment that protects the skin from ultraviolet (UV) rays.

Sebaceous glands produce **sebum**, which moisturizes and protects the skin. Two types of sweat glands are located throughout the skin— eccrine and apocrine glands. **Eccrine glands**, which are also known as merocrine glands, secrete sweat through skin pores in response to the sympathetic nervous system. **Apocrine glands** open into hair follicles in the axillae, scalp, face, and external genitalia.

The skin is home to a complex mixture of normal flora whose composition varies depending on the area of the body. This normal flora consists mostly of bacteria and fungi, which lead to an opportunistic infection when a skin injury occurs. Such superficial opportunistic infections can develop into a severe systemic infection if not managed appropriately.

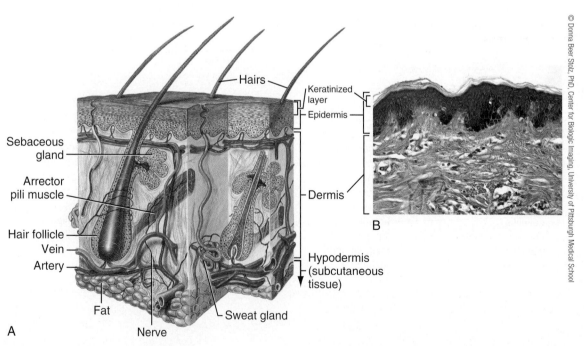

FIGURE 13-1 The layers of the skin.

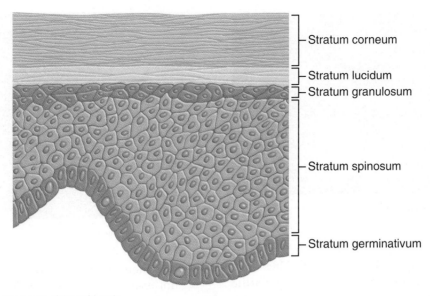

- Stratum corneum
- Stratum lucidum
- Stratum granulosum
- Stratum spinosum
- Stratum germinativum

FIGURE 13-2 The layers of the epidermis.

UNDERSTANDING CONDITIONS THAT AFFECT THE INTEGUMENTARY SYSTEM

When considering alterations of the integumentary system, organizing them based on their basic underlying pathophysiology can increase understanding. With systemic disorders, the primary nursing diagnosis is impaired skin integrity. In such cases, interventions are intended to either prevent such impairment, maintain skin integrity, or improve skin integrity. Because the skin provides a barrier to protect the body from invasion, an additional nursing diagnosis that is relevant is risk for infection. Interventions for this diagnosis are directed at minimizing contamination (e.g., hand washing, wound care) and supporting the immune system (e.g., proper nutrition).

Congenital Integumentary Disorders

Congenital disorders of the integumentary system can vary widely in severity. Many conditions occur because of an error during embryonic development. These errors may occur randomly, due to environmental influences, or because of genetic abnormalities. They may cause either minor conditions with only aesthetic problems (e.g., birthmarks) or life-altering states (e.g., albinism). Occasionally, these seemingly benign conditions may be associated with other, more serious problems that warrant further investigation. Treatment is often unnecessary, but when needed, these options are usually limited.

Birthmarks

Birthmarks are skin anomalies that are present at birth or shortly after. Most are harmless and may even shrink or disappear with age. Birthmarks vary from barely noticeable to disfiguring. These abnormalities may be flat or raised, have regular or irregular borders, and have different shades of coloring including brown, tan, black, pale blue, pink, red, or purple. Birthmarks cannot be prevented and are not the result of anything done or not done during pregnancy. Two types of birthmarks are distinguished—vascular and pigmented.

Vascular birthmarks arise from blood vessels that have not formed correctly; therefore, these birthmarks are generally red. The various types of vascular birthmarks include macular stains, hemangiomas, and port-wine stains.

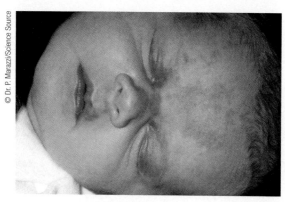

FIGURE 13-3 Macular stain.

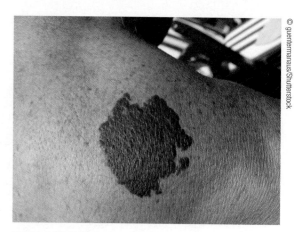

FIGURE 13-5 Port-wine stain.

- **Macular stains**—also called salmon patches, angel kisses, and stork bites—are the most common type of vascular birthmark (FIGURE 13-3). These faint red marks often occur on the forehead, eyelids, posterior neck, nose, upper lip, or posterior head. On a baby, these birthmarks may be more noticeable when crying. Most often these marks fade on their own by 2 years of age, but they sometimes last into adulthood.
- **Hemangiomas**, also referred to as strawberries, are birthmarks that appear as a bright red patch or a nodule of extra blood vessels in the skin (FIGURE 13-4). They may be either superficial or deep. The deep hemangiomas may be bluish because they involve deeper blood vessels. Hemangiomas grow during the first year of life and then usually recede over time. Some hemangiomas, particularly larger ones, may leave scars as they regress; these scars can be corrected by minor plastic surgery. Many hemangiomas are found on the head or neck, although they can appear anywhere on the body. Most are benign and not associated with other medical conditions, but they can cause complications if their location interferes with sight, feeding, breathing, or other bodily functions.
- **Port-wine stains** are discolorations that look like wine was spilled on an area of the body—hence their name (FIGURE 13-5). These birthmarks most often occur on the face, neck, arms, and legs. Port-wine stains can be any size, but they grow only as the child grows. They tend to darken over time and can thicken and have a cobblestone texture in mid-adulthood unless treated. Port-wine stains will not resolve spontaneously, and those occurring near the eye should be assessed for possible complications.

Pigmented birthmarks are made of a cluster of pigment cells, which cause color in skin. These birthmarks can be many different colors, from tan to brown, gray to black, or even blue. The most common pigmented birthmarks are café au lait spots, Mongolian spots, and moles.

- **Café au lait spots** are very common birthmarks that are the color of coffee with milk—hence their name (FIGURE 13-6).

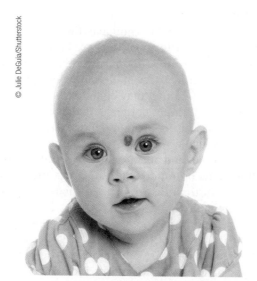

FIGURE 13-4 Hemangioma.

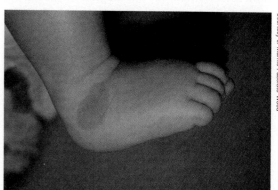

FIGURE 13-6 Café au lait spot.

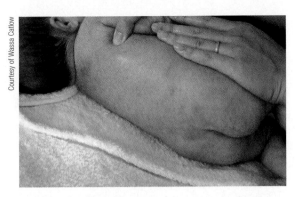

Courtesy of Wassa Catlow

FIGURE 13-7 Mongolian spot.

These birthmarks can appear anywhere on the body and sometimes increase in number as a child gets older. One café au lait spot alone is not usually a concern, but the child should be further evaluated if he or she has several spots larger than a quarter, which can be a sign of neurofibromatosis (see the *Cellular Function* chapter).

- **Mongolian spots** are flat, bluish-gray patches often found on the lower back or buttocks (FIGURE 13-7). These birthmarks are most common on individuals with darker complexions, such as children of Asian, American Indian, African, Hispanic, and Southern European descent. They usually fade, often completely, by school age without treatment.
- **Mole** (congenital nevi, hairy nevi) is a general term for brown nevi (the singular is *nevus*). Most people get moles at some point in life. When present at birth, the mole is called a congenital nevus and will last a lifetime. Large or giant congenital nevi are more likely to develop into skin cancer (melanoma) later in life; however, all moles should be monitored for cancerous changes. Moles can be tan, brown, or black; can be flat or raised; and may have hair growth.

Diagnosis of birthmarks is often made during a physical examination. Treatment strategies vary depending on the type of birthmark, as some birthmarks cannot be treated. With the exception of macular stains, which usually fade away on their own, vascular birthmarks are treatable. Hemangiomas are usually left untreated, as they typically shrink back into themselves by age 9. Larger or more serious hemangiomas often are treated with steroids. Laser therapy is the treatment of choice for port-wine stains. Most port-wine stains lighten significantly after several laser treatments, although some return and need re-treatment. Laser treatment is typically started in infancy when the stain and the blood vessels are smaller. Marks on the head and neck are the most responsive to laser treatment.

Pigmented birthmarks are usually left untreated, with the exception of moles and, occasionally, café au lait spots. Moles (particularly large or giant congenital nevi) are surgically removed. Café au lait spots can be removed with laser treatment but often return.

Some birthmarks can be disfiguring and embarrassing for children. Special opaque makeup can be used to conceal or minimize the appearance of some birthmarks. Additionally, support and coping strategies can be helpful.

Disorders of Melanin

Melanin is a pigment that provides color and protection. Disorders involving melanin result in alterations in skin coloring and can leave the skin vulnerable to the harmful effects of UV light. Melanin disorders include albinism and vitiligo.

Albinism is a recessive condition that results in little or no melanin production. Melanin deficits cause a lack of pigment in the skin, hair, and iris of the eye (FIGURE 13-8). In addition to coloring and protection, melanin plays a role in the development of certain optical nerves. Therefore, all forms of albinism cause problems with eye development and function. Two major types of albinism exist:

- Type 1 albinism—caused by defects that affect melanin production
- Type 2 albinism—caused by a defect in the P gene; children have slight coloring at birth

Myth Busters

A persistent myth about birthmarks warrants discussion: *birthmarks are a result of something the mother did or ate while pregnant.* There is no truth to old wives' tales about stains being caused by something the mother did or ate. The cause of most birthmarks is unknown. Birthmarks can be inherited, but usually are not, and they typically are unrelated to trauma to the skin during childbirth.

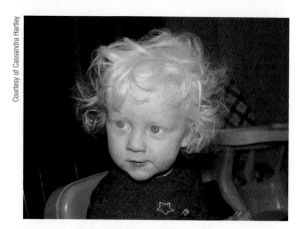

Courtesy of Cassandra Hartley

FIGURE 13-8 Albinism.

The most severe form of albinism is oculocutaneous albinism. People with this form of albinism appear to have white or pink hair, skin, and iris color; they also have vision problems. Another form of albinism, called ocular albinism type 1, affects only the eyes. The affected person's skin and eye colors are usually normal; however, an eye exam will reveal no coloring of the retina. Hermansky-Pudlak syndrome is a form of albinism caused by a single gene; it can occur with a bleeding disorder as well as with lung and bowel diseases. Other complex diseases may lead to color loss in only a certain area (localized albinism):

- Chédiak-Higashi syndrome—lack of coloring all over the skin, but not complete
- Tuberous sclerosis—small areas without skin coloring
- Waardenburg's syndrome—often a lock of hair that grows on the forehead is affected, or no coloring is present in one or both irises

Clinical manifestations of albinism are usually—but not always—apparent in a person's skin, hair, and eye color. Regardless of the effect of albinism on appearance, all people with the disorder experience vision impairments. Manifestations may include the following conditions:

- Skin changes. Although the most recognizable form of albinism results in milky white skin, skin pigmentation can range from white to nearly the same as relatives without albinism. For some people with albinism, skin pigmentation never changes. For others, melanin production may begin or increase during childhood and adolescence, resulting in slight increases in pigmentation. Some people may develop

freckles, moles (with or without pigment), or lentigines (large frecklelike spots) with exposure to the sun.
- Hair changes. Hair color can range from very white to brown. People of African or Asian descent who have albinism may have hair color that is yellow, reddish, or brown. Hair color may also change by early adulthood.
- Eye changes. Eye color can range from very light blue to brown and may change with age. The lack of pigment in the irises makes them somewhat translucent, meaning they cannot completely block light from entering the eye. This translucence can cause very light-colored eyes to appear red in some lighting because of light reflecting off the back of the eye and passing back out through the iris again—similar to the "red eye" that occurs in a flash photograph.
- Vision changes. Multiple vision issues can result from the lack of melanin, including the following problems:
  - Nystagmus (rapid, involuntary back-and-forth eye movement)
  - Strabismus (inability of both eyes to stay directed at the same point or to move in unison, or crossed eyes)
  - Extreme nearsightedness or farsightedness
  - Photophobia (sensitivity to light)
  - Astigmatism (abnormally shaped cornea)
  - Functional blindness

Diagnostic procedures for albinism consist of a history, physical examination (including a thorough ophthalmologic exam), and genetic testing (most accurate). Although there is no cure for albinism, people with this disorder can take steps to improve vision and avoid damage from sun exposure:

- Using sunscreen with a high sun protection factor (SPF) against UVA and UVB rays
- Wearing protective clothing (e.g., long-sleeved shirts, long pants, and hats)
- Limiting time outdoors, especially between 10:00 a.m. and 4:00 p.m., when the sun's UV rays are the most intense
- Wearing sunglasses (UV protected), which may relieve light sensitivity
- Wearing glasses to correct vision problems and eye position
- Having eye muscle surgery to correct abnormal eye movements (i.e., nystagmus)

Albinism does not impair intellectual development, although people with albinism often feel socially isolated and may experience

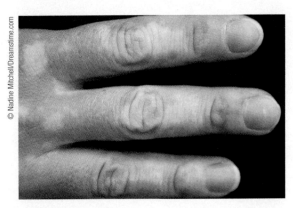

FIGURE 13-9 Vitiligo.

discrimination. Coping strategies and support may be beneficial in addressing these issues. The visual issues may lead to educational challenges. Educational strategies may include sitting at the front of the classroom, using large-print books and notes, and printing materials with high-contrast colors (e.g., black and white).

Vitiligo is a rare condition characterized by small patchy areas of hypopigmentation (FIGURE 13-9). This disorder occurs when the cells that produce melanin die or no longer form melanin, causing slowly enlarging white patches of irregular shapes on the skin. This condition affects people of all races but may be more noticeable and disfiguring in people with dark skin tones. Its exact cause is unknown, but potential causes include an autoimmune condition, genetic influences, sunburn, and emotional stress. Vitiligo has also been associated with pernicious anemia, hypothyroidism, and Addison's disease. Although any area of the body may be affected, depigmentation usually develops first on sun-exposed areas (e.g., hands, feet, arms, face, and lips). While it can start at any age, vitiligo often first appears between 10 and 30 years of age. It generally develops in one of three patterns— focal (depigmentation is limited to one or a few areas of the body), segmental (depigmentation occurs on one side of the body), or generalized (depigmentation is widespread across many parts of the body, often symmetrically).

The natural course of vitiligo is difficult to predict. Sometimes the patches stop forming without treatment. In most cases, pigment loss spreads and can eventually involve most of the skin's surface. In addition to patchy skin depigmentation, clinical manifestations may include depigmentation of the hair, mucous membranes, and retina.

Diagnosis of vitiligo includes a history, physical examination (including a Wood's light exam), skin biopsy, serum autoantibody level measurements, serum thyroid hormone level measurements, and serum vitamin B_{12} level measurements. There is no cure for vitiligo. The goal of treatment is to stop or slow the progression of pigment loss and attempt to return some pigment. Treatment and coping strategies may include the following measures:

- Phototherapy (controlled exposure to intense UV light in a clinic or hospital)
- Pharmacotherapy, including the following medications:
  - Oral synthetic melanizing agents (e.g., trimethylpsoralen [Trisoralen])
  - Topical corticosteroid agents
  - Topical immunosuppressants (e.g., pimecrolimus [Elidel] and tacrolimus [Protopic])
  - Topical repigmenting agents (e.g., methoxsalen [Oxsoralen])
  - Oral or topical photochemotherapy (e.g., psoralen plus UVA radiation)
- Skin graft
- Autologous melanocyte transplant (still experimental)
- Permanent depigmentation of the remaining skin (a last resort reserved for extreme cases)
- Sun safeguards (e.g., sunscreen and protective clothing)
- Coping strategies and support:
  - Makeup or skin dyes
  - Tattooing (most effective around the lips)

Integumentary Changes Associated with Aging

The skin undergoes several changes with aging. Sensations of pain, vibration, cold, heat, pressure, and touch usually decrease over the course of the life span. These changes may be related to decreases in blood flow to touch receptors or the brain that can occur with age. Decreases in these sensations can increase the risk of injury, including falls, decubitus ulcers, burns, and hypothermia.

In addition to sensory changes, the skin undergoes other aging-related changes. It loses elasticity, integrity, and moisture over time. Environmental factors, genetic makeup, and nutrition may all contribute to these changes. The greatest single contributing factor, however, is sun exposure. Natural pigments seem to provide some protection against sun-induced skin damage. Consequently, blue-eyed, fair-skinned people show more of these aging skin changes than people with darker, more heavily pigmented

© Nadine Mitchell/Dreamstime.com

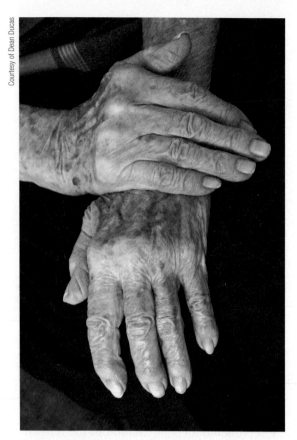

FIGURE 13-10 Lentigo.

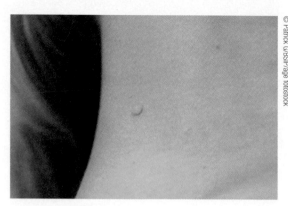

FIGURE 13-11 Skin tags.

skin. With aging, the epidermis thins, even though the number of cell layers remains unchanged. The number of melanocytes decreases, but the remaining melanocytes increase in size. Aging skin thus appears thin, pale, and translucent. Large pigmented spots (called age spots, liver spots, or **lentigos**) may appear in sun-exposed areas (FIGURE 13-10). Changes in the connective tissue reduce the skin's strength and elasticity, especially in sun-exposed areas. Dermis blood vessels become fragile, which can lead to bruising, cherry angiomas, and other similar conditions.

Sebaceous glands also produce less sebum over time. Men experience a minimal decrease in sebum production, usually after the age of 80, whereas women gradually produce less sebum beginning after menopause. This decrease in sebum can make it difficult to maintain skin moisture, resulting in dryness and itching.

The subcutaneous fat layer, which provides insulation and padding, thins with age. This waning subcutaneous layer increases the risk of skin injury and reduces the ability to maintain body temperature. Additionally, this fat layer absorbs some medications, so loss of this layer changes the actions of these medications.

The sweat glands produce less sweat with aging. The resulting decrease in perspiration contributes to difficulty in controlling body temperature.

Aging skin repairs itself more slowly than younger skin. Wound healing may take as much as four times longer to complete. This sluggish repair contributes to decubitus ulcer formation and infections. The presence of chronic diseases (e.g., diabetes mellitus and arteriosclerosis) and other aging-related changes (e.g., impaired immunity and circulatory changes) may further delay healing.

Other skin abnormalities may also develop over time. Abnormalities such as skin tags and other blemishes are more common in older people. **Skin tags** are benign, soft brown or flesh-colored masses that usually occur on the neck (FIGURE 13-11). Most skin tags are painless, but they can become inflamed in the presence of constant friction (e.g., from clothing). Skin tags are more common in persons who are obese or have diabetes mellitus. Skin tags can be removed with surgery, cryotherapy, and cautery.

Inflammatory Integumentary Disorders

Inflammatory skin diseases include a broad group of conditions, ranging in severity from mild itching to serious medical complications. These noncontagious conditions may occur in isolation or in conjunction with other conditions. Most of these disorders can be resolved or managed easily with treatment.

Contact Dermatitis

Contact dermatitis is an acute inflammatory reaction triggered by direct exposure to an irritant or allergen-producing substance (FIGURE 13-12). Contact dermatitis is not contagious or life threatening. It varies in severity depending on the substance, area affected, exposure extent, and individual sensitivity.

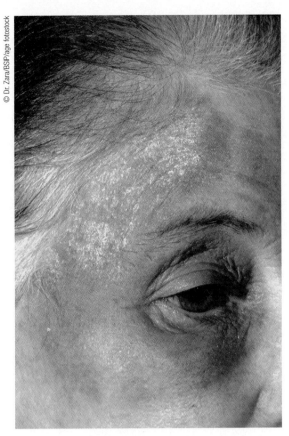

FIGURE 13-12 Contact dermatitis.

Chemicals, acids, rubber gloves, and soaps may all cause irritant contact dermatitis. This type of contact dermatitis does not involve the immune system, but simply triggers the inflammatory response. Irritant contact dermatitis produces a reaction similar to a burn. Manifestations of irritant contact dermatitis typically include erythema and edema but may also include pain, pruritus, and **vesicles** (blisters).

Allergic contact dermatitis results from contact with substances such as metals, chemicals, adhesives, cosmetics, and plants (e.g., poison ivy and poison sumac). Sensitization occurs on the first exposure to the substance, and subsequent exposures to the substance produce manifestations, which is a type IV cell-mediated hypersensitivity (see the *Immunity* chapter). The reaction is usually delayed, with manifestations appearing 24–48 hours after exposure. Typically, manifestations of allergic contact dermatitis include pruritus, erythema, and edema at the site, but small vesicles may also be present.

Diagnostic procedures include a history, physical examination, and allergy testing. Treatment of contact dermatitis centers on identifying and removing the causative agent (e.g., rinsing the affected area). If the offending agent can be avoided, the rash usually resolves

in 2–4 weeks. Self-care measures, such as wet compresses and anti-inflammatory creams (e.g., corticosteroid agents), can help soothe skin and reduce inflammation. Systemic anti-inflammatory agents may be used in severe cases.

Atopic Dermatitis

Atopic dermatitis, also referred to as eczema, is a chronic inflammatory condition (FIGURE 13-13). It has an inherited tendency and may be accompanied by asthma and allergic rhinitis. Atopic dermatitis is most common in infants, but usually resolves by early adulthood. It tends to be characterized by remissions and exacerbations. The exact cause is unknown, but atopic dermatitis may result from an immune system malfunction, similar to hypersensitivity (an elevation of immunoglobulin E is usually present). Atopic dermatitis is thought to be the first of a series of allergic diseases that affect the epithelial surfaces (referred to as the "atopic march" theory)—including food allergies, asthma, and allergic rhinitis (Spergel, 2010).

Complications may include secondary bacterial skin infections, neurodermatitis (permanent scarring and discoloration from chronic scratching), and eye problems (e.g., conjunctivitis). Atopic dermatitis may affect any area, but

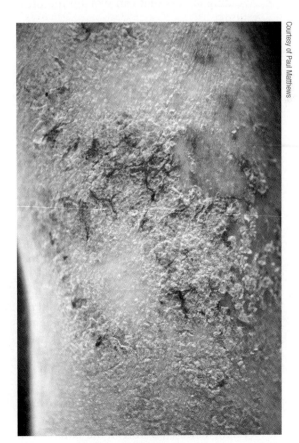

FIGURE 13-13 Atopic dermatitis.

the pattern exhibited tends to be age specific. The skin lesions primarily affect the face, scalp, hands, or feet in young children. The knees and elbows are the most commonly affected sites in older children and adults. Clinical manifestations may be made worse by exposure to allergens (especially to pollen, mold, dust, or animals), cold and dry air, upper respiratory infections, contact with irritants, dry skin, emotional stress, and extreme temperatures. These manifestations include the following signs and symptoms:

- Red to brownish-gray colored skin patches
- Pruritus, which may be severe, especially at night
- Vesicles
- Thickened (lichenified), cracked, or scaly skin
- Irritated, sensitive skin from scratching

Diagnostic procedures for atopic dermatitis include a history, physical examination, allergy testing, and skin biopsy (to rule out other causes). In children, the condition usually improves with age (starting around age 5–6), but flare-ups may occur. Treatment focuses on decreasing the inflammatory process. These strategies may include the following measures:

- Avoiding factors that can worsen manifestations:
    - Long, hot baths or showers
    - Dry skin
    - Stress
    - Sweating
    - Rapid changes in temperature
    - Low humidity
    - Solvents, cleaners, soaps, or detergents
    - Wool or synthetic fabrics or clothing
    - Dust or sand
    - Cigarette smoke
    - Certain foods (e.g., eggs, milk, fish, soy, and wheat)
- Avoiding scratching
    - Moisturizing the skin by applying ointments (e.g., petroleum jelly) 2–3 times per day
    - Using a humidifier
- Employing the following strategies when washing or bathing:
    - Keeping water contact brief and using gentle soap
    - Not excessively scrubbing or drying the skin
    - After bathing, applying lubricating creams, lotions, or ointment on the skin while it is damp to trap moisture in the skin

- Using the following pharmacologic agents:
    - Antihistamine agents (may be topical or oral)
    - Corticosteroid agents (may be topical or oral)
    - Immunomodulators (may be topical or oral)
    - Antibiotics (may be topical or oral if infection is present)
    - Allergen-desensitizing injections
- Receiving phototherapy

Urticaria

Urticaria, or hives, consists of raised erythematous skin lesions (**welts**) (FIGURE 13-14). These lesions are a result of a type I hypersensitivity reaction (see the *Immunity* chapter). This reaction is often triggered by food (e.g., shellfish and nuts) or medicine (e.g., antibiotics) ingestion. Urticaria may also be a result of emotional stress, excessive perspiration, diseases (e.g., autoimmune conditions and leukemia), and infections (e.g., mononucleosis). It occurs when histamine release is initiated by these substances or conditions. The resulting skin lesions are usually short-lived and harmless, but breathing can be

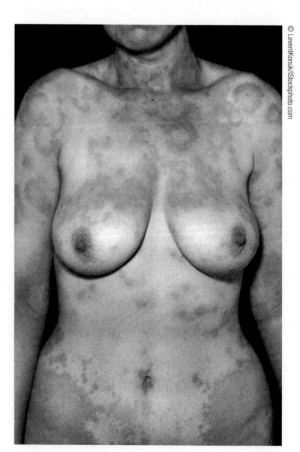

FIGURE 13-14　Urticaria.

impaired when the swelling occurs around the face (angioedema). Additionally, a type I hypersensitivity reaction can progress to an anaphylactic reaction (see the *Immunity* chapter) and shock (see the *Cardiovascular Function* chapter). The diffuse welts may grow large, spread, and fuse together. These welts turn white when pressure is applied (called blanching). In addition to patchy welts, pruritus may be present.

Diagnostic procedures for urticaria include a history, physical examination, allergy testing, and skin biopsy. Treatment focuses on ceasing the inflammatory reaction and maintaining respiratory status (if appropriate). Mild urticaria may disappear without any treatment. Treatment strategies to reduce itching and swelling include the following measures:

- Avoiding hot baths or showers
- Avoiding irritating the area (e.g., with tight-fitting clothing or rubbing)
- Taking antihistamines (e.g., diphenhydramine [Benadryl])

Severe reactions, especially if angioedema is present, may require epinephrine (adrenaline) or corticosteroid injections. Additionally, airway maintenance may be necessary, including an artificial airway, oxygen therapy, and mechanical ventilation. Epinephrine (adrenaline) and other bronchodilator agents can also be administered directly into the respiratory tract to improve ventilation.

Psoriasis

Psoriasis is a common, chronic inflammatory condition that affects the life cycle of the skin cells (FIGURE 13-15). Cellular proliferation is significantly increased in this disorder, such that cells build up too rapidly on the skin's surface (FIGURE 13-16). The process of skin cells growing in the innermost layers of the skin and then rising to the surface normally takes weeks, but with psoriasis, this process occurs over 3–4 days. The ensuing buildup leads to thickening of the dermis and epidermis because the dead cells cannot be shed fast enough.

The exact cause of psoriasis is unknown, but it does seem to be multifactorial in origin, with environmental (e.g., stress, cold, trauma, infections, obesity, excessive alcohol consumption, and certain medications), genetic (e.g., human leukocyte alleles), and immunologic (e.g., high levels of tumor necrosis factor) factors all playing roles in its etiology. This skin condition could be a result of an autoimmune process in which the body—specifically T lymphocytes—mistakes

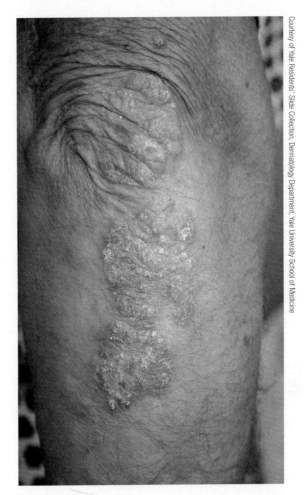

FIGURE 13-15 Psoriasis.

normal skin cells as foreign. Cytokines are then released, which stimulate keratinocyte proliferation.

Psoriasis can affect people of any age, but its onset most frequently occurs between 15 and 35 years of age. The onset may be sudden or gradual, and many patients will experience remissions and exacerbations. The following factors may trigger a psoriasis exacerbation or make the condition more difficult to treat:

- Bacterial or viral infections in any location
- Dry air or dry skin
- Skin injuries (e.g., cuts, burns, and insect bites)
- Use of certain medicines (e.g., antimalaria agents, beta blockers, and lithium)
- Stress
- Too little or too much sunlight
- Excessive alcohol consumption

The severity of psoriasis varies widely, from being a mere nuisance to being disabling; as many as 30% of persons with psoriasis also have

NORMAL SKIN

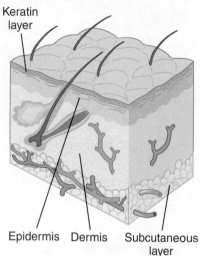

PSORIASIS

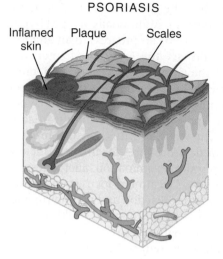

FIGURE 13-16 Cellular changes associated with psoriasis.

arthritis, a combination referred to as psoriatic arthritis. In general, psoriasis may be severe in persons who have a weakened immune system (e.g., those with AIDS, those with autoimmune conditions, or those who are receiving chemotherapy).

Psoriatic lesions begin as a small, red **papule** (firm and solid elevation) that then enlarges. These lesions most often occur on the elbows, knees, and trunk, but can appear anywhere on the body. The early lesions can progress to one of the following types of more advanced psoriatic lesions:

- Erythrodermic—intense erythema that covers a large area
- Guttate—small, pink-red spots
- Inverse—erythema and irritation that occur in the armpits, groin, and skin folds
- Plaque—thick, red patches covered by flaky, silver-white scales (the most common type)
- Pustular—white blisters surrounded by erythema

Other manifestations may include the following signs and symptoms:

- Pruritus
- Genital lesions in males
- Joint pain or aching (psoriatic arthritis)
- Nail changes such as thickening, yellow-brown spots, dents (pits) on the nail surface, and separation of the nail from the base
- Severe dandruff on the scalp

Diagnostic procedures for psoriasis include a history, physical examination, X-rays (if joint pain is present), and skin biopsy (to rule out other causes). Other tests may be conducted to rule out conditions that mimic psoriasis (e.g., seborrheic dermatitis and tinea corporis).

No cure exists for psoriasis, but treatment can improve symptoms significantly in most cases. The goal of psoriasis treatment is to interrupt the process that leads to cell buildup and improve manifestations. Treatment usually requires a multipronged approach and includes three main approaches—topical treatments, phototherapy, and systemic medications:

- Topical treatments:
  - Corticosteroid agents—to slow cell turnover by suppressing the immune system
  - Vitamin D analogues—to slow down the skin cell growth
  - Anthralin (Dritho-Scalp)—to normalize DNA activity in skin cells, remove scales, and smooth skin
  - Retinoids—to normalize DNA activity in skin cells and possibly decrease inflammation
  - Calcineurin inhibitors—to disrupt the activation of T lymphocytes, thereby reducing inflammation and plaque buildup
  - Salicylic acid—to promote shedding of dead skin cells and reduce scaling
  - Coal tar—to reduce scaling, itching, and inflammation, although the mechanism of action remains unknown
  - Moisturizers—to reduce dryness, itching, and scaling; ointment-based moisturizers are the most effective
  - Dandruff shampoo

- Phototherapy:
  - Sunlight—UV light, whether natural or artificial, causes activated T lymphocytes in the skin to die, which slows cell turnover, reduces scaling, and decreases inflammation
  - Broadband ultraviolet B (UVB) phototherapy
  - Narrowband UVB phototherapy—a newer and more effective treatment than broadband UVB treatment
  - Photochemotherapy, or psoralen plus ultraviolet A—administering psoralen, a light-sensitizing medication, before exposure to UVA light to increase the response to the light
  - Excimer laser—a controlled beam of UVB light of a specific wavelength that is directed to only the involved skin
- Oral or injected pharmacotherapy (primarily reserved for severe or resistant cases and used for brief periods because of the potential serious side effects):
  - Retinoids—related to vitamin A; this group of drugs may reduce the production of skin cells
  - Methotrexate—decreases the production of skin cells and suppresses inflammation
  - Cyclosporine—suppresses the immune system similarly to methotrexate
  - Hydroxyurea—suppresses the immune system but not as effectively as methotrexate and cyclosporine
  - Immunomodulator drugs—block interactions between certain immune system cells

In addition to these main strategies, stress management (e.g., coping strategies and support) and avoiding psoriasis triggers may be beneficial.

Infectious Integumentary Disorders

Skin infections are common and may be caused by a number of pathogens (e.g., bacteria, viruses, and parasites). These organisms usually gain access through a breach in the skin or mucous membranes. They often trigger the inflammatory response as well. Such infections can occur in any of the skin layers or structures (e.g., hair follicles); they may be acute or chronic, and vary widely in severity. In most cases, infectious integumentary disorders resolve easily with treatment.

Bacterial Infections

Any number of bacteria present in the body as part of the normal flora or encountered externally may cause bacterial skin infections. These infections can vary in severity from mild to life threatening. Bacteria in the *Staphylococcus* and *Streptococcus* genera are common culprits integumentary infections. These infections can result in numerous conditions:

- **Folliculitis** refers to infections involving the hair follicles. Folliculitis is characterized by tender, swollen areas that form around hair follicles, often on the neck, breasts, buttocks, and face.
- **Furuncles**, or boils, are infections that begin in the hair follicles and then spread into the surrounding dermis. Furuncles most commonly occur on the face, neck, axillae, groin, buttocks, and back. A furuncle lesion starts as a firm, red, painful nodule that develops into a large, painful mass, which frequently drains large amounts of purulent exudate. **Carbuncles** refer to clusters of furuncles.
- **Impetigo** is a common and highly contagious skin infection. Although it can occur without an apparent breach, this infection typically arises from a break in the skin (especially from animal bites, human bites, insect bites, and trauma). Impetigo spreads easily to others by direct contact with skin or contaminated objects (e.g., eating utensils, towels, clothing, and toys). Lesions usually begin as small vesicles that enlarge and rupture, forming the characteristic honey-colored crust (FIGURE 13-17). These lesions can spread throughout the body through self-transfer of the exudate. Impetigo is typically caused by staphylococci; these bacteria produce a toxin that causes impetigo to spread to nearby skin. The toxin attacks collagen, a protein that helps bind skin cells together. Once this protein is damaged, bacteria can spread quickly. Pruritus is common, and lymphadenopathy (swollen lymph nodes) can occur near the lesions.

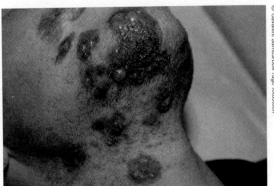

© Cavallini James/BSIP/age fotostock

FIGURE 13-17 Impetigo.

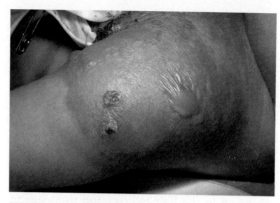

FIGURE 13-18 Cellulitis.

Courtesy of CDC/Allen W. Mathies, MD/California Emergency
Preparedness Office (Calif/EPO), Immunizaiton Branch

- **Cellulitis** refers to an infection deep in the dermis and subcutaneous tissue. It usually results from a direct invasion of the pathogens through a break in the skin, especially those breaches where contamination is likely (e.g., intravenous drug use and bites), or spreads from an existing skin infection. Cellulitis appears as a swollen, warm, tender area of erythema (FIGURE 13-18). Additionally, systemic manifestations of infection are usually present (e.g., fever, leukocytosis, malaise, and arthralgia). If left untreated, cellulitis can lead to necrotizing fasciitis, septicemia, and septic shock.
- **Necrotizing fasciitis** is a serious infection that is generally rare, although its incidence rates are rising. One out of four people who develop this infection will die because of it. Also known as "flesh-eating bacteria," necrotizing fasciitis can aggressively destroy skin, fat, muscle, and other tissue (FIGURE 13-19). This infection typically involves a highly virulent strain of gram-positive, group A, beta-hemolytic *Streptococcus* that invades through a minor cut or scrape. The bacteria begin to grow and release harmful toxins that directly destroy the tissue, disrupt blood flow, and break down material in the tissue. The first sign of infection may be a small, reddish, painful area on the skin. This area quickly evolves into a painful bronze- or purple-colored patch that grows rapidly. The center of the lesion may become black and necrotic. Exudate is often present. The wound may quickly grow, in less than an hour. Systemic manifestations may include fever, tachycardia, hypotension, and confusion. Complications of necrotizing fasciitis include gangrene, multisystem organ failure, and shock.

Diagnostic procedures for all bacterial skin infections center on the identification of the causative organism, usually through cultures. Once the organism is identified, treatment focuses on eradicating the organism with appropriate antibiotic therapy (either systemic or topical). Care should be taken when draining any wounds, as this procedure can spread the infection. Other strategies may include maintaining adequate hydration, wound care, surgical debridement, drainage, hyperbaric oxygen therapy, antipyretic agents, and analgesic agents.

Viral Infections

A number of viruses can cause a multitude of skin issues, each with its own manifestations and treatments. These infections can result in numerous conditions:

- **Herpes simplex type 1** (HSV-1), or a cold sore, is a viral infection typically affecting the lips, mouth, and face. This common infection usually begins in childhood. HSV type 1 can also involve the eyes, leading to conjunctivitis. Additionally, infection with this pathogen can result in meningoencephalitis. The virus is transmitted by contact with infected saliva. The primary infection may be asymptomatic. After the primary infection, the virus remains dormant in the sensory nerve ganglion to the trigeminal nerve until it is reactivated, similar to the pathogenesis of HSV type 2 (see the *Reproductive Function* chapter). Reactivation may be a result of an infection, stress, or sun exposure. When reactivated, HSV type 1 causes painful blisters or ulcerations, which are preceded by a burning or tingling sensation. The lesions resolve spontaneously within 3 weeks, but healing can be accelerated by administration of oral or topical antiviral agents.
- **Herpes zoster**, or shingles, is caused by the varicella-zoster virus. This condition

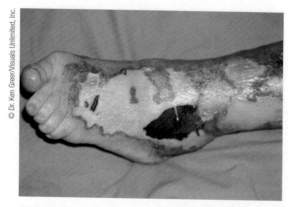

© Dr. Ken Greer/Visuals Unlimited, Inc.

FIGURE 13-19 Necrotizing fasciitis.

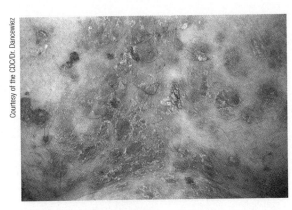

FIGURE 13-20 Herpes zoster.

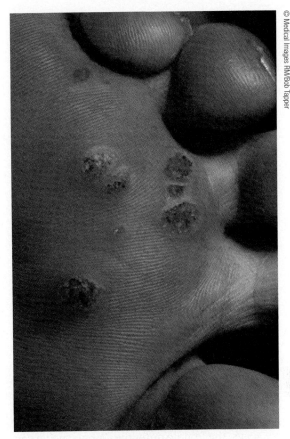

FIGURE 13-21 Verrucae.

appears in the adulthood years after a primary infection of varicella (chickenpox) has occurred in childhood. The virus lies dormant on a cranial nerve or a spinal nerve dermatome until it becomes activated years later. Because the virus affects this nerve only, the condition typically demonstrates unilateral manifestations—for example, pain, paresthesia, and a vesicular rash that develops in a line over the area innervated by the affected nerve (FIGURE 13-20). The rash may appear red or silvery, and it occurs on one side of the head or torso depending on the nerve affected. The skin often becomes extremely sensitive, and pruritus may be present. The rash may persist for weeks to months. In some cases, especially in older persons, neuralgia or pain may continue long after the rash disappears. Blindness may result if the eye is affected. Antiviral agents can limit the condition's duration and severity, and antidepressant and anticonvulsant agents have been beneficial in relieving the neuralgia associated with shingles. Vaccines are available to prevent both varicella and herpes zoster infections.

- **Verrucae**, or warts, are caused by a number of human papillomaviruses. These skin lesions can develop at any age and often resolve spontaneously. They can be transmitted through direct skin contact between people or within the same person. The human papillomavirus replicates in the skin cells, causing irregular thickening. Lesions can appear, which vary in color, shape, and texture depending on their type (FIGURE 13-21). Treatment includes a wide range of local applications such as laser treatments, cryotherapy with liquid nitrogen, electrocautery, and topical medications (e.g., keralytic, cytotoxic, and antiviral agents), but the verrucae may return after treatment.

Parasitic Infections

A number of parasitic infections can occur on the skin, including those caused by fungi and other organisms. These conditions are usually diagnosed through microscopic examination of skin scrapings processed with potassium hydroxide. Many of the causative organisms feed off the dead skin cells of the host and may use the host as a breeding ground. Some of the numerous parasitic skin infections are profiled here:

- **Tinea** causes several types of superficial fungal infections that are described based on the area of the body affected. These fungi typically grow in warm, moist places (e.g., showers). Tinea typically manifests as a circular, erythematous rash (FIGURE 13-22), which is usually associated with pruritus and burning. Tinea capitis is an infection of the scalp commonly encountered in school-aged children. Along with the typical rash associated with tinea, hair loss at the site is common. Tinea corporis, also called ringworm, is an infection of the body. Tinea pedis, also called athlete's foot, involves the feet, especially the toes. Tinea unguium is an infection of the nails, typically the toenails. This infection begins at the tip of one

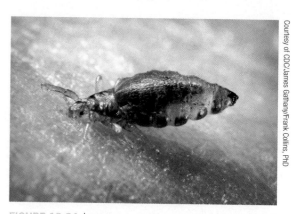

FIGURE 13-22 Tinea.

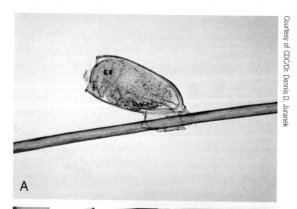

FIGURE 13-24 Louse.

or two nails and then usually spreads to other nails. The nail initially turns white and then brown, causing it to thicken and crack. Several topical and systemic antifungal agents are available to treat tinea infections, but several weeks of treatment may be necessary to resolve the infection.

- **Scabies** is a result of a mite infestation. The male mites fertilize the females and then die. The female mites burrow into the epidermis, laying eggs over a period of several weeks a series of tracts. After laying the eggs, the female mites die. When the larvae subsequently hatch from the eggs, they migrate to the skin's surface. They burrow into the skin in search of nutrients and mature to repeat the cycle. This burrowing appears as small, light brown streaks on the skin (FIGURE 13-23). The burrowing and fecal matter left behind by the mites triggers the inflammatory process, leading to erythema and pruritus. The mites can survive for only short periods without a host, so transmission usually results from close contact. Several topical treatments for scabies are available, but multiple applications are usually needed to successfully eradicate the

infestation. Clothing, linens, and other fabrics will likely require treatment as well.

- **Pediculosis** refers to lice infestation, which can take three forms—*Pediculus humanus corpus* (body louse), *Pediculus pubic* (pubic louse), and *Pediculus humanus capitis* (head louse). Lice are small, brown, parasitic insects that feed off human blood and cannot survive for long without the human host (FIGURE 13-24). The female lice lay eggs (nits) on the hair shaft close to the scalp (FIGURE 13-25). The nits appear as small white, iridescent shells on the hair. After

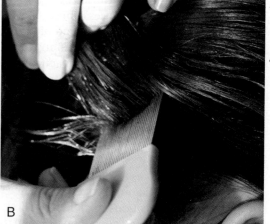

A

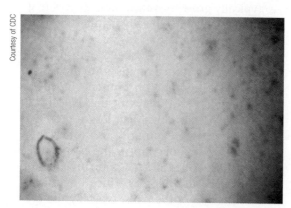

FIGURE 13-23 Scabies.

B

FIGURE 13-25 Nits.

hatching, the lice bite and suck the host's blood; in turn, the site of the bite develops a highly pruritic macule or papule. Pediculosis is easily transmitted through close contact. Several topical treatments are available, but multiple applications are usually needed to successfully eradicate the infestation. Clothing, linens, and other fabrics will likely require treatment as well.

Traumatic Integumentary Disorders

Traumatic integumentary disorders can result from a wide range of injuries. Skin trauma can produce multiple skin conditions, depending on the nature of the injury (FIGURE 13-26). Such injuries may range from mild to life threatening in severity, depending on the location and extent

of the injury. Regardless of the nature or extent of the injury, all traumatic skin conditions increase the risk for infection because they create a breach in the body's protective barrier (see the *Immunity* chapter). Although numerous traumatic skin conditions are possible (e.g., lacerations and abrasions), this section will focus on burns.

Burns

A **burn** is a skin injury that results from exposure to either a thermal (heat) or a nonthermal source. Such sources may include dry heat (e.g., fire), wet heat (e.g., steam or hot liquids), radiation, friction, heated objects, natural or artificial UV light, electricity, and chemicals (e.g., acids, alkaline substances, and paint

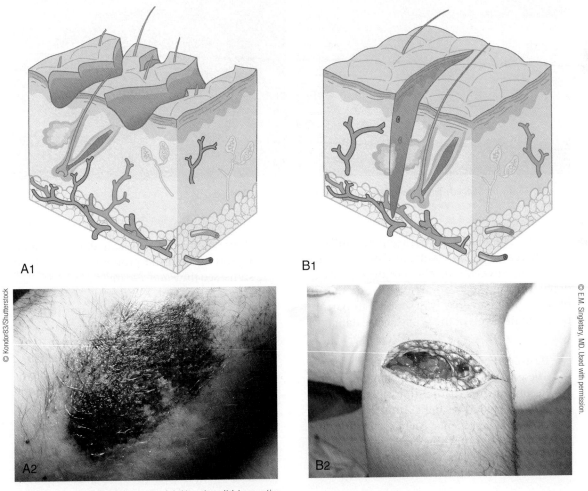

A1

B1

A2

B2

© Kondor83/Shutterstock

© E.M. Singletary, MD. Used with permission.

FIGURE 13-26 Types of wounds. (a) Abrasion. (b) Laceration.

(*continues*)

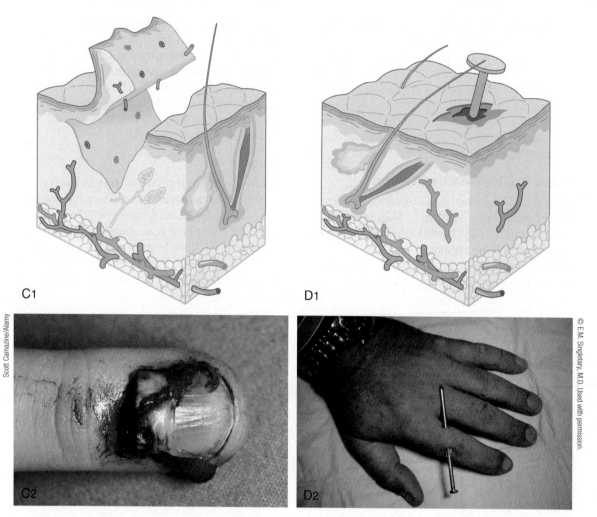

C1

D1

C2

D2

Scott Camazine/Alamy

© E.M. Singletary, M.D. Used with permission.

FIGURE 13-26 (*continued*) Types of wounds. (c) Avulsion. (d) Penetrating wound.

thinner). The burn injury triggers the inflammatory reaction and results in tissue destruction. The severity of the condition varies depending on the location, extent, and nature of the injury. Severity is described, in part, in terms of the levels of the skin that are damaged (**FIGURE 13-27**):

- First-degree burns affect only the epidermis. These burns cause pain, erythema, and edema.
- Second-degree (partial-thickness) burns affect the epidermis and dermis. These burns cause pain, erythema, edema, and blistering.
- Third-degree (full-thickness) burns extend into deeper tissues. These burns cause white or blackened, charred skin that may be numb.

Complication development is usually related to burn severity. Burns may result in any of the following complications:

- Local infection (particularly *Staphylococcus* infection)
- Sepsis

- Hypovolemia (burns can damage blood vessels and plasma proteins, causing fluid shifts; see the *Fluid, Electrolyte, and Acid–Base Homeostasis* chapter)
- Shock (may result from sepsis or hypovolemia)
- Hypothermia (heat is lost through large injuries)
- Respiratory problems (inhaling hot air or smoke can burn the tissues making up the airway, causing inflammation)
- Scarring
- Contractures

Diagnostic procedures consist of a history, physical examination (including determining the percentage of the total body surface area affected), chest X-ray, endoscopy (insertion of a flexible tube with a camera into the trachea and upper airway), complete blood count, and blood chemistry. Burn treatment is complex and varies depending on the location and severity of the injury. Strategies

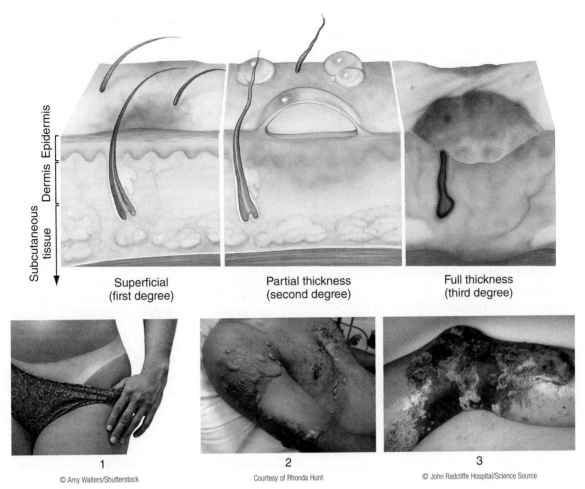

Superficial
(first degree)

Partial thickness
(second degree)

Full thickness
(third degree)

1

© Amy Walters/Shutterstock

2

Courtesy of Rhonda Hunt

3

© John Radcliffe Hospital/Science Source

FIGURE 13-27 Burn classification.

for minor burns may include the following measures:

- Remove the source of the burn.
- If the skin is unbroken, run cool water over the area or soak it in a cool water bath (not ice water). Keep the damaged area submerged for at least 5 minutes. Applying a clean, cold, wet bandage or towel will also help reduce pain.
- After flushing or soaking the burn, cover it with a dry, sterile bandage or clean dressing.
- Protect the burn from pressure and friction.
- Administer analgesics and nonsteroidal anti-inflammatory drugs (NSAIDs) to relieve pain and swelling.
- Apply moisturizing lotion once the skin has cooled.
- If a second-degree burn covers an area more than 2–3 inches in diameter or if it is located on the hands, feet, face, groin, buttocks, or a major joint, treat the burn as a major burn.

For major burns, the following strategies are used:

- Remove the source of the burn.
- If someone is on fire, have the person stop, drop, and roll. Wrap the person in thick material to smother the flames (e.g., a wool or cotton coat, rug, or blanket). Douse the person with water.
- Do not remove burned clothing that is stuck to the skin. The clothing may be soaked with sterile water or saline and then removed, and surgical removal may be necessary in severe cases.
- Ensure the person is breathing. Initiate rescue breathing and cardiopulmonary resuscitation if necessary. Continue to monitor the patient's respiratory status—it can become impaired as edema worsens.
- Maintain respiratory status (e.g., endotracheal intubation with mechanical ventilation and oxygen therapy).
- Cover the burn area with a dry sterile bandage or clean cloth. Do not apply any ointments. Avoid rupturing blisters.

- If fingers or toes are involved, separate them with dry, sterile, nonadhesive dressings.
- Elevate the affected body part above the level of the heart to minimize edema.
- Protect the burn area from pressure and friction.
- Take steps to prevent shock. Place the individual in Trendelenburg position and cover him or her with a coat or blanket. However, do not place the person in this position if a head, neck, back, or leg injury is suspected or if it makes the person uncomfortable.
- Monitor vital signs for signs of shock (e.g., tachycardia and hypotension).
- Administer intravenous fluids (which may include colloids or crystalloids) using specific formulas.
- Administer oral, intravenous, or topical analgesics, sedatives, or antibiotics to reduce pain and to prevent infection.
- Implement reverse isolation (e.g., gowning and limiting visitors).
- Apply meticulous wound care to limit the risk for infection and to promote healing.
- Apply protective dressings.
- Perform skin grafts to promote tissue regeneration, prevent scarring, and aid the healing process.
- Perform surgery as necessary to close the wound, remove dead tissue, or treat related complications (e.g., scarring and contractures).
- Provide physical therapy to reduce the effects of scar tissue.
- Increase dietary intake of protein and carbohydrates to promote healing and support the person's increased metabolic needs.

Chronic Integumentary Disorders

Numerous chronic conditions can affect the integumentary system. These conditions vary in severity. Although most are not life threatening, many can have a significant impact on an individual's appearance.

Acne Vulgaris

Acne vulgaris is a skin condition commonly affecting adolescents, but it can occur at any age. With this condition, the skin's pores become clogged with oil, debris, or bacteria. Pores can become inflamed, developing a pustule, nodule, or cyst. Clogged pores may become either raised with a white top (called a whitehead) or dark (called a blackhead) (FIGURE 13-28). If an infected pore ruptures, the material inside, including oil and bacteria, can spread to the surrounding area and cause an inflammatory reaction. Acne vulgaris commonly appears on the face and shoulders, but may also occur on the trunk, arms, legs, and buttocks. It varies widely in severity, with severe cases sometimes resulting in significant scarring. Risk factors for acne vulgaris include the following:

- Family history
- Hormonal changes (e.g., changes that occur with menstrual periods, pregnancy, birth control pill use, and stress)
- Use of oily cosmetic and hair products
- Use of certain medications (e.g., corticosteroids, testosterone, estrogen, and phenytoin)
- High levels of humidity and sweating

Diagnostic procedures for acne vulgaris include a history and physical examination. Treatment varies depending on the severity, but

Learning Points

Several actions should be avoided with burns:

- Do *not* apply ointment, butter, ice, medications, cream, oil spray, or any household remedy to a severe burn.
- Do *not* breathe, blow, or cough on the burn.
- Do *not* disturb blistered or necrotic skin.
- Do *not* remove clothing that is stuck to the skin.
- Do *not* give the person anything by mouth if there is a severe burn (surgery may be necessary).
- Do *not* immerse a severe burn in cold water because doing so can cause shock.
- Do *not* place a pillow under the person's head if there is an airway burn because this positioning of the head can close the airway.

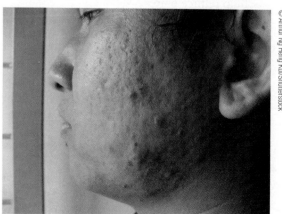

FIGURE 13-28 Acne vulgaris.

these strategies often include the following measures:

- Clean skin gently with a mild, nondrying soap to remove all dirt or makeup once or twice a day, including after exercising; however, avoid excessive or repeated skin washing.
- Shampoo hair daily, especially if it is oily.
- Comb or pull hair back to keep it away from the face, but avoid tight headbands.
- Avoid squeezing, scratching, picking, or rubbing acne because it can lead to skin infections and scarring.
- Avoid touching affected areas.
- Avoid oily cosmetics or creams; use water-based or noncomedogenic formulas.
- Use over-the-counter or prescription acne products containing benzoyl peroxide, sulfur, resorcinol, or salicylic acid.
- Administer oral or topical antibiotics (e.g., erythromycin).
- Apply retinoic acid cream or gel (e.g., Retin-A).
- Administer oral isotretinoin (Accutane).
- Administer oral contraceptives to females.
- Use alternative therapies, including tea tree oil, zinc, guggul, and brewer's yeast.
- Apply photodynamic therapy (laser procedure).
- Apply chemical skin peels.
- Use microdermabrasion or dermabrasion.
- Use soft-tissue fillers (e.g., collagen and fat).
- Limit sun exposure.

Rosacea

Rosacea is a chronic inflammatory skin condition that typically affects the face. It is poorly understood, but is prevalent in persons who are fair skinned, persons who bruise easily, and women. There are four subtypes of rosacea—erythematotelangiectatic type, papulopustular (classic presentation), phymatous, and ocular.

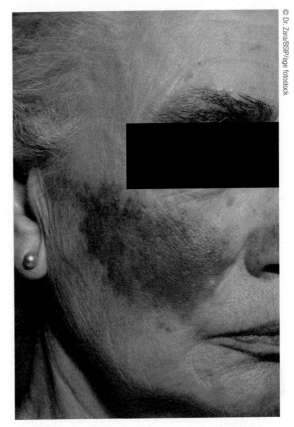

FIGURE 13-29 Rosacea.

© Dr. Zara/BSIP/age fotostock

Rosacea may present as erythema, prominent spiderlike blood vessels (telangiectasia), swelling, or acnelike eruptions (FIGURE 13-29). Additional manifestations may include a thickening of the skin on the nose (rhinophyma), a burning or stinging sensation, and red, watery eyes. If left untreated, rosacea is progressive, but most people with this condition experience remissions and exacerbations. Exacerbation triggers are specific to the individual, but may include sun or wind exposure, sweating, stress, spicy food, alcohol, hot beverages, hot baths, and cold weather.

Myth Busters

There are a couple of myths in regard to acne that warrant clearing up (no pun intended).

Myth 1: Eating greasy foods and chocolate worsens acne.

Contrary to popular belief, greasy foods and chocolate have little effect on acne. Studies are ongoing to determine whether other dietary factors—including high-starch foods (such as bread, bagels, and chips), which increase blood sugar—may play a role in acne.

Myth 2: Acne is a result of the skin being dirty.

Acne is not caused by dirt. In fact, scrubbing the skin too hard or cleansing with harsh soaps or chemicals irritates the skin and can make acne worse. Simple cleansing of the skin to remove excess oil and dead skin cells is all that is required.

Diagnostic procedures for rosacea include a history and physical examination. There is no known cure for rosacea. Instead, treatment strategies center on identifying and avoiding possible triggers, so that affected individuals can reduce exacerbations. These strategies may include the following measures:

- Avoid excessive scrubbing when cleaning.
- Avoid sun exposure (e.g., wear protective hats and clothing, limit exposure time especially between 10:00 a.m. and 4:00 p.m.) and use sunscreen that protects against both UVA and UVB rays every day.
- Avoid prolonged physical exertion in hot weather.
- Manage stress (e.g., through deep breathing and yoga).
- Limit spicy foods, alcohol, and hot beverages.
- Avoid any other triggers.
- Apply topical or oral antibiotics to control skin eruptions.
- Apply retinoic acid cream or gel (e.g., Retin-A).
- Administer oral isotretinoin (Accutane).
- Perform laser surgery to help reduce the redness.
- Perform surgical reduction of enlarged nose tissue.
- Apply green- or yellow-tinted prefoundation creams and powders to reduce the appearance of redness.

Integumentary Cancers

Skin cancer is an abnormal growth of skin cells. According to the Centers for Disease Control and Prevention (CDC, 2016), skin cancer is the most frequently occurring cancer in the United States, and the number of cases continues to rise. Prevalence rates are highest in males, Caucasians, persons with fair complexion, and those with a family history. The overall 5-year survival rate is approximately 92%. UV exposure, either natural or artificial, is by far the most significant risk factor for this type of cancer. For this reason, most skin cancers occur on areas that have the most sun exposure (e.g., the arms and neck).

Three major types of skin cancer are distinguished—basal cell carcinoma, squamous cell carcinoma, and melanoma. Basal cell carcinoma, the most common type, develops from abnormal growth of the cells in the lowest layer of the epidermis. Squamous cell carcinoma involves changes in the squamous cells, which are found in the middle layer of the epidermis. Melanoma develops in the melanocytes; it is the

least common type but the most serious. Basal and squamous cell carcinomas rarely spread, but melanomas often metastasize to other areas.

Skin cancers can vary widely in appearance; they can be small, shiny, waxy, scaly, rough, firm, red, crusty, bleeding, and so on (FIGURE 13-30). Given the many possible presentations, any suspicious skin lesion should be examined by a healthcare professional. The following features may be considered "suspicious":

- Asymmetry—part of the lesion is different from the other parts
- Borders that are irregular
- Color that varies from one area to another with shades of tan, brown, or black (sometimes white, red, or blue)
- Diameter that is usually (but not always) larger than 6 mm in size
- Any skin growth that bleeds or will not heal
- Any skin growth that changes in appearance over time

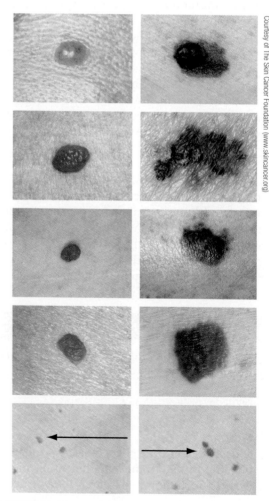

FIGURE 13-30 Skin cancers.

Courtesy of The Skin Cancer Foundation (www.skincancer.org)

Now that we have discussed conditions of the integumentary system, let's put that knowledge into practice. While you are working in a clinic, a patient comes in with multiple lesions. Which lesion should you assess first?

- Raised, tubular, white, snakelike areas on the inner aspects of the wrists
- Irregular blue mole with white specks on the lower leg
- Beige freckles on the backs of both hands

- Large cluster of pustules in the right axilla

Once again, you go through the usual thought process—what would kill the patient first, acute versus chronic conditions, Maslow's hierarchy of needs, and patient safety. First, the lesions on the wrist are likely scars and do not pose any threat. Now, consider the blue mole. Blue is a suspicious color for a mole, and there is color variation in the patient's mole. These findings strongly indicate skin cancer, so keep that lesion on your list. Moving on to the freckles, the color is not suspicious, nor are there any other suspicious indications. These lesions are not likely to pose any threat. Finally, consider the pustules under the axilla. These likely indicate a superficial skin infection. A skin infection is acute but not generally life threatening. After considering all the lesions, you should assess the mole first.

Most skin cancers can be prevented by limiting or avoiding exposure to UV light (e.g., by using sunscreen and wearing protective clothing). Early detection is crucial to positive outcomes; with early detection, even the most aggressive forms can be successfully treated. Diagnostic procedures for skin cancer typically include a history, physical examination, and biopsy. Removal of the cancerous growths offers the best prognosis. Treatment strategies may include the following measures:

- Cryosurgery
- Excisional surgery
- Laser therapy
- Mohs' surgery (the skin growth is removed layer by layer, examining each layer under the microscope, until no abnormal cells remain)
- Curettage and electrodessication (layers of cancer cells are scraped away using a circular blade [curette] and then an electric needle is used to destroy any remaining cancer cells)
- Radiation therapy
- Chemotherapy

Learning Points

All skin lesions, such as moles, should be monitored for any suspicious changes. These changes can be readily identified—their diagnosis is as easy as A, B, C, and D.

A = Asymmetry—part of the lesion is different from the other

B = Borders—irregular

C = Color—varies from one area to another with shades of tan, brown, or black (sometimes white, red, or blue)

D = Diameter—usually (but not always) larger than 6 mm in size (the diameter of a pencil eraser)

CHAPTER SUMMARY

The integumentary system plays a vital role in homeostasis and well-being by protecting the body from invasion by pathogens, maintaining water balance, sensing changes in the environment, and regulating body temperature. Conditions affecting this system can cause issues with any or all of these functions. Some of these conditions can be prevented through measures such as limiting UV light exposure through using sunscreen that protects against UVA and UVB rays, wearing protective clothing, and limiting time outdoors, especially between 10:00 a.m. and 4:00 p.m., when the sun's rays are the most intense. Early diagnosis and treatment of other conditions can improve prognosis.

REFERENCES

AAOS. (2004). *Paramedic: Anatomy and physiology*. Sudbury, MA: Jones & Bartlett.

Centers for Disease Control and Prevention (CDC). (2016). Skin cancer. Retrieved from http://www.cdc.gov/cancer/skin/

Chiras, D. (2011). *Human biology* (7th ed.). Burlington, MA: Jones & Bartlett Learning.

Elling, B., Elling, K., & Rothenberg, M. (2004). *Anatomy and physiology*. Sudbury, MA: Jones and Bartlett.

Gould, B. (2015). Pathophysiology for the health professions (5th ed.). Philadelphia, PA: Elsevier.

Professional guide to pathophysiology (3rd ed.). (2010). Philadelphia, PA: Lippincott Williams & Wilkins.

Spergel, J. (2010). From atopic dermatitis to asthma: The atopic march. *Annuals of Allergy, Asthma, and Immunology*, *105*(2), 107–109.

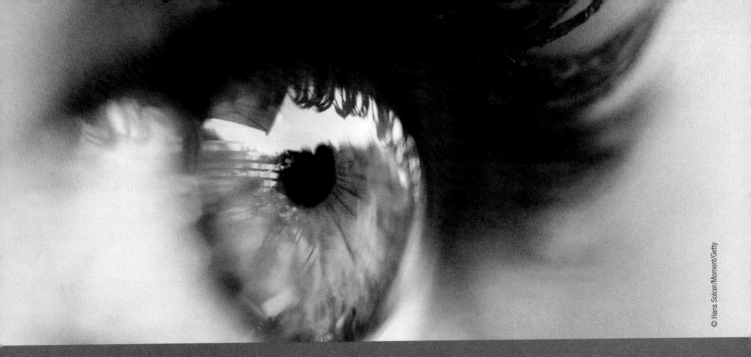

CHAPTER 14
Sensory Function

LEARNING OBJECTIVES

- Discuss normal sensory anatomy and physiology.
- Compare and contrast congenital sensory disorders.
- Describe and discuss sensory conditions associated with aging.
- Compare and contrast infectious and inflammatory sensory disorders.

- Describe and discuss traumatic sensory disorders.
- Describe and discuss chronic sensory disorders.
- Describe and discuss sensory cancers.
- Describe and discuss miscellaneous sensory conditions.

KEY TERMS

amblyopia
anotia
anterior chamber
aqueous humor
atresia
auricle
cataract
choroid
ciliary body
closed-angle (acute)
   glaucoma
cochlea
cone
congenital cataract
congenital glaucoma
congenital hearing loss
conjunctiva
conjunctivitis
cornea
diplopia

ear
eustachian tube
external ear canal
eye
glaucoma
incus
inner ear
intractable pain
iris
keratitis
lacrimal duct
lacrimal gland
lens
macular degeneration
malleus
Meniere's disease
microtia
middle ear
neuropathic pain
nystagmus

open-angle (chronic)
   glaucoma
optic nerve
organ of Corti
ossicle
otitis externa
otitis media
otosclerosis
outer ear
oval window
pain
pain threshold
pain tolerance
phantom pain
pinna
posterior chamber
presbycusis
presbyopia
pupil
referred pain

retina
retinal detachment
rod
saccule
sclera
secondary glaucoma
semicircular canal
somatic pain
stapes
strabismus
tinnitus
tympanic membrane
utricle
vertigo
vestibular apparatus
vestibule
visceral pain
vitreous humor

The human body has a complex surveillance system that senses changes in the internal and external environments. This vigilant system utilizes numerous receptors throughout the body to detect even subtle alterations; these receptors are located in the skin, internal organs, and other tissue. The stimuli perceived by these receptors give rise to sensations, including those related to the general and special senses (**TABLE 14-1**). The general senses include pain, light touch, pressure, temperature, and proprioception (position), while the special senses include taste, smell, sight, hearing, and balance. Disorders of the sensory structures can result in sensory dysfunction. These disorders can result from a wide range of causes including congenital defects, advancing age, infections, and cancers.

Anatomy and Physiology

The ability to sense changes in its ever-changing internal and external environments allows the body to respond to those stimuli and function. Sensations are detected by receptors, which then convert the stimuli into nerve impulses. These impulses travel to the brain by cranial or spinal nerves to be processed and appreciated (**FIGURE 14-1**). The human body contains five types of receptors for the general and special senses: mechanoreceptors (activated by mechanical stimuli such as touch or pressure), chemoreceptors (activated by chemicals in the blood, food, or air), thermoreceptors (activated by heat or cold), photoreceptors (activated by light), and nociceptors (activated by painful stimuli). General sense receptors can occur as exposed or encapsulated nerve endings (**FIGURE 14-2**). The exposed nerve endings detect pain, temperature, and light touch and are located in the skin, bones, and internal organs. One or more layers of cells surround encapsulated nerve endings. A variety of encapsulated nerve endings (e.g., Pacini's corpuscles, Meissner's corpuscles, Krause's end bulbs, and Ruffini's corpuscles) are located throughout the body for a variety of senses. Many of these sensory receptors (especially pain, temperature, and pressure) will stop generating impulses after an extended exposure to stimuli through adaptation.

Pain is associated with many conditions and, therefore, warrants further discussion. Pain is a protective mechanism, warning the body when something is wrong. In addition, pain is the most common reason people seek medical attention and can be used to aid diagnosis. Pain is a subjective feeling, and the perception of pain and the level at which it is sensed (**pain threshold**) can be influenced by affective (emotional), behavior, cognitive (beliefs and attitudes), sensory (perceptual), and physiologic factors. Unrelieved pain can delay healing, stimulate the stress response (see the *Immunity* chapter), and result in **pain tolerance**.

TABLE 14-1	Summary of the General and Special Senses	
Sense	**Stimulus**	**Receptor**
General senses	Pain	Naked nerve endings
	Light touch	Merkel's disks; naked nerve endings around hair follicles; Meissner's corpuscles; Ruffini's corpuscles; end bulbs
	Pressure	Pacinian corpuscles
	Temperature	Naked nerve endings
	Proprioception	Golgi tendon organs; muscle spindles; receptors similar to Meissner's corpuscles in joints
Special senses	Taste	Taste buds
	Smell	Olfactory epithelium
	Sight	Retina
	Hearing	Organ of Corti
	Balance	Crista ampularis in the semicircular canals; maculae in utricle and saccule

GENERALIZED SENSORY PATHWAY

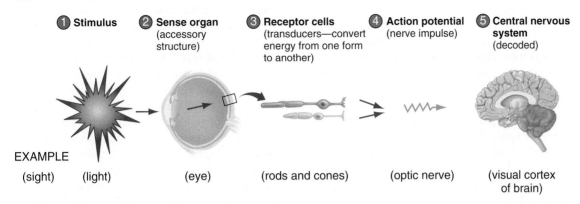

① **Stimulus**   ② **Sense organ** (accessory structure)   ③ **Receptor cells** (transducers—convert energy from one form to another)   ④ **Action potential** (nerve impulse)   ⑤ **Central nervous system** (decoded)

EXAMPLE

(sight)   (light)   (eye)   (rods and cones)   (optic nerve)   (visual cortex of brain)

FIGURE 14-1 The general sensory pathway.

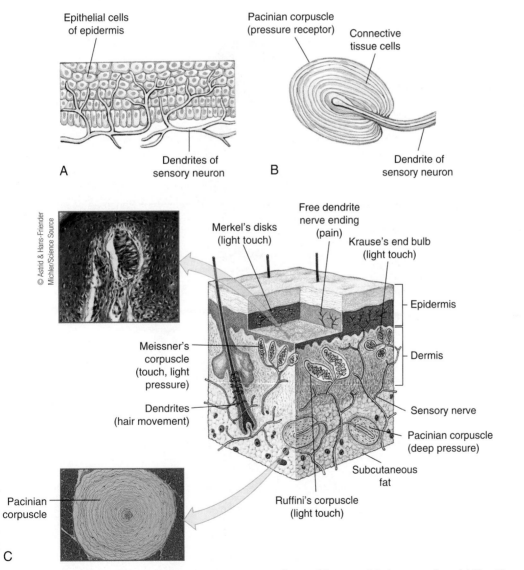

Epithelial cells of epidermis

Pacinian corpuscle (pressure receptor)

Connective tissue cells

Dendrites of sensory neuron

A

Dendrite of sensory neuron

B

© Astrid & Hans-Friender Michler/Science Source

Merkel's disks (light touch)

Free dendrite nerve ending (pain)

Krause's end bulb (light touch)

Epidermis

Dermis

Meissner's corpuscle (touch, light pressure)

Dendrites (hair movement)

Sensory nerve

Pacinian corpuscle (deep pressure)

Subcutaneous fat

Ruffini's corpuscle (light touch)

© Carolina Biological Supply CoVisuals Unlimited, Inc.

Pacinian corpuscle

C

FIGURE 14-2 General sense receptors are either (a) exposed nerve endings or (b) encapsulated nerve endings. (c) The skin houses many of the receptors for the general senses. The Pacinian corpuscle, often located in the dermis of the skin, detects pressure. Meissner's corpuscle, found just beneath the epidermis, detects light touch.

The body perceives two types of pain, each with its own cause, location, and characteristics. **Somatic pain** results from noxious stimuli to the skin, joints, muscles, and tendons. These stimuli may include cutting, crushing, pinching, extreme temperature, and irritating chemicals. Somatic pain is generally easy to pinpoint. In contrast, **visceral pain** results from noxious stimuli to internal organs. These stimuli may include expansion and hypoxia. Visceral pain is usually vague and diffuse. It may even be sensed on body surfaces at distant locations from the originating organ, a phenomenon called **referred pain** (FIGURE 14-3). The exact mechanism by which referred pain arises is unknown, but it is thought to result from the brain's misinterpretation of the visceral impulses as somatic impulses because both types of impulses enter the spinal cord at the same location (see the *Neural Function* chapter). The term **phantom pain** describes pain that exists after the removal of a body part (e.g., amputation). The affected person may feel the discomfort of the removed part. The severing of neurons may result in spontaneous firing of spinal cord neurons because normal sensory input has been lost. This type of pain can be extremely distressing but usually resolves with time. **Intractable pain** describes chronically progressing pain that is unrelenting and severely debilitating. This type of pain does not usually respond well to typical pharmacologic pain treatments (e.g., analgesics and narcotics). Intractable pain is common with severe injuries, especially those crushing in nature. **Neuropathic pain** describes pain that results from

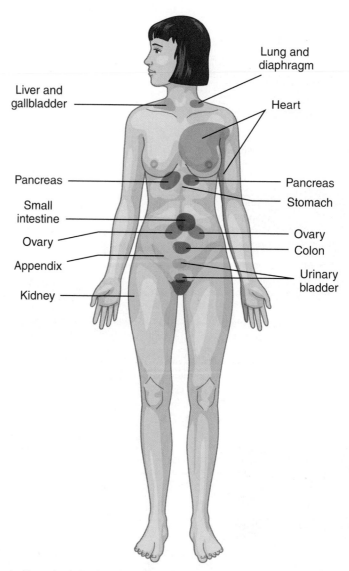

FIGURE 14-3 Referred pain. Visceral pain is often felt on the body surface at the points indicated by the colored areas.

damage to peripheral nerves by disease (e.g., diabetes mellitus) or injury; it tends to be both chronic and intractable. Patients with neuropathic pain also experience losses of the senses of touch and pressure. This condition causes an unusual sensation of paresthesia (numbness) and pain at the same time. The resulting pain is often described as a "prickly," "stabbing," or "burning" sensation.

Eyes

The human **eye** is a remarkable organ that allows us to perceive the environment in which we live. Human eyes are globe-shaped organs located in orbits in the anterior skull. Each eye consists of three distinct layers (**FIGURE 14-4**; **TABLE 14-2**).

The outermost layer of the eye is composed of a durable, fibrous material called the **sclera** (white area) and a clear lens on the anterior side called the **cornea**. Tendons and muscles attach to the sclera to control eye movement. The cornea allows light to enter the eye.

The middle layer of the eye consists of the **choroid**, which contains melanin that absorbs any stray light. The anterior portion of the choroid forms the **ciliary body**, whose smooth muscle fibers control the shape of the lens,

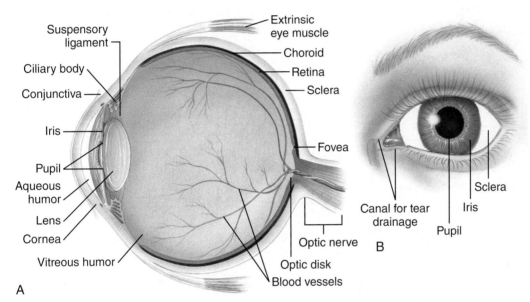

FIGURE 14-4 Anatomy of the eye.

TABLE 14-2	Structures and Functions of the Eye	
Structure		**Function**
Wall		
Outer layer	Sclera	Provides insertion for extrinsic eye muscles
	Cornea	Allows light to enter; bends incoming light
Middle layer	Choroid	Absorbs stray light; provides nutrients to eye structures
	Ciliary body	Regulates the lens, allowing it to focus images
	Iris	Regulates amount of light entering the eye
Inner layer	Retina	Responds to light, converting light to nerve impulses
Accessory structures and components	Lens	Focuses images on the retina
	Vitreous humor	Holds retina and lens in place
	Aqueous humor	Supplies nutrients to structures in contact with the anterior cavity of the eye
	Optic nerve	Transmits impulses from the retina to the brain

allowing it to focus on incoming light. The **iris** is the colored portion of the eye, and the **pupil** is the dark opening in the center of the iris. The choroid layer and the pigmented section of the retina give the pupil its black appearance. The iris contains smooth muscle fibers that control the diameter of the pupil to regulate light entering the eye. The pupil opens and closes reflexively in response to light intensity.

The innermost layer of the eye is the **retina**. It contains an outer, pigmented layer and an inner layer consisting of photoreceptors and nerve cells (**FIGURE 14-5**). The retina is weakly attached to the choroid, making it vulnerable to damage. It contains two types of photoreceptors— rods and cones. The nearly 150 million **rods** in each eye are sensitive to low light and function at night. By comparison, each eye contains approximately 6 million **cones**, which can operate only in bright light and are responsible for visual acuity and color vision.

The axons of the ganglion cells come together at the back of the eye to form the **optic nerve**. This area contains no photoreceptors and is insensitive to light. Visual images are cast

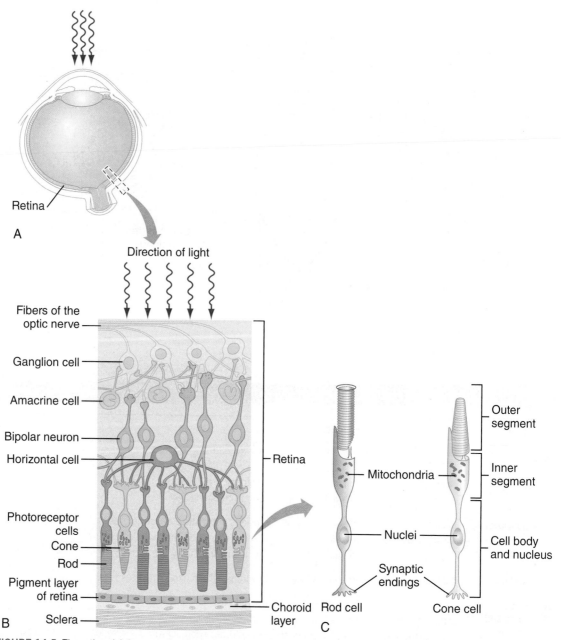

FIGURE 14-5 The retina. (a) Cross section through the wall of the eye, showing (b) the arrangement of the cellular components of the retina. (c) The structure of the rods and cones.

upside down onto the retina, and impulses are transmitted to the visual cortex in the brain. The retina processes some of the image, and then the brain processes the rest.

The **lens** is a transparent, flexible structure that lies behind the iris in the eye. Smooth muscles attached to the lens alter its shape, thereby allowing it to focus on various objects. The lens separates the eye interior into two cavities—the anterior and posterior chambers. The **anterior chamber** is in front of the lens, while the **posterior chamber** is behind the lens. The anterior chamber contains a watery liquid called **aqueous humor** that provides nutrients to the cornea and lens and carries away cellular waste products. A clear, gelatinous material called **vitreous humor** fills the posterior chamber. The pressures exerted by these liquids give the eye its shape.

The inner surface of the eyelid and the exposed surface of the eye are covered by a fragile membrane called the **conjunctiva** and kept moist by the **lacrimal glands**. Blinking cleans the eye by sweeping the fluid across the eye. Tears drain on the inner side of the eye through two **lacrimal ducts**.

Ears

The human **ear** serves to detect and process sound as well as detect body position and maintain balance. The human ear has three separate divisions—outer, middle, and inner ear (**FIGURE 14-6**; **TABLE 14-3**). The **outer ear** consists of the auricle (or **pinna**), ear lobe, and external ear canal. The **middle ear** includes the tympanic membrane and the ossicles. The **inner ear** comprises the cochlea, semicircular canals, saccule, and utricle.

Sound enters the ear through the auricle (**FIGURE 14-7**). The **auricle**, an irregularly shaped cartilage, channels sound into the ear. Sound travels through the **external ear canal** until it reaches the tympanic membrane. The **tympanic membrane**, or eardrum, separates the outer and middle ear. Sound hits the tympanic membrane, creating vibrations that are then transmitted to the ossicles. The **ossicles** consist of three bones—the malleus (hammer), the incus (anvil), and the stapes (stirrup). The **malleus** lies near the tympanic membrane; vibrations from the membranes cause it to rock back and forth. This rocking causes the **incus** to vibrate, which in turn causes the **stapes** to move in and out against the oval window. The **oval window** is the opening to the inner ear, covered with a membrane. The vibrations created by the tympanic membrane are amplified as they are transmitted through the structures to the inner ear. Movement of the oval window causes fluid within the cochlea to vibrate, creating waves. The **cochlea** is a spiral-shaped structure that houses the organ of Corti

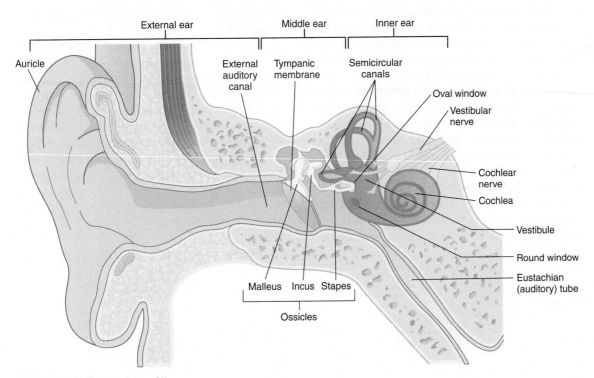

FIGURE 14-6 The structures of the ear.

TABLE 14-3	Structures and Functions of the Ear	
Part	**Structure**	**Function**
Outer ear	Auricle	Funnels sound waves into the external auditory canal
	Ear lobe	No role
	External auditory canal	Directs sound waves to the eardrum
Middle ear	Tympanic membrane, or eardrum	Vibrates when struck by sound waves
	Ossicles	Transmit sound to the cochlea in the inner ear
Inner ear	Cochlea	Converts fluid waves to nerve impulses
	Semicircular canals	Detect head movement
	Saccule and utricle	Detect head movement and linear acceleration

(FIGURE 14-8). The **organ of Corti** contains hearing receptors, in the form of hair cells. Vibrations at the organ of Corti stimulate hair movement. Dendrites wrap the bases of these hair cells. Hair movement causes the dendrites to form nerve impulses that travel to the brain via the vestibulocochlear nerve, which is also known as cranial nerve VIII (see the *Neural Function* chapter).

The inner ear also holds the **vestibular apparatus** (FIGURE 14-9), which consists of two parts—the semicircular canals and the vestibule. The **semicircular canals** are three ringlike, fluid-filled structures that house receptors for body position and movement. The fluid in the semicircular canals works much like a carpenter's level. Movement of the head causes the fluid in the semicircular canal to move; this movement then stimulates dendrites to send impulses to the brain to report the movement. The **vestibule** is a bony chamber positioned between the cochlea and the semicircular canals; it houses receptors that respond to body position and movement. The vestibule contains the **utricle** and the **saccule**, both of which have receptor organs. Nerve impulses generated in the vestibular apparatus travel to a cluster of nerve cell bodies in the brain stem. At the brain stem, these impulses are combined with input from the eyes, skin, joints, and muscles. This center then directs the information to many areas of the brain (see the *Neural Function* chapter). The majority of the information travels on a pathway to the cerebral cortex, increasing awareness of position and movement. Another pathway leads to the muscles of the limbs and torso; information sent via this pathway enables them to maintain balance and correct body position if necessary.

The middle ear also opens into the pharynx via the **eustachian tube**. The eustachian tube acts as a pressure valve. Normally, it remains closed, but the tube may open up with activities such as yawning and swallowing. Opening the eustachian tube allows air to flow in and out of the middle ear, equalizing the internal and external pressures on the tympanic membrane. The function of the eustachian tube becomes apparent when the ears "pop" while taking off in an airplane. This popping sensation is a result of pressure being released from the eustachian tubes.

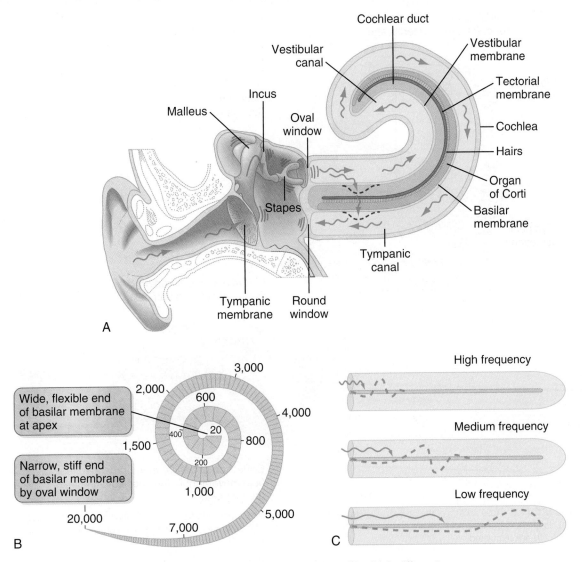

A

B

C

The numbers indicate the frequencies with which different
regions of the basilar membrane maximally vibrate.

FIGURE 14-7 Transmission of sound through the ear. The cochlea is unwound here to simplify matters. (a) Vibrations are transmitted from the stirrup (stapes) to the oval window. Fluid pressure waves are established in the vestibular canal and pass to the tympanic canal, causing the basilar membrane to vibrate. (b) A representation of the basilar membrane, showing the points along its length where the various wavelengths of sound are perceived. Notice that the basilar membrane is narrowest at the base of the cochlea at the oval window end and widest at the apex. (c) High-frequency sounds set the basilar membrane near the base of the cochlea into motion. Hair cells send impulses to the brain, which interprets the signals as a high-pitch sound. Low-frequency sounds stimulate the basilar membrane where it is widest and most flexible.

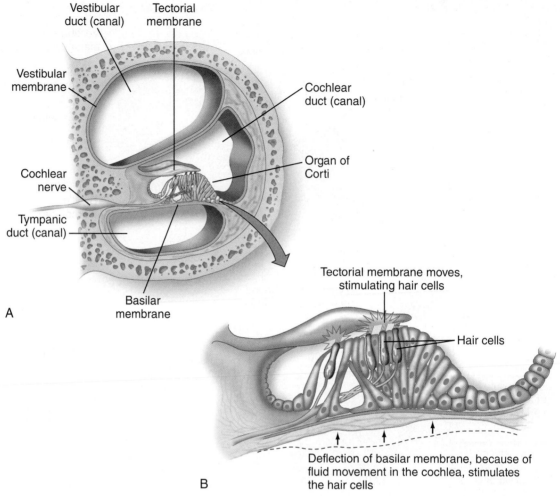

Vestibular duct (canal)

Tectorial membrane

Vestibular membrane

Cochlear duct (canal)

Cochlear nerve

Organ of Corti

Tympanic duct (canal)

Basilar membrane

A

Tectorial membrane moves, stimulating hair cells

Hair cells

Deflection of basilar membrane, because of fluid movement in the cochlea, stimulates the hair cells

B

FIGURE 14-8 Cross section of the cochlea. (a) Notice the three fluid-filled canals and the central position of the organ of Corti. (b) Hair cells of the organ of Corti are embedded in the overlying tectorial membrane. When the basilar membrane vibrates, the hair cells are stimulated.

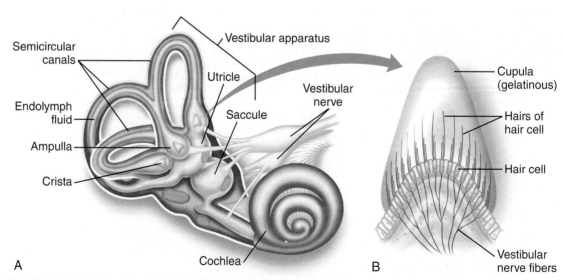

Semicircular canals

Vestibular apparatus

Utricle

Endolymph fluid

Vestibular nerve

Ampulla

Saccule

Crista

Cupula (gelatinous)

Hairs of hair cell

Hair cell

Vestibular nerve fibers

A

Cochlea

B

FIGURE 14-9 Vestibular apparatus. (a) This illustration shows the location of the cristae in the ampullae of the semicircular canals. The semicircular canals are filled with endolymph. (b) When the head spins, the endolymph is set into motion. This action deflects the gelatinous cupula of the crista, thereby stimulating the receptor cells.

UNDERSTANDING CONDITIONS THAT AFFECT THE SENSES

When considering sensory conditions, organizing them based on their basic underlying pathophysiology can increase understanding. In sensory disorders, the primary nursing diagnosis is altered sensory perception. Interventions focus on overcoming those deficits. Because the senses receive and process environmental information, an additional nursing diagnosis that is relevant is risk for injury. Interventions directed at minimizing injury are specific to the sensory deficit.

Congenital Sensory Disorders

Congenital sensory disorders vary widely in severity. Many different conditions may arise when an error occurs during embryonic development. These errors may occur randomly, due to environmental influences, or because of genetic abnormalities. They may result in minor conditions with only aesthetic problems (e.g., microtia) or life-altering states (e.g., congenital cataracts). Treatment is often unnecessary, but when needed, treatment options are usually limited.

Eyes

Congenital eye conditions are rare. These conditions vary widely in severity, but vision impairment is present to some degree in most cases. These conditions seldom happen in isolation and are often associated with other disorders.

Congenital Cataracts

Congenital cataracts involve a clouding of the lens that is present at birth. This clouding of the usually clear lens results in hazy vision. In most cases, no specific cause can be identified. However, congenital cataracts have been associated with several genetic and chromosomal conditions (e.g., Down syndrome, Turner's syndrome, and galactosemia) as well as intrauterine infection exposure (e.g., congenital rubella, syphilis, toxoplasmosis, and herpes simplex).

In addition to clouding of the lens, clinical manifestations usually include a failure of the affected infant to demonstrate visual awareness and the presence of **nystagmus** (rapid, involuntary back-and-forth eye movement). Diagnostic procedures for congenital cataracts consist of a history and physical examination (including a thorough ophthalmology exam). Additional tests may be necessary to determine other associated conditions.

In some cases, congenital cataracts are mild and do not affect vision; these cases require no treatment. Moderate to severe cataracts that affect vision will require cataract extraction surgery, followed by placement of an artificial intraocular lens. Patching to force the child to use the weaker eye may be required to prevent amblyopia (lazy eye). Treatment for any underlying disorder may also be needed.

Ears

Congenital conditions affecting the ears usually result from an absence or malformation of the external ear. These conditions may or may not affect hearing. **Anotia** refers to the absence of the auricle, while **microtia** refers to an underdeveloped, small auricle (**FIGURE 14-10**). Persons with anotia and microtia may also lack an external ear canal (**atresia**). These conditions are more common in males than in females and are often associated with other congenital conditions affecting the head (e.g., hemifacial microsomia, Goldenhar syndrome, and Treacher-Collins syndrome). Such congenital ear conditions may be unilateral or bilateral. In addition to these structural abnormalities, **congenital hearing loss** can occur because of damage associated with maternal rubella and syphilis infection during pregnancy.

Sensory Conditions Associated with Aging

The way in which the body senses and responds to sensory input changes with age. In general, the senses become less acute and less able to distinguish details. These sensory changes vary in severity but can have a tremendous impact on lifestyle and quality of life. Aging increases

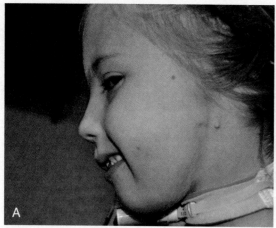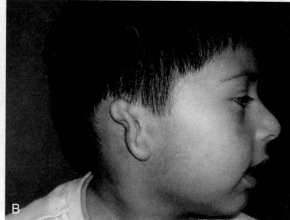

FIGURE 14-10 (a) Anotia. (b) Microtia.

Courtesy of Dr. Arturo Bonilla, Microtia—Congenital Ear Deformity Institute (http://microtia.org)

the threshold needed to perceive sensory input, so the amount of sensory input needed to be aware of the sensation becomes greater. Physical changes in the body part related to the sensation account for most of the other sensation changes. Hearing and vision changes can be the most dramatic, but all senses can be affected by aging. Equipment such as glasses and hearing aids or changes in lifestyle can compensate for many of the sensory aging changes.

Eyes

Age-related eye changes may begin as early as 30 years of age. Such changes include less tear production as well as structural deteriorations. All of the eye structures change to some degree with aging. The cornea becomes less sensitive, so injuries may go unnoticed. By age 60, pupils decrease to about one-third of the size they were at age 20. The pupil may also react more slowly in response to darkness or bright light than it did in one's youth. The lens becomes yellowed, less flexible, and slightly cloudy. The fat pads supporting the eye decrease and the eye sinks back into the skull. The eye muscles weaken, decreasing the ability to rotate the eye fully and limiting the visual field. Visual acuity also may gradually decline.

Glasses or contact lenses may help correct these age-related vision changes. Nearly all persons 55 years of age or older need glasses at least part of the time. However, the severity of changes varies. Only 15–20% of elderly persons have vision deficits severe enough to impair driving ability, and only 5% become unable to read.

The most common eye problem associated with aging is difficulty focusing the eyes, a condition called **presbyopia**. Additionally, intolerance to glare as well as difficulty adapting to darkness and brightness may be experienced, making driving at night difficult. Inability to distinguish colors can also become more pronounced with age. Keeping a red light on in darkened rooms (such as the hallway or bathroom) may make it easier to see than using a regular night light because it produces less glare than a white light bulb.

Ears

All of the ear structures thicken and change with aging, affecting balance and hearing. Hearing may decline slightly, especially in regard to high-frequency sounds. This hearing loss is accelerated in people who were exposed to excessive noise or smoking when they were younger. Such age-related hearing loss is called **presbycusis**. Some hearing loss is almost inevitable, but an estimated 30% of all people older than age 65 have significant hearing impairment. Hearing acuity (sharpness) may decline slightly beginning at about 50 years of age, possibly caused by changes in the auditory nerve. In addition, the brain may have a slight decreased ability to process or translate sounds into meaningful information. Impacted cerumen is another cause of impaired hearing and is more common with increasing age.

Sensorineural hearing loss involves damage to the inner ear, auditory nerve, or the brain. This type of hearing loss may or may not respond to treatment, but hearing aids can improve function. Conductive hearing loss occurs when an individual has problems transmitting sound through the outer and middle ear to the inner ear. Surgery or a hearing aid may be helpful for this type of hearing loss, depending on the specific cause.

Persistent, abnormal ear noise (tinnitus) is another common hearing problem, especially for older adults. Tinnitus may be described as a ringing, buzzing, roaring, or humming sound. It is usually a result of mild hearing loss.

Infectious and Inflammatory Sensory Disorders

Infectious sensory disorders can result from a wide range of causative agents, often triggering the inflammatory response. These conditions may be acute or chronic and vary widely in severity. In most cases, infectious sensory disorders usually resolve with treatment.

Eyes

Eye infections can result from a variety of pathogenic organisms, usually bacteria and viruses. Many of these infections are self-limited, and most respond well to treatment. However, severe or untreated infections can lead to visual impairment. These conditions can also be caused by other events that can trigger the inflammatory process (e.g., trauma, allergens, and irritants).

Conjunctivitis

Conjunctivitis, or pink eye, refers to an infection or inflammation of the conjunctiva, the lining of the eyelids and sclera (**FIGURE 14-11**). Conjunctivitis may be caused by viruses (most common), bacteria (e.g., *Staphylococcus*, *Chlamydia*, and gonorrhea), allergens (e.g., pollen and dust), chemical irritants, and trauma. Each cause produces slightly different manifestations. Regardless of its cause, conjunctivitis can generate edema, blurry vision, photophobia, and pain. Viral infections normally produce a watery or mucuslike exudate. Bacterial infections usually produce a yellow-green exudate. Allergens and irritants typically produce redness, itching, and excessive tearing. Risk factors for developing conjunctivitis include wearing contact lenses as well as using contaminated makeup or ophthalmic medications. Bacterial and viral conjunctivitis are highly contagious through direct contact, and steps are necessary to prevent transmission of the infection (e.g., hand washing, limiting contact, proper eye hygiene, and discarding contaminated ophthalmic products).

Diagnostic procedures for conjunctivitis focus on identifying the causative agent and include a history, physical examination (including an ophthalmic examination, often conducted by an ophthalmologist), and drainage culture. Many cases of conjunctivitis will resolve without treatment. Treatment may vary depending on the underlying cause. These strategies may include ophthalmic or oral antibiotics, antihistamines, corticosteroid agents, and artificial tears. Additionally, warm moist compresses can soothe the discomfort associated with conjunctivitis. Cool compresses can improve edema if present. Maternal transmission of sexually transmitted infections to the infants eyes can occur during vaginal delivery. Because those infections can potentially causing blindness, infants are generally treated with ophthalmic antibiotics shortly after birth.

Keratitis

Keratitis refers to an inflammation of the cornea that can be triggered by an infection or trauma (**FIGURE 14-12**). Common causes of keratitis include trauma (e.g., artificial ultraviolet exposure, welding, contact lens overuse, and abrasions) and viral infections (e.g., herpes simplex, varicella zoster, Epstein-Barr, and cytomegalovirus). Herpes simplex type 1 virus can

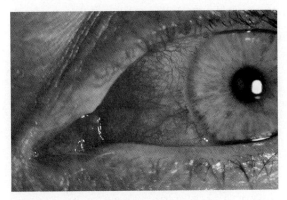

FIGURE 14-11 Conjunctivitis.

Courtesy of John T. Halgren, MD, University of Nebraska Medical Center

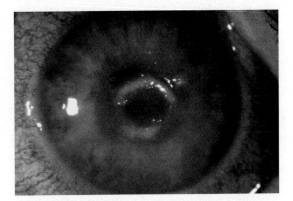

FIGURE 14-12 Keratitis.

Courtesy of Christopher J. Rapuano, MD, Cornea Service, Wills Eye, Professor, Jefferson Medical College of Thomas Jefferson University, Philadelphia, PA

be self-transmitted from the mouth and cause an ulcerated form of keratitis. Clinical manifestations reflect the inflammatory process and include severe pain, erythema, drainage (clear or mucopurulent), excessive tearing, photophobia, and visual disturbances.

Diagnostic procedures for keratitis focus on identifying the causative agent and include a history, physical examination (including an ophthalmic examination, often conducted by an ophthalmologist), and drainage culture. Treatment varies depending on the underlying etiology, but strategies often include ophthalmic or oral antibiotics and corticosteroid agents.

Ears

Ear infections can result from a variety of pathogens, usually bacterial or viral. These conditions are classified based on the area of the ear infected and typically resolve with treatment.

Otitis Media

Otitis media describes an infection or inflammation of the middle ear. Otitis media is a common condition in young children. The eustachian tubes of young children are narrower, straighter, and shorter than those of adults and older children—a developmental variation in anatomy that decreases the ability of fluid to drain from the young child's middle ear adequately. In addition to these structural differences, a young child's immune system is less equipped to manage infections (see the *Immunity* chapter) than that of an adult or older child. Another cause of fluid accumulation in the middle ear is adenoid enlargement, usually due to inflammation. Because of their close proximity to the eustachian tubes, enlargement of the adenoids can compress the tubes.

Typically, otitis media begins as a viral upper respiratory infection, so it is more common in the winter months than in the rest of the year. The viral infection migrates to the middle ear, causing accumulation of fluid behind the tympanic membrane. This fluid buildup provides a prime medium for secondary bacterial growth. Additional risk factors include child care in group settings, feeding infants in the supine position, environmental smoke exposure, pacifier use, a history of allergic rhinitis, and presence of orofacial deformities (e.g., cleft lip or palate). *Streptococcus pneumoniae* and *Haemophilus influenzae* are frequent bacterial causes of otitis media.

Otitis media can lead to rupture of the tympanic membrane, scar tissue formation, and conductive hearing loss. Additionally, the infection can spread to nearby structures and cause mastoiditis, cholesteatoma (a benign epithelial cell tumor on the tympanic membrane), meningitis, and osteomyelitis.

Clinical manifestations can vary depending on age; in some cases, the infection may be asymptomatic. When present, manifestations frequently include the following signs and symptoms:

- Ear pain (related to pressure in the middle ear)
- Crying or irritability
- Rubbing or pulling at the ear
- Mild hearing deficits
- Sleep disturbances
- Red, bulging tympanic membrane
- Indications of infection (e.g., fever, malaise, and chills)
- Purulent or clear exudate from the external ear canal (if the tympanic membrane ruptures)
- Nausea, vomiting, and diarrhea
- Headache

Diagnostic procedures for otitis media consist of a history, a physical examination (including an otologic examination), drainage culture (if drainage is present), and hearing test (if the individual has recurrent infections). The otologic examination usually includes visualization of the tympanic membrane, tympanometry (which measures tympanic membrane movement), and acoustic reflectometry (reflection of sound).

Treatment focuses on eradicating any infection present, decreasing the amount of fluid in the middle ear, and managing pain. Strategies may include oral or otologic (usually not effective unless the tympanic membrane has ruptured) antibiotics and analgesics. Additionally, oral decongestant and antihistamine agents may be administered. Antipyretics may be necessary to control fever. Drainage tubes (tympanostomy tubes) can be inserted to facilitate fluid drainage for children with recurrent otitis media (**FIGURE 14-13**). Removal of the adenoids may also be performed with the placement of tympanostomy tubes.

Otitis Externa

Otitis externa, or swimmer's ear, refers to an infection or inflammation of the external ear canal or auricle. Otitis externa is usually bacterial in origin (often *Pseudomonas aeruginosa*) but may also be fungal. It generally arises from moisture in the ear that creates an environment for

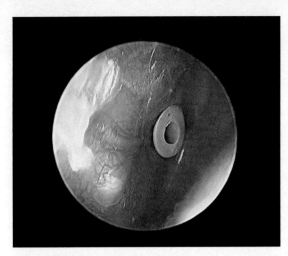

FIGURE 14-13 Tympanostomy tubes.

Courtesy of Andrew Heaford and Richard Smith, University of Iowa

bacterial or fungal growth or introduction of the organisms from external sources. Risk factors include swimming in contaminated water, scratching the outside or inside of the ear, and insertion of foreign objects (e.g., cotton swabs, earphones, and ear plugs) into the ears. Most cases of otitis externa are mild and respond well to treatment, but occasionally this condition can lead to hearing loss, cellulitis, necrosis, osteomyelitis, and meningitis. Clinical manifestations of otitis externa include ear pain that worsens with auricle movement, purulent exudate, pruritus, a sensation of fullness in the ear, and hearing deficits.

Diagnostic procedures typically consist of a history, physical examination (including an otologic examination), and exudate analysis (e.g., culture and sensitivity). Because of the easy access to the external ear canal, treatment strategies are typically applied locally. These strategies may include otologic antibiotic, antifungal, corticosteroid, and analgesic agents. Additionally, the external ear canal may be cleaned (e.g., via lavage of warm saline) and a cotton wick may be inserted to increase medication penetration and absorb drainage. Prevention strategies include drying the ears after swimming or bathing with an alcohol-based product, avoiding insertion of foreign objects into the ear, wearing ear plugs, and treating pools properly.

Traumatic Sensory Disorders

Traumatic sensory disorders can result from a wide range of injuries, and can vary widely in severity. Often the patient's prognosis depends on prompt treatment.

Eyes

Eye trauma can result from numerous types of injuries. These injuries may result from direct physical trauma or chemical burns. Any of the eye structures can be involved, including the eyelid, cornea, or the entire eye globe. These conditions may vary in severity from mild (e.g., black eye) to sight threatening (e.g., corneal abrasions and closed-angle glaucoma). The eye is highly vulnerable to injury, and vision deficits often result from such damage. Clinical manifestations vary depending on the nature of the injury, but may include eye pain, edema, blurry vision, **diplopia** (double vision), dry eyes, photophobia, floaters, pupil dilation, and pupils that are unresponsive to light.

Early diagnosis and treatment can prevent or limit the severity of visual deficits. Diagnostic procedures consist of a history and physical examination (including an ophthalmic examination, often by an ophthalmologist). Treatment strategies may include the following measures:

- Flushing the irritant out of the eye with sterile saline
- Avoiding rubbing the eye (can worsen the damage)
- Leaving an embedded object in the eye
- Covering the eye with a sterile dressing or cloth
- Applying eye patches to protect the eye during the healing process
- Repairing any damage surgically

Ears

Ear trauma can result from a variety of injuries to any of the internal or external ear structures. These injuries may stem from direct physical trauma (e.g., foreign objects and insects) or exposure to excessively loud noises (e.g., explosions and gunshots). Such events can result in permanent hearing deficits. Clinical manifestations of ear trauma may include bloody or clear exudate, tinnitus, dizziness, ear pain, hearing deficits, nausea, vomiting, edema, and a sensation that an object is in the ear.

Treatment strategies vary depending on the nature of the injury. These strategies may include the following measures:

- Removing the object if it is visible and easily removed
- Flushing the ear with sterile water or saline to remove small objects (alcohol or mineral oil may be used for insects to kill them, limiting the trauma during their removal)

One night Tammy, a 24-year-old female, was cleaning her ears with a cotton swab as she does every night as a part of her hygiene routine. She was in a hurry to go out on a date. Her hand slipped as she was cleaning her ears with the cotton swab, and the swab went deep into her right ear. Her ear immediately began to bleed. She continued to get dressed for her date, assuming the bleeding would stop, but it did not. She decided to cancel the date and have her ear checked by a healthcare provider at the after-hours clinic.

At the clinic, the healthcare provider told Tammy that she had probably perforated her tympanic membrane, and it would likely heal in a few weeks. The bleeding continued for the next 24 hours, so Tammy called the clinic again. The healthcare provider at the clinic referred her to an ear, nose, and throat specialist the next day. During her visit with the specialist, Tammy explained the incident with the cotton swab, and the specialist reminded her—as she had heard many times before—"Never put anything smaller than your elbow in your ear." Upon examination, the specialist determined that Tammy had a severe perforation of her tympanic membrane that required surgical repair with skin grafting to prevent permanent severe hearing loss.

Post surgical repair, Tammy continues to have significant hearing loss in her right ear. The risk for graft rejection remains. Steps to protect her hearing are vital and include limiting exposure to excessive noise and avoiding ototoxic medications.

- Performing surgery to remove objects or repair the damage
- Limiting exposure to loud sounds as structures heal

Chronic Sensory Disorders

Numerous chronic conditions can affect the sensory organs. These conditions are often mild and easily managed. In some cases, however, they may cause significant sensory deficits.

Eyes

Many chronic conditions affecting the eyes are progressive and can result in visual deficits. Most of these conditions can be prevented. With early treatment, most cases can be managed effectively.

Glaucoma

Glaucoma refers to a group of eye conditions that lead to damage to the optic nerve. This damage is often caused by increased intraocular pressure, but it can also result from decreased blood flow to the optic nerve (FIGURE 14-14). Pressures inside the eye can climb when the outflow of aqueous humor becomes blocked or when production of aqueous humor increases to an abnormal level. These increased pressures cause ischemia and degeneration of the optic nerve.

Glaucoma is the second leading cause of blindness (after diabetic retinopathy) in the United States. There are four types of glaucoma:

- **Open-angle (chronic) glaucoma**. Open-angle glaucoma is the most common type. For reasons that are unclear, intraocular pressure increases gradually over an extended period. This type of glaucoma tends to run in families, and rates are six to eight times higher among African American individuals than among people of other races. Clinical manifestations typically include painless, insidious, bilateral changes in vision (e.g., tunnel vision, blurred vision, halos around lights, and decreased color discrimination). Because the vision changes are gradual and there are typically no other manifestations, open-angle glaucoma can often be overlooked or misdiagnosed as presbyopia.
- **Closed-angle (acute) glaucoma**. Closed-angle glaucoma, which is a medical emergency, results from a sudden blockage of aqueous humor outflow. This blockage can be caused by trauma, sudden pupil dilation (e.g., exposure to bright light after prolonged exposure to darkness), prolonged pupil dilation (e.g., medications for eye examinations), and emotional stress. Closed-angle glaucoma is typically unilateral, but may affect both eyes. Clinical manifestations are usually sudden in onset and worsen quickly. These manifestations may include severe eye pain, headache, nausea, vomiting, a nonreactive pupil, erythema, haziness of the cornea, and vision changes (e.g., halos around lights and cloudy vision).

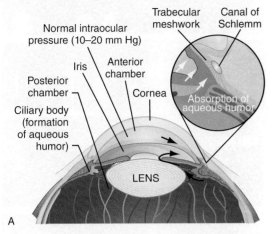

Normal flow of aqueous humor

Normal intraocular pressure (10–20 mm Hg)

Trabecular meshwork

Canal of Schlemm

Iris

Anterior chamber

Posterior chamber

Cornea

Ciliary body (formation of aqueous humor)

Absorption of aqueous humor

LENS

A

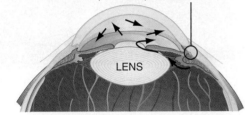

Chronic (open-angle) glaucoma

Degeneration and obstruction of trabecular meshwork and canal of Schlemm decreases absorption of aqueous humor

LENS

B

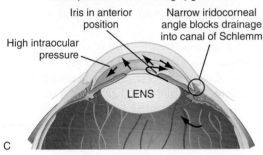

Acute (narrow or closed-angle) glaucoma

Iris in anterior position

Narrow iridocorneal angle blocks drainage into canal of Schlemm

High intraocular pressure

LENS

C

FIGURE 14-14 Types of glaucoma.

- **Congenital glaucoma.** This type of glaucoma is present at birth. It results from abnormal development of outflow channels (trabecular meshwork) of the eye. Congenital glaucoma follows an X-linked, recessive hereditary pattern. It may go unnoticed for a few months after birth. Clinical manifestations may include excessive lacrimation, photophobia, corneal edema, gray-white appearance to the cornea, enlarged eye globe, and vision deficits.
- **Secondary glaucoma.** Secondary glaucoma may result from the use of certain medications (e.g., corticosteroids and anticholinergic agents), eye diseases (e.g., uveitis and nearsightedness), systemic diseases (e.g., arteriosclerosis and diabetes mellitus), and trauma.

Diagnostic procedures for glaucoma consist of a history and physical examination (including an ophthalmic examination). The ophthalmic examination typically involves a gonioscopy (use of a special lens to see the outflow channels of the angle), tonometry (which measures intraocular pressure), optic nerve imaging, pupillary reflex response, retinal examination, slit lamp examination (using a microscope and light to examine the anterior eye structures), visual acuity testing, and visual field measurement.

Treatment focuses on decreasing intraocular pressure. Early detection and treatment are crucial to preserve vision, so those persons at risk for glaucoma should be routinely screened for this condition (usually once a year). Treatment strategies vary depending on the type.

Strategies for open-angle glaucoma may include the following measures:

- Ophthalmic medications (usually a combination of two or three types), including the following:
  - Beta blockers (to reduce aqueous humor production)
  - Alpha agonists (to reduce production and increase drainage of aqueous humor)
  - Carbonic anhydrase inhibitors (to reduce aqueous humor production)
  - Prostaglandin-like compounds (to increase aqueous humor outflow)
  - Miotic or cholinergic agents (to increase aqueous humor outflow)
  - Epinephrine compounds (to increase aqueous humor outflow)
  - Alpha$_2$-adrenergic agonists (to protect the optic nerve)
  - Oral medications (not generally effective when used alone), including carbonic anhydrase inhibitors
  - *N*-methyl-D-aspartate receptor antagonists (may protect the optic nerve)
- Laser surgery to open aqueous humor outflow
- Filtering surgery (to remove a small section of the trabecular meshwork)
- Drainage implants

The main strategy for treating closed-angle glaucoma is iridotomy (a surgical laser procedure to open a new channel in the iris).

The main strategy for treating congenital glaucoma is surgery to open the aqueous humor outflow channels (e.g., laser, filtering, and drainage implants).

Strategies to treat secondary glaucoma include the following measures:

- Chronic disease management
- Treatment or elimination of the underlying causes
- Previously discussed glaucoma pharmacologic and surgical treatments

Cataracts

A **cataract** is opacity or clouding of the lens (**FIGURE 14-15**). Cataracts can occur as a congenital condition (previously discussed) or develop later in life. Over time, proteins in the lens break down, making the lens cloudy. Risk factors for adult-onset cataracts include family history, advancing age, smoking, ultraviolet (UV) light exposure (natural or artificial), metabolic conditions (e.g., diabetes mellitus), certain medications (e.g., corticosteroids), and eye injury (e.g., trauma and infection). Cataracts may affect one or both eyes and do not necessarily affect eyes symmetrically. In addition to the cloudy appearance of the lens, clinical manifestations may include the following signs and symptoms:

- Cloudy, fuzzy, foggy, or filmy vision (**FIGURE 14-16**)
- Color intensity loss
- Diplopia
- Impaired night vision, gradually progressing to impaired day vision
- Halos around lights
- Photosensitivity
- Frequent changes in eyeglass or contact prescription

Diagnostic procedures for cataracts consist of a history and physical examination (including an ophthalmic examination). The ophthalmic examination typically involves visual acuity

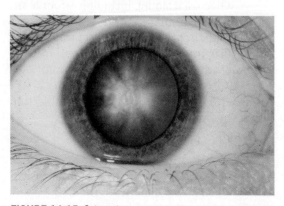

FIGURE 14-15 Cataracts.
Courtesy of National Eye Institute/NIH

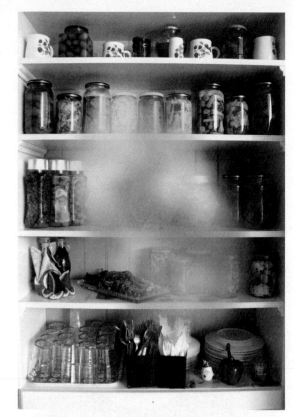

FIGURE 14-16 Visual changes associated with cataracts.
Modified from photo © Effrosyni Labropoulou/Dreamstime.com

testing, retinal examination, and slit lamp examination.

Surgery is the only effective treatment for cataracts. Surgical procedures may include removal of the cataract (e.g., phacoemulsification) or a lens transplant. Surgery is typically performed one eye at a time, as an outpatient procedure with a local anesthetic. Recovery time is usually short, and the prognosis is good. Additional strategies may include managing or eliminating contributing factors.

Macular Degeneration

Macular degeneration refers to a deterioration of the macular area of the retina. Macular degeneration is caused by impaired blood supply to the macula that results in cellular waste accumulation and ischemia. The most significant risk factor for this condition is advancing age. Macular degeneration has a tendency to run in families and is most prevalent in females and Caucasians. Additional risk factors include smoking, increased UV light exposure (natural or artificial), high-fat diet, decreased carotenoid intake, and obesity.

Two types of macular generation are distinguished—dry and wet. Dry macular degeneration—the most common form—occurs when the blood vessels under the macula become thin and brittle. Small yellow deposits (drusen) form under the macula. These deposits increase in size and number, blurring vision and creating a dim spot in the central vision. Wet macular degeneration occurs in only approximately 10% of people with macular degeneration. In this type, brittle vessels break down, and new, abnormal, fragile blood vessels grow under the macula (choroidal neovascularization). These vessels leak blood and fluid, leading to macula damage. Although not as common as dry macular degeneration, this form causes more vision loss. Dry macular degeneration progresses gradually (over years) in contrast to the wet form, which results in a sudden, rapid vision loss (over weeks or months).

Macular degeneration is often asymptomatic initially. The most common manifestation of the dry form is blurry vision with a loss of central vision. The most frequent manifestations of the wet form are distortion of straight lines, dark spots in central vision, and sudden loss of central vision.

Diagnostic procedures for macular degeneration consist of a history and physical examination (including an ophthalmic examination). The ophthalmic examination usually involves visual acuity using the Amsler grid, retinal examination, fluorescein angiogram (uses dye and a camera to evaluate retinal blood flow), and optical coherence tomography (noninvasive retinal imaging).

No treatment exists for dry macular degeneration. However, a combination of vitamins, antioxidants, and zinc—often called the Age-Related Eye Disease Study 2 formula (Chew et al., 2013)—may slow the disease's progression. Smokers should not use this treatment. The recommended supplements contain the following nutrients:

- 500 milligrams (mg) of vitamin C
- 400 international units of vitamin E
- 80 mg of zinc
- 2 mg of copper
- 10 mg of lutein
- 2 mg of zeaxanthin

Although there is no cure for wet macular degeneration, the following treatment strategies may be used:

- Laser surgery—specifically, laser photocoagulation (lasers destroy the abnormal blood vessels)
- Photodynamic therapy (light activates an injected drug to destroy leaking blood vessels)
- Antiangiogenesis or antivascular endothelial growth factor therapy (medications injected into the eye that slow the formation of new blood vessels in the eye)

Low-vision aids (e.g., magnifying glasses and large print) and occupational therapy can also improve independence and quality of life.

Ears

Many chronic conditions affecting the ears are progressive and can result in hearing deficits. Some of these conditions are preventable. With early treatment, most cases can be managed.

Otosclerosis

Otosclerosis refers to an abnormal bone growth in the middle ear, usually involving an imbalance in bone formation and resorption. The cause of otosclerosis is unknown, but it appears to have a hereditary component. In this condition, an abnormal spongelike bone grows in the middle ear, preventing the ear structures from vibrating in response to sound waves. As the abnormal bone grows, hearing loss progressively worsens. Nerve loss can occur in conjunction with the conductive hearing loss. Otosclerosis is most common in young adults, women, and Caucasians. Pregnancy may also trigger otosclerosis. Typically, otosclerosis affects both ears. Tinnitus and vertigo may be present as well.

Diagnostic procedures consist of a history, physical examination (including a hearing test), and temporal-bone computed tomography (CT). Treatment for otosclerosis focuses on minimizing hearing loss or improving hearing. These strategies may include the following measures:

- Medications such as oral fluoride, calcium, or vitamin D, which may help to control the hearing loss, although their efficacy remains in question
- Hearing aids to treat hearing loss
- Surgery to remove the stapes (stapedectomy) and replace it with a prosthesis to cure the condition
- Laser surgery to create an opening in the stapes (stapedotomy) with or without the placement of the prosthetic device

Meniere's Disease

Meniere's disease is a disorder of the inner ear that results from endolymph swelling. This swelling stretches the membranes and interferes with the hair receptors in the cochlea and vestibule. The exact cause is unknown, but Meniere's disease may be associated with metabolic disturbances, hormonal imbalances, autoimmune diseases (e.g., systemic lupus erythematosus, and rheumatoid arthritis), head injuries, otitis media, and syphilis. Additional risk factors include allergic rhinitis, alcohol abuse, stress, fatigue, certain medications (e.g., aspirin), and respiratory infections. Clinical manifestations of Meniere's disease typically occur in waves of acute episodes that last several months, followed by brief periods of relief. The attacks may be triggered by changes in barometric pressure or any of the risk factors. These manifestations include intermittent episodes of vertigo, tinnitus, unilateral hearing loss, and a sensation of ear fullness. Other manifestations include nausea, vomiting, diarrhea, headache, and uncontrollable eye movement. Repeated episodes can lead to permanent hearing loss.

Diagnostic procedures for Meniere's disease consist of a history, physical examination (including a neurologic assessment), hearing test, balance test, electrocholeography (which measures fluid accumulation in the ear), electronystagmography (balance sensors are placed in the inner ear to assess balance in relation to eye movement), caloric stimulation (instillation of warm or cold solution into the inner ear to test eye reflexes), head CT, and head magnetic resonance imaging (MRI). There is no cure for Meniere's disease. Instead, treatment focuses on relieving inner ear pressure and relieving symptoms. Strategies may include the following measures:

- Antihistamine agents (to decrease fluid accumulation)
- Benzodiazepines (to improve vertigo)
- Anticholinergic agents (to decrease fluid accumulation)
- Diuretics (to decrease fluid accumulation)
- Antiemetic agents (to improve nausea and vomiting)
- Limiting dietary sodium intake (to decrease fluid retention)
- Avoiding triggers (e.g., alcohol and stress)
- Middle ear injections of gentamicin (an ototoxic antibiotic that can reduce balance structures) or corticosteroids (to reduce swelling)
- Partial or complete surgical removal of the endolymph or inner ear
- Vestibular nerve resection
- Hearing aids
- Meniett device (for difficult-to-treat vertigo; it improves fluid exchange by applying pulses of pressure to the ear canal through a ventilation tube)
- Physical therapy to improve balance

Sensory Organ Cancers

Any of the sensory organs can develop cancer, but such disease is rare. The severity varies depending on the type of cancer, and treatment often follows the typical cancer management regimens (e.g., chemotherapy, radiation, and surgery) (see the *Hematopoietic Function* chapter). Ear cancer is extremely rare and typically involves skin cancer (see the *Integumentary Function* chapter) of the auricle. For this reason, ear cancer will not be included in this discussion.

Eyes

An uncommon condition, eye cancer can affect any part of the eye, from the eyelid to the intraocular structures. The most common intraocular cancers in adults are melanoma and lymphoma. The most frequent eye cancer in children is retinoblastoma. Cancer can also metastasize to the eye from other parts of the body. According to the American Cancer Society (2014), eye cancer is most common in Caucasians, and has an overall 5-year survival rate of nearly 80%. Clinical manifestations of eye cancer typically include some sort of visual disturbance (e.g., losing part of the visual field and seeing flashing lights).

Most cases of eye cancer are found during a routine ophthalmic examination (e.g., finding dark spots on the iris). Additional diagnostic procedures may include a history, ultrasound, fluorescein angiography (imaging of blood vessels in the eye using contrast dye), biopsy, and other tests to detect and evaluate metastasis (e.g., CT and MRI).

Treatment varies depending on the cancer type, location, and size. Surgery is the foundation of most eye cancer treatment. It may entail removal of all (enucleation) or part of the eye (e.g., iridectomy and choroidectomy). Additionally, radiation may be used (e.g., teletherapy and brachytherapy). A prosthetic eye may be used if the entire eye is removed.

Miscellaneous Sensory Organ Conditions

Several sensory organ conditions that do not fall under the previously discussed categories warrant discussion.

Eyes

A few eye conditions that do not fit previously discussed categories can occur. These conditions may be manifestations of other problems or happen alone. Some of these conditions are minor, causing minimal deficits. Other conditions can cause severe visual deficits.

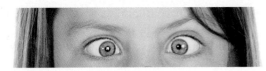

FIGURE 14-17 Strabismus.
© Justin Paget/Shutterstock

Strabismus

Strabismus, or cross-eyes, is a gaze deviation of one eye (**FIGURE 14-17**). With strabismus, the eyes do not coordinate to focus on the same object together, resulting in diplopia. This condition most often appears at birth or shortly after. In children, the brain will begin to ignore the input from one of the eyes. If the brain continues to ignore one eye, the eye will never function properly, and permanent visual deficits may result (e.g., amblyopia). A weak or hypertonic eye muscle, a short muscle, or a neurologic deficit can cause strabismus. These defects are often associated with chromosomal defects (e.g., Down syndrome), intrauterine infection exposure (e.g., congenital rubella), eye cancers (e.g., retinoblastoma), and traumatic brain injuries.

Diagnostic procedures for strabismus consist of a history and physical examination (including an ophthalmic examination and a neurologic examination). Treatment focuses on strengthening the weak eye and realigning the eyes. It often involves resting the normally aligned eye to strengthen the misaligned eye. Strategies usually include glasses (e.g., prism glasses), eye muscle exercises, eye patching, and surgery.

Amblyopia

Amblyopia, or lazy eye, is the loss of one eye's ability to see details. It is the most common cause of vision problems in children. Amblyopia occurs when the brain and the eyes do not work together properly; that is, the brain favors one eye. The preferred eye has normal vision, but because the brain ignores the other eye, vision does not develop normally. The normal eye attempts to compensate for the affected eye, creating a vicious cycle in which the normal eye becomes stronger and the affected eye becomes weaker. The brain stops growing between 5 and 10 years of age, at which time the condition becomes permanent. Strabismus is the most frequent cause of amblyopia. Other causes include a family history, bilateral astigmatism, congenital cataracts, farsightedness, and nearsightedness.

Diagnostic procedures for amblyopia consist of a history and physical examination (including an ophthalmic examination). Much like with strabismus, treatment focuses on strengthening the weak eye and realigning the eyes. It often involves resting the normal eye to strengthen the weaker eye. Strategies usually include wearing glasses (e.g., prism glasses), eye muscle exercises, eye patching, ophthalmic medication (atropine may be used to dilate the pupil of the normal eye to "chemically patch" it), and surgery.

Retinal Detachment

Retinal detachment is an acute condition that occurs when the retina separates from its supporting structures. This separation can happen spontaneously or because of severe nearsightedness (myoplia), trauma, diabetes mellitus, inflammation, degenerative aging changes, and scar tissue. Retinal detachment occurs when vitreous humor leaks through a retinal tear and accumulates underneath the retina. Leakage can also occur through tiny holes where the retina has thinned due to aging or other retinal disorders. Less commonly, fluid can leak directly underneath the retina without a tear or break. As vitreous humor collects underneath it, the retina peels away from the underlying choroid. These detached areas may expand over time, like wallpaper that, once torn, slowly peels off a wall. In turn, the retina becomes ischemic and stops functioning, causing vision loss.

Retinal detachment is typically painless. Clinical manifestations often include flashes of light in the peripheral visual field, blurred vision, floaters, and darkening vision (like a curtain drawing across a visual field). Diagnostic procedures consist of a history and physical examination (including an ophthalmic examination, often performed by an ophthalmologist). The ophthalmic examination may involve an electroretinogram (a record of the electrical currents in the retina produced by visual stimuli), fluorescein angiography, intraocular pressure measurements, ophthalmoscopy, a refraction test, retinal photography, color discrimination, visual acuity testing, slit lamp examination, and eye ultrasound.

Retinal detachment is a medical emergency requiring immediate treatment. Surgery is often the best treatment option. Surgical options include a cryopexy (intense cold application to the area with an ice probe to form scar tissue, which holds the retina to the underlying layer), laser surgery (to seal the tears or holes in the retina), pneumatic retinopexy (placing a gas bubble in the eye to help the retina float back into place), scleral buckle (indents the eye wall), and vitrectomy (removes gel or scar tissue pulling on the retina). These procedures may be performed alone or in combination with each other.

Ears

A few ear conditions that do not fit previously discussed categories can occur. These conditions may be manifestations of other problems or happen alone. Most of these conditions are mild, causing only minor issues.

Tinnitus

Tinnitus describes hearing abnormal noises in the ear. These noises may be described as a ringing, buzzing, humming, whistling, roaring, or blowing. Tinnitus is a common problem, affecting approximately 45 million Americans (American Tinnitus Association, 2013). It is not a condition itself, but rather a symptom of an underlying issue. Although tinnitus can be bothersome, it does not usually warrant significant concern. Tinnitus may be associated with presbycusis, exposure to excessive noise, cerumen impaction, otosclerosis, Meniere's disease, stress, head injury, acoustic neuroma (a benign tumor on the acoustic nerve), atherosclerosis, hypertension, carotid stenosis, arteriovenous malformation, caffeine, and ototoxic medications (e.g., many antibiotics, aspirin, chemotherapies, and diuretics).

Diagnostic procedures for tinnitus focus on identification of the underlying cause. These procedures may consist of a history, physical examination (including a complete hearing test and otoscopic examination), and additional tests as necessary to identify the cause. Treating the underlying disorder (e.g., removing cerumen and controlling blood pressure) will resolve tinnitus in most cases. If needed, additional strategies may include the following measures:

- Tricyclic antidepressants to reduce tinnitus symptoms
- Alprazolam (Niravam, Xanax), a benzodiazepine, to reduce tinnitus symptoms

- Acamprosate (Campral), a drug used to treat alcoholism, to relieve tinnitus
- Masking tinnitus symptoms with white noise machines and hearing aids
- Avoiding factors that can worsen tinnitus (e.g., caffeine, smoking, and ototoxic medications)

Vertigo

Vertigo refers to an illusion of motion. Vertigo is not the same as dizziness. Dizziness is feeling "lightheaded," or as though one might faint. In contrast, people experiencing vertigo have a sensation that they or the room is spinning or moving. In addition to the sensation of movement, clinical manifestations may include nausea and vomiting.

Two types of vertigo are distinguished—peripheral and central. Peripheral vertigo occurs when there is a problem with the vestibular labyrinth, semicircular canals, or vestibular nerve. Certain medications (e.g., aminoglycoside antibiotics), head injury, Meniere's disease, nerve compression, infection, and inflammation may cause this type of vertigo. Central vertigo occurs when there is a problem in the brain, particularly in the brain stem or cerebellum. Arteriosclerosis, certain medications (e.g., antiseizure agents and aspirin), alcohol, migraines, multiple sclerosis, and seizures may cause this type of vertigo.

Diagnostic strategies for vertigo include a history, physical examination, and other tests to determine the underlying etiology (e.g., head CT and MRI). Pharmacology is the mainstay of treatment. The medications used for this purpose include anticholinergic agents, antihistamines (especially meclizine [Antivert]), benzodiazepines, and antiemetics. Safety precautions should also be taken to prevent injury from falls (e.g., changing positions slowly and mobility assistance).

application to practice

Now that we have discussed conditions of the sensory function system, let's put that knowledge into practice. While working in a clinic, you encounter the following patients. Which patient would at greatest risk for developing significant vision problems?

- A postpartum woman
- A young man who has diabetes mellitus
- A middle-aged adult who takes aspirin daily
- An older man with mild presbyopia

When determining who is at greatest risk, start by counting risk factors. The postpartum woman has no significant risk factors that would damage vision. Now, consider the young man with diabetes. Diabetic retinopathy is the number one cause of blindness. The fact that the patient is young means he could have the condition longer, increasing his likelihood of developing vision problems. Moving on to the middle-aged man taking aspirin, this patient has no significant risk factors for vision issues. Finally, consider the older man with mild presbyopia. Increased age is a risk factor for many eye conditions. Mild presbyopia is part of normal aging, however, and does not increase risk of other conditions. In contrast, severe presbyopia does increase risk of vision problems. Considering all of these patients, the young man with diabetes is at the highest risk for vision problems. Knowing that, the patient should have an annual eye exam.

CHAPTER SUMMARY

The sensory organs work together to sense changes in the body's internal and external environment. This information is then relayed to the nervous system for interpretation and response. Disorders of these organs can significantly affect the body's sensory function and can even be life altering. Some of these conditions can be prevented by restricting noise exposure (e.g., wearing protective ear coverings and minimizing music volume) and shielding the eyes (e.g., by wearing protective eye goggles and UV-protective sunglasses). Early diagnosis and treatment of other conditions can improve prognosis.

REFERENCES

AAOS. (2004). *Paramedic: Anatomy and physiology*. Sudbury, MA: Jones & Bartlett.

American Cancer Society. (2014). Eye cancer. Retrieved from http://www.cancer.org/cancer/eyecancer/

American Tinnitus Association. (2013). Demographics. Retrieved from https://www.ata.org/understanding-facts/demographics

Chew, E., Clemons, T., Agron, E., Sperduto, R., Sangiovanni, J., Kurinij, N., & Davis, M. (2013). Long-term effects of vitamins C and E, beta-carotene, and zinc on age-related macular degeneration: AERDS report no. 35. *Ophthalmology, 120*, 1604–1611.

Chiras, D. (2011). *Human biology* (7th ed.). Sudbury, MA: Jones & Bartlett Learning.

Elling, B., Elling, K., & Rothenberg, M. (2004). *Anatomy and physiology*. Sudbury, MA: Jones and Bartlett.

Gould, B. (2015). Pathophysiology for the health professions (5th ed.). Philadelphia, PA: Elsevier.

Professional guide to pathophysiology (3rd ed.). (2010). Philadelphia, PA: Lippincott Williams & Wilkins.

Normal Lab Values

Cardiac Packet	
CPK-MB/CPK relative index	< 2.5%
CPK—total	WM: 60–320 units/L
	WF: 50–200 units/L
	BM: 130–450 units/L
	BF: 60–270 units/L
Glucose	70–110 mg/dL
LDH—total	100–190 units/L
LDH-1	14–26%
Troponin 1	Negative

CBC	
RBC count	M: 4.5–6.0 million/cc
	F: 4.0–5.5 million/cc
Hct	M: 40–50%
	F: 35–45%
Hgb	M: 14–18 g/dL
	F: 12–16 g/dL
RBC indices	
MCV	80–95 μm^3
MCH	27–31 pg
MCHC	32–36 g/dL
RDW	11–15%
WBC count	5,000–10,000/mm^3
Granulocytes	
Neutrophils	2,500–8,000/mm^3
Eosinophils	50–500/mm^3
Basophils	25–100/mm^3
Agranulocytes	
Lymphocytes	1,000–4,000/mm^3
Monocytes	100–700/mm^3
Platelet count	150,000–400,000/mm^3

Chem 7, Chem 12, Chem 20, Hepatic Function Panel, Renal Function Panel, Abdominal Pain Panel

ALP	30–100 units/L
ALT (SGPT)	5–40 units/L
Amylase	50–190 units/L
AST (SGOT)	5–40 units/L
Bilirubin—total	0.1–1.25 mg/dL
Direct	0.1–0.3 mg/dL
Indirect	0.2–1.0 mg/dL
BUN	8–20 mg/dL
Ca^{++}—total	9–11 mg/dL
Ionized	4.25–5.25 mg/dL

Coagulation Tests

Coagulation factors	
I (fibrinogen)	200–400 mg/dL
II (prothrombin)	80–120%
D-Dimer	< 250 mcg/L
FDPs	< 10 mcg/mL
Platelet count	150,000–400,000/mm³
PT	11–15 s
PTT	60–80 s
aPTT	25–40 s
Thrombin time	10–13 s

CSF

Pressure	70–200 mm H_2O
Color	Clear
Protein	10–45 mg/dL
Glucose	45–78 mg/dL
WBCs—total	< 5 cells/mm³
Neutrophils	0–4%
Lymphocytes	60–80%
Monocytes	20–50%

Electrolyte Panel

Na^+	135–145 mEq/L
K^+	3.5–5 mEq/L
Cl	91–110 mEq/L
CO_2	20–30 mEq/L

Lipid Profile

HDL	M: > 45 mg/dL
	F: > 55 mg/dL
LDL	60–180 mg/dL
VLDL	25–50%
Total cholesterol	< 200 mg/dL
Triglycerides	M: 40–60 mg/dL
	F: > 35–135 mg/dL

Toxicology: Toxic Levels

Drug Serum Screen

Acetaminophen	> 250 mcg/mL
Alcohol	
Intoxicated	0.1–0.4%
Stuporous	0.4–0.5%
Comatose	> 0.5%
ASA	> 300 mcg/mL
Barbitals	
Sedatives	> 10 mcg/mL
Anticonvulsants	> 40 mcg/mL
Carboxyhemoglobin	> 20%
Dilantin	> 20 mcg/mL
Lead	> 40 mcg/mL
Lithium	> 2.0 mEq/L

Drug Urine Screen

Amphetamine	> 3 mcg/mL
Diet suppressants	> 15 mcg/mL
Dextroamphetamine phenmetrazine	> 50 mcg/mL
Methamphetamine	> 40 mcg/mL
Mercury	> 100 mcg/day

Urinalysis

Volume	750–1,800 cc/day
pH	4.6–8.0
Appearance	Clear
Color	Amber
Specific gravity	1.003–1.030
Osmolality	250–1,000 mOsm/L
Albumin	10–100 mg/day

(continues)

Urinalysis (*continued*)

Amylase	< 17 units/h
Calcium	< 250 mg/day
Creatinine	0.75–1.5 g/day
Glucose	< 500 mg/day
Potassium	25–125 mEq/day
Protein	0–8 mg/dL
Sodium	40–220 mEq/day
Urea nitrogen	10–20 g/day
Uric acid	250–750 mg/day

Root Words and Combining Forms

Root Word	Combining Form	Definition	Example
A			
abdomen	abdomin/o	abdomen	abdominocentesis
acanth		thorn	acanthosis
achilles	achill/o	Achilles' heel	achillobursitis
acid	acid/o	acid (pH)	acidosis
acoust	acoust/o	hearing	acoustics
acr	acr/o	extremity	acroarthritis
actin	actin/o	ray	actinodermatitis
acu	acul/o	needle	acupuncture
aden	aden/o	gland	adenosis
adip	adip/o	fat	adipocyte
adren	adren/o	adrenal gland	adrenomegaly
aer	aer/o	air	aerophore
agglutinat	agglutinat/o	clumping	agglutination
albin	albin/o	white	albinuria
albumin	albumin/o	protein	albuminuria
alkali	alkali/o	basic (pH)	alkalosis
all	all/o	other	allochromasia
alveoli	alveol/o	small hole, air sac	alveoloclasia
ambly	ambly/o	dull	amblyopia
ambul	ambul/o	walk	ambulate
ametr	ametr/o	disproportionate	ametropia
amnion	amni/o	amnion	amniocentesis
amyl	amyl/o	starch	amylorrhea
andr	andr/o	man (male)	androgenus
angi	angi/o	vessel	angioplasty
angina	angin/o	choke	anginose

Root Word	Combining Form	Definition	Example
A			
aniso	anis/o	unequal	anisocytosis
ankyl	ankyl/o	stiffened, crooked	ankylosis
anthrac	anthrac/o	coal	anthracosis
antr	antr/o	cavity	antroscopy
anus	an/o	anus	anoscope
aort	aort/o	aorta	aortography
append	append/o	appendix	appendectomy
arachn	arachn/o	spider	arachnoid
arteri	arteri/o	artery	arterial
arthr	arthr/o	joint	arthroscopy
atel	atel/o	imperfect, incomplete	atelectasis
ather	ather/o	fatty	atherosclerosis
atri	atri/o	atrium, chamber	atriomegaly
audi	audi/o	hear	audiology
aur	aur/o	ear	aural
axill	axill/o	armpit	axillary
B			
bacteri	bacteri/o	bacteria	bacteriuria
balan	balan/o	glans	balanitis
bas	bas/o	base (pH)	basophyl
bil	bil/i	gall, bile	biliary
bilirubin	bilirubin/o	bilirubin	hyperbilirubinism
bio	bi/o	life	biosphere
blephar	blephar/o	eyelid	blepharitis
bol	bol/o	cast, throw	anabolic
brachy	brachy/o	arm	brachyocephalic
bronch	bronch/o	bronchi	bronchitis
bucc	bucc/o	cheek	buccocclusion
burs	burs/o	pouch	bursitis
C			
cac	cac/o	bad, diseased	cachexia
calc	calc/i	calcium	calciuria
calcane	calcane/o	heel bone	calcaneodynia
capn	capn/i	smoke, carbon dioxide	hypercapnia
carcin	carcin/o	cancer	carcinoma

Root Word	Combining Form	Definition	Example
cardi	cardi/o	heart	cardioplagia
carp	carp/o	wrist	carpopedal
cata	cat/a	down, downward	catatonic
caud	caud/o	tail	caudal
caus	caus/o	heat	causalgia
cecum	cec/o	cecum	cecoileostomy
celi	celi/o	abdomen	celioma
centr	centr/i	center	centrilobular
cephal	cephal/o	head	cephalhydrocele
cerebell	cerebell/o	little brain (cerebellum)	cerebellospinal
cerebr	cerebr/o	brain (cerebrum)	cerebromalacia
cerumin	cerumin/o	wax	ceruminolysis
cervic	cervic/o	neck	cervicofacial
cheil	cheil/o	lip	cheilosis
chem	chem/o	chemical	chemotherapy
cholangi	cholangi/o	bile vessel	cholangioma
chole	chole/o	gall, bile	cholecystogram
choledoch	choledoch/o	common bile duct	choledochotomy
cholester	cholester/o	cholesterol, fat	cholesterosis
chondr	chondr/o	cartilage	chondrocarcinoma
chori	chori/o	chorion	chorioadenonia
choroid	choroid/o	choroid	choroiditis
cine	cine/o	motion	cineradiography
cinemato	cinemat/o	motion	cinematoradiograph
cirrho	cirrh/o	yellow, tawny	cirrhosis
cis	cis/o	cut	excision
cistern	cistern/o	reservoir, cavity	cisternography
clavic	clavic/o	clavicle	clavicotomy
clavicul	clavicul/o	clavicle	clavicular
cleid	cleid/o	clavicle	cleidorrhexis
clon	clon/o	turmoil	clonogenic
coagul	coagul/o	clot	coagulopathy
coccidioid	coccidioid/o	fungus	coccidioidmycosis
coccyx	coccyg/o	tail bone	coccygodynia
cochle	cochle/o	snail	cochleotopic

(continues)

Root Word	Combining Form	Definition	Example
C			
coit	coit/o	coming together	coitis
coll	coll/o	glutinous, jelly-like	colragenitis
colon	colon/o	colon	colonoscopy
colp	colp/o	vagina	colporrhapy
condyl	condyl/o	knuckle	condyloma
coni	coni/o	dust	coniosis
copr	copr/o	feces, excrement	coprostasis
cord	cord/o	cord	cordotomy
coria	cori/o	pupil (eye)	diplocoria
cortic	cortic/o	cortex	corticosterone
cost	cost/o	rib	costosternal
cox	cox/o	hip	coxalgia
crani	crani/o	skull	craniotomy
cretin	cretin/o	cretin	cretinism
crin	crin/o	secrete	endocrinology
crypt		hidden	cryptorchism
culd	culd/o	cul-de-sac	culdocentesis
cutane	cutan/o	skin	subcutaneous
cycl	cycl/o	ciliary body	cycloplegia
cyst	cyst/o	bladder	cystistaxia
cyt	cyt/o	cell	cytoplasm
D			
dacry	dacry/o	tear	dacryoma
dactyl	dactyl/o	finger, toe	dactylospasm
dem	dem/o	people	endemic
dendr	dendr/o	branched	dendritis
dent	dent/i	tooth	dentifrice
derm	derm/o	skin	dermomycosis
dermat	dermat/o	skin	dermatitis
didym	didym/o	testis	didymalgia
dilat	dilat/o	widen	dilation
dipl	dipl/o	double	diplopia
dips	dips/o	thirst	dipsomania
disk	disk/o	disk	diskectomy
diverticul	diverticul/o	diverticula	diverticulitis

Root Word	Combining Form	Definition	Example
dont	dont/o	tooth	oligodontia
dos	dos/i	giving	dosimeter
duoden	duoden/o	duodenum	duodenostomy
dur	dur/o	hard	duroarachnitis

E

Root Word	Combining Form	Definition	Example
electr	electr/o	electricity	electrocardiogram
embol	embol/o	throwing in	embolism
emmetr	emmetr/o	ideal	emmetropia
emphys	emphys/o	inflate	emphysema
encephal	encephal/o	brain	encephalogram
enter	enter/o	intestine	enteritis
epidem	epidem/o	upon people	epidemic
epididym	epididym/o	epididymis	epididymectomy
episi	episi/o	vulva, pudenda	episiotomy
erythrocyt	erythrocyt/o	red blood cell	erythrocytosis
esophage	esophag/o	esophagus	esophagocele
esthesi	esthesi/o	feeling	anesthesia

F

Root Word	Combining Form	Definition	Example
fasci	fasci/o	hand	fasciodis
fibr	fibr/o	fiber	fibroma
fibrin	fibrin/o	fiber	fibrinogen
fibul	fibul/o	fibula	fibular
fluor/o	fluor/o	fluorescence	fluoroscopy
foramin	foramin/o	foramen, opening	foraminoctomy
format	format/o	formation	malformation

G

Root Word	Combining Form	Definition	Example
galact	galact/o	milk	galactorrhea
gangli	gangli/o	knot	ganglionectomy
gastr	gastr/o	stomach	gastritis
gen	gen/o	beginning, origin	genesis
genet	genet/o	producing	genetics
genit	genit/o	genitals	genitourinary
genital	genital/o	genitals	hypogenitalia
ger	ger/o	old age	geriatric
geront	geront/o	aged	gerontology

(*continues*)

Root Word	Combining Form	Definition	Example
G			
gigant	gigant/o	giant	gigantism
gingiv	gingiv/o	gums	gingivitis
glandul	glandul/o	little acorn, gland	glandular
glomerul	glomerul/o	little ball	glomerulitis
gloss	gloss/o	tongue	glossopharyngeal
gluc	gluc/o	glucose, sugar	glucocorticoid
glyc	glyc/o	sugar	glycogenesis
gonad	gonad/o	ovaries, testes	gonadotropin
goni	goni/o	angle	gonioscope
granul	granul/o	granular	granulocyte
gravid	gravid/o	pregnant	primigravida
gynec	gynec/o	female	gynecology
H			
halat	halat/o	breathe	inhalation
hem	hem/o	blood	hemoglobin
hemat	hemat/o	blood	hematocrit
hepat	hepat/o	liver	hepatoma
herni	herni/o	hernia	herniotomy
hidr	hidr/o	sweat	anhidrosis
hirsut	hirsut/o	hair	hirsutism
hist	hist/o	tissue	histology
hol	hol/o	whole	holography
humer	humer/o	humerus	humeral
hydr	hydr/o	water	hydrocele
hymen	hymen/o	hymen	hymenectomy
hypn	hypn/o	sleep	hypnosis
hyster	hyster/o	womb, uterus	hysterectomy
I			
ichthy	ichthy/o	fish (scaly)	ichthyosos
icter	icter/o	jaundice	icterogenic
ile	ile/o	ileum	ileostomy
ili	ili/o	ilium	iliosacral
immun	immun/o	safe, protect	immunotherapy
insul	insul/o	pancreatic islets	insuloma
insulin	insulin/o	insulin	insulinogenic

Root Word	Combining Form	Definition	Example
ion	ion/o	ion	ionoradioscope
irid	irid/o	iris	iridomalacia
ischem	ischem/o	hold back	ischemic
ischi	ischi/o	hip	ischiodynia
J			
jejun	jejun/o	jejunum	jejunotomy
K			
kary	kary/o	nucleu (cell)	karyotype
kel	kel/o	tumor	keloid
kerat	kerat/o	cornea	keratitis
ket	ket/o	ketone	ketosis
kinesi	kinesi/o	motion	bradykinesia
kinet	kinet/o	motion	kinetosis
kyph	kyph/o	hump	kyphosis
L			
labyrinth	labyrinth/o	maze	labyrinthitis
lacrim	lacrim/o	tear	lacrimotomy
lamin	lamin/o	shin plate	laminectomy
lapar	lapar/o	flank, abdomen	laparotomy
laryng	laryng/o	larynx	laryngoscope
later	later/o	side	lateroflexion
laxat	laxat/o	loosen	laxative
lei	lei/o	smooth	leiomyosarcoma
letharg	letharg/o	drowsiness	lethargy
lingu	lingu/o	tongue	nigralingua
lip	lip/o	fat	lipoatrophy
lith	lith/o	stone	lithotripsy
lob	lob/o	lobe	lobotomy
log	log/o	word, study	logomania
lord	lord/o	bending, curvature	lordosis
lumb	lumb/o	loin	lumbodynia
lymph	lymph/o	lymph, lymph gland	lymphoma
M			
mamm	mamm/o	breast	mammogram
mandibul	mandibul/o	lower jaw	mandibular

(*continues*)

Root Word	Combining Form	Definition	Example
M			
mast	mast/a	breast	mastectomy
maxill	maxill/o	upper jaw	maxillotomy
meat	meat/o	passage	meatotomy
mediastin	mediastin/o	mediastinum	mediastinits
medull	medull/o	marrow, spinal	medulloepithelioma
melan	melan/o	black	melanoma
men	men/o	month, menstruate	dysmenorrhea
mening	mening/o	membrane	meningitis
menisc	menisc/o	crescent shape	meniscitis
metr	metr/o	uterus	metritis
micturit	micturit/o	urinate	micturition
mitr	mitr/o	mitral valve	mitral
morph	morph/o	form, shape	morphology
muc	muc/o	mucus	mucositis
muscul	muscul/o	muscle	musculoskelectal
my	my/o	muscle	myoblast
myc	myc/o	fungus	mycosis
myel	myel/o	spinal cord	myeloma
myring	myring/o	membrane, mucus	myringoplasty
N			
narc	narc/o	night, sleep	narcosis
nas	nas/o	nose	nasogastric
necr	necr/o	death	necrosis
nephr	nephr/o	kidney	nephrema
neur	neur/o	nerve	neuroma
neutr	neutr/o	neither, neutral (pH)	neutrophyl
noct	noct/o	night	nocturia
nucle	nucle/o	nucleus, central	nuclear
nyct	nyct/o	night	nyctalgia
nyctal	nyctal/o	blind, night	nyctalopia
O			
ocul	ocul/o	eye	oculopupillary
olecran	olecran/o	elbow	olecranarthopathy
oment	oment/o	omentun	omentectomy
omphal	omphal/o	umbilicus	omphalitis

Root Word	Combining Form	Definition	Example
onc	onc/o	tumor	oncology
onych	onych/o	nail	onychitis
oophor	oophor/o	ovary	oophoritis
ophthalm	ophthalm/o	eye	ophthalmopathy
opt	opt/o	eye	optomyometer
orchi	orchi/o	testicle	orchitis
orchid	orchid/o	testicle	orchidopexy
organ	organ/o	organ	organomegaly
oscill	oscill/o	swing	oscillopsia
osm	osm/o	smell	anosmia
oste	oste/o	bone	osteorrhapy
ot	ot/o, ov/i, ov/o	ear, egg	otosclerosis, oviduct, ovoplasm
ovul	ovul/o	egg, ovum	ovulate
ox	ox/o	oxygen	anoxia
oxy	oxy/o	oxygen	oxytoxin

P

palat	palat/o	palate	palatitis
pancreat	pancreat/o	pancreas	pancreatitis
papill	papill/o	papilla	papilledema
par	par/o	bear	paroxism
parathyr	parathyr/o	parathyroid gland	parathyroidism
patell	patell/o	patella, kneecap	patellapexy
path	path/o	disease	pathology
ped	ped/o	foot	pedal
ped	ped/i	child	pediatrics
pedicul	pedicul/o	louse	pediculosis
pen	pen/o	penis	penitis
pept	pept/o	digest	peptogenic
perine	perine/o	perineum	perineocele
phac	phac/o	lens	phacosclerosis
phag	phag/u	eat, engulf	phagocyte
phalange	phalang/o	finger, toe	phalangectomy
pharmac	pharmac/o	drug	pharmacotherapy
pharyng	pharyng/o	pharynx	pharyngitis
phe	phe/o	dusky, muzzle	pheochromocytoma

(continues)

Root Word	Combining Form	Definition	Example
P			
phim	phim/o	muscle	phimosis
phleb	phleb/o	vein	phlebitis
phon	phon/o	sound, voice	phonopathy
phragm	phragm/o	partition	diaphragm
phragma	phragmat/o	partition	diaphragmatocele
phren	phren/o	diaphragm	phrenoplegia
physi	physi/o	nature	physiology
physic	physic/o	nature	physician
pin	pin/o	drink, pinlitary gland	pinocytosis
pineal	pineal/o	pineal body	pinealoma
pituitar	pituitar/o	pituitary gland	pituitarism
pleur	pleur/o	pleura	pleuritis
pneum	pneum/o	air	pneumothorax
pneumon	pneumon/o	lung	pneumonitis
poikil	poikil/o	irregular shape, passage	poikilocytosis
por	por/o	passage	poroma
porphyr	porphyr/o	porphyrin, purple	porphyrinuria
presby	presby/o	old	presbycusis
proct	proct/o	rectum, anus	proctatestomy, proctalgia
prostat	prostat/o	prostate	prostatectomy
psych	psych/o	mind	psychology
pteryg	pteryg/o	winglike	pterygomandibular
ptyal	ptyal/o	salvia	ptyalorrhea
pub	pub/o	pubis	pubovesical
pulm	pulm/o	lung	pulmometer
pulmon	pulmon/o	lung	pulmonectomy
pupill	pupill/o	pupil	pupillary
py	py/o	pus	pyorrhea
pyel	pyel/o	renal pelvis	pyelonephritis
pylor	pylor/o	pyloris	pyloroplasty
pyr	pyr/o	fire	pyrogenic
pyret	pyret/o	fever	pyretogenic
R			
rachi	rachi/o	spine	rachiomyelitis
radi	radi/o	ray, radius	radionecrosis

Root Word	Combining Form	Definition	Example
radiat	radiat/o	radiant	radiation
radic	radic/o	root	radicotomy
radicul	radicul/o	root	radiculitis
rect	rect/o	rectum, loosen	rectocele, relaxation
ren	ren/o	kidney	renogastric
reticul	reticul/o	net, network	reticulocyte
retin	retin/o	retina	retinitis
rhabd	rhabd/o	rod	rhabdomyoma
rhin	rhin/o	nose	rhinorrhagia
rhythm	rhythm/o	rhythm	arrhythmia
rhytid	rhytid/o	wrinkle	rhytidectomy

S

Root Word	Combining Form	Definition	Example
sacr	sacr/o	sacrum	sacrodynia
salping	salping/o	tube	salpingopexy
sanguin	sanguin/o	blood	consanguinity
sarc	sarc/o	flesh	sarcoma
scapul	scapul/o	scapula	scapulopexy
schiz	schiz/o	split	schizophrenia
scler	scler/o	hard, fibrous	scleroderma
scoli	scoli/o	curvature	scoliosis
scot	scot/o	dark	scotoma
seb	seb/o	oil	seborrhea
senil	senil/o	old	senilism
ser	ser/o	serum	serology
sial	sial/o	saliva	sialadenitis
sid	sid/o	iron	sideropenia
sigmoid	sigmoid/o	sigmoid, colon	sigmoidoscope
sin	sin/o	curve	sinoatrial
sit	sit/o	foot	sitotherapy
somat	somat/o	body	somatotrophic
somn	somn/o	sleep	somnambulism
son	son/o	sound	sonogram
sperm	sperm/o	seed	spermolysis
spermat	spermat/o	seed	spermatocyst
sphincter	sphincter/o	closure	sphincteroplasty

(*continues*)

Root Word	Combining Form	Definition	Example
S			
sphygm	sphygm/o	pulse	sphygmomanometer
spin	spin/o	thorn, spine	spinocerebellar
spir	spir/o	breath	spirometer
spir	spir/o	coil	spiradenoma
splen	splen/o	spleen	splenectomy
spondyl	spondyl/o	vertebra	spondylitis
staped	staped/o	stapes, stirrup	stapedectomy
staphyl	staphyl/o	cluster, uvula	staphyloplasty
steat	steat/o	fat	steatolysis
sten	sten/o	narrowing	stenosis
stern	stern/o	sternum	sternalgia
steth	steth/o	chest	stethoscope
stigmat	stigmat/o	point	stigmatism
stomat	stomat/o	mouth, opening	stomatitis
strept	strept/o	chain	streptococcus
sympath	sympath/o	sympathy	sympathectomy
syphil	syphil/o	syphilis	syphilopsychosis
T			
tars	tars/o	ankle bone	tarsectomy
ten	ten/o	tendon	tenorrhagia
tendin	tendin/o	tendon	tendinitis
tendon	tendon/o	tendon	tendonitis
terat	terat/o	monster	teratoma
test	test/o	testis	testalgia
thalass	thalass/o	sea	thalassemia
than	than/o	death	euthanasia
thel	thel/o	nipple	thelorrhagia
therm	therm/o	heat	hydrothermic
thromb	thromb/o	blood clot	thrombosis
thym	thym/o	thymus	thymopexy
thyr	thyr/o	thyroid	thyroptoss
tibi	tibi/o	tibia	tibial
tinnit	tinnit/o	jingling	tinnitus
toc	toc/o	birth	tocology
tom	tom/o	cut	tomography

Root Word	Combining Form	Definition	Example
ton	ton/o	tone, tension	tonography
tonsill	tonsill/o	tonsil	tonsillitis
top	top/o	place	topography
torti	torti/o	twisted	torticollis
toxic	toxic/o	poison	toxicology
trache	trache/o	trachea	tracheostomy
traumat	traumat/o	wound, injure	traumatology
trephinat	trephinat/o	bore	trephination
trich	trich/o	hair	trichomycosis
trigon	trigon/o	trigone	trigonitis
trop	trop/o	turn	neurotropism
tubercul	tubercul/o	swelling	tuberculosis
tympan	tympan/o	drum	tympanitis
U			
ul	ul/o	scar	ulectomy
ulcer	ulcer/o	surface excavation	ulcerogenic
uln	uln/o	elbow	ulnad
ungu	ungu/o	nail	ungula
ur	ur/o	urine	uremia
ureter	ureter/o	ureter	ureterolith
urethr	urethr/o	urethra	urethrocystitis
urin	urin/i	urine	uriniparous
urinat	urinat/o	urine	urination
uter	uter/o	uterus	uteralgia
uve	uve/o	uvea	uveitis
V			
vag	vag/o	vagus nerve, wandering	vagotomy
vagin	vagin/o	vagina	vaginectomy
varic	varic/o	twisted vein	varicocele
vas	vas/o	vessel, duct	vasotripsy
vascul	vascul/o	small vessel	vasculopathy
vector	vector/o	carrier	vectorcardiogram
ven	ven/o	vein	venostasis
vener	vener/o	desire, love (sexual intercourse)	venereal
veni	veni/o	vein	venisuture

(*continues*)

Root Word	Combining Form	Definition	Example
V			
ventricul	ventricul/o	ventricle	ventriculitis
vertebr	vertebr/o	vertebra	vertebrectomy
vertig	vertig/o	dizziness, vesicle	vertigo
vesic	vesic/o	vesicle	vesicocele
vesicul	vesicul/o	vesicle	vesiculotomy
vir	vir/o	virus	viruria
viril	viril/o	masculine	virilism
viscer	viscer/o	body organs	visceroenic
vitamin	vitamin/o	vitamin	hypervitaminosis
vitre	vitre/o	vitreous humor	vitreous
vulv	vulv/o	vulva	vulvovaginitis
X			
xanth	xanth/o	yellow	xanthemia
xen	xen/o	alien, foreign	xenophobia
xiph	xiph/o	sword	xiphoid
Z			
zo	zo/o	animal	zooderma
zon	zon/o	encircling area	zonesthesia
zyg	zyg/o	joined	zygodactyly

© Y. H. Hui, PhD

Glossary

achlorhydria Decrease in stomach acid production, occasionally because of atrophic gastritis.

acne vulgaris A skin condition that commonly affects adolescents, but can occur at any age. In this condition, the skin's pores become clogged with oil, debris, or bacteria. The pore can become inflamed, developing a pustule, nodule, or cyst.

acquired immunity Immunity that results from subsequent exposures to an antigen because memory cells recall the antigen as foreign, and antibody production is rapid.

acromegaly Increase in bone size caused by excessive growth hormone levels in adulthood.

actin One of two types of myofilament. It is involved in muscular contractions, cellular movement, and cell shape maintenance.

action potential The creation of neural charges.

active acquired immunity The immunity gained by actively obtaining an antigen through invasion or vaccination. In active immunity, a person makes his or her own antibodies, and protection is usually long term.

active infection Phase that occurs when the primary infection can no longer be controlled. During this phase, tuberculosis can spread throughout the lungs and to other organs.

active transport The movement of a substance from an area of lower concentration to an area of higher concentration, against a concentration gradient.

acute In regard to disease, a condition that is short term in nature, occurring and resolving quickly.

acute bronchitis An inflammation of the tracheobronchial tree or large bronchi, most commonly caused by a wide range of viruses. The airways become inflamed and narrowed due to the results of the inflammatory process.

acute gastritis Type of gastritis that usually develops suddenly and is likely to be accompanied by nausea and epigastric pain. It can be a mild, transient irritation, or it can be a severe ulceration with hemorrhage.

acute lung injury (ALI) A slightly less severe form of acute respiratory distress syndrome.

acute renal failure (ARF) A sudden loss of renal function. This loss is generally reversible and is most common in critically ill, hospitalized patients. Also called acute kidney injury.

acute respiratory distress syndrome (ARDS) A sudden failure of the respiratory system often occurring from fluid accumulation in the alveoli. ARDS has many other names, such as shock lung, wet lung, and stiff lung.

acute respiratory failure (ARF) A serious, life-threatening condition that can be the result of many pulmonary disorders. Oxygen levels become dangerously low, or carbon dioxide levels become dangerously high. The low oxygen levels are unable to meet the body's metabolic needs.

acute tissue rejection The most common and treatable type of tissue rejection. This type of rejection usually occurs between 4 days and 3 months following a transplant. Acute reactions are cell mediated and result in transplant cell destruction (lyses) or necrosis.

adaptation Method by which cells attempt to prevent their own death from environmental changes. They may modify their size, numbers, or types in an attempt to manage these changes and maintain homeostasis.

adaptive or acquired defenses Immunity that results in antibody development in response to antigen.

Addison's disease A deficiency of adrenal cortex hormones.

adrenal gland Gland with an inner portion and an outer portion that is located on a kidney.

afferent arteriole Point at which the blood enters the glomerulus.

afferent nerve A type of nerve of the peripheral nervous system, which carries impulses from the body to the brain. Also called sensory nerve.

afferent tract Fibers that carry sensory information in the form of action potentials from the periphery back to the brain. Also called ascending fibers.

afterload The pressure the left ventricle must exert to get the blood out of the heart and into the aorta. The higher the afterload, the harder it is for the heart to eject the blood, thus lowering stroke volume. Both afterload and preload can affect blood pressure. As afterload and preload increase, blood pressure increases.

AIDS dementia complex Dementia that occurs in the later stages of AIDS. The human immunodeficiency virus invades the brain tissue and may be exacerbated by other infections and tumors that are frequently associated with AIDS. Also called HIV-associated encephalopathy.

alarm The first stage of the general adaptation syndrome, which includes the generalized stimulation of the sympathetic nervous system, resulting in the release of catecholamines and cortisol, also known as the fight-or-flight response.

albinism A recessive condition that results in little or no melanin production.

aldosterone A hormone secreted by the adrenal cortex that increases blood volume by increasing the reabsorption of sodium in the kidneys; sodium attracts water. Increasing water reabsorption will increase blood volume. Aldosterone is the principal mineralocorticoid.

allele One gene that may have many variants, which determines a characteristic.

allogeneic Type of transplant in which tissue is used from the same species and is of similar tissue type, but is not identical. Most transplants use allogeneic tissue.

alpha cell One of five types of cells in the islets of Langerhans; it secretes glucagon.

alveolus (plural: alveoli) A hollow, saclike structure that is the final branching of the respiratory tree and acts as the primary gas exchange unit of the lung.

Alzheimer's disease (AD) The most common form of dementia. The disease causes healthy brain tissue to degenerate and atrophy.

amblyopia The loss of one eye's ability to see details. Amblyopia is the most common cause of vision problems in children. It occurs when the brain and eyes do not work together properly; the brain favors one eye. Also called lazy eye.

amenorrhea The absence of menstruation.

ammonia A metabolic waste managed by the kidneys. This highly toxic product results from the breakdown of amino acids in the liver.

amphiarthrose A slightly moveable joint that can be seen in the vertebral column.

ampulla A pouch that joins the seminal vesicles to form the ejaculatory duct.

amylin Substance that is released from the beta cells along with insulin. Amylin has a synergistic relationship with insulin to control glucose.

amyotrophic lateral sclerosis (ALS) A disease that involves damage of the upper motor neurons of the cerebral cortex and lower motor neurons of the brain stem and spinal cord. Also called Lou Gehrig's disease after the famous baseball player who died of it.

anaphase Phase of mitosis in which chromosomes separate and move to opposite poles.

anaphylactic shock Type of distributive shock that is a consequence of an allergic reaction. The allergic reaction leads to a cascade of events similar to that of septic shock, except the mediators differ. Additionally, bronchospasms and laryngeal edema that can impair the patient's respiratory status occur.

anaplasia The loss of differentiation that occurs with cancer.

anasarca Edema that is generalized throughout the body.

anemia A common acquired or inherited disorder of the erythrocytes that impairs the oxygen-carrying capacity of the blood.

aneurysm Condition in the walls of an artery caused by high pressures, plaque, and infections. These walls weaken and balloon outward.

angina Chest pain with a cardiac origin.

anion A negatively charged electrolyte.

anion gap The difference between the sum of cations and anions found in plasma.

ankylosing spondylitis A progressive inflammatory disorder affecting the sacroiliac joints, intervertebral spaces, and costovertebral joints.

ankylosis Joint fixation and deformity.

anotia The absence of the auricle.

anteflexed Tilted forward.

anterior chamber The cavity of the eye interior that is in front of the lens.

antibody-producing cell Type of B cell that produces millions of antibody molecules during its 24-hour life span.

antidiuretic hormone (ADH) Hormone secreted by the posterior pituitary gland that increases water reabsorption in the kidney, which in turn increases blood volume and blood pressure. Antidiuretic hormone is a vasoconstrictor.

antigen A foreign agent.

aorta The largest artery in the body, which originates from the left ventricle.

aortic valve A three-leaflet valve that guides the passage of blood from the left ventricle to the aorta and prevents the backward flow of blood.

apocrine gland Gland that opens into hair follicles in the axillae, scalp, face, and external genitalia.

apoptosis Mechanism of programmed cell death that occurs because of morphologic changes in cells.

appendicitis An inflammation of the vermiform appendix. The inflammation can be life threatening and is most often caused by an infection.

appendicular skeleton One of two divisions of the human skeleton. It consists of bones that form the arms, shoulders, pelvis, and legs.

appendix A small, wormlike structure attached to the cecum with seemingly no function but plenty of potential to cause harm if it becomes inflamed.

aqueous humor Watery liquid in the anterior chamber of the eye that provides nutrients to the cornea and lens and carries away cellular waste products.

arachnoid layer The middle layer of the meninges, named for its spider web–like vascular system.

areola An area of pigmentation surrounding the nipple of the breast.

areolar gland Gland that produces secretions that protect and lubricate the nipple and areola of the breast during breastfeeding.

arrhythmia Deviations from normal electric conduction in the heart. Arrhythmias vary in severity and are classified according to their origins. Also called dysrhythmia.

arterial blood gas (ABG) The long-standing, principal diagnostic tool for evaluating acid–base balance.

arteriole Small blood vessel that branches off arteries that are near the heart.

artery A blood vessel that carries blood away from the heart.

ascending fibers Fibers that carry sensory information in the form of action potentials from the periphery back to the brain. The ascending fibers have a variety of tracts that communicate specific sensory input. Also called afferent tracts.

ascending testicle A testicle that has returned to the lower abdomen and cannot easily be guided back into the scrotum. Also called acquired undescended testicle.

ascites Fluid that accumulates in the peritoneal cavity.

aspiration The entrance of food into the trachea and lungs.

aspiration pneumonia Type of pneumonia that frequently occurs when the gag reflex is impaired because of a brain injury or anesthesia. Aspiration pneumonia can also occur because of impaired lower esophageal sphincter closure secondary to nasogastric tube placement or disease (e.g., gastroesophageal reflux disease).

asthma A chronic pulmonary disease that produces intermittent, reversible airway obstruction. It is characterized by acute airway inflammation, bronchoconstriction, bronchospasm, bronchiole edema, and mucus production. Asthma is the most common chronic illness in children.

atelectasis Incomplete alveolar expansion or collapse of the alveoli. It occurs when the walls of the alveoli stick together.

atherosclerosis A chronic inflammatory disease characterized by thickening and hardening of the arterial wall. Lesions (or plaques) composed of lipids develop on the vessel wall and calcify over time. Development of these lesions causes vessel obstruction, platelet aggregation, and vasoconstriction.

atopic dermatitis A chronic inflammatory skin condition triggered by an allergen.

atresia A condition in which a body passage is closed or missing. It includes lack of the valve opening in the heart to allow blood flow (pulmonary atresia) and lack of an external ear canal (aural atresia).

atrial natriuretic peptide A hormone released when the atria of the myocardium is overstretched, indicating increased fluid volume.

atrioventricular (AV) node The area of the heart located between the atria and the ventricles that receives impulses from the sinoatrial node. The impulses are delayed or move slowly through the atrioventricular node to allow for complete ventricular filling. This area can initiate impulses if the sinoatrial node begins failing.

atrophic gastritis Stomach condition caused by shrinkage and inflammation of the stomach lining.

atrophy State that occurs because of decreased work demands on a cell. When cellular work demands decrease, the cells decrease in size and number.

aura An unusual sensation (e.g., smells, tastes, or visual hallucinations) that occurs just prior to an impending seizure. Some people with focal seizures, especially complex focal seizures, may experience auras. These auras are actually simple focal seizures in which the person maintains consciousness.

auricle The irregularly shaped cartilage that channels sound into the ear. Also referred to as the pinna.

autoimmune Type of reaction in which the body's normal defenses become self-destructive—recognizing self as foreign.

autologous Type of transplant in which the host and the donor are the same person, such as when someone donates his or her own blood prior to a scheduled surgery and then receives it during the surgery.

automaticity A process whereby cardiac cells generate an impulse to contract even with no external nerve stimulus.

automatism Strange, repetitive behavior exhibited by a person having a complex focal seizure.

autonomic hyperreflexia A massive sympathetic response that can cause headaches, hypertension, tachycardia, seizures, stroke, and death; most commonly associated with spinal cord injuries above the sixth thoracic vertebra.

autonomic nervous system System that controls smooth muscles and is responsible for the fight-or-flight response.

autoregulation A mechanism to maintain tissue perfusion in which the blood vessels dilate to increase blood flow and constrict if the intracranial pressure is increased.

autosomal dominant Type of disorder in which a single gene mutation is passed from an affected parent to an offspring regardless of sex. Autosomal dominant disorders occur with homozygous and heterozygous allele pairs.

autosomal recessive Type of disorder in which single gene mutations are passed from an affected parent to an offspring regardless of sex, but they occur only in homozygous allele pairs.

autosome A paired set of chromosomes in DNA.

axial skeleton One of two divisions of the human skeleton. It forms the long axis of the body and includes the skull, vertebral column, and rib cage.

axon A projection of a neuron that makes connections with nearby cells. Axons transmit impulses away from the cell body.

azotemia A buildup of waste products.

B cell A cell that is a major part of the body's third line of defense. B cells mature in the bone marrow, where they differentiate into memory cells or immunoglobulin-secreting (antibody) cells. B cells eliminate bacteria, neutralize bacterial toxins, prevent viral reinfection, and produce immediate inflammatory response. Each B cell has receptor sites for a specific antigen; when it encounters the antigen, the B cell activates and multiplies into either an antibody-producing cell or a memory cell.

bacterial pneumonia A form of pneumonia that is more severe than viral pneumonia and can result from viral pneumonia.

baroreceptor Receptor in the carotid artery that detects the pressure in the heart and arteries.

Bartholin's glands Glands that lie just within the labia minor and provide lubrication during sexual intercourse.

basal ganglion (plural: ganglia) A key structure deep within the cerebrum, diencephalon, and midbrain. The basal ganglia play a pivotal role in coordination, motor movement, and posture.

base excess/deficit The concentration of buffer—in particular, bicarbonate. Positive values indicate an excess of base or a deficit of acid. Negative values indicate a deficit of base or an excess of acid.

basilar skull fracture A skull fracture located at the base of the skull and usually accompanied by cerebrospinal fluid leakage.

benign Near-normal, differentiated condition of a cell or tumor, which causes fewer problems than an abnormal cell or tumor. Benign cells are usually encapsulated and are unable to metastasize.

benign prostatic hyperplasia (BPH) A common, nonmalignant enlargement of the prostate gland that occurs as men age.

beta cell One of five types of cells in the islets of Langerhans; it secretes insulin.

bicarbonate–carbonic acid system A buffer mechanism that is the largest system in the extracellular fluid. Carbonic acid and bicarbonate (base) are the key players in this system.

bile A green or yellowish liquid that contains water, bile salts (formed from cholesterol), conjugated bilirubin, cholesterol, and electrolytes (including bicarbonate).

birthmark A skin anomaly that is present at birth or shortly after.

bladder A reservoir where urine is held until excretion.

bladder cancer Any cancer that forms in the tissue of the bladder.

blue bloaters Nickname given to those patients with chronic bronchitis, who are unable to increase ventilatory effort to maintain adequate gas exchange. These patients eventually develop cyanosis and edema.

bone A specialized form of connective tissue. This living, metabolically active tissue is the site of fat and mineral storage (especially calcium) as well as hematopoiesis.

bone marrow Soft, fatty tissue found inside bones.

Bowman's capsule A double-membrane chamber that surrounds the glomerulus.

brain Organ located within the skull that contains billions of neurons.

brain stem Part of the central nervous system that includes the pons, cerebellum, and medulla. It connects the brain to the spinal cord. The brain stem is crucial for many basic body functions, and injury to the brain stem can easily result in death.

breast cancer Cancer of the breast; the most common malignancy in women, and the second leading cause of cancer death in women.

bronchiole Part of the lung that controls airflow.

bronchiolitis A common viral infection of the bronchioles most frequently caused by the respiratory syncytial virus. The infection most often occurs in children younger than 1 year of age, and incidence increases in the fall and winter months.

bronchopneumonia The most frequent type of pneumonia. It is generally a patchy pneumonia throughout several lobes.

bronchus (plural: bronchi) Large tube leading from the trachea to the lungs that carries air to and from the lungs.

bundle branches Specialized cardiac muscle cells that branch off the bundle of His to conduct electrical impulses through the ventricles.

bundle of His Collection of specialized cardiac muscle cells that conduct electrical impulses from the atrioventricular node.

burn A skin injury that can result from a thermal or a nonthermal source. These sources may include dry heat, wet heat, radiation, friction, heated objects, natural or artificial UV light, electricity, and chemicals.

café au lait spot Common type of birthmark that is the color of coffee with milk.

calcitonin Hormone secreted by the thyroid that regulates serum calcium levels. It alters serum calcium levels by inhibiting osteoclast activity and stimulating osteoblast activity.

calcium The most abundant mineral in the body. It is necessary for bone and teeth formation, muscle contractility, coagulation, and other body processes.

callus A mass of cells and fibers that bridges broken bone ends together inside and outside.

calyx (plural: calyces) Tube through which urine drains from the renal pyramid of the medulla to the renal pelvis for excretion through the ureters.

cancer The disease state associated with uncontrolled cellular growth. Key features include rapid, uncontrolled proliferation and a loss of differentiation.

candidiasis A yeast infection caused by the common fungus *Candida albicans*.

capillary A branch of an arteriole. It has thin walls to allow oxygen and nutrients to pass out of the capillaries into the cells. Additionally, carbon dioxide and waste products are passed from the cells into the capillaries.

carbuncle A cluster of boils.

carcinogenesis The process by which cancer develops. It occurs in three phases: initiation, promotion, and progression.

cardiac muscle Type of muscle that constitutes the heart and is under involuntary control.

cardiac output The amount of blood the heart pumps in 1 minute. Cardiac output is determined by stroke volume and heart rate ($CO = SV \times HR$, where CO is cardiac output, SV is stroke volume, and HR is heart rate).

cardiac tamponade Condition that results when fluid accumulates in the pericardial cavity to the point that it compresses the heart. This compression prevents the heart from filling during diastole, resulting in decreased cardiac output.

cardiogenic shock Type of shock in which the left ventricle cannot maintain adequate cardiac output. Compensatory mechanisms of heart failure are triggered; however, these mechanisms increase cardiac workload and oxygen consumption, resulting in decreased contractility. Consequently, tissue and organ perfusion decrease, leading to multisystem organ failure.

cardiomyopathy A group of conditions affecting the myocardium. Cardiomyopathies are classified into three groups: dilated, hypertrophic, and restrictive.

cartilage A shiny connective tissue that is tough and flexible. Several types of cartilage can be found throughout the body in the ears, nose, bones, and joints.

caseous necrosis Type of necrosis that occurs when the necrotic cells disintegrate, but the cellular debris remains for months or years.

cataract Opacity or clouding of the lens of the eye.

cation A positively charged electrolyte.

cauda equina Individual nerve roots of the spinal cord at the vertebral canal.

cauda equina syndrome Injury to the nerve roots in the area of the cauda equina.

cecum A pouch at the end of the small intestine.

celiac disease An inherited, autoimmune, malabsorption disorder. Also called celiac sprue.

cell membrane The semipermeable boundary containing the cell and its components.

cellulitis An infection deep in the dermis and subcutaneous tissue. Cellulitis usually results from a direct invasion through a breach in the skin, especially those breaches where contamination is likely.

central nervous system (CNS) Body system made up of the brain and spinal cord.

cerebellum Part of the brain stem that communicates with other regions of the brain to coordinate the synergistic motion of muscle movement and balance as well as cognition.

cerebral aneurysm A localized outpouching of a cerebral artery. This weakening of the artery may occur as a congenital defect or develop later in life.

cerebral contusion A bruising of the brain with rupture of small blood vessels and edema. Most contusions result from a blunt blow to the head that causes the brain to make a sudden impact with the skull.

cerebral palsy (CP) A group of nonprogressive disorders that appear in infancy or early childhood and permanently affect motor movement and muscle coordination. In addition to motor dysfunction, other cerebral functioning may be affected.

cerebral vascular accident (CVA) An interruption of cerebral blood supply. A CVA is an infarction of the brain, so it is often referred to as a brain attack. Also called stroke.

cerebrospinal fluid (CSF) A plasmalike liquid that fills the space between the arachnoid and pia mater layers of the brain to provide additional cushioning and support to the central nervous system.

cerebrum The largest region of the brain; it controls the higher thought processes.

cervical cancer Cancer of the cervix. The Pap smear can detect precancerous changes. Procedures can be performed to remove these precancerous cells, limiting the likelihood of these changes progressing to permanent malignant changes.

cervix The narrow opening from the uterus to the vagina.

chancre An infected, ulcerative lesion often associated with sexually transmitted infections such as syphilis.

chemoreceptor A receptor that detects chemical changes in the blood.

chlamydia One of the most prevalent sexually transmitted infections; caused by *Chlamydia trachomatis*.

chloride A mineral electrolyte and the major extracellular anion. Chloride assists in fluid distribution by attaching to sodium or water.

cholecystitis Inflammation or infection in the biliary system caused by calculi.

cholelithiasis Gallstones; a common condition that affects both genders and all ethnic groups relatively equally.

chondrosarcoma A slow-growing tumor that begins in cartilage cells that are commonly found on the ends of bones.

chordee A downward curvature of the penis.

chorea Uncontrolled, rapid, jerky movements.

choroid The part of the middle layer of the eye that contains melanin, which absorbs stray light.

chromosome A nucleotide in DNA.

chronic State that occurs when an acute disease does not resolve in a short period of time. A chronic disease often has fewer notable signs than an acute disease,

and it occurs over a longer period of time. Chronic diseases might not ever resolve but may become manageable.

chronic bronchitis An obstructive respiratory disorder characterized by inflammation of the bronchi, a productive cough, and excessive mucus production. Chronic bronchitis differs from acute bronchitis in that the chronic type is not necessarily caused by an infection, and symptoms persist longer.

chronic gastritis Type of gastritis that develops gradually and is likely to be accompanied by a dull epigastric pain and a sensation of fullness after minimal intake. It can be asymptomatic.

chronic kidney disease A gradual loss of renal function that is irreversible.

chronic obstructive pulmonary disease (COPD) A group of chronic respiratory disorders characterized by irreversible, progressive tissue degeneration and airway obstruction.

chronic overdistention Condition caused by a perceived inability to interrupt work to void. This chronic avoidance of emptying the bladder results in detrusor muscle areflexia and overflow incontinence. Also called nurse's bladder and teacher's bladder.

chronic tissue rejection Type of tissue rejection that occurs from about 4 months to years after the transplant. This reaction is most likely due to an antibody-mediated immune response. Antibodies and complements become deposited in the transplanted tissue vessel walls, resulting in decreased blood flow and ischemia.

chronotropic The rate of contraction.

Chvostek's sign An indicator of hypocalcemia in which a spasm or brief contraction of the corner of the mouth, nose, eye, and muscles in the cheek results from tapping the facial nerve in front of the ear.

chyme A mixture of food that has been chemically digested and churned in the stomach.

ciliary body The part of the middle layer of the eye that contains smooth muscle fibers that control the shape of the lens to focus on incoming light.

cilium (plural: cilia) Organelle that moves in a wavelike motion to propel mucus and trapped particles upward to the mouth where they can be expectorated.

cirrhosis Chronic, progressive, irreversible, diffuse damage to the liver resulting in decreased liver function.

cleft lip Congenital defect that results from failure of the maxillary processes and nasal elevations or upper lip to fuse during development. It may occur with a cleft palate. A cleft lip and palate can affect the appearance of one's face and may lead to problems with feeding, speech, ear infections, and hearing.

cleft palate An opening between the oral cavity and the nasal cavity. It may occur with a cleft lip. A cleft lip and palate can affect the appearance of one's face and may lead to problems with feeding, speech, ear infections, and hearing.

clitoris Part of the vulva formed by the connection of the two labia minor. The clitoris is sensitive to stimulation and becomes filled with blood during sexual arousal. It contains two corpora cavernosa, similar to the penis.

closed-angle (acute) glaucoma Type of glaucoma that results from a sudden blockage of aqueous humor outflow; it is a medical emergency.

closed fracture Type of fracture in which the skin is intact.

coagulative necrosis Type of necrosis that usually results from an interruption in blood flow.

cochlea A spiral-shaped structure in the inner ear that houses the organ of Corti.

colon Part of the lower gastrointestinal tract that makes up most of the large intestine. The colon has three relatively straight sections (ascending, transverse, and descending). It absorbs 90% of the water and electrolytes that enter this structure.

colorectal cancer Cancer of the colon and/or rectum.

comminuted fracture A fracture characterized by multiple fracture lines and bone pieces.

comminuted skull fracture A skull fracture characterized by several fracture lines.

communicating hydrocephalus Cerebrospinal accumulation that occurs when the fluid is not properly absorbed by the bloodstream.

community-acquired pneumonia Pneumonia that is acquired outside the hospital or healthcare setting.

compact bone The hard outer surface of a bone.

compartment syndrome A serious condition that results from pressure increases in a compartment, usually the muscle fascia in the case of fractures. The pressure impinges on the nerves and blood vessels contained within the compartment, potentially compromising the distal extremity.

compensatory mechanism Physiologic response to homeostatic imbalance in attempt to maintain normalcy.

complete fracture Type of fracture in which the bone is broken into two or more separate pieces.

complication A new problem that arises as a result of a disease.

compound skull fracture A skull fracture where brain tissue is exposed.

compression fracture A fracture in which the bone is crushed or collapses into small pieces.

concussion A momentary interruption of brain function. Concussions usually result from a mild blow to the head that causes sudden movement of the brain, disrupting neurologic functioning. Concussions may or may not lead to a loss of consciousness. Amnesia, confusion, sleep disturbances, and headaches may follow a concussion for a period of weeks or months.

conductivity The ability of cells to conduct electrical impulses.

condyloma acuminatum (plural: condylomata acuminata) Benign genital wart caused by the group of viruses called human papillomaviruses.

cone A photoreceptor in the eye that operates in bright light and is responsible for visual acuity and color vision. There are approximately 6 million cones in the human eye.

congenital Conditions involving defects or damage to a developing fetus.

congenital cataract A clouding of the usually clear lens of the eye that is present at birth. It results in hazy vision.

congenital glaucoma Type of glaucoma that is present at birth. It is a result of abnormal development of outflow channels (trabecular meshwork) of the eye.

congenital hearing loss Loss of hearing that can occur because of damage associated with maternal rubella and syphilis infection during pregnancy.

conjunctiva A fragile membrane that covers the inner surface of the eyelid and the exposed surface of the eye.

conjunctivitis An infection or inflammation of the conjunctiva, the lining of the eyelids and sclera.

constipation A change in bowel pattern characterized by infrequent passage of stool.

constrictive pericarditis Condition that results from chronic inflammation of the pericardium. The pericardium becomes thick and fibrous and adheres to the heart. The loss of elasticity restricts cardiac filling, which causes systemic congestion and decreases cardiac output.

contact dermatitis An acute inflammatory reaction triggered by direct exposure to an irritant or allergen-producing substance.

convalescence The stage of recovery following a disease that may last for days or months.

cornea A clear lens on the anterior side of the outermost layer of the eye that allows light to enter the eye.

coronary artery disease (CAD) Disease that occurs when atherosclerosis develops in the arteries supplying the myocardium. Blood flow temporarily diminishes in the coronary arteries, causing subsequent oxygen reduction to the cardiac muscle.

cortex The outer portion of an adrenal gland that is regulated by negative feedback involving the hypothalamus and adrenocorticotropic hormones.

cortisol The principal glucocorticoid, which increases serum glucose levels.

contrecoup The second area of damage in a traumatic brain injury. Where the brain first impacts the skull is the coup; the brain then rebounds and impacts the opposite side of the skull, which is the contrecoup.

coup The initial area that the brain impacts in the skull in a traumatic brain injury.

Cowper's glands Two pea-sized glands adjacent to the urethra that secrete another alkaline fluid into the urethra to neutralize acidity caused by urine transportation. Cowper's gland secretions can sometimes be seen at the meatus before ejaculation. This secretion aids in lubrication of the penis during sexual intercourse and may contain some sperm leftover from a previous ejaculation.

cranial nerves Set of nerves through which the brain accomplishes a variety of physiologically vital functions and cognitive activities. Twelve pairs branch directly from the base of the brain.

crenation Shrinkage of a cell as a result of too much water moving out of the cell.

crepitus A grating sound.

Creutzfeldt-Jakob disease (CJD) A rare, but rapidly progressive form of dementia caused by an infectious prion.

Crohn's disease An insidious, slow-developing, progressive condition that often develops in adolescence. It is characterized by patchy areas of inflammation involving the full thickness of the intestinal wall and ulcerations.

cryptorchidism A congenital condition in which one or both testes do not descend from the abdomen to the scrotum prior to birth.

curative A goal of treatment aimed at eradicating disease.

Curling's ulcer Stress ulcer associated with a burn.

Cushing's reflex A mechanism to maintain tissue perfusion in which a complex cascade of events results in increased blood pressure.

Cushing's syndrome Excessive cortisol levels that result from the increased corticotropin levels.

Cushing's triad Increased blood pressure, bradycardia, and changes in respiratory pattern that result from unresolved vasoconstriction, increased cardiac contractility, and increased cardiac output.

Cushing's ulcer Stress ulcer associated with a head injury.

cystic fibrosis A common inherited respiratory disorder that presents at birth. This life-threatening condition causes severe lung damage and nutrition deficits.

cystitis Inflammation of the bladder.

cystocele Condition that occurs when the bladder protrudes into the anterior wall of the vagina.

cytoplasm A colorless, viscous liquid inside the cell that contains water, nutrients, ions, dissolved gases, and waste products; it is where the cellular work takes place.

cytotoxic cell Type of T cell that destroys cells infected with viruses by releasing lymphokines that destroy cell walls. Also called killer cell and effector cell.

deamination The process of stripping amino groups from molecules.

defecation The expulsion of the feces from the rectum.

degenerative Related to conditions that cause parts of the body to deteriorate.

dehydration Fluid deficit.

delta cell One of five types of cells in the islets of Langerhans; it secretes somatostatin.

dementia A group of conditions in which cortical function is decreased, impairing cognitive skills and motor coordination. Issues with memory are common with dementia and include short-term memory losses as well as confusion of historical events.

dendrite A projection of a neuron that makes connections with nearby cells. Dendrites transmit impulses toward the cell body.

deoxyribonucleic acid (DNA) A double-stranded chain of nucleotides called chromosomes.

depolarization An increase in electrical charge through the exchange of ions across the cell membrane caused by the rapid inflow of positively charged sodium ions.

depressed (skull) fracture Type of fracture that occurs in the skull when the broken piece is forced inward on the brain.

dermatome The area of the skin innervated by a given pair of spinal sensory nerves. Each spinal nerve, with the exception of the first cervical vertebra, has a specific body surface area from which it obtains sensory information.

dermis The middle layer of the skin, which is composed of dense, irregular connective tissue and little fat tissue. The dermis includes nerves, hair follicles, smooth muscle, glands, blood vessels, and lymphatic vessels.

descending fibers Fibers that carry motor impulses in the form of action potentials from the brain to the fibers of the peripheral nervous system. Also called efferent tracts.

detrusor hyperreflexia Increased contractile activity of the detrusor muscle of the bladder, resulting in urinary incontinence.

developmental Arising during embryonic or fetal development.

diabetes insipidus Excessive fluid excretion in the kidneys caused by deficient antidiuretic hormone levels.

diabetes mellitus (DM) A group of conditions characterized by hyperglycemia (high serum glucose levels) resulting from defects in insulin production, insulin action, or both.

diabetic ketoacidosis A pH imbalance characterized by increased ketones in the urine caused by insufficient insulin; if cells are starved for energy, the body may begin to break down fat-producing toxic acids (ketones).

diagnosis Identification of disease.

diaphragm A dome-shaped muscle that separates the thoracic and abdominal cavities and aids in respiration.

diaphysis The body of a bone.

diarrhea A change in bowel pattern characterized by an increased frequency, amount, and water content of the stool.

diastole The bottom number in a blood pressure reading, which indicates rest or relaxation by the ventricles.

diastolic dysfunction Type of heart failure characterized by decreased ventricular filling resulting from abnormal myocardial relaxation and increased left ventricular pressure. This type of heart failure is caused by conditions that stiffen the myocardium, such as coronary artery disease, hypertrophic and restrictive cardiomyopathy, and pericardial disease.

diencephalon Part of the brain that includes the thalamus and hypothalamus.

differentiation A process by which cells become specialized in terms of cell type, function, structure, and cell cycle. This process does not begin until approximately 15–60 days after the sperm and ova unite.

diffusion The movement of solutes (particles dissolved in a solvent) from an area of higher concentration to lower concentration.

dilated cardiomyopathy Type of cardiomyopathy that affects systolic function. It is the most common type of cardiomyopathy.

diplopia Double vision.

disease The state in which a bodily function is no longer occurring normally. Diseases range from merely causing temporary stress to causing life-changing complications.

dislocation The separation of two bones where they meet at a joint.

dissecting aneurysm A false aneurysm in which weakening occurs in the inner layers of a blood vessel.

disseminated intravascular coagulation (DIC) A life-threatening disorder that occurs as a complication of other diseases and conditions. Clotting factors become abnormally active, often because of an inappropriate immune reaction. Hypercoagulation is followed by hemorrhaging as the clotting factors are completely utilized.

distributive shock Type of shock in which vasodilation causes hypovolemia.

diverticula An outwardly bulging pouch of the intestinal wall that occurs when mucosa sections or large intestine submucosa layers herniate through a weakened muscular layer.

diverticular disease Conditions related to the development of diverticula.

diverticulitis A state in which diverticula have become inflamed, usually because of retained fecal matter. Diverticulitis can result in potentially fatal obstructions, infection, abscess, perforation, peritonitis, hemorrhage, and shock.

diverticulosis Asymptomatic diverticular disease. Usually there are multiple diverticula present.

dominant More powerful. In genetics, the dominant allele is more likely to be expressed in the offspring than the recessive one.

dorsal root Root formed from about 6–8 dorsal rootlets. The roots combine to form the spinal nerve.

dromotropic The rate of electrical conduction.

drug-induced asthma A type of asthma that is frequently caused by aspirin and can be fatal. Reactions can be delayed up to 12 hours after drug ingestion.

dry gangrene Type of gangrene that occurs when bacterial presence is minimal, and the skin has a dry, dark brown or black appearance.

duodenal ulcer Type of ulcer that is commonly associated with excessive acid or *H. pylori* infections. Manifestations typically include epigastric pain that is relieved in the presence of food.

dura mater The tough outer layer of the central nervous system.

dwarfism Short stature caused by deficient levels of growth hormone, somatotropin, or somatotropin-releasing hormone.

dyslipidemia An increased level of lipids in the blood. These lipids include cholesterol and triglycerides, which are necessary for cellular membrane formation. Also called hyperlipidemia.

dysmenorrhea Painful menstruation, to the extent that it impairs usual daily activities.

dysphagia Difficulty swallowing.

dysplasia The final cellular adaptation, in which cells mutate into cells of a different size, shape, and appearance.

dysrhythmia Deviations from normal electric conduction in the heart. Dysrhythmias vary in severity and are classified according to their origins. Also called arrhythmia.

ear Organ that detects and processes sound, detects body position, and maintains balance.

eccrine gland Gland that secretes sweat through skin pores in response to the sympathetic nervous system. Also called merocrine gland.

eclampsia An acute and life-threatening complication of pregnancy, characterized by tonic–clonic seizures, usually occurring in a patient who had developed preeclampsia.

ectopic pregnancy Pregnancy in which the zygote does not reach the uterus, but rather implants outside the uterus.

ectopic testes Undescended testes that deviate from the path of descent.

edema Excess fluid in the interstitial space. Edema is a problem of fluid distribution, not necessarily of fluid overload.

effector cell One of two major types of T cells that work to destroy antigens. Also called killer cell.

efferent arteriole Point at which blood exits the glomerulus.

efferent nerve A type of nerve that carries impulses from the brain to the corresponding muscle receptor, resulting in muscle contraction and movement. Also called motor nerve.

efferent tracts Tracts that carry motor impulses in the form of action potentials from the brain to the fibers of the peripheral nervous system. Also called descending fibers.

ejaculation Propulsion of sperm-containing fluid.

ejaculatory duct Canal in the male reproductive tract formed by union of the vas deferens and the duct from the seminal vesicle.

electrolyte A chemical that is a charged conductor when it is dissolved in water.

embolus A portion or all of a thrombus that breaks loose and travels through the circulatory system until it embeds in a smaller vessel. Any other traveling bodies (e.g., air, fat, tissue, bacteria, amniotic fluid, tumor cells, and foreign substances) can become emboli as well.

emesis The involuntary or voluntary forceful ejection of chyme from the stomach up through the esophagus and out the mouth. It is a common event that can result from a wide range of conditions. Also called vomiting.

emphysema An obstructive respiratory disorder that results in the destruction of the alveolar walls, leading to large, permanently inflated alveoli.

encephalitis An inflammation of the brain and spinal cord, usually resulting from an infection.

endocardium The inner epithelial layer of the heart that makes up the valves.

endocytosis The act of bringing a substance into a cell.

endometrial cancer Cancer of the uterus; a common malignancy in women.

endometriosis Condition in which the endometrium begins growing in areas outside the uterus.

endometrium The inner mucosal lining of the uterine wall that undergoes hormonal changes to facilitate and maintain pregnancy.

enuresis The involuntary urination by a child after the age of 4–5 years, when bladder control is expected.

enzyme Protein that facilitates chemical reactions in cells.

epidemic Increasing cases of a disease in a group.

epidemiology Tracking patterns of diseases in a group of people. This tracking includes occurrence, incidence, prevalence, transmission, and distribution of the disease.

epidermis The outermost layer of the skin, which is composed of squamous epithelia.

epididymis Structure in the male reproductive tract that stores sperm until ejaculation, up to 6 weeks.

epididymitis An inflammation of the epididymis, the duct connecting the testes to the vas deferens.

epidural hematoma Hematoma that results from bleeding between the dura and skull, usually caused by an arterial tear.

epiglottis Part of the respiratory system that closes the larynx when food is swallowed.

epiglottitis A life-threatening inflammation of the epiglottis, the protective cartilage lid covering the trachea opening.

epilepsy A disorder that results from spontaneous firing of abnormal neurons; it is characterized by recurrent seizures for which there is no underlying or correctable cause.

epinephrine Hormone produced by the medulla during times of stress. With norepinephrine, it mediates the fight-or-flight response of the sympathetic nervous system.

epiphysis The growth plates at either end of a bone.

epispadias The urethral meatus occurring on the dorsal surface of the penis instead of the end.

epithalamus Dorsal posterior segment of the diencephalon, which includes the habenula, the stria medullaris, and the pineal body.

epsilon cell One of five types of cells in the islets of Langerhans; it secretes ghrelin.

erectile dysfunction (ED) The inability to attain or maintain a penile erection sufficient to complete sexual intercourse. Also called impotence.

erythrocyte Red blood cell.

erythropoietin Hormone produced by the kidney that promotes the formation of red blood cells in the bone marrow.

esophageal cancer Cancer of the esophagus; usually a squamous cell carcinoma.

esophagus Part of the upper gastrointestinal system that has muscular rings to move the food toward the stomach.

essential hypertension Type of hypertension in which there is no identifiable cause, which occurs in 90–95% of hypertension cases in adults. This type of hypertension tends to develop gradually over many years. Also called primary hypertension.

etiology The cause of a disease.

eustachian tube A pressure valve for the tympanic membrane.

Ewing's sarcoma An aggressive tumor for which the origin is unknown. Ewing's sarcoma may begin in nerve tissue within the bone.

exacerbation Disease state that occurs when the manifestations increase after a period of remission.

excitability The ability of the cells to respond to electrical impulses.

exercise-induced asthma Common type of asthma that usually occurs 10–15 minutes after activity ends. Symptoms can linger for an hour with exercise-induced asthma.

exhaustion The third stage of the general adaptation syndrome. This stage is initiated if the stressor is prolonged or overwhelms the body. During the exhaustion phase, the body becomes depleted and damage may appear as homeostasis can no longer be maintained. As the body's defenses are utilized, disease or death results.

exocytosis The release of materials from a cell, usually with the assistance of a vesicle.

exophthalmos Protruding eyes with decreased blinking and movement.

expiration Exhalation; one of the two phases of breathing.

expiratory reserve volume The amount of air beyond tidal volume that can be exhaled forcefully, which is beyond the normal passive exhalation.

exsanguination The spillage of blood out of the circulatory system as the result of a ruptured aneurysm.

external ear canal Part of the ear through which sound travels until reaching the tympanic membrane.

extracellular fluid Fluid found outside the cells.

extrinsic asthma A condition caused by increased immunoglobulin E synthesis and airway inflammation, resulting in mast cell destruction and inflammatory mediator release. Extrinsic triggers include allergens such as food, pollen, dust, and medications. This type of asthma usually presents in childhood or adolescence.

eye One of two globe-shaped organs located in orbits in the anterior skull that allow the brain to perceive the environment.

facilitated diffusion The movement of substances from an area of lower concentration to an area of higher concentration with the assistance of a carrier molecule.

fallopian tubes Two cylinders that extend from the fundus of the uterus to near the ovaries.

fascia Fibrous connective tissue that surrounds muscles. It may also surround muscle groups.

fat embolism Condition that occurs when fatty marrow enters the bloodstream after a fracture to one of the long bones. The emboli can travel to vital organs such as the lungs, brain, or heart.

fat necrosis Type of necrosis that occurs when lipase enzymes break down intracellular triglycerides into free fatty acids.

fatty streaks Early stages of atherosclerosis. These streaks are made up of macrophages, and cholesterol accumulates within the macrophages.

feces Mixture of the undigested or unabsorbed remnants in the colon, along with bacteria (one-third of the feces). Feces also introduce mucus (approximately 300 mL daily) to aid in bowel movements, even in times of decreased dietary intake.

fibrocystic breast disease The presence of numerous benign nodules in the breast.

fibromyalgia A syndrome predominately characterized by widespread muscular pain and fatigue. Fibromyalgia affects muscles, tendons, and surrounding tissue, but not the joints.

fibrous plaque A lesion associated with atherosclerosis; a pearly, white area within an artery that causes the intimal surface to bulge into the lumen. It is composed of lipid, cell debris, smooth muscle cells, collagen, and, in older persons, calcium.

flat bone Strong, flat plate of bone that protects the body's vital organs and provides a base for muscular attachment. Anterior and posterior surfaces of flat bones are formed from compact bone to provide strength, and the center consists of spongy bone and varying amounts of bone marrow.

flexor reflex A withdrawal reflex in response to touching an unpleasant stimulus. The flexor reflex causes the muscles of a limb to withdraw the limb from the source of the stimulus without any conscious action.

fluid deficit Condition that occurs when total body fluid levels are not sufficient to meet the body's needs.

fluid excess Condition that occurs when total body fluid levels are greater than the body's needs.

fluid volume deficit Fluid deficit of the intravascular compartment. Also called hypovolemia.

fluid volume excess Excess fluid in the intravascular compartment. Also called hypervolemia.

focal seizure One of two categories of seizure; it occurs in just one part of the brain. Also called partial seizure.

follicle One of several functional units of the thyroid gland. These follicles produce thyroxine (T_4), triiodothyronine (T_3), and thyrocalcitonin (calcitonin).

folliculitis Infections involving the hair follicles. Folliculitis is characterized by tender, swollen areas that form around hair follicles, often on the neck, breasts, buttocks, and face.

foramen magnum The large and only opening in the skull.

forced expiratory volume in 1 second The amount of air that can be forcibly exhaled from the lungs in the first second of a forced exhalation.

forced vital capacity The amount of air that can be forcibly exhaled from the lungs after a forced inspiration.

foreskin A sheath of loose skin that covers the glans penis at birth. The foreskin is often surgically removed for hygienic, cultural, or religious reasons.

fracture A break in the rigid structure of the bone.

frank blood Blood that is bright red.

free radicals Injurious, unstable agents that can cause cell death.

frontal lobe Lobe of the brain that facilitates voluntary motor activity and plays a role in personality traits.

fully compensated A pH level that has returned to normal.

functional incontinence Type of incontinence that occurs in many older adults, especially people in nursing homes, in which a physical or mental impairment prevents them from making it to the toilet in time.

furuncle An infection that begins in the hair follicles and then spreads into the surrounding dermis. The lesion starts as a firm, red, painful nodule that develops into a large, painful mass, which frequently drains large amounts of purulent exudate. Also called boil.

fusiform aneurysm An aneurysm that occurs around the entire circumference of a blood vessel. One of two major types of true aneurysm.

gallbladder A small, saclike organ located on the undersurface of the liver that serves as a reservoir for bile. In addition to storing bile, the gallbladder concentrates the bile by removing water.

gangrene A form of coagulative necrosis that is characterized by a combination of impaired blood flow and bacterial invasion.

gas gangrene Type of gangrene that develops because of *Clostridium*, an anaerobic bacterium. This type of gangrene is the most serious and has the greatest potential for being fatal.

gastric cancer Cancer of the stomach, which occurs in several forms.

gastric ulcer Type of stomach ulcer that is uncommon but deadly. Gastric ulcers typically are associated with malignancy and nonsteroidal anti-inflammatory drug use. Pain associated with gastric ulcers typically worsens with eating.

gastritis An inflammation of the mucosal lining of the stomach that can be either acute or chronic.

gastroenteritis Inflammation of the stomach and intestines, usually because of an infection or allergic reaction.

gastroesophageal reflux disease (GERD) A condition in which chyme periodically backs up from the stomach into the esophagus. Occasionally, bile can back up into the esophagus. The presence of these gastric secretions irritates the esophageal mucosa.

gene A segment of deoxyribonucleic acid (DNA) that serves as a template of protein synthesis.

general adaptation syndrome A cluster of systemic manifestations resulting from body modifications made in an attempt to cope with a stressor.

generalized seizure A seizure that results from abnormal neuronal activity on both sides of the brain. It may cause loss of consciousness, falls, or massive muscle spasms.

genetic Related to the passage of physical, biochemical, and physiologic traits from biological parents to their children.

genetics The study of heredity—the passage of physical, biochemical, and physiologic traits from biological parents to their children.

genital herpes A sexually transmitted infection that causes blisters on the genitals and in the reproductive tract.

gestation The support of fetal development from conception to birth by the female reproductive system.

gestational diabetes A form of glucose intolerance diagnosed during pregnancy.

ghrelin Substance secreted by the epsilon cells; it stimulates hunger.

gigantism Tall stature caused by excessive growth hormone levels prior to puberty.

glaucoma A group of eye conditions that lead to damage to the optic nerve. This damage is often caused by increased intraocular pressure, but can also be caused by decreased blood flow to the optic nerve.

glomerular filtration rate (GFR) The best measure of renal functioning; it measures the speed at which blood moves through the glomerulus. GFR can be calculated using a formula that incorporates serum creatinine levels, age, gender, and ethnicity. Usual GFR is approximately 125 mL/min.

glomerulonephritis A bilateral inflammatory disorder of the glomeruli that typically follows a streptococcal infection.

glomerulus A cluster of capillaries in the kidneys through which blood passes.

glucagon Substance secreted by alpha cells that is released when serum glucose levels fall. Glucagon stimulates the breakdown of glycogen to glucose, which raises serum glucose levels.

glucocorticoid Steroid that is secreted by the middle region of the adrenal cortex.

glucose A sugar molecule that provides energy.

goiter A visible enlargement of the thyroid gland.

gonadocorticoid Sex hormone secreted by the innermost region of the adrenal cortex.

gonorrhea Sexually transmitted infection caused by *Neisseria gonorrhoeae*. Referred to colloquially as the clap.

gout An inflammatory disease resulting from deposits of uric acid crystals in tissues and fluids within the body.

grading System used to measure cell appearance in tumors and other neoplasms by classifying the degree of cellular differentiation. The grading score is from G1 to G4, with G4 indicating high differentiation.

graft-versus-host rejection Type of tissue rejection in which the graft fights the host. This potentially life-threatening type of reaction occurs *only* with bone marrow transplants. The immunocompetent graft cells recognize the host cells as foreign and organize a cell-mediated attack. The host is usually immunocompromised and unable to fight the graft cells.

Graves' disease An autoimmune condition that stimulates thyroid hormone production.

greenstick fracture An incomplete fracture in which the bone is bent and only the outer curve of the bend is broken.

gross total incontinence A continuous leaking of urine, day and night, or the periodic uncontrollable leaking of large volumes of urine. In these cases, the bladder has no storage capacity.

gyrus (plural: gyri) A fold that increases the surface area of the cerebrum. At birth, these folds are minimal, but they increase as the brain develops into adulthood.

Hashimoto's thyroiditis The most common cause of thyroid gland failure. Also called autoimmune thyroiditis.

HCO₃ Bicarbonate. Part of the body's buffer system, it is secreted by the kidneys.

health The absence of disease. This definition can be expanded to include wellness of mind, body, and spirit. It is one's normal state.

heart failure A condition in which the heart is unable to pump an adequate amount of blood to meet metabolic needs. This pump inadequacy leads to decreased cardiac output, increased preload, and increased afterload. These three events result in decreased contractility and stroke volume. Often referred to as heart failure.

helper cell A type of regulator cell that activates, or calls up, B cells to produce antibodies.

hemangioma A vascular birthmark that appears as a bright red patch or a nodule of extra blood vessels in the skin. Also called a strawberry.

hematemesis Blood in the vomitus. It has a characteristic brown, granular appearance like coffee grounds.

hematocrit A laboratory expression of how much of the blood volume is being occupied by the erythrocytes.

hematoma A collection of blood in the tissue that develops from ruptured blood vessels. Hematomas can develop immediately or slowly and are classified by their location.

hematopoiesis The process of blood formation; it occurs primarily in the bone marrow.

hemoglobin Part of an erythrocyte. It binds to oxygen, giving blood its red color.

hemoglobin system Buffer mechanism in the erythrocytes that works by binding to or releasing hydrogen and carbon dioxide.

hemoglobin S An abnormal type of hemoglobin that distorts the shape of erythrocytes, especially in a setting of low oxygen. These fragile, sickle-shaped cells deliver less oxygen to the body's tissues. Such cells also can easily clog small blood vessels and break into pieces that disrupt blood flow.

hemolysis Excessive destruction of erythrocytes that causes hemolytic anemia.

hemophilia A An X-linked recessive bleeding disorder that involves a deficit or abnormality of clotting factor VIII. Also called classic hemophilia.

hemorrhagic stroke The deadliest kind of stroke; it occurs when blood vessels rupture inside the brain.

hepatic artery Part of the liver's dual blood supply; it carries oxygenated blood from the general circulation to the liver at a rate of approximately 300 mL/min to nourish the liver.

hepatitis An inflammation of the liver that can be caused by infection (usually viral), alcohol, medications, or autoimmune disease.

hepatobiliary system The liver, gallbladder, and pancreas, collectively. They are called a system because of their close proximity to one another and their complementary functions.

hereditary Transmitted before birth.

herniated intervertebral disk A state in which the nucleus pulposus protrudes through the annulus fibrosus. Also called slipped disk and ruptured disk.

herniation The displacement of brain tissue.

herpes simplex type 1 A viral infection typically affecting the lips, mouth, and face. This common infection usually begins in childhood. Also called cold sore.

herpes simplex virus (HSV) One of a family of more than 70 herpes viruses; the cause of genital herpes.

herpes zoster A viral infection caused by the varicella-zoster virus. The condition appears in adulthood years after a primary infection of varicella (chickenpox) in childhood. The virus lies dormant on a cranial nerve or a spinal nerve dermatome until it becomes activated years later; it affects this nerve only. Also called shingles.

heterozygous Allele pair in which one allele is dominant and the other allele is recessive for a particular gene.

hiatal hernia Condition in which a section of the stomach protrudes upward through an opening in the diaphragm toward the lung.

high-density lipoprotein (HDL) A type of lipid that assists with removing cholesterol from the body. Also called good cholesterol.

homeostasis Equilibrium, balance, consistency, or stability. In the body, this self-regulating, give-and-take system responds to minor changes in the body's status through compensation mechanisms. Compensation mechanisms attempt to counteract those changes and return the body to its normal state.

homozygous Identical allele pair for a particular gene.

host-versus-graft rejection The most common type of tissue rejection, in which the host fights the graft.

human papillomavirus (HPV) A virus that causes benign warts, and sometimes genital warts. There are more than 70 different types of HPV. HPV infection can also lead to the development of reproductive (e.g., cervical and penile) and anal cancers.

Huntington's disease (HD) A condition caused by a genetically programmed degeneration of neurons in the brain. It is an autosomal dominant disorder involving a defect on chromosome 4. Also called Huntington's chorea.

hyaline cartilage The type of cartilage most associated with bone, often found in joints.

hydrocele Fluid accumulation between the layers of the tunica vaginalis or along the spermatic cord.

hydrocephalus A condition in which excess CSF accumulates within the skull, which dilates the ventricles and compresses the brain and blood vessels. The pressure from the excess CSF thins the cortex, causing severe brain damage.

hydronephrosis An abnormal dilation of the renal pelvis and the calyces of one or both kidneys that occurs secondary to a disease.

hymen A thin connective tissue that covers the external vaginal opening to some degree.

hyperacute tissue rejection Type of tissue rejection that occurs immediately to 3 days after a transplant. Hyperacute reactions occur due to a complement response in which the recipient has antibodies against the donor. This complement response triggers a systemic inflammatory reaction. The response is so quick that often the tissue has not had a chance to establish vascularization; as a result, the tissue becomes permanently necrotic.

hypercalcemia Condition in which ionizing calcium levels climb above 5 mEq/L. Hypercalcemia results from excessive intake of ionizing calcium or release of ionizing calcium from the bone as well as inadequate excretion.

hyperchloremia An excess amount of chloride in the blood (more than 108 mEq/L). It is usually a result of an underlying condition and without its own clinical manifestations.

hyperglycemia An excess amount of glucose in the blood (more than 180 mg/dL). It can be a result of an underlying condition (e.g., diabetes mellitus) or use of medications (e.g., corticosteroid agents).

hyperkalemia Serum potassium level greater than 5 mEq/L. Hyperkalemia is unusual in the healthy individual and may be a medical emergency.

hypermagnesemia Condition in which magnesium levels increase to more than 2.5 mEq/L. This rare electrolyte imbalance usually results from renal failure or excessive laxative or antacid use.

hypernatremia Condition that results from high serum sodium levels (more than 145 mEq/L). The excessive sodium levels generally lead to high serum osmolality (more than 295 mOsm/kg) because of the imbalance between sodium and water.

hyperparathyroidism A condition of excessive parathyroid hormone production by the parathyroid glands.

hyperphosphatemia Condition in which phosphorus levels climb above 4.5 mg/dL.

hyperpituitarism A condition in which the pituitary gland secretes excessive amounts of one or all of the pituitary hormones.

hyperplasia An increase in the number of cells in an organ or tissue. This increase occurs only in cells that have the ability to perform mitotic division, such as epithelial cells.

hyperprolactinemia Excessive prolactin levels that result in menstrual dysfunction and galactorrhea (inappropriate lactation).

hypersensitivity An inflated or inappropriate response to an antigen. The result is inflammation and destruction of healthy tissue. Hypersensitivity reactions may be immediate, occurring within minutes to hours of reexposure, or delayed, occurring several hours after reexposure.

hypertension A prolonged elevation in blood pressure.

hyperthyroidism Hypermetabolic state caused by excessive thyroid hormones that result from increased thyrotropin levels.

hypertonic solution An intravascular solution that has a higher concentration of solutes than those in the intravascular compartment. Hypertonic solutions cause fluid to shift from the intracellular space to the intravascular space.

hypertrophic cardiomyopathy Type of cardiomyopathy that mainly affects diastolic function.

hypertrophy Condition in which cells increase in size in an attempt to meet the body's increased work demand. This change may be a result of normal or abnormal changes.

hypervolemia Excess fluid in the intravascular compartment.

hypocalcemia Condition in which ionized calcium levels fall below 4 mEq/L. Hypocalcemia occurs from increased losses or decreased intake of ionized calcium.

hypochloremia Condition in which chloride levels fall below 98 mEq/L. Hypochloremia rarely occurs in the absence of other electrolyte abnormalities and, therefore, does not have its own set of clinical manifestations.

hypodermis The innermost layer of the skin. It is composed of soft, fatty tissue as well as blood vessels, nerves, and immune cells. Also called subcutaneous tissue.

hypoglycemia A low serum glucose level.

hypokalemia Condition in which potassium levels drop below 3.5 mEq/L. Usually, hypokalemia results from excessive loss, inadequate intake, or increased potassium cellular uptake.

hypomagnesemia Condition in which magnesium levels drop below 1.8 mEq/L.

hyponatremia Condition that results from low serum sodium levels (less than 135 mEq/L). Serum osmolality levels also fall below 275 mOsm.

hypoparathyroidism Condition in which the parathyroid gland does not produce sufficient amounts of parathyroid hormone.

hypophosphatemia Condition in which phosphorus levels drop below 2.5 mg/dL.

hypopituitarism A rare, complex condition in which the pituitary gland does not produce sufficient amounts of some or all of its hormones.

hypospadias Condition in which the urethral meatus is found on the ventral surface of the penis instead of the end.

hypothalamic–pituitary axis Hormones produced by the anterior pituitary gland and regulated by the hypothalamus.

hypothalamus The basal portion of the diencephalon, which regulates the pituitary gland. The hypothalamus connects the nervous and endocrine systems; it regulates many bodily functions.

hypothyroidism Condition in which the thyroid does not produce sufficient amounts of the thyroid hormones.

hypotonic solution An intravascular solution that has a lower concentration of solutes than that found in the intravascular compartment. Administration of hypotonic solutions causes fluid to shift from the intravascular space to the intracellular space.

hypovolemia Fluid deficit of the intravascular compartment.

hypovolemic shock Type of shock in which venous return declines because of external blood volume losses. Preload drops, decreasing ventricular filling and stroke volume.

iatrogenic Caused by an unintended effect of a medical treatment.

idiopathic Unknown.

idiopathic thrombocytopenic purpura (ITP) A hypocoagulopathy state as a result of the immune system destroying its own platelets. It can be either acute or chronic.

immunodeficiency A diminished or absent immune response that increases susceptibility to infections.

impacted fracture Type of fracture in which one end of the bone is forced into the adjacent bone.

impetigo A common and highly contagious skin infection. Although it can occur without an apparent break, it typically arises from a breach in the skin. Impetigo spreads easily to others by direct contact with skin or contaminated objects. Lesions usually begin as a small vesicle that enlarges and ruptures, forming the characteristic honey-colored crust.

impregnation The fertilization of eggs.

incomplete fracture Type of fracture in which the bone is partially broken.

increased intracranial pressure Increased volume in the limited space of the cranial cavity. Increased intracranial pressure may occur because of a traumatic brain injury or because of other conditions that would increase the volume in the skull.

incus Bone in the ear that vibrates as a result of the malleus rocking, which in turn causes the stapes to move in and out against the oval window. Also called anvil.

infantile hypertrophic pyloric stenosis (IHPS) A narrowing and obstruction of the pyloric sphincter due to enlargement (hypertrophy) of the pyloric muscle that occurs within the first few months of life.

infarction Permanent damage to tissue.

infectious mononucleosis A disease caused by the Epstein-Barr virus, a common virus of the herpes family. Most people are exposed to the virus as children, and because of the exposure, they develop immunity to the virus and do not ever develop infectious mononucleosis. Also known as mono and the kissing disease.

infectious rhinitis The common cold, a viral upper respiratory infection. The most frequent culprit is the rhinovirus, but it can be caused by many viruses.

infective endocarditis An infection of the endocardium. It was previously called bacterial endocarditis.

inferior vena cava Large vein that carries deoxygenated blood from the lower half of the body to the right atrium.

infertility A biologic inability to contribute to reproduction.

inflammatory Triggering the inflammatory response.

inflammatory bowel disease (IBD) Chronic inflammation of the gastrointestinal tract, usually the intestines.

inflammatory response A series of reactions triggered by damage or trauma to body tissue.

influenza A viral infection that may affect the upper and lower respiratory tract. There are three strains: A, B, and C. The virus is highly adaptive and constantly mutates, preventing the development of any long-term immune defense.

initiation Phase of carcinogenesis in which the exposure of the cell to a substance or event causes DNA damage or mutation.

innate immunity Nonspecific defense mechanisms that are activated immediately or within a few hours in the presense of an antigen. These mechanisms include physical barriers, chemicals, the general immune response (e.g., inflammatory response, complement system, phagocytes). These mechanisms respond to antigens in a generic way and do not provide long-term protection against specific antigens.

inner ear Division of the ear that consists of the cochlea, semicircular canals, saccule, and utricle.

inotropic The strength of contraction.

insidious Onset of a disease with vague symptoms.

inspiration Inhalation. One of the two phases of breathing. Inspiration is an active neural process that begins with nerve impulses traveling from the brain to the diaphragm.

inspiratory reserve volume The amount of air beyond the tidal volume that can be taken in with the deepest inhalation.

insulin Hormone secreted by beta cells that is released when serum glucose levels increase. Insulin stimulates cellular uptake of glucose, which decreases serum glucose levels.

interferon A small protein that is released from cells infected by viruses. It prevents the virus from replicating and boosts the immune system.

interneuron A neuron that connects the sensory and motor neurons in the spinal cord.

interstitial A fluid compartment between the cells.

interstitial pneumonia A type of pneumonia that occurs in the areas between the alveoli. Interstitial pneumonia is usually caused by viruses (e.g., influenza type A and B) or by uncommon bacteria (e.g., *Legionella*). Also called atypical pneumonia.

intestinal obstruction Blockage of intestinal contents in the small intestine or large intestine.

intracellular fluid Fluid found inside the cells.

intracerebral hematoma A hematoma that results from bleeding in the brain tissue. Intracerebral hematomas are caused by contusion or shearing injuries but can also result from hypertension, cerebral vascular accidents (strokes), aneurysms, or vascular abnormalities.

intractable pain Chronically progressing pain that is unrelenting and severely debilitating. This type of pain does not usually respond well to typical pharmacologic pain treatments. Intractable pain is common with severe injuries, especially crushing injuries.

intrarenal condition Cause of acute renal failure that directly damages the structures of the kidneys.

intravascular A fluid compartment inside the blood vessels.

intrinsic asthma Type of asthma that usually presents after age 35 and is not an allergic reaction. Intrinsic triggers include upper respiratory infections, air pollution, emotional stress, smoking, exercise, and cold exposure.

iris The colored portion of the eye. The iris contains smooth muscle fibers that control changes in the diameter of the pupil so as to regulate the amount of light entering the eye.

irregular bone One of the five types of bones found within the skeleton. Irregular bones do not fall into any other category, due to their nonuniform shape. They primarily consist of spongy bone, with a thin outer layer of compact bone.

irritable bowel syndrome (IBS) A chronic gastrointestinal condition characterized by exacerbations associated with stress. Irritable bowel syndrome includes alterations in bowel pattern and abdominal pain not explained by structural or biochemical abnormalities.

ischemia Decreased blood flow to tissue or an organ. It essentially strangles the tissue or organ by limiting the supply of necessary nutrients and oxygen.

ischemic stroke The most common type of stroke. It is caused by an interruption in blood flow, often resulting from a thrombus or emboli.

islet of Langerhans Area situated among the many small acini in the pancreas that carries out endocrine functions. The human pancreas contains approximately 1 million islets of Langerhans, and each islet of Langerhans contains five types of cells.

isotonic solution An intravascular solution that has concentrations of solutes equal to those in the intravascular compartment. Because of these solute concentrations, isotonic solutions allow fluid to move equally between compartments.

isthmus A thin band of tissue that connects the two lobes of the thyroid gland by extending across the anterior aspect of the trachea.

jaundice A yellowish discoloration of the skin and sclera caused by an excessive amount of bilirubin in the bloodstream. It can result from bile entering the bloodstream or erythrocyte lysis.

joint A structure that connects bones of the skeleton. Joints are classified by their degree of movement: moveable, slightly moveable, and immoveable.

joint capsule The saclike envelope enclosing the cavity of a synovial joint.

karyotype A representation of a person's individual set of chromosomes.

keratin A protein that strengthens skin.

keratitis An inflammation of the cornea that can be triggered by an infection or trauma.

killer cell A type of T cell that destroys cells infected with viruses by releasing lymphokines that destroy cell walls. Also called cytotoxic cell and effector cell.

kyphosis An increase in the curvature of the thoracic spine outward. Also called hunchback.

labia majora The two large, fatty skin folds that protect the perineum and aid in lubrication.

labia minora Two small, firm skin folds located just inside the labia majora.

lacrimal duct The duct through which tears drain on the inner side of each eye.

lacrimal gland The gland that keeps the inner surface of the eyelid and the exposed surface of the eye moist.

lactation The production and secretion of milk for the feeding of offspring.

lamella (plural: lamellae) A thin layer of osteocytes.

large intestine Part of the lower gastrointestinal tract. It is 5 feet long in adults and contains the cecum, colon, and rectum.

laryngitis An inflammation of the larynx that is usually a result of an infection, increased upper respiratory exudate, or overuse. With laryngitis, the vocal cords become irritated and edematous because of the inflammatory process. This inflammation distorts sounds, leading to hoarseness and in some cases making the voice undetectable.

laryngotracheobronchitis A common viral infection in children 1–2 years of age, although older children and adults may also contract it. It usually begins as an upper respiratory infection with nasal congestion and cough. The larynx and surrounding area swell, leading to airway narrowing and obstruction. This swelling can lead to respiratory failure. Also called croup.

larynx The voice box. The larynx is made of cartilage and plays a central role in swallowing and talking.

latent herpes genitalis The second stage of genital herpes, which begins once the antibodies are formed.

latent syphilis The final stage of syphilis. The early latency stage begins when the secondary symptoms disappear and lasts 1–4 years. The late latency stage can last for years as the infection spreads to the brain, nervous system, heart, skin, and bones. Also called tertiary syphilis.

left atrium Receiving chamber on the left side of the heart. It receives blood from the pulmonary circulation; after leaving this chamber, blood travels to the left ventricle.

left-sided heart failure Type of heart failure that results from ineffective left ventricular contractility. As cardiac output falls, blood that is not being pumped out into the body backs up first in the left atrium and then in the pulmonary circulation.

left ventricle Pumping chamber on the left side of the heart. This chamber pumps blood to the systemic circulation.

Legionnaires' disease A specific type of pneumonia that is caused by *Legionella pneumophila*. The bacteria thrive in warm, moist environments, particularly air-conditioning systems and spas. Legionnaires' disease is not contagious. Most people acquire this type of pneumonia from inhaling the bacteria as they are spread by an air-conditioning system or spa.

leiomyoma A uterine fibroid; a firm, rubbery growth of the myometrium.

lens A transparent, flexible structure that lies behind the iris of the eye. Smooth muscles attached to the lens alter its shape, allowing the lens to focus on objects.

lentigo A large, pigmented spot that may appear in a sun-exposed area. Also called age spot or liver spot.

leukemia A cancer of the leukocytes. With leukemia, the bone marrow makes abnormal leukocytes. Leukemia cells do not die when they should, so they sometimes crowd out normal leukocytes, erythrocytes, and thrombocytes. This crowding makes it difficult for normal blood cells to do their work.

leukocyte White blood cell.

leukocytopenia Decreased white blood cell level; it can indicate an immune deficiency state (e.g., bone marrow suppression).

leukocytosis Increased white blood cell level; it can indicate an active infectious process.

ligament A bundle of dense connective tissue that connects bones to bones in a joint and provides support to the joint.

linear skull fracture A simple crack in the skull.

lipid A broad group of naturally occurring molecules that includes fats, fat-soluble vitamins (such as vitamins A, D, E, and K), monoglycerides, diglycerides, phospholipids, and others. The main biological functions of lipids are as energy storage locations, as structural components of cell membranes, and as important signaling molecules.

lipid bilayer A fatty double covering that makes up the membrane of a cell. The interior surface of the bilayer is uncharged and primarily consists of lipids. The exterior surface of the bilayer is charged and is less fatty than the interior surface.

liquefaction necrosis Type of necrosis that occurs when caustic enzymes dissolve and liquefy necrotic cells.

liver An organ that performs as many as 500 different functions. Some of the liver's primary roles are vital for homeostasis.

liver cancer Cancer of the liver. It most commonly occurs as a secondary tumor that has metastasized from the breast, lung, or other gastrointestinal structures.

lobar pneumonia Type of pneumonia confined to a single lobe in the lung and described based on that affected lobe (e.g., right upper lobe).

lobe Subdivision of a bodily organ or part, delineated by shape or connective tissue. Examples can be seen in the lung and brain.

local adaptation syndrome The localized version of general adaptation syndrome. In this syndrome, the body attempts to limit the damage associated with a stressor by confining the stressor to one location.

long bone One of the five types of bones found within the skeleton. A long bone has a body that is longer than it is wide, growth plates at either end, a hard outer surface, and an inner region that is less dense than the outer region and contains bone marrow.

longitudinal fissure The dividing point of the cerebrum into right and left hemispheres.

lordosis An exaggerated concave of the lumbar spine. Also called swayback.

low-density lipoprotein (LDL) A lipid that is a major contributor to the plaque formation associated with atherosclerosis. Also called bad cholesterol.

lower esophageal sphincter (LES) Part of the upper gastrointestinal system that relaxes to allow food to enter the stomach and that prevents the stomach contents from refluxing into the esophagus.

lung Organ responsible for gas exchange.

lung cancer Cancer of the lung. The third most common neoplasm, which can arise as either a primary or secondary tumor.

lymph Fluid that drains from the lymph capillaries into larger vessels and ducts that empty into large veins at the base of the neck. The movement of lymph occurs much in the same way that blood moves through veins, with the assistance of valves and movement.

lymphatic system An extensive network of vessels and glands that returns excess fluid in body tissue to the circulatory system and works with the immune system.

lymphedema Swelling, usually in the arms and legs, because of lymph obstruction. Lymphedema can occur on its own or as a result of another disease or condition.

lysis Bursting of a cell that occurs if too much water enters the cell membrane, causing excessive swelling.

macular degeneration A deterioration of the macular area of the retina caused by impaired blood supply to the macula that results in the cellular waste accumulation and ischemia.

macular stain The most common type of vascular birthmark. These faint red marks often occur on the forehead, eyelids, posterior neck, nose, upper lip, or posterior head. Also called salmon patch, angel kiss, and stork bite.

magnesium An intracellular cation that is mostly stored in the bone and muscle.

malignant State of a tumor that is usually made up of undifferentiated, nonfunctioning cells that are reproducing rapidly. Malignant tumors often penetrate surrounding tissue and spread to secondary sites.

malignant hypertension An intensified form of hypertension that may not respond well to treatment efforts.

malleus A bone that lies near the tympanic membrane of the ear. Vibrations from the membrane cause the malleus to rock back and forth. Also called hammer.

mammary glands Glands that are located in the breast of the male and female, but function only in females. They produce milk when stimulated to do so.

manifestation The clinical effects or evidence of a disease. Manifestations may include both signs (what can be seen or measured) and symptoms (what the patient describes).

mastication Chewing.

mastitis An inflammation of the breast tissue that can be associated with infection and lactation.

matrix Extracellular material in which osteocytes are embedded. The matrix consists of calcium phosphate crystals that make the bones hard and strong. It also contains collagen fibers that reinforce the bone, giving it flexible strength.

meatus An opening or passageway.

medulla 1. The part of the brain stem that acts as the conduction pathway for ascending and descending nerve tracts. The medulla coordinates heart rate, peripheral vascular resistance, breathing, swallowing, vomiting, coughing, and sneezing. 2. The inner portion of an adrenal gland. It is regulated by nerve impulses from the hypothalamus and produces epinephrine and norepinephrine during times of stress.

meiosis A form of cell division that occurs only in mature sperm and ova.

melanin A pigment that provides color to the skin as well as protection from ultraviolet rays. Disorders involving melanin result in alterations in skin coloring and can leave the skin vulnerable to the harmful effects of UV light. Melanin disorders include albinism and vitiligo.

melena Dark, tarry stool associated with a significant amount of bleeding high in the gastrointestinal tract.

memory cell Type of B cell that aids in the body's quick response to subsequent exposures to an antigen because memory cells recall the antigen as foreign, and antibody production is rapid.

Meniere's disease A disorder of the inner ear that results from endolymph swelling, which stretches the membranes and interferes with the hair receptors in the cochlea and vestibule.

meninges A set of three tough membranes that encase the central nervous system.

meningitis An inflammation of the meninges, usually resulting from an infection.

meningocele A rare form of spina bifida that involves a bony defect, but where the meninges protrude through the vertebral opening.

menopause The complete and permanent cessation of the menstrual cycle.

menorrhagia Increased menstrual blood flow amount and duration.

menstrual cycle A series of monthly changes in females that begin at puberty and continue through the reproductive years.

menstruation Shedding of the endometrium. It generally occurs on a regular basis (usually every 28 days) during the reproductive years of women. Also called period.

mesentery A double-layer peritoneum containing blood vessels and nerves that supplies the intestinal wall.

metabolic Related to the body's metabolism.

metabolic acidosis Condition that results from a deficiency of bicarbonate or an excess of hydrogen.

metabolic alkalosis Condition that results from an excess of bicarbonate or a deficiency of hydrogen.

metabolic syndrome A cluster of risk factors occurring together—hyperglycemia, high blood pressure, hypercholesterolemia, and increased waist circumference. Metabolic syndrome increases a person's risk for developing cardiovascular disease, diabetes mellitus, and stroke.

metaphase Phase of mitosis in which the spindle fibers attach to centromeres and chromosomes align.

metaplasia The process of one adult cell being replaced by another cell type.

metastasize To spread (e.g., cancer cells).

metrorrhagia Vaginal bleeding between menstrual periods in premenopausal women.

microtia An underdeveloped, small auricle.

micturition Urination.

midbrain The smallest region of the brain, which acts as a sort of relay station for auditory and visual information. The midbrain controls the visual and auditory systems as well as eye movement.

middle ear Division of the ear that includes the tympanic membrane and the ossicles.

Middle East respiratory syndrome An emerging illness caused by a coronavirus family. It is currently isolated to four countries in the Arabian Peninsula.

mineralocorticoid Steroid produced by the outermost region of the adrenal cortex.

minute respiratory volume The amount of air inhaled and exhaled in 1 minute. It is determined by the tidal volume multiplied by the respirations per minute.

mitosis The most common form of cell division, in which the cell divides into two separate cells. In mitosis, the division of one cell results in two genetically identical and equal daughter cells. This process occurs in four phases: prophase, metaphase, anaphase, and telophase.

mitral valve A bicuspid valve that guides the passage of blood from the left atria to the left ventricle and prevents the backward flow of blood.

mixed dysfunction A categorization of heart failure that is a combination of systolic and diastolic dysfunction.

mixed incontinence Type of incontinence in which symptoms of more than one type of urinary incontinence are experienced.

mole A brown nevus. Moles can be tan, brown, or black; can be flat or raised; and may have hair growth.

Mongolian spot Type of birthmark that is a flat, bluish-gray area often found on the lower back or buttocks. These birthmarks are most common on individuals with darker complexions.

Monro-Kellie hypothesis A supposition that states the cranial cavity cannot be compressed, and the volume inside the cavity is fixed (normal intracranial pressure is 60–200 mm H_2O or 4–15 mm Hg). The skull and its components create a state of volume equilibrium, such that any increase in volume of one component must be compensated by a decrease in volume of another component.

mons pubis The pad of fat over the symphysis pubis that becomes covered with hair after puberty.

morbidity The disease rate within a group.

mortality The death rate from a particular disease.

motor nerve A type of nerve that carries impulses from the brain to the corresponding muscle receptor, resulting in muscle contraction and movement. Also called efferent nerve.

mucosa The innermost of four layers of the walls of the gastrointestinal tract. The mucosa produces mucus.

mucus A thick, sticky substance produced by the goblet cells in the epithelial lining of the nose, trachea, and bronchi.

multifactorial disorder A result of an interaction between genes and environmental factors. Such a disorder does not follow a clear-cut pattern of inheritance. Multifactorial disorders may be present at birth, as with cleft lip or palate, or they may be expressed later in life, as with hypertension.

multiple myeloma A cancer of the plasma cells that most often affects older adults. Multiple myeloma is characterized by excessive numbers of abnormal plasma cells in the bone marrow crowding out the blood-forming cells and causing Bence Jones proteins to be excreted in the urine.

multiple sclerosis (MS) A debilitating autoimmune condition that involves a progressive and irreversible demyelination of brain, spinal cord, and cranial nerve neurons. This damage occurs in diffuse patches throughout the nervous system and slows or stops nerve impulses.

muscle fiber Muscle cell that is a cylinder with multiple nuclei.

muscle layer One of the four layers of the walls of the gastrointestinal tract. It includes circular and longitudinal smooth muscle layers. This layer contracts in a wavelike motion to propel food through the gastrointestinal tract.

muscular dystrophy (MD) A group of inherited disorders characterized by degeneration of skeletal muscle. Muscles become weaker as damage worsens. There are nine different forms of muscular dystrophy.

myasthenia gravis An autoimmune condition in which acetylcholine receptors are impaired or destroyed by immunoglobulin G autoantibodies, leading to a disruption of normal communication between the nerve and muscle at the neuromuscular junction.

myasthenic crisis A potentially life-threatening complication of myasthenia gravis that occurs when the muscles become too weak to maintain adequate ventilation.

Mycoplasma pneumoniae A common type of pneumonia that usually affects people younger than 40 years of age.

myelin sheath Covering that surrounds axons to increase the rate of impulse transmission.

myelomeningocele The most severe form of spina bifida. In this form, the spinal canal remains open along several vertebrae in the lower or middle back. Also called open spina bifida.

myocardial infarction (MI) Death of the myocardium from sudden blockage of coronary artery blood flow. Other names for a myocardial infarction include heart attack and acute coronary syndrome.

myocarditis An inflammation of the myocardium. This is an uncommon condition, in which there is a period of at least several weeks (in some cases a decade) between exposure of the causative agent and the development of symptoms.

myocardium The middle layer of the heart; the muscle portion of the organ.

myofibril A threadlike structure that extends the entire length of the muscle fiber.

myofilament Protein fibers found in muscle fibers.

myometrium The middle layer of the uterine wall, made up of smooth muscle and a vascular system. During pregnancy, the vascular system radically increases to support the fetus.

myosin One of two types of myofilament—the darker and thicker of the two types. Myosin myofilaments are fibrous globulins that work with actin to form actomyosin.

myxedema Advanced hypothyroidism. This condition is rare, but when it occurs, it can be life threatening. Clinical manifestations include marked hypotension, respiratory depression, hypothermia, lethargy, and coma.

nausea A subjective urge to vomit that may precede vomiting.

necrosis A cell's inability to survive due to the extent of damage.

necrotizing fasciitis A rare, serious infection that can aggressively destroy skin, fat, muscle, and other tissue. One out of four people with this infection will die because of it. Also called flesh-eating bacteria.

negative feedback system One of two types of feedback systems that maintain homeostasis (the other is a positive feedback system). The negative feedback system, which is the most common type, works to maintain a deficit in the system. Examples of negative feedback systems include temperature and glucose regulation.

neoplasm A cellular growth that is no longer responding to normal regulator processes, usually because of a mutation. Also called a tumor.

neoplastic Related to abnormal or uncontrolled cellular growth.

nephritic syndrome Inflammatory injury to the glomeruli that can occur when antibodies interact with normally occurring antigens in the glomeruli.

nephrolithiasis The presence of renal calculi (kidney stones).

nephron One of 1–2 million microscopic filtering units in the kidney. Each is similar to a long-stemmed funnel and has multiple sections, and each section is responsible for excreting or reabsorbing specific substances.

nephrotic syndrome Condition that results from antibody–antigen complexes lodging in the glomerular membrane, triggering the complement system.

nerve Part of the peripheral nervous system that consists of bundles of nerve fibers, where each fiber is part of the neuron.

neurogenic bladder All types of bladder dysfunction caused by an interruption of normal bladder nerve innervation.

neurogenic shock Type of distributive shock in which a loss of sympathetic tone in vascular smooth muscle and autonomic function lead to massive vasodilation. Blood pools in the venous system, leading to decreased venous return, cardiac output, and hypotension.

neuroglia Type of cells that play several important supportive roles in the nervous system. Neuroglia cells scaffold neural tissue as well as isolate and protect neuron cell membranes. Additionally, they regulate interstitial fluid, defend the neuron against pathogens, and assist with neural repair.

neuromelanin A specialized, dark pigment found in the brain.

neuron The fundamental unit of the nervous system. Neurons generate bioelectric impulses and transmit them from one area of the body to another.

neuropathic pain Pain that results from damage to peripheral nerves by disease or injury. This type of pain tends to be chronic and intractable.

neurotransmitter Chemical that is released from the presynaptic terminal and crosses the synaptic cleft in one direction to stimulate an electrical reaction in nearby neurons.

neutropenia An insufficient number of circulating neutrophils (fewer than 1,500 cells/µL; the normal range is 2,000–7,500 cells/µL). With fewer of these first responders, the body is poorly equipped to fight infections. The degree to which the body can fight infections, especially bacterial infections, is related to the severity of the neutropenia.

neutrophil An infection-fighting agent. Usually the first cells to arrive on the scene of an infection, neutrophils are attracted by various chemicals released by infected tissue. Neutrophils escape from the capillary wall and migrate to the site of infection. Once they get to the site, neutrophils phagocytize microorganisms, preventing the infection from spreading.

nipple Part of the breast, which is surrounded by the areola.

nocturnal asthma Type of asthma that usually occurs between 3:00 a.m. and 7:00 a.m. and is thought to be related to circadian rhythms. At night, cortisol and epinephrine levels decrease, while histamine levels increase.

nocturnal enuresis Bed-wetting.

node of Ranvier Node that separates Schwann cells.

non-small-cell carcinoma An aggressive type of lung cancer; the most common type of malignant lung cancer. It has several subgroups—squamous cell carcinoma, adenocarcinoma, and bronchioalveolar carcinoma. Often referred to as bronchogenic carcinoma.

noncommunicating hydrocephalus Type of hydrocephalus that occurs when the cerebrospinal fluid flow is disrupted or not properly absorbed by the bloodstream. Also called obstructive hydrocephalus.

nonvolatile acid An acid produced from sources other than carbon dioxide, which is not excreted by the lungs.

norepinephrine Hormone produced by the medulla during times of stress. With epinephrine, it mediates the fight-or-flight response of the sympathetic nervous system.

nosocomial pneumonia Pneumonia that develops more than 48 hours after a hospital admission.

nucleotides Molecules that join together to form RNA and DNA.

nucleus The control center of the cell, which contains all the genetic information (DNA) for the cell and is surrounded by a double membrane. The nucleus regulates cell growth, metabolism, and reproduction.

nystagmus Rapid, involuntary back-and-forth eye movement.

oblique fracture A fracture at an angle to the bone shaft.

obstructive hydrocephalus A type of hydrocephalus that occurs when cerebrospinal fluid flow is disrupted or not properly absorbed by the bloodstream. Also called obstructive hydrocephalus.

occipital lobe Lobe of the brain that processes visual information.

occult blood Blood that occurs in small amounts and is not usually apparent.

occupational asthma A type of asthma that is caused by a reaction to substances encountered at work. Symptoms develop over time, worsening with each exposure and improving when one is away from work.

oligomenorrhea Infrequent menstruation; a long menstrual cycle.

oncogene Gene that activates cell division and influences embryonic development.

oogenesis The generation of eggs.

open-angle (chronic) glaucoma Type of glaucoma in which intraocular pressure increases gradually over an extended period. It is the most common type.

open fracture Type of fracture in which the skin is broken. The bone fragments or edges may be angled and protrude out of the skin. Open fractures are associated with more damage to soft tissue and carry a greater risk for infection.

opportunistic infection An infection caused by pathogens that do not normally cause disease in healthy individuals.

optic nerve The nerve formed at the back of the eye by axons of the ganglion cells coming together. This area contains no photoreceptors and is insensitive to light.

oral cancer Cancer anywhere in the mouth. Most are squamous cell carcinomas of the tongue and mouth floor. Approximately 75% of cases can be attributed to use of smoked and smokeless tobacco.

organ of Corti Part of the cochlea that contains hearing receptors, the hair cells. Vibrations at the organ of Corti stimulate hair movement.

organelle An internal cellular structure. Organelles perform the work that maintains the cell's life.

orgasm The climax of pleasurable sensations.

osmolarity Solute concentration.

osmosis The movement of water or another solvent across the cellular membrane from an area of low solute concentration to an area of high solute concentration.

osmotic pressure The tendency of water to move by osmosis.

ossicle Part of the ear consisting of three bones—malleus, incus, and stapes.

osteoarthritis (OA) A localized joint disease characterized by deterioration of articulating cartilage and its underlying bone as well as bony overgrowth. The surface of the cartilage becomes rough and worn, interfering with joint movement. Also called wear-and-tear arthritis and degenerative joint disease.

osteoblast Cell on the outer surface of the periosteum that aids in remodeling and repair by rebuilding new compact bone to increase bone strength.

osteochondroma A type of benign tumor that consists of cartilage and bone.

osteoclast A cell that breaks down some spongy bone.

osteocyte Osteoblast that has become surrounded by calcified extracellular material.

osteomalacia A softening and weakening of bones in adults, usually because of an extreme and prolonged vitamin D, calcium, or phosphate deficiency.

osteomyelitis An infection of the bone tissue.

osteonecrosis Death of bone tissue due to a loss of blood supply. Also called avascular necrosis.

osteopenia Bone mass that is less than expected for age, ethnicity, or gender.

osteoporosis A condition characterized by a progressive loss of bone calcium that leaves the bones brittle.

osteosarcoma An aggressive tumor that begins in the bone cells, usually in the femur, tibia, or fibula.

otitis externa An infection or inflammation of the external ear canal or auricle. Also called swimmer's ear.

otitis media An infection or inflammation of the middle ear. It is a common condition in young children.

otosclerosis An abnormal bone growth in the middle ear, usually involving an imbalance in bone formation and resorption.

outer ear Division of the ear that consists of the auricle (or pinna), ear lobe, and external ear canal.

oval window The opening to the inner ear covered with a membrane. Movement of the oval window causes fluid within the cochlea to vibrate, creating waves.

ovarian cancer Cancer of the ovaries. There is no reliable screening test, it is difficult to treat, and it often has metastasized at the time of diagnosis. However, advances in treatment are improving the survival rates.

ovarian cyst A benign, fluid-filled sac on the ovary. Often the cyst forms in the ovulation process. Instead of the follicle releasing the egg, the fluid stays in the follicle, creating a cyst.

ovaries Paired, almond-shaped organs located on each side of the uterus.

overactive bladder Urge incontinence with no known cause.

overflow incontinence Incontinence as a result of an inability to empty the bladder.

ovulation The transportation of the eggs.

pacemaker Cells that create the rhythmic, chemical impulses that in turn cause contraction of the heart muscle. The rate at which these impulses fire controls the heart rate.

PaCO$_2$ Partial pressure of carbon dioxide; it indicates the adequacy of pulmonary ventilation.

Paget's disease A progressive condition characterized by abnormal bone destruction and remodeling, which results in bone deformities.

pain A subjective feeling that serves as a protective mechanism, warning the body when something is wrong. In addition, pain is the most common reason why people seek medical attention and can be used to aid diagnosis.

pain threshold The perception of pain.

pain tolerance The amount of pain that an individual can physically and emotionally withstand.

palliative Treatment aimed at increasing comfort.

pancreas An organ with exocrine digestive functions and endocrine functions. The pancreas lies underneath the stomach and liver and between the two kidneys in the retroperitoneum.

pancreatic cancer An aggressive malignancy (most commonly adenocarcinoma) of the pancreas that can quickly spread to structures nearby.

pancreatic polypeptide Substance secreted by cells that is thought to regulate some of the pancreatic activities.

pancreatitis An inflammation of the pancreas that can be acute or chronic.

pancytopenia A lack of erythrocytes, leukocytes, and platelets.

pandemic An epidemic that has spread to a larger population.

panhypopituitarism A condition consisting of an inadequate or absent production of the anterior pituitary hormones.

papule A small, red, elevated area of the skin.

paralysis A lack of voluntary use of the affected limbs.

paralytic ileus A functional intestinal obstruction.

paraphimosis A condition in which the foreskin is retracted and cannot be returned over the glans penis.

paraplegia Loss of lower-extremity function.

parasympathetic nervous system Subdivision of the autonomic nervous system that is responsible for the rest-and-digest response.

parathyroid gland A gland located on the posterior surface of the thyroid. There are usually four of these glands, each of which secretes parathyroid hormone.

parathyroid hormone (PTH) A hormone that works in opposition to calcitonin to regulate serum calcium levels.

parietal lobe The lobe of the brain that receives and interprets sensory input, with the exception of smell, hearing, and vision.

parietal peritoneum layer The outer layer of the peritoneum that covers the abdominal wall as well as the top of the bladder and uterus.

Parkinson's disease A progressive condition involving the destruction of the substantia nigra in the brain. This destruction results in a lack of dopamine, a chemical messenger that allows smooth, coordinated muscle movement.

partial pressure of oxygen The concentration of oxygen in the blood.

partially compensated A pH level that is abnormal.

parturition The birth of the fetus.

passive acquired immunity The protection gained by receiving antibodies made outside the body by another person, animal, or recombinant DNA. In passive immunity, the person is not actively producing antibodies, and protection is short lived. Examples of passive immunity include mother-to-fetus transfer through placenta or breastfeeding transference.

pathogenesis The development of a disease.

pathologic fracture A type of fracture that results from a weakness in the bone structure secondary to conditions such as tumors or osteoporosis.

pathophysiology The study of changes in normal anatomy and physiology that go wrong.

pediculosis A lice infestation that can take three forms—*Pediculus humanus corpus* (body louse), *Pediculus pubic* (pubic louse), and *Pediculus humanus capitis* (head louse). Lice are small, brown, parasitic insects that feed off human blood and cannot survive for long without the human host.

pelvic inflammatory disease (PID) An infection of the female reproductive system.

penile cancer Cancer of the penis. The exact cause is unknown, but risk is thought to be increased by the presence of smegma, being uncircumcised, poor hygiene, phimosis, and human papillomavirus infection.

penis Part of the male external genitalia; it contains erectile tissue that fills with blood during sexual arousal.

peptic ulcer disease (PUD) Erosive lesions affecting the lining of the stomach or duodenum.

perfusion The process of delivering oxygen and nutrients with arterial blood to tissue.

pericardial effusion Fluid accumulation between the pericardium and the heart.

pericarditis An inflammation of the pericardium. The fluid may be serous, purulent, serosanguineous, or hemorrhagic. As the pericardial tissue becomes inflamed, the swollen tissue rubs together, creating friction.

pericardium Sac that encloses, protects, and supports the heart.

perimetrium The outer, serous layer of the uterine wall that covers all of the fundus and part of the corpus, but none of the cervix.

periosteum A layer of connective tissue that covers compact bone surfaces. It serves as the site of muscle attachment (via tendons).

peripheral nerve A nerve that branches from a plexus and supplies sensory and motor functions to many areas of the body.

peripheral nervous system (PNS) A division of the nervous system made up of the nerves.

peripheral vascular disease (PVD) A narrowing in the peripheral vessels. Most often this condition is caused by atherosclerosis, but it can also be caused by thrombus, inflammation (e.g., thromboangiitis obliterans), or vasospasms (e.g., Raynaud's disease and Raynaud's phenomenon).

peripheral vascular resistance (PVR) The force opposing the blood in the peripheral circulation. PVR increases as the diameter and elasticity of the blood vessels decreases.

peristalsis The wavelike contraction of the muscle layer of the gastrointestinal tract that propels food through the gastrointestinal tract.

peritoneal cavity The space between the parietal peritoneum layer and the visceral peritoneum layer. It contains serous fluid that decreases friction and facilitates movement of the peritoneum.

peritoneum The large serous membrane that lines the abdominal cavity.

peritonitis An inflammation of the peritoneum that can be life threatening.

pH A measure of hydrogen concentration in the plasma. It is a negative logarithm that reflects hydrogen concentrations; the higher the hydrogen concentration, the lower the pH number.

phagocytosis Endocytosis that involves solid particles. Also called cell eating.

phantom pain Pain that exists after the removal of a body part. The affected person may feel the discomfort of the removed part. The severing of neurons may result in spontaneous firing of spinal cord neurons because normal sensory input has been lost. This type of pain can be very distressing but usually resolves with time.

pharynx Passageway that connects the oral and nasal cavities to the larynx.

phenotype The outward, physical expression of genes, such as eye color.

pheochromocytoma A rare tumor of the adrenal medulla. The tumor excretes epinephrine and norepinephrine and can be life threatening because of the effects of epinephrine and norepinephrine.

phimosis Condition that occurs when the foreskin cannot be retracted from the glans penis.

phosphate system Buffer mechanism that acts much like the bicarbonate–carbonic acid system. Buffering in this system primarily takes place in the kidneys by moving hydrogen.

phosphorus An ion that is a component of phosphate. It is found in the bones and, in smaller quantities, in the bloodstream.

pia mater The innermost layer of the meninges; it rests directly on the brain and spinal cord.

pigmented birthmark A birthmark made of a cluster of pigment cells, which cause color in skin. These birthmarks can be many different colors, from tan to brown, gray to black, or even blue.

pink puffers Nickname given to patients with emphysema, who often hyperventilate, giving a pink appearance to their skin.

pinna The irregularly shaped cartilage that channels sound into the ear. Also referred to as the auricle.

pinocytosis Endocytosis that involves a liquid. Also called cell drinking.

pituitary gland Pea-sized gland located at the base of the brain. It can be divided into two parts—the anterior and posterior pituitary gland. The pituitary gland is often referred to as the master gland. Despite its small size, this gland secretes several hormones that influence many different body functions.

placenta A vascular organ that develops during pregnancy to nourish the fetus through the umbilical cord.

plasma Liquid portion of the blood, primarily composed of protein.

plasma membrane The semipermeable boundary of a cell containing the cell and its components. Also called cell membrane.

plasmin An enzyme that dissolves clots once healing has occurred.

pleural effusion The accumulation of excess fluid in the pleural cavity that can compress the lungs and limit their expansion during inhalation.

pleurisy Inflammation of the pleural membranes, which leads to swollen and irregular tissue. This inflammation is often associated with pneumonia and creates friction in the pleural membranes.

plexus An organized collaboration of several intersected nerves.

***Pneumocystis jiroveci* pneumonia** A specific type of pneumonia that is caused by a yeastlike fungus, *Pneumocystis jiroveci*. It occurs as an opportunistic infection and can be fatal to immunocompromised individuals (e.g., children or those with AIDS or cancer).

pneumonia An inflammatory process caused by numerous infectious agents (e.g., bacteria, viruses, and fungi) and injurious agents or events (e.g., aspiration and smoke). *Streptococcus pneumoniae* is responsible for 75% of all cases of pneumonia.

pneumothorax Air in the pleural cavity. The presence of atmospheric air in the pleural cavity and the separation to pleural membranes can lead to atelectasis. The pressure can cause a partial or complete collapse of a lung.

polycystic kidney disease (PKD) An inherited disorder characterized by numerous grape-like clusters of fluid-filled cysts in both kidneys.

polycystic ovary syndrome A condition in which the ovary becomes enlarged and contains numerous cysts.

polydipsia Excessive thirst.

polymenorrhea Frequent menstruation due to a short menstrual cycle.

polyphagia An increase in the hunger sensation.

polyuria An increase in the amount of water that is excreted.

pons The part of the brain stem that contains the nerves that regulate sleep and breathing.

port-wine stain Vascular birthmark that looks like wine was spilled on an area of the body. These birthmarks most often occur on the face, neck, arms, and legs.

portal hypertension Increase in vessel pressures in the hepatic artery and the portal vein. This increased pressure is often associated with liver disease.

portal vein Part of the liver's dual blood supply; it carries partially deoxygenated blood from the stomach, pancreas, and spleen, as well as from the small and large intestines, to the liver, at a rate of approximately 1,000 mL/min, so that the liver can process nutrients and digestion by-products.

positive feedback system One of two types of feedback systems that maintain homeostasis (the other is a negative feedback system). The positive feedback system works to increase an output in the system. An example of a positive feedback system is a blood clot.

posterior chamber The cavity of the eye interior that is behind the lens.

postictal period The period following a generalized seizure, during which the individual may be confused, be fatigued, and fall into a deep sleep.

postrenal condition Cause of acute renal failure that interferes with the urine excretion.

postsynaptic cell membrane The membrane that receives and responds to a signal (binds neurotransmitter) from the presynaptic cell.

potassium The primary intracellular cation. Potassium plays a crucial role in electrical conduction, acid–base balance, and metabolism (carbohydrate, protein, and glucose).

PP cell One of five types of cells in the islets of Langerhans; it secretes a pancreatic polypeptide.

predisposing factor Tendency that puts an individual at risk for developing certain diseases.

pregnancy-induced hypertension (PIH) Hypertension that occurs for the first time during pregnancy. It occurs in 5–8% of all pregnancies.

preload The amount of blood returning to the heart, which the heart has to manage. Both afterload and preload can affect blood pressure. As afterload and preload increase, blood pressure increases.

premenstrual dysphoric syndrome A severe form of premenstrual syndrome that is characterized by severe depression, tension, and irritability.

premenstrual syndrome (PMS) A group of physical and emotional symptoms that affect many women prior to menstruation for reasons not fully understood.

prerenal condition Cause of acute renal failure that disrupts blood flow on its way to the kidneys.

presbycusis Age-related hearing loss.

presbyopia Difficulty focusing the eyes resulting from age-related changes.

presynaptic terminal Terminal bouton or some similar structure. It is a specialized area within the axon of the presynaptic cell that contains neurotransmitters enclosed in small membrane-bound spheres.

prevention Strategies used to avoid the development of disease in individuals or groups.

priapism A prolonged, painful erection.

primary deficit Type of immunodeficiency that involves basic developmental failures, many resulting from genetic or congenital abnormalities (e.g., hypogammaglobulinemia).

primary herpes genitalis The first stage of genital herpes. It usually occurs within 2–10 days of exposure and is characterized by blisters or open lesions, fever, headache, muscle aches, swollen lymph nodes in the groin area, painful urination, and vaginal discharge.

primary hypertension Type of hypertension in which there is no identifiable cause. It occurs in 90–95% of hypertension cases in adults and tends to develop gradually over many years. Also called essential hypertension.

primary syphilis The first stage of syphilis. Painless chancres (usually one) form at the site of infection about 2–3 weeks after initial infection.

primary tuberculosis infection One of two stages of tuberculosis pathogenesis. In this stage, infection occurs when the bacillus first enters the body.

prion An abnormal protein particle that causes proteins to fold abnormally, especially in nervous tissue.

prodrome In infection with the herpes simplex virus, a tingling or burning sensation at the site just before a lesion appears.

prognosis An individual's likelihood of surviving, making a full recovery, or regaining normal functioning after developing a disease.

programmed cell death The process of eliminating unwanted cells. Also called apoptosis.

progression Phase of carcinogenesis in which the tumor invades, metastasizes, and becomes drug resistant. The final phase of carcinogenesis, it is irreversible.

progressive stage State of shock that begins when the compensatory mechanisms fail to maintain cardiac output. Tissues become hypoxic, cells switch to anaerobic metabolism, lactic acid builds up, and metabolic acidosis develops.

prolactin A hormone from the anterior pituitary gland that stimulates milk production.

proliferation The regulated process by which cells divide and reproduce.

promotion Phase of carcinogenesis in which the mutated cells are exposed to factors that promote their growth. It may occur just after initiation or years later, and it can be reversible if the promoting factors are removed.

prophase Phase of mitosis in which the chromosomes condense and the nuclear membrane disintegrates.

prophylactic Treatment aimed at preventing disease.

prostate cancer Cancer of the prostate. It is the most common cancer among men. The slow-growing tumor is often confined to the prostate, improving the prognosis.

prostate gland A chestnut-shaped gland at the base of the urethra in men; it produces fluid that mixes with the sperm and secretions of the seminal vesicles. This prostate fluid further deceases acidity, increases sperm motility, and prolongs sperm life.

prostatitis Inflammation of the prostate, which can be either acute or chronic.

protein system The most abundant buffering system. Proteins can act as an acid or a base by binding to or releasing hydrogen. Proteins exist in intracellular and extracellular fluid but are most abundant inside the cell.

protoplasm A colorless, viscous liquid containing water, nutrients, ions, dissolved gases, and waste products, where the cellular work takes place. Also called cytoplasm.

psoriasis A common chronic inflammatory condition that affects the life cycle of the skin cells.

pulmonary artery Vessel that carries deoxygenated blood from the right ventricle to the lungs for oxygenation.

pulmonary circulation The portion of the cardiovascular system that carries oxygen-depleted blood away from the heart and to the lungs, and then returns oxygenated blood back to the heart.

pulmonary vein Vessel that carries oxygenated blood from the lungs to the left atrium.

pulmonic valve A three-leaflet valve that guides the passage of blood from the right ventricle to the pulmonary artery and prevents the backward flow of blood.

pulse pressure The difference between the systolic and diastolic blood pressures.

pupil The dark opening in the center of the iris that opens and closes reflexively in response to light intensity.

Purkinje network of fibers Area of specialized cells in the heart that receives impulses from the bundle branches and stimulates ventricular contraction.

pus Yellowish-white wound drainage.

pyelonephritis An infection that has reached one or both kidneys.

pyloric sphincter A muscular ring through which chyme passes as it leaves the stomach in small, varying amounts. The pyloric sphincter prevents reflux of bile from the small intestines into the stomach.

pyloric stenosis A narrowing and obstruction of the pyloric sphincter.

pyrogen A molecule released by macrophages that have been exposed by bacteria.

quadriplegia Loss of all or most function in all four limbs; also known as tetraplegia.

Raynaud's disease A condition that is result of vasospasms of arteries—most often of the hands—that occurs because of sympathetic stimulation.

recessive Less influential. In genetics, the recessive allele is less likely to be expressed in the offspring than the dominant one.

rectocele Condition that occurs when the rectum protrudes through the posterior wall of the vagina.

rectum A reservoir to store feces.

recurrent herpes genitalis The fourth stage of genital herpes; characterized by the reactivation of the virus and clinical manifestations.

red marrow Bone marrow that serves as the blood-cell factory (hematopoiesis). As humans age, this red marrow is slowly replaced by fat, creating yellow marrow.

reduce A fracture treatment in which the broken bone fragments are brought together to promote healing. Reduction can be accomplished by manual manipulation or surgery.

referred pain Pain at distant locations from the originating organ.

reflex incontinence Urinary incontinence caused by trauma or damage to the nervous system.

regulator cell One of two major types of T cells that work to destroy antigens. Regulator cells include helper T cells and suppressor T cells.

regurgitation Insufficiency or incompetence. In the heart, it occurs when the valve leaflets do not completely close. Incompetent valves allow blood to flow in both directions.

remission Disease state that occurs when the manifestations subside.

renal artery The artery that supplies each kidney with blood.

renal capsule Connective tissue that surrounds the kidneys.

renal cell carcinoma The most frequently occurring kidney cancer in adults. It is most common in individuals 50–70 years of age.

renal cortex The area immediately beneath the renal capsule that contains the functional units of the kidney.

renal hilum The opening in the kidney that the renal artery and nerves enter and the renal vein and ureter exit.

renal pelvis Funnel-like area in the center of the kidney in which urine drains.

renal sinus A cavity into which the renal hilum opens.

renin–angiotensin–aldosterone system A vital control and compensatory mechanism that is activated when renal blood flow is decreased, often in hypotensive states. When blood flow is decreased to the kidneys, renin is released from the kidneys, which in turn activates angiotensin I to become converted to angiotensin II (a vasoconstrictor) and stimulates aldosterone secretion. In hypotensive states, this mechanism raises blood pressure and maintains vital organs. In chronic disease states such as hypertension, it is inappropriately activated because of vasoconstriction to the kidneys, further contributing to the hypertension.

repolarization 1. The recovery of the ventricles, represented by T waves. Repolarization of the atria does not appear on an electrocardiogram because it is hidden by the other more prominent waveforms. 2. Restoration of the resting potential of the cell membrane.

residual volume Volume of air left in the lungs after maximum exhalation.

resistance The second stage of the general adaptation syndrome. In this stage, the body chooses the most effective and advantageous defense. Cortisol levels and the sympathetic nervous system return to normal, causing the fight-or-flight symptoms to disappear. The body will either adapt or alter its functioning in an attempt to limit problems or become desensitized to the stressor.

respiratory acidosis Condition that results from carbon dioxide retention, which leads to increased carbonic acid and, in turn, decreased pH.

respiratory alkalosis Condition that results from excess exhalation of carbon dioxide, which leads to carbonic acid deficits and pH increases.

resting potential A slight charge that the plasma side of the neuron membrane has at rest because of the sodium ions concentrated on the outside of the cell.

restrictive cardiomyopathy Type of cardiomyopathy that is characterized by rigidity of the ventricles leading to diastolic dysfunction.

retching A strong, unproductive effort to vomit.

retention An inability to empty the bladder.

reticular activation system Specialized nerve fibers through which the reticular formation sends impulses to the cerebral cortex. The reticular formation and reticular activation system are responsible for alertness during the day and can prevent sleeping at night.

reticular formation A region of the brain stem in which most of the branches of the many nerve fibers passing through the brain stem terminate. The reticular formation acts like a gatekeeper, receiving all incoming and outgoing information. It sends impulses to the cerebral cortex through specialized nerve fibers.

retina The innermost layer of the eye. It contains an outer, pigmented layer and an inner layer consisting of photoreceptors and nerve cells. The retina is weakly attached to the choroid, making it vulnerable to damage.

retinal detachment An acute condition in which the retina separates from its supporting structures.

retractile testicle A testicle that moves back and forth between the scrotum and the lower abdomen. Such a testicle is easily returned to the scrotum through gentle manipulation.

retroflexed Tilted backward. Often used in reference to the uterus.

rheumatoid arthritis (RA) A systemic, autoimmune condition involving multiple joints. In RA, the inflammatory process primarily affects the synovial membrane, but it can also affect other organs.

rhinosinusitis An inflammation of the sinus cavities, most often caused by a viral infection. Previously referred to as sinusitis.

rickets A softening and weakening of bones in children, usually because of an extreme and prolonged vitamin D, calcium, or phosphate deficiency.

right atrium Receiving chamber on the right side of the heart. It receives blood from the peripheral circulation, and blood leaves this chamber and travels to the right ventricle.

right-sided heart failure Type of heart failure that results from an ineffective right ventricular contractility. As a result, blood does not move appropriately out of the right ventricle. Blood backs up first into the right atrium and then into the peripheral circulation, causing increased pressures in the capillary bed.

right ventricle Pumping chamber of the left side of the heart. It pumps blood to the pulmonary circulation.

rod A photoreceptor in the eye that is sensitive to low light and that functions at night. There are nearly 150 million rods in the human eye.

rootlet A small nerve along the dorsal and ventral surfaces of the spinal cord from which spinal nerves arise.

rosacea A chronic inflammatory skin condition that typically affects the face. Rosacea is poorly understood, but it is prevalent in persons who are fair skinned, persons who bruise easily, and women. It may present as erythema, prominent spiderlike blood vessels (telangiectasia), swelling, or acnelike eruptions.

rugae Wrinkles in the stomach that unfold as the stomach fills.

saccular aneurysm A bulge on the side of a blood vessel. One of two major types of true aneurysm.

saccule A bed of sensory cells situated in the inner ear. It translates head movements into neural impulses that the brain can interpret.

sarcomere Repeated structural unit into which myofilaments are organized.

scabies A result of a mite infestation. The female mites burrow into the epidermis, laying eggs over a period of several weeks. The larvae hatch from the eggs and then migrate to the skin's surface. The larvae burrow in search of nutrients and mature to repeat the cycle. The burrowing and fecal matter left by the mites triggers the inflammatory process, leading to erythema and pruritus.

Schwann cell A cell that produces the myelin sheath.

sciatica A radiating, aching pain, sometimes with tingling and numbness, that starts in the buttock and extends down the back or side of one leg.

sclera White, fibrous material of the outermost layer of the eye.

scoliosis A lateral deviation of the spine. This lateral curvature may affect the thoracic or lumbar area, or both. Scoliosis may also include a rotation of the vertebrae on their axis.

scrotum A sac of skin just below the penis that contains the testes, epididymis, and lower spermatic cords.

sebaceous gland A gland that produces sebum.

sebum Secretion of the sebaceous gland that moisturizes and protects the skin.

second line of defense Part of the immune system that responds to antigen invasions that occur as the result of tiny breaks in the skin or in the lining of the respiratory, digestive, or genitourinary tracts.

secondary glaucoma Type of glaucoma that is a result of certain medications, eye diseases, and systemic diseases.

secondary hypertension Type of hypertension that tends to appear suddenly and cause higher blood pressure than primary hypertension does.

secondary immunodeficiency An acquired immunodeficiency that involves a loss of immune function because of a specific cause (e.g., infection, splenectomy, malnutrition, hepatic disease, drug therapy, or stress).

secondary syphilis Stage of syphilis that occurs about 2–8 weeks after the first chancres form. Approximately 33% of those individuals who do not have their primary syphilis treated will develop this second stage. A generalized brown-red rash that does not itch characterizes this stage.

secondary tuberculosis infection A condition that occurs when the primary TB infection can no longer be controlled, such that the TB spreads throughout the lungs and other organs.

seizure A transient physical or behavior alteration that results from an abnormal electrical activity in the brain.

selectively permeable Condition that allows a cell to maintain internal balance or homeostasis.

semen Fluid made up of ejaculatory fluid and sperm. It flows from the ejaculatory duct to the urethra, where it is released from the penis during sexual intercourse.

semicircular canal A ringlike, fluid-filled structure that houses receptors for body position and movement. Movement of the head causes the fluid in the semicircular canal to move. Fluid movement stimulates dendrites to send impulses to the brain to report this movement. There are three semicircular canals in each human ear.

seminal vesicles A pair of pouches that secrete an alkaline ejaculatory fluid containing sugar, protein, and prostaglandins. The seminal vesicles join with the ampulla to form the ejaculatory duct.

sensory nerve A type of nerve of the peripheral nervous system. It carries impulses from the body to the brain. Also called afferent nerve.

septic shock Type of distributive shock in which a bacterium's endotoxins activate an immune reaction. Inflammatory mediators are triggered, increasing capillary permeability and fluid shifts from the vascular compartment to the tissue. Falling cardiac output leads to multisystem organ failure.

serosa The outermost of the four layers of the walls of the gastrointestinal tract.

sesamoid bone One of the five types of bones found within the skeleton. Sesamoid bones are usually short or irregular bones embedded in a tendon. They are typically present in a tendon where it passes over a joint and serve to protect the tendon.

severe acute respiratory syndrome (SARS) A rapidly spreading respiratory illness that presents similarly to atypical pneumonia. Prevalence rates are higher in Asian countries. SARS is caused by a coronavirus, SARS-CoV. Transmission occurs through inhalation of respiratory droplets, close contact, or oral–fecal contact. SARS has high mortality and morbidity rates.

sex-linked Type of genetic disorder that is caused by genes located on the sex chromosomes.

sexually transmitted infection (STI) Any of a broad range of infections that can be contracted through sexual contact. Sometimes referred to as sexually transmitted disease (STD).

shedding herpes genitalis The third stage of herpes, wherein the virus is reactivated but produces no symptoms.

shock A clinical syndrome resulting from inadequate tissue and organ perfusion because of decreased blood volume or circulatory stagnation.

short bone One of the five types of bones found within the skeleton. Short bones are approximately as wide as they are long, and their primary function is to provide support and stability with little movement. Short bones contain only a thin layer of compact bone, along with spongy bone and relatively large amounts of bone marrow.

signs Clinical manifestations that can be seen or measured.

simple fracture A fracture with a single break in the bone and bone ends that maintain their alignment and position.

sinoatrial (SA) node Area of the heart where the conduction pathway originates. All impulses originating in the sinoatrial node travel through the right and left atria, resulting in atrial contraction. The sinoatrial node automatically generates impulses ranging from 60 to 100 beats per minute (sinus rhythm).

sinusitis An inflammation of the sinus cavities, most often caused by a viral infection. More recently referred to as rhinosinusitis.

skeletal muscle Muscle that connects to bone. The most frequently occurring muscle type, it makes up approximately 40% of the body's weight.

skeleton The 206 bones of varying shapes and sizes in the human body. The skeleton provides support and protection for vital organs such as the heart, lungs, and brain.

Skene's gland Gland in the mucosal lining of the vagina that secretes a protective, lubricating fluid during sexual intercourse.

skin Outer covering of the body that is composed of three layers—endodermis, dermis, and epidermis.

skin cancer An abnormal growth of skin cells.

skin tag A benign, soft brown or flesh-colored growth, usually on the neck.

small-cell carcinoma A type of lung cancer that occurs almost exclusively in heavy smokers and is less frequent than non-small-cell cancers. Also called oat-cell carcinoma.

small intestine The longest section of the gastrointestinal tract (approximately 20 feet long in adults). This length allows for adequate nutrient absorption as the small intestine continues the digestion process. In the small intestine, the enzymes that have been secreted into the gastrointestinal tract break the large food molecules into smaller molecules, which are then absorbed.

smegma An oily secretion produced by the glans that can combine with dead skin to form a cheesy substance. If the smegma is not regularly removed from under the foreskin, the penis can become irritated and infected.

smooth muscle Type of muscle that lines the walls of hollow organs and tubes and is found in the eyes, skin, and glands. Smooth muscles are involuntary.

sodium The most significant cation. Sodium is the most prevalent electrolyte of extracellular fluid, and its primary function is to control serum osmolality and water balance.

somatic pain One of two types of pain the body perceives. It results from noxious stimuli to the skin, joints, muscles, and tendons. These stimuli may include cutting, crushing, pinching, extreme temperature, and irritating chemicals. Somatic pain is generally easy to pinpoint.

somatostatin Hormone secreted by delta cells that regulates insulin and glucagon.

spermatic cord A cordlike structure, consisting of the vas deferens and its accompanying arteries, veins, nerves, and lymphatic vessels, that passes from the abdominal cavity through the inguinal canal down into the scrotum to the back of the testicle.

spermatocele A sperm-containing cyst that develops between the testes and the epididymis.

spermatogenesis The generation of sperm.

spina bifida A neural tube defect that can vary in severity from mild to debilitating. Neural tube development begins early in pregnancy, starting at the cervical area and progressing toward the lumbar area, and the neural tube usually closes by the fourth week of gestation. In spina bifida, the posterior spinous processes on the vertebra fail to fuse. This opening permits the meninges and spinal cord to herniate, resulting in neurologic impairment.

spina bifida occulta The mildest form of spina bifida. It results in a small gap in one or more of the vertebrae. The spinal nerves and meninges do not usually protrude through the opening, so most children with this form have no clinical manifestations and experience no neurologic deficits.

spinal cord A long, thin, tubular bundle of nervous tissue that exits the skull through the large and only opening in the skull, called the foramen magnum.

spinal cord injury (SCI) Injury that occurs directly to the spinal cord or indirectly to surrounding bones, tissues, or blood vessels.

spinal reflex arc The process that creates an unconscious response to stimuli.

spinal shock A temporary suppression of neurologic function because of spinal cord compression. In spinal shock, neurologic function gradually returns.

spiral fracture A fracture that twists around the bone shaft.

spongy bone The inner region of a bone, which is less dense than the outer region.

spontaneous pneumothorax Type of pneumothorax that develops when air enters the pleural cavity from an opening in the internal airways.

sprain An injury to a ligament that often involves stretching or tearing of the ligament.

stable angina pectoris Type of cardiac chest pain that is a result of ischemia that is initiated by increased demand (activity) and relieved with the reduction of that demand (rest).

stapes One of the three ossicles in the middle ear. Also called stirrup.

status asthmaticus A life-threatening, prolonged asthma attack that does not respond to usual treatment.

status epilepticus Seizures that last longer than 20 minutes or subsequent seizures that occur before the individual has fully regained consciousness from previous seizures.

stenosis A narrowing of a tubular structure, such as the heart valves. When the heart valves are stenosed, blood moving through the valves is reduced, causing blood to back up in the chamber just before the valve.

stomach An expandable food and liquid reservoir. When empty, the stomach wall shrinks, forming wrinkles called rugae. As the stomach fills, the rugae unfold and the wall stretches to accommodate a volume of as much as 2–4 liters.

strabismus A gaze deviation of one eye. With strabismus, the eyes do not coordinate to focus on the same object together, resulting in diplopia. Also called cross-eyes.

strain An injury to a muscle or tendon that often involves stretching or tearing of the muscle or tendon.

stress fracture Type of fracture that occurs from repeated excessive stress. Also called fatigue fracture.

stress incontinence Loss of urine from pressure exerted on the bladder by coughing, sneezing, laughing, exercising, or lifting something heavy. Stress incontinence occurs when the sphincter muscle of the bladder weakens.

stress ulcer Type of peptic ulcer disease that develops because of a major physiologic stressor on the body.

stroke volume The amount of blood ejected from the heart with each contraction. In addition to afterload, stroke volume is affected by preload.

subarachnoid hemorrhage A hemorrhage that results from bleeding in the space between the arachnoid and the pia mater in the brain. The primary clinical presentation is a severe headache with a sudden onset that is worse near the back of the head.

subdural hematoma A hematoma that develops between the dura mater and the arachnoid in the brain, frequently caused by a small venous tear. Because it is a result of a venous tear, a subdural hematoma generally develops slowly.

submucosa layer One of four layers of the walls of the gastrointestinal tract. It is composed of connective tissue that includes blood vessels, nerves, lymphatics, and secretory glands.

substantia nigra A brain structure located in the mesencephalon (midbrain) that plays an important role in reward, addiction, and movement. *Substantia nigra* is Latin for "black substance," as parts of the substantia nigra appear darker than neighboring areas due to high levels of neuromelanin. Parkinson's disease is caused by the death of dopaminergic neurons in the substantia nigra pars compacta.

subthalamus Part of the thalamus that participates in motor activities.

sulcus (plural: sulci) The grooves in between the gyri of the brain.

superior vena cava Large vein that carries deoxygenated blood from the upper half of the body to the right atrium.

suppressor cell A type of regulator cell that turns antibody production off.

surfactant A substance on the surface of the alveoli. Surfactant is a lipoprotein produced by alveoli cells and has a detergent-like quality. This watery substance produces surface tension on the alveoli, which enhances pulmonary compliance and prevents the alveoli from collapsing.

suture An immoveable joint in the skull.

sympathetic nervous system (SNS) Subdivision of the autonomic nervous system. It is responsible for the fight-or-flight response.

symptoms Clinical manifestations that are described by the patient.

synapse The gap between the neurons. This gap includes the presynaptic terminal, the synaptic cleft (space between neurons), and a postsynaptic cell membrane.

synaptic cleft Space between neurons.

synarthrose An immoveable joint.

syndrome A group of signs and symptoms that occur together.

syndrome of inappropriate antidiuretic hormone (SIADH) Condition of increased renal water retention caused by excessive antidiuretic levels.

syngenic Type of transplant in which tissue from the identical twin of the host is used.

synovial fluid A transparent viscous fluid secreted by the synovial membrane that lubricates cartilage in the synovial joints.

synovial joint A freely moveable joint; it is the most common type of joint. Synovial joints contain cartilage that is lubricated by a transparent viscous fluid secreted by the synovial membrane.

syphilis An ulcerative sexually transmitted infection caused by *Treponema pallidum*, a spiral-shaped (spirochete) bacterium that requires a warm, moist environment to survive.

systemic circulation The part of the cardiovascular system that carries oxygenated blood away from the heart to the body, and returns deoxygenated blood back to the heart.

systemic lupus erythematosus (SLE) A chronic, autoimmune, inflammatory disorder that can affect any connective tissue. It is thought that B cells are activated for unknown reasons to produce autoantibodies and autoantigens that combine to form immune complexes.

systole The top number in a blood pressure reading, which indicates work done by the ventricles.

systolic dysfunction Type of heart failure characterized by decreased cardiac output due to decreased contractility.

T$_3$ Triiodothyronine; a hormone produced by the follicles of the thyroid gland to regulate cellular metabolism and growth and development.

T$_4$ Thyroxine; a hormone produced by the follicles of the thyroid gland to regulate cellular metabolism and growth and development.

T cell A cell that is a major part of the body's third line of defense. It is produced in the bone marrow and matures in the thymus, which is why it is called a T cell. Two major types of T cells work to destroy antigens—regulator cells and effector cells.

telophase Phase of mitosis in which chromosomes arrive at each pole and new membranes are formed.

temporal lobe The lobe of the brain that plays an essential role in hearing and memory.

tendon Specialized tough cord or band of dense connective tissue that is a continuous extension of the periosteum.

tension pneumothorax The most serious type of pneumothorax; it occurs when the pressure in the pleural space is greater than the atmospheric pressure. This increased pressure is due to trapped air in the pleural space or entering air from a positive-pressure mechanical ventilator.

teratogen A birth defect–causing agent.

terminal bouton Miniscule bulge into which several small fibers terminate. These terminal boutons communicate with neurons, muscle fibers, or glands.

tertiary syphilis The final stage of syphilis. The early latency stage begins when the secondary symptoms disappear and lasts 1–4 years. The late latency stage can last for years as the infection spreads to the brain, nervous system, heart, skin, and bones. Also called latent syphilis.

testes Gonads; organs that produce sperm and the sex hormones.

testicular cancer Cancer of the testicles. Testicular cancer can occur as a slow-growing or fast-growing tumor. Risk for developing testicular cancer is thought to be increased by family history, infection, trauma, and cryptorchidism. Testicular cancer usually affects one testicle, but can affect both.

testicular torsion An abnormal rotation of the testis on the spermatic cord.

testosterone Hormone that gives males their classic secondary sex characteristics and sex drive. Testosterone also regulates metabolism and protein anabolism, inhibits pituitary secretion of the gonadotropins, and promotes potassium excretion and renal sodium reabsorption.

thalamus Part of the diencephalon that receives and relays most of the sensory input, affects mood, and initiates body movements (especially those associated with fear or anger).

third line of defense The body's specific immune system that includes T cells and B cells.

third spacing Significant fluid increases in compartments where fluid does not normally collect (e.g., peritoneum). Fluid is not easily exchanged among the other extracellular fluids.

thromboangiitis obliterans An inflammatory condition of the arteries. Also known as Buerger's disease.

thrombocyte A blood platelet.

thrombocytopenia Decreased platelet levels; a condition that increases the risk of bleeding and infection.

thrombocytosis Increased platelet levels; a condition that increases the risk of thrombus formation.

thromboplastin A factor in blood clotting, which is stimulated by the release of thromboplastin from damaged cells lining blood vessels.

thrombotic thrombocytopenic purpura (TTP) A coagulation disorder that is a result of a deficiency of an enzyme necessary for cleaving von Willebrand's factor.

thrombus A blood clot that consists of platelets, fibrin, and red and white blood cells. These clots can form anywhere in the circulatory system.

thyroid gland A gland located at the base of the neck below the larynx that consists of two lobes, one on either side of the trachea.

thyroid-stimulating hormone (TSH) Hormone produced by the pituitary gland that promotes the thyroid to produce T$_3$ and T$_4$.

thyrotoxicosis Thyroid crisis; a sudden worsening of hyperthyroidism symptoms that may occur with infection or stress. Fever, decreased mental alertness, and abdominal pain may occur. Thyrotoxicosis is a medical emergency.

tidal volume The amount of air involved in one normal inhalation and exhalation.

tinea A parasite that causes several types of superficial fungal infections described by the area of the body affected. Tinea corporis, or ringworm, is an infection of the body. Tinea pedis, or athlete's foot, involves the feet, especially the toes. Tinea unguium is an infection of the nails, typically the toenails.

tinnitus Persistent, abnormal noises in the ear. This noise may be described as a ringing, buzzing, humming, whistling, roaring, or blowing.

TNM staging Method of expressing the extent of cancer by evaluating the tumor size, nodal involvement, and metastatic progress.

tonicity The osmotic pressure of two solutions separated by a semipermeable membrane.

tophus (plural: tophi) A large, hard nodule consisting of uric acid crystals deposited in soft tissues, usually in cooler areas of the body.

trachea The windpipe; it carries air from the oral and nasal cavities to the lungs.

transcellular A third compartment of fluid in the body, in addition to the interstitial and intravascular compartments.

transient incontinence Urinary incontinence resulting from a temporary condition.

transient ischemic attack (TIA) A temporary episode of cerebral ischemia that results in symptoms of neurologic deficits. Transient ischemic attacks are often called ministrokes because these neurologic deficits mimic a cerebral vascular accident or stroke except that these deficits resolve within 24 hours (1–2 hours in most cases).

transverse fracture A fracture straight across the bone shaft.

traumatic brain injury (TBI) Injury that is usually caused by a sudden and violent blow or jolt to the head (called a closed injury) or a penetrating (known as an open injury) head injury that disrupts the normal brain function.

traumatic pneumothorax Type of pneumothorax that is caused by any blunt or penetrating injury to the chest. These injuries can inadvertently occur during certain medical procedures.

treatment Strategies used to manage or cure a disease.

trichomoniasis Infection caused by *Trichomonas vaginalis*, a one-celled anaerobic organism. This extracellular parasite can burrow under the mucosal lining. Colloquially referred to as trick.

tricuspid valve A three-leaflet valve that guides the passage of blood from the right atria to the right ventricle and prevents the backward flow of blood.

Trousseau's sign An indicator of hypocalcemia in which a strategically placed blood pressure cuff elicits a carpal spasm.

tuberculosis (TB) A potentially serious infectious disease that is increasing globally after declining in previous decades.

tumor A cellular growth that is no longer responding to normal regulator processes. Also called neoplasm.

tumor grading system The degree of differentiation of a malignancy. The grading system determines the degree of differentiation on a scale of 1 to 4 in order of clinical severity, with grade 1 cancers being well differentiated and less likely to cause problems and grade 4 cancers being undifferentiated, meaning they are highly likely to cause problems because they do not resemble any characteristics of the original tissue.

tunica adventitia The outer layer of the blood vessels, which consists of elastic and fibrous connective tissue.

tunica intima The smooth, thin, inner layer of the blood vessels.

tunica media The middle layer of the blood vessels, which is composed of elastic tissue and smooth muscle that is responsible for the vessel's ability to constrict and dilate.

tympanic membrane Part of the ear that separates the outer ear and the middle ear. Sound hits the tympanic membrane, creating vibrations. Also called eardrum.

type 1 diabetes Type of diabetes mellitus that develops when the body's immune system destroys pancreatic beta cells. To survive, people with type 1 diabetes must have insulin delivered by injection or a pump. This form of diabetes usually strikes children and young adults, although disease onset can occur at any age. Previously called insulin-dependent diabetes and juvenile-onset diabetes.

type 2 diabetes Type of diabetes that usually begins as insulin resistance, a disorder in which the cells do not use insulin properly. As the need for insulin rises, the pancreas gradually loses its ability to produce it. Previously called non-insulin-dependent diabetes and adult-onset diabetes.

type I hypersensitivity Immunoglobulin E–mediated type of hypersensitivity, in which an allergen activates T cells, which then bind to mast cells. Repeated exposure to relatively large doses of the allergen is usually necessary to cause this response.

type II hypersensitivity Tissue-specific type of hypersensitivity, which generally involves the destruction of a target cell by an antibody-directed, cell-surface antigen. Immunoglobulin G or M reacts with an antigen on the cell, activating the complement system. The effects of type II reactions include cell lysis and phagocytosis.

type III hypersensitivity Immune complex–mediated type of hypersensitivity, in which circulating antigen–antibody complexes accumulate and are deposited in the tissue. This accumulation triggers the complement system, causing local inflammation and increased vascular permeability, so more complexes accumulate.

type IV hypersensitivity Cell-mediated type of hypersensitivity, which involves a delayed processing of the antigen by the macrophages. Once processed, the antigen is presented to the T cells, resulting in the release of lymphokines that cause inflammation and antigen destruction.

type A influenza The most common type of influenza virus. It includes several subtypes, including H1N1. Type A influenza is usually responsible for the most serious epidemics and global pandemics.

type B influenza Type of influenza virus that can cause regional epidemics, but the disease it produces is generally milder than that caused by type A influenza.

type C influenza Type of influenza virus that causes sporadic cases and minor, local outbreaks. Type C has never been connected with a large epidemic.

ulcerative colitis A progressive condition of the rectum and colon mucosa that usually develops in the second or third decade of life. Inflammation causes epithelium loss, surface erosion, and ulceration.

uncompensated A pH level that is still normal.

unstable angina A change in cardiac chest pain; the pain becomes unpredictable, occurs at rest, or increases in frequency or intensity. It is considered a preinfarction state.

urea One of the three most significant metabolic wastes managed by the kidneys.

uremia Waste accumulation due to renal impairment.

ureter Part of the urinary system that transports the urine using peristaltic actions to the bladder for storage.

urethra Tube that empties the urinary bladder.

urge incontinence A sudden, intense urge to urinate, followed by an involuntary loss of urine.

uric acid A metabolism by-product managed by the kidneys that is a result of the breakdown of nucleotides, the building blocks of DNA.

urinary incontinence Involuntary loss of urine.

urinary tract infection (UTI) Infection of the urinary tract that often ascends from the urinary meatus. It is typically caused by *Escherichia coli* and occurs more frequently in females.

urination The voluntary contraction of the bladder and relaxation of the external sphincter, forcing urine out through the urethra.

urticaria Raised erythematous skin lesions that are a result of a type I hypersensitivity reaction. Also called hives.

uterine prolapse The descent of the uterus or cervix into the vagina.

uterus A hollow, pear-shaped organ held in place by the broad, round, and uterosacral ligaments.

utricle A division of the inner ear that detects motion and position.

vagina A hollow, tunnel-like structure that extends from the cervix to the external genitalia.

varicocele A dilated vein in the spermatic cord.

varicose vein A dilated, tortuous, engorged vein that develops because of improper venous valve function. The most common location in which varicose veins occur is the legs, but they can be found in the esophagus (esophageal varices) and the rectum (hemorrhoids). Also called varicosity.

vas deferens Part of the male duct system that carries sperm out of the testes.

vascular birthmark Birthmark that consists of blood vessels that have not formed correctly; therefore, these birthmarks are generally red.

vein A blood vessel that carries blood back to the heart.

ventilation The transportation of air from the atmosphere to the lungs and out again.

ventilation/perfusion ratio A measurement used to assess the efficacy and adequacy of ventilation and perfusion. Also called VQ ratio.

ventral root A root formed from approximately 6–8 ventral rootlets. The roots combine to form the spinal nerve.

ventricle A hollow area. In the brain, ventricles are interconnected, and cerebrospinal fluid fills and flows freely between them. In the heart, they are pumping chambers.

venule A blood vessel that is larger than a capillary. Venules merge together to form veins.

verruca (plural: verrucae) A viral infection caused by any of a number of the human papillomaviruses. Verrucae can develop at any age and often resolve spontaneously. They can be transmitted through direct skin contact between people or within the same person.

vertebral canal Part of the central nervous system through which the spinal cord extends to the second lumbar vertebra.

vertigo An illusion of motion. People experiencing vertigo have a sensation that they or the room is spinning or moving.

vesicle A blister.

vestibular apparatus Part of the inner ear that includes the semicircular canals and the vestibule.

vestibule **1.** A bony chamber positioned between the cochlea and semicircular canals of the ear. The vestibule houses receptors that respond to body position and movement. **2.** The area of the vagina that contains the urethral and vaginal opening.

viral pneumonia A form of pneumonia that is usually mild and heals without intervention, but that can lead to a virulent bacterial pneumonia.

visceral pain One of two types of pain the body perceives. It results from noxious stimuli to internal organs and may include expansion and hypoxia. Visceral pain is usually vague and diffuse. It may even be sensed on body surfaces at distant locations from the originating organ.

visceral peritoneum layer The inner layer of the peritoneum that encases the abdominal organs.

vital capacity The sum of the tidal volume and reserves in the lungs.

vitiligo A rare condition characterized by small patchy areas of hypopigmentation. Vitiligo occurs when the cells that produce melanin die or no longer form melanin, leading to slowly enlarging white patches of irregular shapes on the skin.

vitreous humor A clear, gelatinous material that fills the posterior chamber of the eye.

volatile acid Acid that can be excreted via the lungs.

volatile gas Gas that can be excreted via the lungs.

vomiting The involuntary or voluntary forceful ejection of chyme from the stomach up through the esophagus and out of the mouth. It is a common event that often results from a wide range of conditions. Also called emesis.

vomitus The stomach contents ejected beyond the mouth during vomiting.

von Willebrand's disease A common bleeding disorder caused by a defect or deficiency of a blood clotting protein, called von Willebrand factor.

vulva The structures of external female genitalia. These structures include the mons pubis, the labia majora, the labia minora, the clitoris, and the vestibule.

water intoxication Fluid excess that occurs in the intracellular space.

welt A raised erythematous skin lesion.

wet gangrene Type of gangrene that occurs with liquefaction necrosis. Extensive damage from bacteria and white blood cells combine to produce a liquid wound.

white matter Bundles of myelinated nerves.

Wilms' tumor A rare kidney cancer that primarily affects children. Also called nephroblastoma.

xenogenic Type of transplant in which tissue is used from a different species.

yellow marrow Bone marrow that begins to form during adolescence and is present in most bones by adulthood. Yellow marrow can be reactivated to produce blood cells under certain circumstances.

Zika virus disease Condition resulting from an infection of the Zika virus, a member of the virus family *Flaviviridae*. The virus spreads mostly by the bite of an infected *Aedes* species mosquito, but it can also be transmitted from mother to fetus and through sexual contact.

zygote A fertilized egg.

Index